MANUAL
EQUINE
PRACTICE

REUBEN J. ROSE

DVSc, PhD, FRCVS, DipVetAn, MACVSc

Professor of Veterinary Clinical Studies
Department of Veterinary Clinical Sciences
University of Sydney, Sydney, Australia

formerly Appleton Professor of Equine Surgery
College of Veterinary Medicine
University of Florida, Gainesville, Florida

DAVID R. HODGSON

BVSc, PhD, FACSM, Diplomate ACVIM

Superintendent, Rural Veterinary Centre
Department of Animal Health
University of Sydney
Camden, Australia

formerly Associate Professor of Equine Medicine
College of Veterinary Medicine
Washington State University
Pullman, Washington

W.B. SAUNDERS COMPANY

A Division of Harcourt Brace & Company

Philadelphia • London • Toronto • Montreal • Sydney • Tokyo

W.B. SAUNDERS COMPANY
A Division of
Harcourt Brace & Company

The Curtis Center
Independence Square West
Philadelphia, Pennsylvania 19106

Drug Notice

Equine medicine is an ever-changing field. But as new research and clinical experience grow, changes in treatment and drug therapy become necessary or appropriate. The authors and editors of this work have carefully checked and verified drug dosages to assure that dosage information is precise and in accord with standards accepted at the time of publication. Readers are advised, however, to check the product information currently provided by the manufacturer of each drug to be administered to be certain that changes have not been made in the recommended dose or in the contraindications for administration. This is of particular importance in regard to new or infrequently used drugs. Recommended dosages for animals are sometimes based on adjustments in the dosage that would be suitable for humans. Some of the drugs mentioned have been given experimentally by the authors. Others have been used in dosages greater than those recommended by the manufacturer. In these kinds of cases, the authors have reported on their own considerable experience. It is the responsibility of those administering a drug, relying on their professional skill and experience, to determine dosages, the best treatment for the patient, and whether the benefits of giving a drug justify the attendant risk. The editors cannot be responsible for misuse or misapplication of the material in this work.

THE PUBLISHER

Library of Congress Cataloging-in-Publication Data

Rose, R. J. (Reuben J.)
    Manual of equine practice / Reuben J. Rose, David R. Hodgson.
       p.   cm.
    ISBN 0–7216–3739–6
    1. Horses—Diseases—Handbooks, manuals, etc.   2. Horses—
Diseases—Diagnosis—Handbooks, manuals, etc.   I. Hodgson, David
R.   II. Title.
    SF951.R688   1993
    636.1′089—dc20   92–21745

MANUAL OF EQUINE PRACTICE   ISBN 0–7216–3739–6

Printed in the United States of America.

Last digit is the print number: 9   8   7   6   5   4   3   2

Dedicated to our parents,

Ben and Kit Rose and John and Judy Hodgson,

for their encouragement and love

as well as assistance through the battles of life.

Contributors

DAVID R. HODGSON, B.V.Sc., Ph.D., Diplomate A.C.V.I.M.

Superintendent, Rural Veterinary Centre, University of Sydney, Camden, Australia

JOHN KOHNKE, B.V.Sc., R.D.A.

Technical Services Manager, Vetsearch International Pty. Ltd., North Rocks, Australia

DARIA N. LOVE, D.V.Sc., Ph.D., M.R.C. Path.

Associate Professor in Veterinary Pathology, Department of Veterinary Pathology, University of Sydney, Sydney, Australia

REUBEN J. ROSE, D.V.Sc., Ph.D., F.R.C.V.S.

Professor of Veterinary Clinical Sciences, Department of Veterinary Clinical Sciences, University of Sydney, Sydney, Australia

Acknowledgments

We are grateful to Dr. Daria Love and Dr. John Kohnke for their superb contributions to this book. Dr. Michelle LeBlanc provided excellent advice and amendments to the section on reproduction and we are grateful for her assistance. Dr. Jennifer Hodgson provided advice and amendments to the section on clinical bacteriology, and her assistance is much appreciated. Mr. Kevin Dennes undertook all the photography, and Ms. Bozena Jantulik did all the artwork. We would like to acknowledge their great care and attention to detail; we are particularly grateful for their expertise and cooperation in achieving the desired results. Dr. Ruth Davis, Ms. Shirley Ray, Dr. Aasha Sinha, and Ms. Louise Southwood helped with compiling drug dosages, editing of material, and collation of references. We thank our wives, Suzette and Jenny, for their support and forbearance. Our thanks also go to the Saunders editorial staff and particularly to Ms. Linda Mills for her advice and expert editorial assistance. Finally, we enjoyed working with Mr. John Fitzpatrick of Editorial Services of New England, Inc., on the final stages of book editing and thank him for his contribution and attention to detail.

Preface

Over the past 5 years there has been a great increase in the number of books available to the equine practitioner. In general these are multi-author books dealing with the medical and surgical disorders of horses or technical books providing "how to do" instructions for specific surgical techniques. There is therefore no shortage of well referenced information relating to diseases of horses. The difficulty for the equine practitioner is sorting the wood from the trees in the daily grind of practice life, which often revolves around stomach tubing, cortisone injections, and lameness examinations rather than ACTH stimulation tests and arthroscopic surgery.

This book is written for both students and equine–mixed practice veterinarians to distill important information about the main body systems in an accessible form. Between us, we have had considerable experience in equine practice, having worked in Australia, New Zealand, Europe, North America, and the United Kingdom. Our main aim in writing the book was to provide practical information in a form which could be easily accessed and could travel with the veterinarian. This handbook developed from a small book written in 1983 by Reuben Rose and published by the Sydney University Postgraduate Committee in Veterinary Science, called the *Vade Mecum* (Latin, translated literally as "go with me"). This book was very well received by veterinarians and the feedback provided has resulted in the current updated and considerably expanded version called *Manual of Equine Practice*. The book is organized into body systems and within these systems follows a similar format. We have particularly emphasized the area of diagnosis, which in the busy life of the equine practitioner can be overlooked in favor of treatment. The old adage of "when all else fails, do a clinical examination" is one that consistently haunts us.

Within each system, we have tried to organize the book in a way that is useful to a practitioner. Each body system is subdivided into important clinical areas and individual conditions are listed alphabetically within these areas. We have included a few references that should be readily available to most practitioners. With treatment, any drug used in the book is referenced to a section in the back of the book which provides details of the forms of the drug available and the trade names, as well as the dose rates.

The usefulness of a book like this depends on feedback from veterinarians in practice. We welcome any criticisms or suggestions that will permit the next edition to more completely meet the needs of the equine veterinarian.

Reuben J. Rose
David R. Hodgson

Contents

Physical Examination

A detailed physical examination is the cornerstone of equine practice. One of the difficulties that most equine practitioners face is the pressure of time, with the result that priority is given to treatment rather than to diagnosis. When a wrong diagnosis is made, it is often because key aspects of the physical examination are neglected. Sometimes this is something obvious, such as failure to auscultate the right side of the chest so that a heart murmur is missed. Other cases may be presented with one problem, for example, a foreleg lameness, but the most significant problem may be low-grade pulmonary disease that remains undetected because only the leg was examined and a general physical examination was not done. It is unrealistic to expect that a full physical examination will be undertaken on every horse seen in a busy equine practice because there are not enough hours in the day. However, it is essential to obtain an accurate history from the owner or trainer and to perform a basic examination on every horse seen. In most circumstances this involves only an extra 2 to 3 minutes, but it can be of great value in saving later embarrassment or litigation.

One of the temptations when examining a horse for a particular problem is to stop the examination when a problem is discovered that matches the history. However, the importance of conducting a logical and sequential standardized examination cannot be overemphasized. First, a database of normal findings for the various body systems will be established, and second, familiarity and expertise develop in the expeditious performance of the examination. This helps to avoid the possibility of overlooking an important problem.

KEY POINT ▶ Important steps in establishing an initial diagnosis are:

- Determine the presenting complaint and establish the history relating to the particular problem.
- Undertake a complete physical examination in an attempt to define or localize the problem(s).
- Compile a specific problem list.

- Establish a series of differential diagnoses based on the problems identified.
- Undertake diagnostic tests, such as radiology, hematology, or blood biochemistry, that will assist in establishing a definitive diagnosis.

It is essential to establish the most likely differential diagnoses prior to performing diagnostic tests, because the tests should support the clinical findings. Too frequently, clinicians will perform a complete blood count and blood biochemical profile in the hope that something will show up. Not only is this poor veterinary medicine, but it also can divert attention from the real problem to a laboratory finding that may be of little clinical relevance.

Once these basic diagnostic steps are taken, therapy can be commenced, except in the case of emergencies that demand immediate treatment, for example, severe hemorrhage, shock, and colic. However, even in acute problems, a brief clinical examination that includes vital signs (heart rate, respiratory rate, rectal temperature, pulse quality, mucous membrane color, and capillary refill time) should be performed quickly prior to initial therapy.

SIGNALMENT

Diagnosis may be assisted by considering the age, breed, sex, and purpose for which the horse is used. Some specific details of signalment are included in the next chapter, which outlines various presenting problems. Considering breed, sex, age, and use allows certain diseases to be placed at the top of the list of differential diagnoses. One of the problems in colleges of veterinary medicine is that a rather exotic range of cases is presented that may not reflect the types of cases found in practice. For example, a student on equine rotation in some North American veterinary schools could easily get the impression that most horses presenting with colic require surgery. The reality is, of course, that in equine practice, many cases of colic will recover with minimal therapy.

KEY POINT ▶ It should be remembered that "common diseases occur commonly."

For example, the horse at pasture with an acute hindleg lameness probably has a subsolar abscess rather than a hip luxation. Some details relating to signalment will be discussed with examples related to specific diseases.

Age
Musculoskeletal Disease

Certain conditions, for example, multifocal septic arthritis, osteochondritis dissecans, and angular limb deformities, are more common in young horses. In contrast, degenerative joint disease is more common in older horses and is also affected by degree of use.

Respiratory Disease

Age is important in determining the extent and severity of various respiratory disorders. Infectious respiratory disease tends to be more severe in the very young and in the aged. This may be related to reduced immunocompetence. In contrast, chronic obstructive pulmonary disease (COPD) is found most commonly in middle-aged horses that have had repeated exposure to specific allergens. Horses with COPD usually have had prolonged exposure to a stable environment where there is poor ventilation.

Cardiovascular Disease

With cardiac disease, although congestive heart failure is most commonly found in older horses, congenital heart disease may not be manifested until athletic endeavors are required. Horses are usually presented because of exercise intolerance or dyspnea.

Gastrointestinal Disease

Age contributes to the incidence and type of gastrointestinal abnormalities. Gastric ulceration, pyloric stenosis, and ascarid impaction must be considered when a foal is presented with clinical signs of colic. Volvulus and intussusception of the small intestine occur more commonly in horses less than 3 years of age. Conversely, pedunculated lipomas are more common in older horses, as is gastric neoplasia.

Neurologic Disease

Neonatal maladjustment syndrome is the most common cause of neurologic disturbances in foals, whereas in yearlings and 2-year-olds, cervical vertebral malformation is a common cause of spinal cord ataxia. Neurologic diseases more common in older horses include nigropallidal encephalomalacia and protozoal myeloencephalitis.

Skin Disease

Ringworm is a common cause of pruritus and focal alopecia in young horses, whereas *Culicoides* hypersensitivity is more common in older horses.

Breed
Musculoskeletal Disease

Breed predilections exist for some conditions causing lameness. "Bucked shins" is a common problem of young thoroughbred and quarter horses in training. Chip fractures of the dorsal aspect of the carpal bones are more frequently diagnosed in thoroughbreds and quarter horses than in standardbreds. Standardbreds tend to have a greater incidence of hindleg lameness and fractures of the pedal bone than thoroughbreds or quarter horses. Quarter horses appear to have a very high incidence of navicular disease, whereas the incidence is lower in Arabians. In ponies, upward fixation of the patella and laminitis are more common than in other breeds.

Respiratory Disease

Although few breed-specific associations have been found for respiratory disease, combined immunodeficiency is primarily found in Arabian foals. Many of these foals are presented with chronic respiratory infections that are unresponsive to therapy. In the thoroughbred, laryngeal hemiplegia is more common than in other breeds and is generally first noticed between 2 and 3 years of age. Laryngeal hemiplegia is also very common in draft horses.

Cardiovascular Disease

Atrial fibrillation appears to be found more commonly in standardbred trotters and pacers than in other performance horses. Congenital cardiovascular disease is more common in Arabian horses than in other breeds.

Gastrointestinal Disease

Atresia ani may be more common in Appaloosa horses. Entrapment of the epiploic foramen is more common in thoroughbred horses than in other breeds.

Neurologic Disease

Breed can be important in neurologic disease. Thoroughbreds have a higher incidence than other breeds of cervical vertebral malformation, whereas Arabians have an assortment of congenital problems, including cervical malformations and cerebellar abiotrophy.

Skin Disease

Pemphigus foliaceus is found more commonly in Appaloosa horses than in other breeds. There is a condition known as "curly coat" that is an inherited condition in Percheron horses. A depigmenting condition known as "pinky syndrome" or Arabian fading syndrome occurs in Arabian horses.

Sex

Sex of the horse is less important than age, breed, and use in predisposing to or determining disease states. However, it is obvious that some conditions, for example, inguinal hernias, will occur only in colts or stallions. In contrast, in mares the hormonal changes associated with pregnancy and lactation may play a role in the onset of some diseases. Both osteochondritis dissecans and idiopathic laryngeal hemiplegia are more common in males than in females.

Purpose for Which the Horse Is Used

Use of the horse is of major importance in determining the likelihood of various types of abnormalities. This will clearly interact with the horse's breed.

Musculoskeletal Disease

Fractures of the phalanges, sesamoids, and carpal bones, together with tendon strains, are more common in athletic horses, whereas long bone fractures appear to be more likely in horses in groups at pasture. Back problems are more common in jumping and hunting horses. Navicular disease is more common in horses used for cutting, roping, and barrel racing.

Respiratory Disease

Respiratory disease is more common in horses stabled in crowded and stressful environments. Because thoroughbred, quarter horse, and standardbred racehorses are often transported long distances, pneumonia and pleuritis are more common than in pleasure horses. Some functional upper airway disorders (e.g., laryngeal hemiplegia) will be of little or no significance in dressage horses, whereas such afflictions will severely limit horses performing at high exercise intensities.

Cardiovascular Disease

Minor cardiovascular problems and some major ones (e.g., valvular incompetence and atrial fibrillation) will only result in clinical manifestations in horses required to perform competitive athletic activities.

Gastrointestinal Disease

Various types of colic appear to be more common in horses kept at pasture than in horses in stable environments. For example, sand colic and enteroliths are more common in pastured horses.

Neurologic Disease

Traumatic neurologic disease is common in showjumping, eventing, and steeplechasing horses.

Skin Disease

Ringworm is more common in horses kept in racing stables, because there is a predominance of young horses under these circumstances.

KEY POINT ► Management, husbandry, and geography can be important in determining the types and incidence of various diseases.

For example, pneumonia and septicemia are more common on stud farms where there is overcrowding. *Rhodococcus equi* infections usually have a higher incidence in specific geographic areas. This may well be related to soil type, since infections are more common in foals kept on sandy soils. Other examples include sand colic, which tends to occur most commonly in drier sandy regions, and equine protozoal myeloencephalitis, with greatest incidence in the eastern regions of North America.

HISTORY

Prior to any examination, a thorough and accurate history should be obtained. History taking is a skill that has to be developed and is an art rather than a science. The ability to ask the right question can sometimes be important in indicating the most likely differential diagnoses. In obtaining the history, leading questions should be avoided. These are questions where the owner is led to provide the answer that the veterinarian wants rather than the one that reflects the history of the horse's problem. Misleading histories are quite common because many owners make their own diagnosis of their horse's problem prior to its presentation to the veterinarian. This often results in a selective history that reflects the owner's or trainer's bias.

History taking has two major components: past and present. These are equally important in obtaining the correct diagnosis and in determining the approach to therapy.

KEY POINT ► The current history begins with questions relating to the presenting signs and should seek the owner's or trainer's assessment of the problem as static, worsening, or improving.

The detail and extent of the history collected will depend on the duration of the problem and need for any immediate therapy. For example, many details of history have little relevance to the immediate treatment of a horse that has severe colic and shows signs of shock.

KEY POINT ▶ The past history should begin with questions about the horse's condition immediately before the onset of the problem, followed by selective details.

The details sought will vary from months to years prior to presentation, depending on the nature of the problem. For example, in a horse presented for colic, it is of great significance that the problem is recurrent over several years rather than a single, isolated event. Chronic problems, probably involving the blood supply from the cranial mesenteric artery, have a more guarded prognosis than isolated events related to changes in feed or exercise state. Changes in appetite and demeanor together with alterations in body condition are important features of a variety of diseases.

Some specific questions that will provide important information relating to the problem being investigated are provided in the next chapter on presenting problems.

KEY POINT ▶ Despite careful and detailed history collection, the clinician should view the information with healthy skepticism.

It is common for conflicting details to be given when a second veterinarian questions the same client. It is also important to avoid any scientific jargon, because many owners will be reluctant to tell you that they do not understand. This also applies when discussing a diagnosis or deciding which option should be used in therapy. It may be useful to confirm an important detail later in the examination by asking a previous question in a slightly different manner.

PHYSICAL EXAMINATION

This section discusses the broad approach to a physical examination. Specific information is provided in each of the chapters on body systems, which include diagnostic aids. In the initial examination, the main consideration is to determine or confirm from the history provided which body system(s) is involved.

A number of approaches may be used when the initial examination is undertaken. While many problem-oriented record systems work through a system approach to examination, it is probably more common in practice to start the examination at the front of the horse and work to the rear. The time spent on a specific region will be dictated by the history and presenting complaint. However, many problems involve multiple body systems. For example, in a thoroughbred horse presented for exercise intolerance, it is quite common to find that the horse has a low-grade lameness, abnormal respiratory sounds on auscultation of the chest, evidence of atrophy of the left dorsal cricoarytenoid muscle, and a cardiac arrhythmia. Therefore, it is important, even with the most obvious problem, to perform as thorough a physical examination as the circumstances allow.

General Overview

The initial part of the examination should involve an overview of the horse. This brief evaluation should be conducted at a distance of 2 to 3 m (6 to 10 feet), and the horse should be viewed from the front, left and right sides, and rear. Of particular importance is the demeanor, which can indicate if the horse is showing signs of systemic disease or is in pain. Note should be made of whether the horse is alert or depressed.

KEY POINT ▶ During this brief examination, any asymmetries, swellings, or other irregularities should be noted prior to commencing a more detailed examination.

Evidence of scars, rub marks, or localized hair loss may be more evident at this stage of the examination. After taking note of obvious abnormalities, the more detailed examination should begin.

Examination of the Head and Neck

- *The nostrils should be checked* for symmetry and airflow. Additionally, the air from the nostrils should be smelled for any abnormal odors, which could indicate infection of the nasal conchae, sinuses, guttural pouches, or lower respiratory tract.
- *The incisor teeth are inspected* for evidence of malocclusion (Fig. 1-1), after which digital pressure is applied to the mucous membrane above the corner incisor teeth to determine the capillary refill time (Fig. 1-2).
- *Normal capillary refill time is 1 to 2 seconds,* and this is increased in horses with shock due to a decrease in peripheral perfusion.

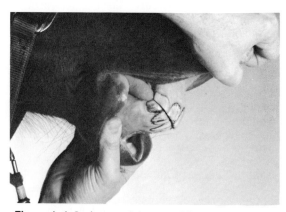

Figure 1-1. Incisor teeth inspected for malocclusion.

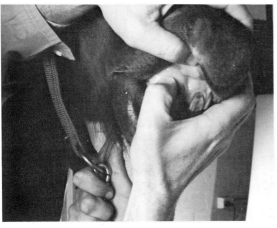

A

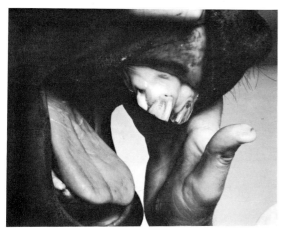

B

Figure 1–2. A. Digital pressure applied to the gums above the corner incisor teeth to determine capillary refill time. B. Blanching of mucous membrane following digital pressure applied to the gums.

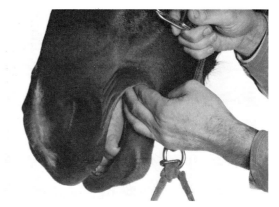

Figure 1–3. Introduction of the left hand into the left interdental space for a one-handed tooth examination.

■ *After examination of the nasal contours for swelling, percussion of the maxillary and frontal sinuses should be performed* (Figs. 1-8 and 1-9). This ensures that there is no evidence of pain or a dull sound, which could indicate sinusitis or the presence of fluid within the sinus cavities. The sound obtained is more distinctive if a thumb is placed in the interdental space so that the mouth is slightly open during percussion.

■ *The eyes should be examined* for signs of corneal scarring, conjunctivitis, immune-mediated uveitis (periodic ophthalmia), or cataracts. A menace response should be elicited (Fig. 1-10) and a direct pupillary light response (Fig. 1-11) should be determined, as well as a consensual response. The third eyelid also should be examined by applying digital pressure to the eyeball via the upper eyelid (Fig. 1-12).

■ *The pulse should be felt in the facial artery* as it turns around the angle of the mandible (Fig.

■ *The teeth should be examined* using a one-hand technique (Figs. 1-3 and 1-4), with the back of the hand inserted via the interdental space and used to push the tongue between the teeth on the opposite side of the mouth. This means that the horse will have to bite its tongue before it crushes your fingers. Alternatively, a mouth gag can be used, as shown in Figures 1-5 to 1-7. Of the various gags available, we prefer the Swale's gag (Figs. 1-6 and 1-7) because it is easy to apply and is well tolerated by most horses. Abnormalities of tooth wear and sharp edges on the labial side of the upper cheek teeth and the lingual side of the lower cheek teeth should be noted. Sharp edges on the teeth can contribute to a range of problems because of lacerations to the mucous membranes of the mouth when the bit is applied. At this stage, the age of the horse also can be determined.

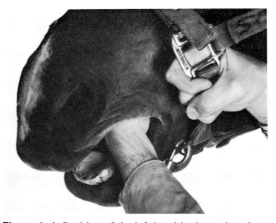

Figure 1–4. Position of the left hand in the oral cavity, forcing the tongue to the right occlusal surfaces of the cheek teeth so that palpation of left cheek teeth can be done.

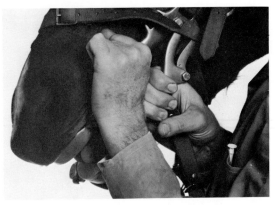

Figure 1–5. Application of a Hausmann mouth gag showing opening of the gag prior to examination of the mouth and teeth.

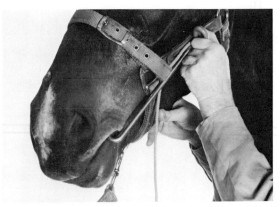

Figure 1–7. Swale's mouth gag in place.

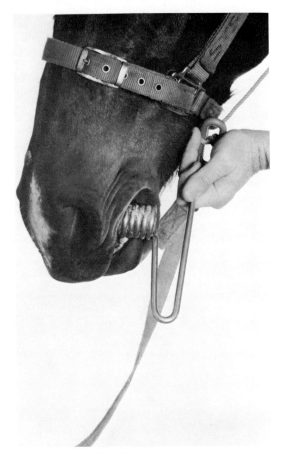

Figure 1–6. Insertion of a Swale's mouth gag via the left interdental space to allow examination of the right dental arcades.

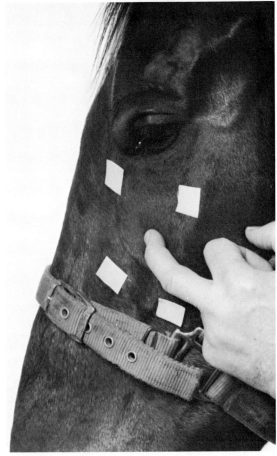

Figure 1–8. Percussion over the maxillary sinus. The white tape shows the boundaries of the sinus.

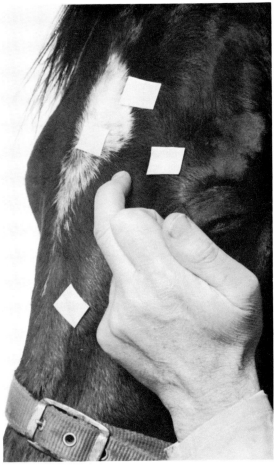

Figure 1-9. Percussion over the frontal sinus. The white tape shows the boundaries of the sinus.

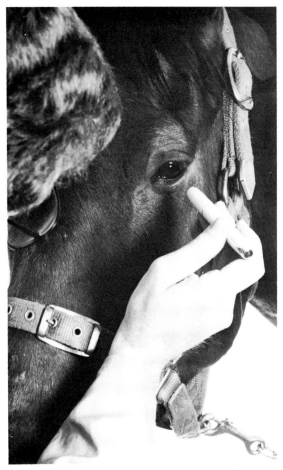

Figure 1-11. Evaluation of a direct pupillary light response.

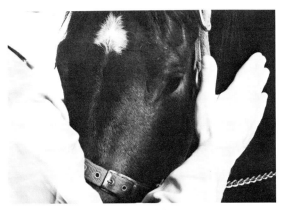

Figure 1-10. Evaluation of the menace response.

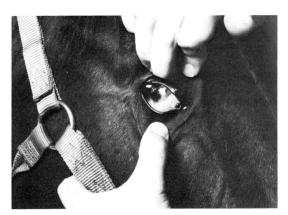

Figure 1-12. Protrusion of the third eyelid (nictitating membrane) by pressure applied to the eyeball via the upper eyelid.

1-13*a*). Other sites for determining the pulse rate and quality are shown in Figure 13*b* to *d*. The important things to note are the pulse character, amplitude, and regularity.

■ *Palpation for lymph node enlargement* should be performed between the rami of the mandibles and in the region of Viborg's triangle to determine if enlargement of the mandibular and pharyngeal lymph nodes is present.

■ *The larynx also should be palpated* at this stage to determine if atrophy of the dorsal cricoarytenoid muscle can be felt (Fig. 1-14). If present, as in horses with idiopathic left laryngeal hemiplegia, the muscular process of the left arytenoid cartilage will be more prominent than on the right side. Any scarring or thickening of skin that could suggest a previous laryngoplasty or laryngotomy should be noted.

KEY POINT ▶ If there is any indication of more prominence of the left muscular pro-

cess of the arytenoid cartilage, a laryngeal adductor ("slap test") should be performed while palpating the muscular process on left and right sides.

Slapping the left thorax gently with the open hand should result in the right muscular process adducting, and this can be felt as a flicking or movement of the process. Similarly, slapping of the right thorax should result in the muscular process of the left arytenoid cartilage "flicking." In horses with idiopathic left laryngeal hemiplegia, the flicking of the left muscular process does not occur or is reduced in response to the slap test. The slap-test response also may be lost in horses with cervical spinal cord disease.

■ *Palpation of the lateral processes of the cervical vertebrae* is done (Fig. 1-15), and the range of lateral movement and degree of neck flexion are noted, together with any indications of pain.

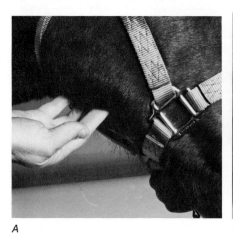
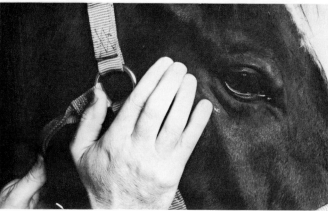

A *B*

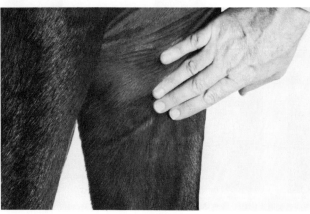
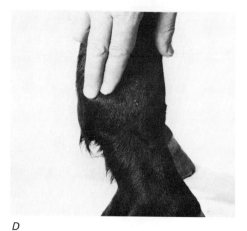

C *D*

Figure 1–13. *A*. Palpation of the pulse in the right facial artery over the right horizontal ramus of the mandible. *B*. Palpation of the pulse in the transverse facial artery just caudal to the lateral canthus of the right eye. *C*. Palpation of the pulse in the median artery of the left foreleg. (Note that it may be difficult to detect a pulse in this location because the artery is quite deep.) *D*. Palpation of the pulse in the digital (palmar) artery of the right foreleg.

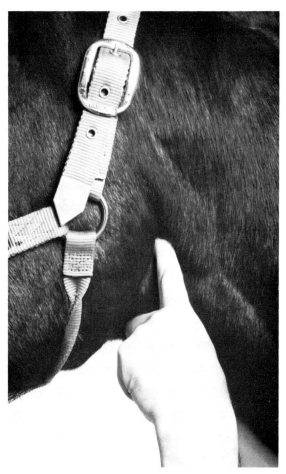

Figure 1–14. Palpation for prominence of the left muscular process indicating atrophy of the left dorsal cricoarytenoid muscle. The left index finger is shown ventral to the tendon of the sternocephalicus muscle. The muscular process is palpated on the dorsum of the larynx. This position is also used when evaluating the "slap test" for laryngeal adductor function.

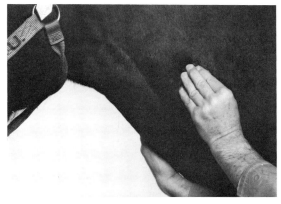

Figure 1–15. Palpation of the transverse processes of the cervical vertebrae shown on the left side of the neck.

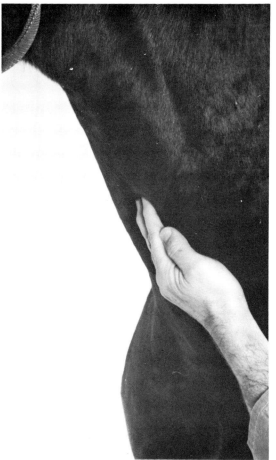

Figure 1–16. Palpation of the cervical trachea for signs of stenosis.

■ *The trachea also should be palpated* (Fig. 1-16) in the cervical region, and any narrowing should be noted. Both jugular veins should be checked for patency so that thrombophlebitis can be diagnosed. This problem is common in racehorses that receive regular intravenous injections. Evidence of an increased jugular pulse also should be noted because this could indicate congestive heart failure.

Examination of the Forelegs

■ *The forelegs should be inspected* for any swellings, particularly from the carpus distally, because most forelimb lamenesses are found in the lower part of the leg. Note particularly the proximal carpal and mid-carpal joints, the second metacarpal bone, the flexor tendons, the interosseous (suspensory) ligament, and the fetlock joint, including the palmar pouch. It is important to compare any response with that in the opposite foreleg.

KEY POINT ▶ Figures showing detailed examination of the forelimb are shown in Chapter 3, pages 49 to 54.

- *Examination of the foreleg should commence at the foot,* and after checking for signs of increased heat around the hoof wall and coronary band, hoof testers should be applied around the foot and across the frog to determine if pain can be elicited (see Chap. 3). With the leg held up, the lateral cartilages should be palpated to check for any ossification, and the pastern region should be flexed and rotated to determine whether a painful response can be produced. This is shown by the horse withdrawing its leg in response to flexion.
- *The fetlock joint is flexed* to examine the range of movement and to ascertain if there are signs of pain. Note should be made of any dorsal enlargement of the joint or distension of the palmar pouch, located in the distal metacarpus between the suspensory ligament and the palmar aspect of the third metacarpal bone.
- *The flexor tendons and interosseous (suspensory) ligament are palpated,* with weight off the leg, for evidence of heat, swelling, and pain. Note that firm pressure on the interosseous ligament near its point of bifurcation will produce a painful reaction in normal horses. The area of the inferior check ligament, just distal to the carpus on the palmar aspect of the proximal third metacarpal bone, also should be palpated.
- *The second and fourth metacarpal bones are palpated* to determine if any swellings ("splints") are present proximally or for swelling and callus associated with a fracture of the distal part of one of the small metacarpal bones.
- *The dorsal aspect of the third metacarpal bone is palpated* to determine if pain resulting from "bucked shins" is present.
- *The carpus should be examined closely* because carpal injuries are common in athletic horses. Any distension of the joint capsule over the dorsal aspect of the proximal carpal (radiocarpal) and middle carpal (intercarpal) joints should be noted and the joints carefully palpated and flexion tests performed. In some acute injuries, pain can be elicited by firm digital pressure being applied over the affected carpal bone. The carpus should then be flexed so that the foot is taken up past the point of the elbow. In many chronic carpal injuries, pain will not be evoked until the last few degrees of carpal flexion. A normal horse will not show any response to extreme carpal flexion, and therefore, an adverse response should be treated with suspicion. The area above the carpus is difficult to examine, particularly with regard to localizing signs. Flexion, extension, and abduction of the upper forelimb can be carried out to check for signs of pain and the musculature palpated.

Examination of the Chest

- *When examining the chest,* the most important part of the initial assessment is to *note the character and frequency of the respirations.* This is best done at a distance so that the degree of respiratory effort can be noted. In the absence of lower respiratory disease, a horse at rest will have a slow respiratory rate (8–16 breaths/min) with very little evidence of chest-wall movement. Any prolongation of inspiration or expiration should be observed. In addition, if the abdominal component of expiration is pronounced, a lower airway problem can be suspected. Initially, the heart should be auscultated using a stethoscope, with the bell placed under the triceps muscles at a level just ventral to an imaginary line through the point of the shoulder (Fig. 1-17). Auscultation is carried out from both the left and right sides of the chest. The heart should be auscultated for at least 1 minute, noting disturbances of rhythm or the presence of murmurs.

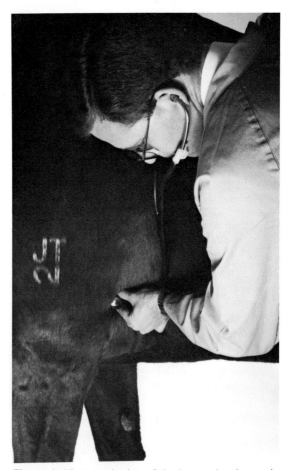

Figure 1–17. Auscultation of the heart, showing position of bell of the stethoscope under the triceps musculature.

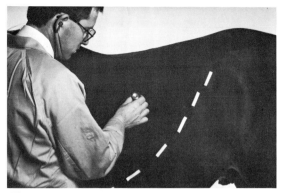

Figure 1–18. Auscultation of the lung fields showing outline of the diaphragm with white tape.

KEY POINT ► The normal heart rate at rest ranges from 28 to 36 beats/min in the adult horse and 70 to 100 beats/min in foals during the first few days of life.

■ *Auscultation of both the left and right lung fields is carried out* (Fig. 1-18), but in most normal horses breathing quietly at rest, few sounds will be detected. The exception to this is auscultation over the hilar region and the trachea. If there is any suspicion of abnormal sounds (gurgles or wheezes), a plastic bag can be placed over the horse's nose to stimulate respiration due to the combination of hypoxia and rebreathing of carbon dioxide (see Chap. 4). This technique will increase both the frequency and depth of respiration and thus permit abnormal lung sounds to be heard more easily.
■ *Percussion of the chest wall should be undertaken* if there is any indication of a respiratory abnormality. This is achieved using a plexor and pleximeter. Alternatively, a dessert spoon can be used as a pleximeter and a patellar hammer as a plexor. The spoon is placed over the dorsal aspect of one of the ribs, and the hammer is used to tap on the spoon as it is moved ventrally (see Chap. 4). A dull sound may indicate the presence of fluid in the chest. Alternatively, using the thumb and third finger, the back of the fingernail can be flicked against the chest wall (Fig. 1-19). The area of the thorax over the lung fields should be percussed from dorsal to ventral and from cranial to caudal.

Examination of the Abdomen

Detailed examination of the abdomen is difficult, and if an abdominal problem is suspected, various specialized procedures may be necessary. However, at the initial examination, note should be taken of the abdominal outline to determine if there

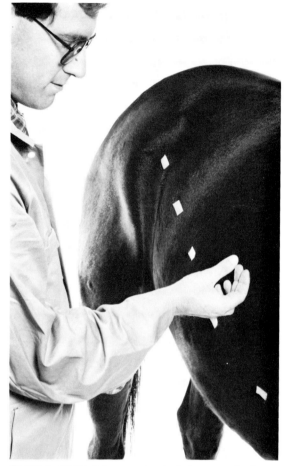

Figure 1–19. Digital percussion technique over the lung fields to determine areas of dullness. The middle finger is flicked against the chest wall.

is abdominal distension, which may be found in certain types of colic where there is tympany of the large bowel.

■ *Auscultation of the abdomen should be performed* on the left and right sides, over both the paralumbar fossae and lower flank regions (Figs. 1-20 and 1-21). Over the right paralumbar fossa, ileocecal valve sounds (these sound like a toilet flushing) may be heard approximately every 30 to 60 seconds. It is important to determine whether the gut sounds are normal, increased, or decreased.
■ *If abdominal distension is present,* percussion while listening with a stethoscope placed over the area of distension can be useful to determine if there is a gas-filled viscus.
■ *The rectal temperature should be taken* at this stage. Normal values are in the range 98 to 102°F (36.5–38.5°C) for adult horses. Foals tend to be at the high end of this range.

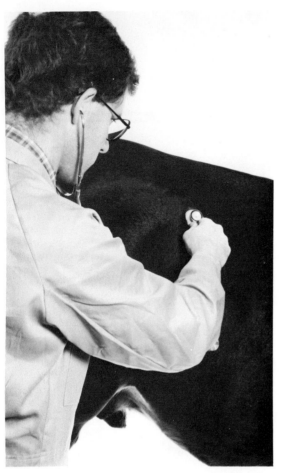

Figure 1–20. Auscultation of the abdomen showing examination of the right paralumbar fossa.

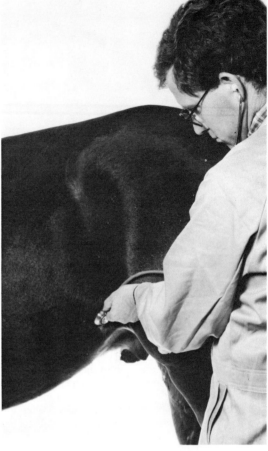

Figure 1–21. Auscultation of the abdomen showing examination over the left lower flank region.

Examination of the Back

Structural or anatomic abnormalities of the back, including scoliosis, lordosis, and kyphosis, can be best appreciated by standing behind (but not too close) the horse that is weight bearing evenly on the hindlegs. It is useful to have something to stand on, so the horse's back can be viewed from above.

- *The dorsal spinous processes should be palpated* over the thoracic and lumbar regions, and firm pressure should be applied over the tuber sacrale. In horses with hindleg weakness or sacroiliac pain, mild pressure at this site will result in the horse crouching away from the examiner (Fig. 1-22).
- *Stroking, with the blunt end of a ballpoint pen,* over the thoracolumbar area results in the horse dipping its back, whereas doing so at the caudal sacral region will cause the horse to arch its back. Some horses are hypersensitive to this examination, and the reaction found should be assessed

and differentiated from a response to a pathologic process involving soft tissue or vertebrae.

Examination of Genitalia

- *Unless the history indicates* the possibility of a urogenital problem, a *detailed examination of the genitalia is not necessary.*
- *In both stallions and geldings, the preputial area should be examined* for any signs of discharge, which could indicate an infection, squamous cell carcinoma, or habronemiasis. In a stallion, the testicles should be palpated to make sure that the horse is not a cryptorchid.
- *In fillies and mares, the perineal conformation should be noted* to determine the likelihood of pneumovagina causing a clinical problem. The presence of current or previous Caslick's operations also should be noted. If there are any signs of discharge from the vulva or "scalding" around the hindlegs, a more detailed reproductive or uri-

Examination of the Gait

After completing the general examination, the history will indicate whether the gait should be assessed. This is most likely to be necessary where there is a musculoskeletal or neuromuscular problem. The basic examination should include walking and trotting the horse on a hard surface to detect any signs of lameness or ataxia. It also may be useful to lunge the horse if a musculoskeletal problem is suspected because some lamenesses are more obvious when the animal is trotted in a tight circle.

Rectal Examination

A rectal examination is not usually considered to be part of the normal examination procedure, but it should be undertaken where there is a history of a gastrointestinal problem, an unusual hindleg lameness, or an internal reproductive disorder. It is important that the horse be adequately restrained and, if necessary, tranquilized. Propantheline, given at a dose rate of 0.1 to 0.2 mg/kg intravenously, is also worthwhile if relaxation of the rectum is required. However, propantheline may also result in ileus, and therefore care should be taken with its use. Restraint is best and most safely achieved in stocks, although the use of tail restraint with or without a sideline is also quite effective.

Details of how to perform a rectal examination are presented in Chapter 7. For general examination, we have found the following sequence to be useful: After introduction of the arm, the pelvis is examined for any swelling or crepitus. If a pelvic problem is suspected, different regions of the pelvis can be palpated while an assistant gently rocks the horse by pushing against the tuber coxa on either the left or right side. After examining the pelvis, the bladder and reproductive organs (in the mare) should be examined. Next, the left lateral abdominal wall is palpated. With further anterior exploration, the caudal border of the spleen is felt, and dorsally, the caudal border of the left kidney is evident. Although variable, the pelvic flexure of the large colon may be palpable on the left side of the ventral caudal abdomen. On the right side of the abdomen, the small colon can be determined by the presence of fecal balls and its mobility. Depending on the degree of distension of the cecum, different portions can be palpated. If it is severely distended with gas or impacted with food, the base can be felt toward the dorsal abdominal wall. However, in most conditions, the only reliable finding is the ventral taenia. Palpation of the mesenteric root, cranial mesenteric artery, and lymph nodes is difficult in most large horses, particularly if there is abdominal pain present. In stallions, it is always wise to check the integrity of the internal inguinal rings, which can be felt on the lateral part of the ventral abdominal wall just cranial to the femoral canal. In some conditions, enlargement of the inguinal lymph nodes can be detected. After completing a rectal

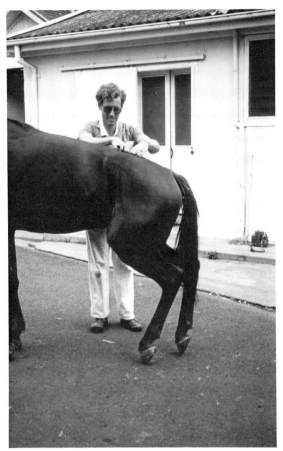

Figure 1–22. Horse showing sacroiliac pain on palpation over the tuber sacrale.

nary examination is required, together with possible catheterization of the bladder and a rectal examination.

Examination of the Hindlegs

The distal part of the hindlegs is examined in a similar manner as for the forelegs.

- *The hock is the most common site of chronic hindleg lameness* and therefore should be inspected carefully for swelling.
- *The stifle should be examined* by palpating between the three patellar ligaments. The medial femoropatellar pouch is found between the medial and middle patellar ligaments, whereas the lateral femoropatellar pouch is found between the middle and lateral patellar ligaments. In gonitis, it is common to find distension of one or both femoropatellar pouches.
- *Hindleg symmetry* should be checked because in some chronic hindleg lamenesses, atrophy of the gluteal muscles on the affected side will be evident.

TABLE 1–1. Prepurchase Examination Form, American Association of Equine Practitioners

Name of Horse	Breed	Tattoo	Sex	Color	Age	Markings

Seller's statement before examination:

Seller's Name	Address	Phone number

How long have you been acquainted with this animal? _____

How long have you had this animal under your personal care? _____

Do you have knowledge of present or past _____ Diseases _____ Lameness _____

Treatments _____ Vices (stable or being ridden) _____ Disabilities _____

Medications _____ Eccentricities _____

Do you have knowledge of past performances of this animal for the proposed use? _____

Do you have a personal estimate of the suitability of this animal for this purpose?

Unique _____ Exceptional _____ Adequate _____ No opinion _____

Signature of Seller _____ Date _____

Address _____

Buyer's Statement of the Purchase of this Horse:

Buyer's Name	Address	Phone number

To what use do you intend to put this horse (degree of work, hours to be used)? _____

What is the age, size, ability, and experience of the intended rider?

How long have you been acquainted with this animal? _____

How long have you tried this animal? _____

How many of the proposed uses have you tried? _____

Of what relative importance are the following to you?

Appearance of the horse including (and any) blemishes _____

Performance _____ Temperament _____

How do you rate the suitability of this horse for the intended purpose?

Unique _____ Exceptional _____ Adequate _____

What type of care (stabling) is anticipated for this horse? _____

Intensive (continual care and supervision) _____

Average (stabled daily for feeding, etc.) _____

Casual (on pasture most of the time) _____

Signature of Buyer _____ Date _____

Address _____

PHYSICAL EXAMINATION

Place _____ Date _____ Time _____

Weather _____

GENERAL HEALTH AND APPEARANCE

Approximate height _____ Approximate weight _____

Cert. of height (pony) _____ Temperature (rectal) _____

Complete the following with N = normal, AB = abnormal, NE = not examined.

A. Bilateral symmetry
  1. Head and neck _____
  2. Body _____
  3. Legs _____
  4. Feet _____
B. Eyes
  1. Symmetry _____
  2. Reflexes _____
  3. Lids _____
  4. Mucous membranes _____
  5. Cornea _____
  6. Ophthalmoscopic exam _____
C. Mouth
  1. Lips _____
  2. Tongue _____
  3. Teeth _____
  4. Gums _____
  5. Mucous membrane _____
  6. Odor _____
  7. Bite _____
D. Nasal and paranasal
  1. Symmetry _____
  2. Airflow _____
  3. Odor _____
  4. Mucous membranes _____
  5. Percussion _____
  6. Exudate _____
E. Pharynx, larynx, trachea
  1. Palpation _____
  2. Cough induction (reflex) _____
  3. Auscultation at rest _____
     After exercise _____
     After recovery _____
F. Cardiovascular
  1. Palpation (heart and pulse) _____
  2. Auscultation at rest _____
     After exercise _____
     After recovery _____
  3. Pulse rate and quality _____
G. Pulmonary
  1. Percussion _____
  2. Auscultation at rest _____
     After exercise _____
     After recovery _____
  3. Respiratory (rate rest) _____

H. Digestive
  1. Percussion _____
  2. Auscultation _____
  3. Inspection of feces _____
I. Genital–urinary
  1. External _____
  2. Inspection and palpation _____
     (a) Breeding soundness, mares
          Barren _____ Maiden _____
          Foaling _____
  1. Rectal examination _____
  2. Speculum examination _____
  3. Culture _____
     (b) Breeding soundness, stallions
  1. Rectal examination _____
  2. Test breeding _____
  3. Culture _____
  4. Semen examination _____
  5. Inspection and palpation _____
J. Integument
  Note especially "used" marks (interference with the saddle, girth sores, firing or other treatment, dermatoses, etc.). Insignificant scars need not be enumerated.
K. Musculoskeletal
     (a) Vertebral column
  1. Symmetry _____
  2. Palpation _____
  3. Manipulation _____
     (b) Limbs
  1. Symmetry _____
  2. Palpation _____
  3. Manipulation _____
     (c) Gaits
  1. Symmetry _____
  2. Freedom of movement on hard surface _____
  3. On soft surface _____
  4. On a straight way _____
  5. Turning both ways _____
L. Vices: Cribbing ___ Weaving ___
  Digging ___ Savaging ___ Other ___
  1. Stable manners _____
  2. Field manners _____
M. Nervous system
  1. Inspection _____
  2. Has horse been nerved _____
  3. If so, where _____

Conditions other than normal found in the animal (list by title):
_____
_____
_____

SPECIAL PROCEDURES
ECG _____
Endoscopy _____
Radiographs _____
Rectal examination _____
Nerve blocks _____
Laboratory studies _____
Other _____
  _____

Signature: _____
Address: _____
Date: _____

examination, it is very important to inspect the glove to ensure that there is no blood present, which could indicate mucosal damage or a rectal tear.

Prepurchase Examination

The prepurchase examination, also referred to by some as the "soundness examination" or "vet check," has great potential for conflict. Many vendors sell horses with problems that they hope will not be detected before money changes hands. The veterinarian may unwittingly be caught in the middle of a dispute, which may result in litigation. There are some important points about prepurchase examinations that can help in preventing these problems:

- The examination should only be performed on behalf of the purchaser, not the seller. Veterinarians should resist any attempt by a vendor to get them to examine a horse that is for sale because there is inevitably a conflict of interest.
- Written statements from both the seller and purchaser may be helpful and prevent misunderstandings in the future about the reasons for the examination. The American Association of Equine Practitioners has a format for history collection and the examination that is useful (see Table 1-1).
- It should be clarified with the client exactly what is included in the examination. In many cases, problems arise because the client has not understood the nature of the examination.
- A prepurchase examination is a detailed physical examination without the use of any diagnostic aids such as radiography, endoscopy, and electrocardiography. The latter specialized techniques may be offered as additional aids to the routine examination. The term *complete physical examination* should be avoided.
- A written report must be provided that clearly identifies the horse examined and lists the problems found. The terms *sound* and *unsound* are best avoided.
- The report should contain a clear description and markings (preferably a diagram) of the horse together with the time, date, and place of examination. The American Association of Equine Practitioners advises that no opinion be given as to the suitability of the horse, which is the sole responsibility of the buyer. However, the report should provide an opinion as to the functional significance of any abnormal findings listed.
- It is easy to overlook a body system if a checklist is not used. The format set out in Table 1-1 is that suggested by the American Association of Equine Practitioners, and we have found it very helpful in ensuring a detailed examination.

Physical Restraint

With better drugs available for restraint of horses, physical restraint is less important than in the past. However, there are a range of techniques that are of considerable use in equine practice. It is important to be confident when approaching horses because they can detect nervousness and are often more difficult to handle if they sense this emotion in the handler. Most horses are used to being approached from the left or near side.

KEY POINT ► The most common mistake that we have seen in students and clinicians used to working with horses in stocks is that they stand in front of horses when performing tasks such as stomach tubing and teeth examination.

This is a certain way to be struck by the front feet of a horse. All examinations and procedures performed in the unrestrained horse should be done standing beside and close to the horse. The simplest restraint procedures for temporary diversion of the horse to allow insertion of a needle or injection include grasping a fold of skin on the neck (Fig. 1-23) and twisting an ear (Fig. 1-24). If further restraint is required, the use of a twitch is useful (Figs. 1-25 and 1-26). However, it should be noted that many clients, particularly those with pleasure horses, do not like to see their horses twitched, and therefore, the twitch should be used only where necessary. Once the twitch is applied, several half hitches should be made around the handle of the twitch using the lead rope, and the person holding the twitch should stand at the level of the shoulder (Fig. 1-27). In some cases, horses will try to strike when the twitch is applied or when a procedure such as stomach tubing is undertaken. In these horses, it may be helpful to use the horse's blanket, with the lining on the outer side, around the neck like a table napkin

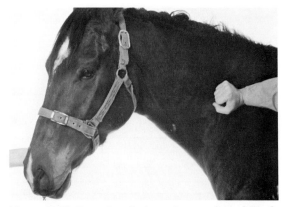

Figure 1–23. Restraint of a horse by grasping a fold of skin on the left side of the neck.

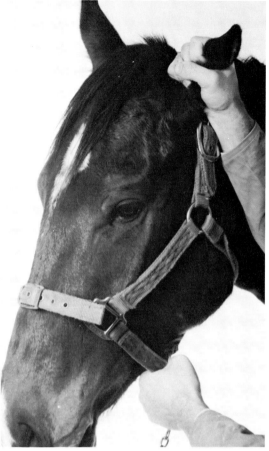

Figure 1–24. Twisting of an ear for restraint in a horse.

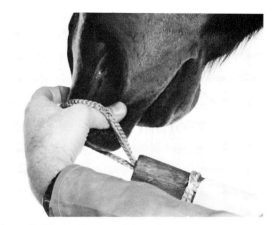

Figure 1–26. Application of the twitch to the upper lip.

(Fig. 1-28). This not only quiets most horses but also prevents them from inflicting trauma on the examiner if the horses attempt to strike. The other useful restraint technique is the single sideline (Figs. 1-29 to 1-32). A single sideline will assist in restraint of difficult horses and may be useful for performing rectal examinations where stocks are not available and for performing standing castrations. Protection for the examining veterinarian also can be achieved if rectal examinations are performed around the door of a box stall or with the horse backed up to several bales of hay.

Other simple forms of restraint include covering the horse's eyes (Fig. 1-33), which may be useful in horses that are reactive to needles, and the use of a stallion chain placed over the dorsum of the nose (Fig. 1-34). With the latter technique, care must be

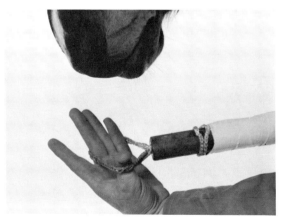

Figure 1–25. A rope twitch showing the position of the fingers in the twitch loop prior to grasping the upper lip.

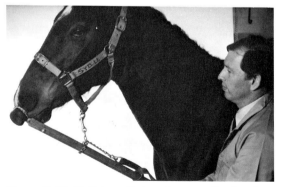

Figure 1–27. Twitch applied to the upper lip showing half hitches around the twitch handle and position in which the handler should stand.

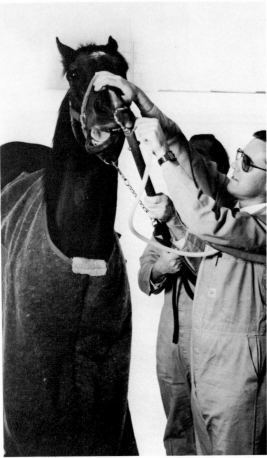

Figure 1–28. Demonstration of a horse's blanket being used to assist in preventing the horse from striking. The blanket is placed inside out and fastened around the horse's neck.

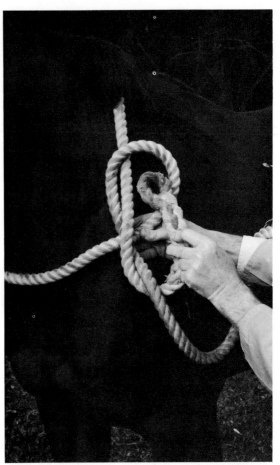

Figure 1–30. Completion of the bowline knot for a single sideline. The free end of the rope is passed through the loop, around the rope, and passed back into the loop.

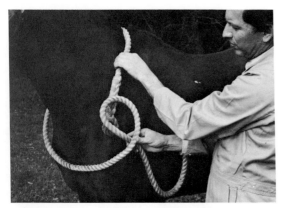

Figure 1–29. Beginning of a bowline knot for application of a single sideline. A loop is made in the rope through which the free end of the rope is passed.

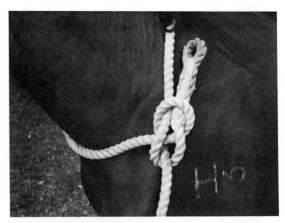

Figure 1–31. Bowline knot tied for a single sideline. This type of knot will not slip.

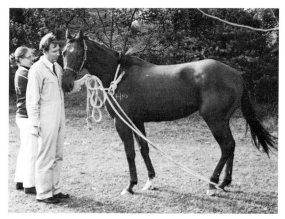

Figure 1–32. Single sideline applied for restraint.

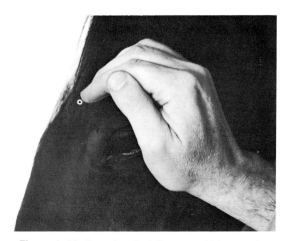

Figure 1–33. Covering the left eye to aid in restraint.

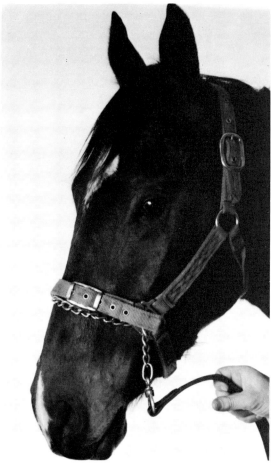

Figure 1–34. Use of a stallion chain applied over the dorsum of the nose to aid in restraint.

taken to ensure that excessive tension is not placed on the lead, but rather a short, sharp jerk is given where needed. Because some horses object to a twitch, an alternative is the placement of a stallion chain under the top lip (Fig. 1-35). The chain is attached to the right side of the headstall and, after passing under the upper lip, is taken through the D ring on the headstall.

Lifting one of the forelegs or hindlegs may be useful to aid in restraint and must be undertaken to examine the limbs. The correct techniques for lifting the foreleg and hindleg are shown in Figures 1-36 to 1-43.

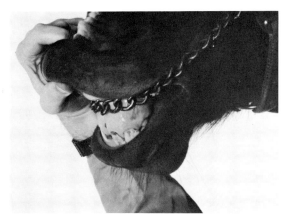

Figure 1–35. Use of a stallion chain applied under the top lip to aid in restraint.

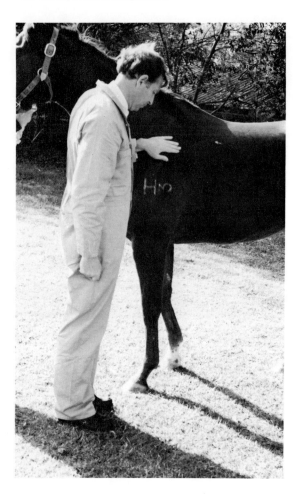

Figure 1–36. Commencing position for picking up the left foreleg with the examiner facing toward the rear of the horse.

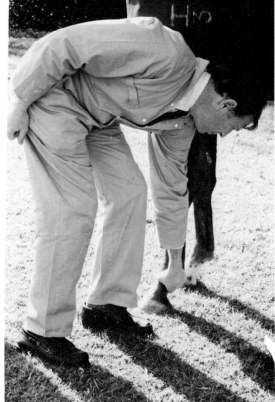

Figure 1–37. To pick up the left foreleg, the left hand is run distally down the leg until the area of the pastern is reached. The pastern is grasped with the hand, and the left shoulder of the examiner is used to push against the horse and shift weight off the left leg.

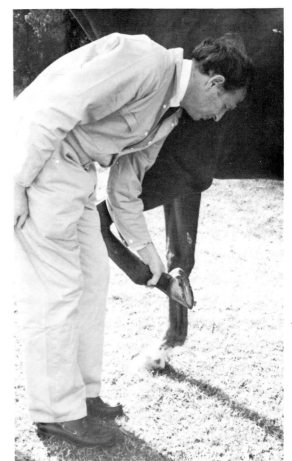

Figure 1–38. The left leg is picked up.

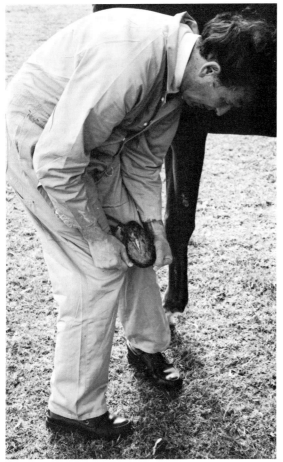

Figure 1–39. To examine the horse's foot, it is held between the knees of the examiner. This is most easily done if the examiner's toes are pointed inward.

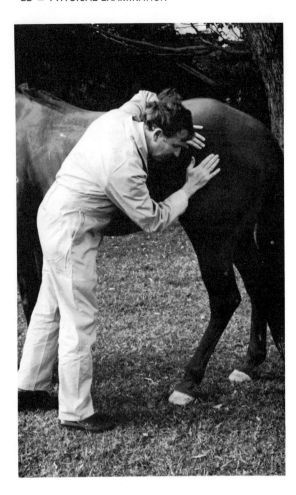

Figure 1–40. Commencing position for picking up the left hindleg.

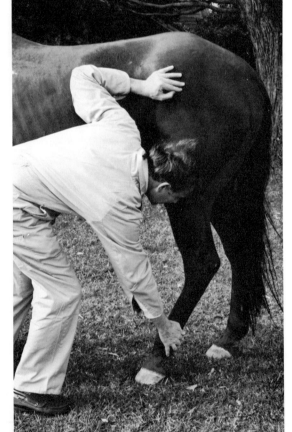

Figure 1–41. With the left hand placed on the tuber coxa, the right hand is run distally to the plantar aspect of the pastern.

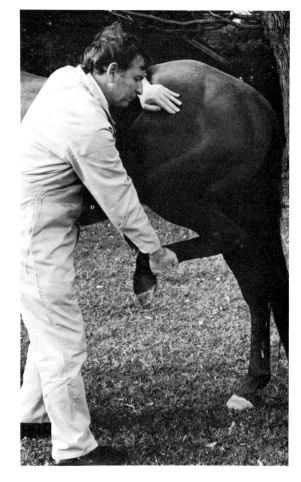

Figure 1–42. Using the left hand, weight is shifted onto the right hindleg of the horse, and the left hindleg is pulled cranially.

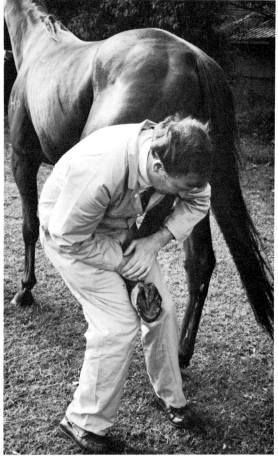

Figure 1–43. The examiner walks caudally, stepping between the hindlegs, so that the leg is moderately extended, and the left hind foot is rested on the knees.

CHAPTER 2

Protocols for Common Presenting Complaints

LIST OF PROTOCOLS

ABDOMINAL PAIN: COLIC

Signalment
  Age of the Horse
    Parasites—young horses
    Gastrointestinal ulcers—young horses
    Intussusception—young horses
    Large intestine impaction—older horses
    Anterior enteritis—adult horses
    Lipomas—older horses
    Enteroliths—older horses
    Epiploic foramen entrapment—young
      horses
  Breed and Use
    Thoroughbred and Quarter Horse Racehorse
      Spasmodic colic
      Cecal dilatation
      Large intestine impaction
      Anterior enteritis
      Gastroduodenal ulcers
      Small intestine volvulus and torsion
      Pleuritis
      Peritonitis

      Colitis
      Sand colic
      Herniation of small intestine through the epi-
        ploic foramen
      Entrapment of bowel through the nephro-
        splenic ligament
    Standardbred Trotter and Pacer
      Spasmodic colic
      Cecal dilatation
      Large intestine impaction
      Anterior enteritis
      Gastroduodenal ulcers
      Small intestine volvulus and torsion
      Pleuritis
      Peritonitis
      Colitis
      Sand colic
      Entrapment of bowel through the nephro-
        splenic ligament
    Working Quarter Horse
      Spasmodic colic
      Impaction colic
      Sand colic

Thromboembolic cranial mesenteric arteritis
Grain overload
Enteroliths
Cystic urolithiasis
Entrapment of bowel through the nephro-
splenic ligament
Pleasure Horses
Sand colic
Spasmodic colic
Impaction colic
Thromboembolic cranial mesenteric arteritis
Strangulating lipoma
Enteroliths
Grain overload
Abdominal tumors
Cystic urolithiasis
Entrapment of bowel through the nephro-
splenic ligament
Cholelithiasis
Peritonitis
Pleuritis
Foals
Retained meconium
Gastroduodenal ulcers
Small intestine intussusception
Rupture of urinary bladder
Sex
Inguinal herniation of the small bowel–stal-
lions
Large bowel torsion—postpartum mares
Uterine torsion—pregnant mares
Cystic urolithiasis—geldings and stallions
Retailed meconium—male foals
Rupture of urinary bladder—male foals
History
How long has the pain been present?
Is the horse straining?
Has the horse been rolling?
What is the horse's deworming history?
What medication has the horse received?
Is this an acute onset or has the horse been
slowly developing signs?
What has the horse been eating, and when did
it last eat?
Is the horse exposed to sand at pasture?
Have the teeth been checked recently?
Is the pain continuous or intermittent?
How long is it since feces were passed?
Are the feces normal in appearance and con-
sistency?
Have there been any other episodes of abdom-
inal pain?
Physical Examination
General Inspection
Attitude—depressed or bright
Behavior—pawing, attempting to roll, glancing
at flanks, frequent urination
Abdominal distension
Detailed Inspection
Vitals: HR, RR, temperature, pulse quality
Gut sounds
Capillary refill time

Mucous membrane color
Temperature of extremities
Diagnostic Procedures
Stomach Intubation
Presence/absence of excess fluid
Gastric reflux (Spend 5 minutes to ensure that
no reflux is present. Backflush tube with
water, and try to siphon off fluid.)
Rectal Examination
Impaction of the large bowel
Displaced bowel
Distended small bowel loops
Check nephrosplenic space, inguinal canal
(stallions)
Abdominocentesis
Fluid color
Fluid turbidity
Presence of blood
Presence of ingesta
Clinical Pathology
Hematocrit and total serum/plasma protein
White cell count and differential
Plasma and abdominal fluid lactate determina-
tions
Venous or arterial acid–base status
Abdominal fluid: cytology, total protein, bac-
teriology
Serum/plasma electrolyte values
Plasma/serum fibrinogen
Liver function: GGT, SDH, AP, bile acids
Ultrasound
Examination of the liver
Examination of the kidneys
Differential Diagnoses
Spasmodic colic*
Large intestine impaction*
Anterior enteritis*
Large intestine displacement/torsion
Gastroduodenal ulcers
Sand colic
Small intestine volvulus and torsion
Small intestine intussusception
Cecal dilatation
Peritonitis
Colitis
Herniation of small intestine through the epi-
ploic foramen
Grain overload
Thromboembolic cranial mesenteric arteritis
Enteroliths
Strangulating lipoma
Abdominal tumors
Abdominal abscess
Cystic urolithiasis
Hepatitis
Cholelithiasis
Pleuritis

*Denotes most likely diagnosis.

ALOPECIA

Signalment

Age of the Horse

Seborrheic alopecia—older horses

Hormonal disturbances—older horses

Breed and Use

Pemphigus foliaceus (Appaloosa)

Sex

No significant effect

History

How long has the problem been present?

Has the diet recently been changed?

Is pruritus associated with the alopecia?

Has the alopecia been treated?

What was the response to treatment?

Is the horse eating normally?

Is the horse losing weight?

Physical Examination

General Inspection

General body condition

Attitude—depressed or bright

Note distribution of alopecia

Detailed Inspection

Vitals: HR, RR, temperature, gut sounds, capillary refill time

Determine whether the lesions are localized or generalized

Note if any evidence of pruritus

Evidence of self-trauma

Clipping of hair in a pruritic region and examination of skin with a hand lens

Clinical Pathology

CBC

Total plasma protein

Examination of the Skin

Skin scrapings

Impression smears

Intradermal skin testing

Acetate tape preparations

Bacterial/fungal cultures

Skin biopsies (histopathology, fluorescent antibody testing)

Differential Diagnoses

Dermatophilosis*

Dermatophytosis*

Culicoides hypersensitivity

Cutaneous habronemiasis

Anhidrosis

Sarcoid

Pemphigus foliaceus

Seborrheic dermatosis

Equine linear keratosis

Cutaneous onchocerciasis

Ectoparasites (e.g., biting flies, lice, ticks, harvest mites or "chiggers," mosquitoes)

Folliculitis/furunculosis

Urticaria due to inhaled allergens or drug administration

Mercury blister

Contact dermatitis

Photosensitization, primary and secondary

Scratches ("grease heel")

Phycomycosis

Habronemiasis

Neurologic diseases (e.g., rabies, polyneuritis equi, self-mutilation syndrome)

ANEMIA

Signalment

Age of the Horse

Neonatal isoerythrolysis—newborn foals

Equine infectious anemia—mature horses

Guttural pouch mycosis—mature horses

Piroplasmosis (babesiosis)—mature horses

Ehrlichiosis—mature horses

Breed and Use

Thoroughbred and Quarter Horse Racehorse

Anemia of chronic disease

Blood loss anemia

Gastrointestinal parasitism

Gastrointestinal ulcer disease

Nonsteroidal anti-inflammatory drug toxicity

Phlebotomy

Neoplasia

Vasculitis

Equine viral arteritis

Standardbred Trotter and Pacer

Anemia of chronic disease

Blood loss anemia

Gastrointestinal ulcer disease

Gastrointestinal parasitism

Nonsteroidal anti-inflammatory drug toxicity

Phlebotomy

Neoplasia

Vasculitis

Equine viral arteritis

Working Quarter Horse

Anemia of chronic disease

Blood loss anemia

Gastrointestinal parasitism

Gastrointestinal ulcer disease

Nonsteroidal anti-inflammatory drug toxicity

Neoplasia

Vasculitis

Equine viral arteritis

Pleasure Horses

Anemia of chronic disease

Nutritional (starvation)

Blood loss anemia

Gastrointestinal ulcer disease

Gastrointestinal parasitism

Nonsteroidal anti-inflammatory drug toxicity

Transfusion reactions

Equine infectious anemia

---

*Denotes most likely diagnosis.

Neoplasia
Equine viral arteritis
Piroplasmosis
Leptospirosis
Chronic liver disease
Gastrointestinal parasites
Thrombocytopenia
Oxidant toxicosis (e.g., drugs, onions, red maple leaf)
Vasculitis (purpura hemorrhagica)
Disseminated intravascular coagulation
Coagulopathies
Dicoumarin poisoning (sweet clover)
Aplastic anemia
Autoimmune anemia
Guttural pouch mycosis
Foals, All Breeds
Neonatal isoerythrolysis
Septicemia
Congenital disorders
Transfusion reactions
Aplastic anemia
Trauma
Hemophilia
Sex
No significant effect

History
Is there a history or evidence of hemorrhage or injury?
Is the horse receiving any medication?
Is the horse regularly dewormed?
Does the horse have evidence of intercurrent disease or malnutrition?
What are the constituents of the diet?
Is the horse housed in an area where viral or parasitic causes of anemia are common? If so, has the horse been infested with ticks?
What is the status of Coggins testing?
Is there evidence of exercise intolerance?
Are there other horses with similar signs?

Physical Examination
General Inspection
Note general condition of horse
Mental status of the horse
Evidence of edema
Detailed Examination
Vital signs: HR, RR, rectal temperature, mucous membrane color, capillary refill time, presence of icterus
Examination of mucous membranes for petechial and echymotic hemorrhage
Examine regional lymph nodes for enlargement
Examination of feces
Rectal examination
Examination of urine for hematuria
Examination for evidence of epistaxis

Diagnostic Procedures
Clinical Pathology
CBC and fibrinogen
Thrombocyte count
Coagulation profile

Presence of Heinz bodies
Serum biochemistry: GGT, SDH, AST, AP, creatinine, urea, electrolytes
Protein electrophoresis
Methemoglobin quantitation
Fecal occult blood determination
Blood smears for equine piroplasmosis and erhlichiosis
Bone Marrow Aspiration
Cytology
Myeloid–erythroid ratio
Serology
Coggins test
Coombs test
Equine viral arteritis titers and virus isolation
Complement fixation test for equine piroplasmosis
Endoscopic Examination
Blood from the guttural pouch openings
Blood from the ethmoid region
Presence of blood in the trachea

Differential Diagnoses
Anemia of chronic disease*
Gastrointestinal parasitism*
Blood loss anemia
Nutritional (starvation)
Nonsteroidal anti-inflammatory drug toxicity
Aplastic anemia
Autoimmune anemia
Equine infectious anemia
Gastrointestinal ulcer disease
Transfusion reactions
Neoplasia
Coagulopathies (e.g., disseminated intravascular coagulation)
Piroplasmosis
Leptospirosis
Chronic liver disease
Thrombocytopenia
Oxidant toxicosis (e.g., drugs, onions, red maple leaf)
Vasculitis
Dicoumarin poisoning (sweet clover)
Guttural pouch mycosis
Neonatal isoerythrolysis
Septicemia
Congenital disorders
Transfusion reactions

ATAXIA

Signalment
Age of the Horse
Cerebellar abiotrophy—foals
Neonatal maladjustment syndrome—foals
Septicemia—foals

---

*Denotes most likely diagnosis.

Cervical vertebral malformation—young
horses
Viral encephalomyelitides—mature horses
Protozoal myeloencephalitis—mature
horses
Atlanto-occipital malformation—young
horses (Arabians)
Discospondylitis—foals
Equine degenerative myeloencephalopa-
thy—young horses
Idiopathic vestibular syndrome—mature
horses
Otitis media/interna—mature horses
Rabies—mature horses
Vertebral osteomyelitis—foals
Arabian idiopathic epilepsy—foals
Breed and Use
Thoroughbred Racehorse
Cervical vertebral malformation
Head/spinal cord trauma
Protozoal myeloencephalitis
Herpesvirus myeloencephalitis
Idiopathic vestibular syndrome
Viral encephalomyelitides
Equine degenerative myeloencephalopathy
Rabies
Otitis media/interna
Standardbred Trotter and Pacer
Cervical vertebral malformation
Head/spinal cord trauma
Protozoal myeloencephalitis
Herpesvirus myeloencephalitis
Idiopathic vestibular syndrome
Viral encephalomyelitides
Equine degenerative myeloencephalopathy
Rabies
Otitis media/interna
Working Quarter Horse
Cervical vertebral malformation
Head/spinal cord trauma
Protozoal myeloencephalitis
Herpesvirus myeloencephalitis
Idiopathic vestibular syndrome
Viral encephalomyelitides
Equine degenerative myeloencephalopathy
Rabies
Otitis media/interna
Pleasure Horses
Cervical vertebral malformation
Head/spinal cord trauma
Protozoal myeloencephalitis
Herpesvirus myeloencephalitis
Idiopathic vestibular syndrome
Viral encephalomyelitides
Equine degenerative myeloencephalopathy
Rabies
Neuritis of the cauda equina
Hepatoencephalopathy
Lead poisoning
Botulism
Organophosphate toxicosis

Otitis media/interna
Locoweed toxicosis
White snakeroot poisoning
Narcolepsy/epilepsy
Verminous myelitis
Foals, All Breeds
Head/spinal cord trauma
Neonatal maladjustment syndrome
Septicemia
Idiopathic epilepsy (Arabians)
Vertebral osteomyelitis
Toxoinfectious botulism
Sex
Epilepsy (mares), increased incidence when
in estrus

History
How long have the signs been present?
Are there other neurologic signs?
Is there a history of trauma?
Is there a history of intercurrent infectious dis-
ease?
Are other horses affected?
Has the horse's diet altered recently?
Is the horse insured?
Are the signs progressive?
Were the signs sudden or insidious in onset?
Has the horse received any medication? (Note:
Ivermectin administration)

Physical Examination
General Inspection
Note mental status and behavior
Signs of trauma
Signs of asymmetry
Detailed Examination
Vitals: HR, RR, temperature, capillary refill
time, gut sounds
Neurologic examination
Assessment of cranial nerves
Assessment of gait and spinal cord function
Palpation of the neck and back
Laryngeal adductor ("slap") test by palpation
of the larynx

Diagnostic Procedures
Endoscopy
Examination of the nasopharynx, larynx, and
trachea
Laryngeal adductor ("slap") test
Radiography
Head and neck
Myelography
CSF Collection
Lumbosacral collection, standing
Atlanto-occipital collection, general anesthesia
(except foals)
Clinical Pathology
Hematology: CBC and fibrinogen
Liver enzymes
CSF: cytology, protein, color
Serology
EEE, WEE, herpesvirus

Differential Diagnoses
    Head/spinal cord trauma*
    Cervical vertebral malformation*
    Protozoal myeloencephalitis*
    Herpesvirus myeloencephalitis*
    Viral encephalomyelitides
    Equine degenerative myeloencephalopathy
    Hepatoencephalopathy
    Idiopathic vestibular syndrome
    Lead poisoning
    Botulism
    Organophosphate toxicosis
    Rabies
    Otitis media/interna
    Neuritis of the cauda equina
    Locoweed toxicosis
    White snakeroot poisoning
    Narcolepsy/epilepsy
    Neonatal maladjustment syndrome
    Septicemia
    Idiopathic epilepsy (Arabians)
    Vertebral osteomyelitis
    Toxoinfectious botulism
    Verminous myelitis
    Idiopathic polyneuropathy

COLLAPSE

Signalment
  Age of the Horse
    Congenital cardiovascular disorders—foals
    Acquired cardiovascular disease—mature horses
    Hepatoencephalopathy—mature horses
    Idiopathic convulsive syndrome—foals
    Rabies—mature horses
  Breed and Use
    Thoroughbred and Quarter Horse Racehorse
      Ruptured aorta or pulmonary artery
      Trauma
      Acquired cardiovascular disease
      Seizure disorders
    Standardbred Trotter and Pacer
      Ruptured aorta or pulmonary artery
      Trauma
      Acquired cardiovascular disease
      Seizure disorders
    Working Quarter Horse
      Cardiovascular disease
      Trauma
      Seizure disorders (e.g., epilepsy, convulsions)
      Narcolepsy
      Hyperkalemic periodic paralysis
    Pleasure Horses
      Cardiovascular disease

---

*Denotes most likely diagnosis.

      Seizure disorders (e.g., epilepsy, convulsions)
      Narcolepsy
    Foals, All Breeds
      Congenital cardiac disease
      Narcolepsy
      Idiopathic epilepsy (Arabians)
      Neonatal maladjustment syndrome
      Septicemia
      Trauma
  Sex
    Mares are more commonly affected by epilepsy when in estrus.
History
    How long have the signs been present?
    Is the collapse related to exercise or excitement?
    Is the collapse related to feeding?
    Are signs exacerbated by external stimuli (e.g., noise, light)?
    Is the collapse a regular or isolated event?
    Is there a recent history of trauma?
    Are there any warning signs prior to collapse?
    Does the horse show signs of distress prior to or after collapse?
    Are siblings or close relatives affected similarly?
    Are signs exacerbated by administration of phenothiazine tranquilizers?
Physical Examination
  General Inspection
    Behavior of the horse
    Mental status of the horse
    Signs of trauma
    Head posture
  Detailed Examination
    Vitals: HR, RR, temperature, capillary refill time, evidence of jugular pulse or edema
    Presence of icterus
    Auscultation of the heart
    Neurologic examination
Diagnostic Procedures
  Clinical Pathology
    CBC, fibrinogen, electrolytes
    Liver enzymes
  Electrocardiography
    Conduction disturbances
    Arrhythmias
  Ultrasound
    Chamber enlargement
    Valvular lesions
    Papillary muscle rupture
  Hyperkalemic Periodic Paralysis Challenge Test
    Potassium chloride by stomach tube
Differential Diagnoses
  Adults
    Ruptured aorta or pulmonary artery (death)*
    Trauma*
    Acquired cardiovascular disease
    Seizure disorders
    Narcolepsy

Foals
Congenital cardiac disease*
Narcolepsy*
Idiopathic epilepsy (Arabians)*
Neonatal maladjustment syndrome
Septicemia
Trauma

COUGHING

Signalment
Age of the Horse
Rhodococcus equi infections—foals
Viral respiratory disease—young horses
Herpesvirus—young horses
Influenza—young horses
Strangles infections—young horses
Allergic respiratory disease (COPD)—mature horses
Upper respiratory problems—young horses
Breed and Use
Thoroughbred and Quarter Horse Racehorse
Viral respiratory disease
Bacterial pneumonia/pleuritis
Upper respiratory tract problems
Exercise-induced pulmonary hemorrhage (EIPH) ("bleeders")
Pharyngitis
Standardbred Trotter and Pacer
Viral respiratory disease
Bacterial pneumonia/pleuritis
Upper respiratory tract problems
Exercise-induced pulmonary hemorrhage (EIPH) ("bleeders")
Pharyngitis
Working Quarter Horse
Strangles
Viral respiratory disease
Herpesvirus
Influenza
Bacterial bronchitis/pneumonia
Allergic respiratory disease (COPD)
Pleasure Horses
Strangles
Viral respiratory disease
Herpesvirus
Influenza
Bacterial bronchitis/pneumonia
Allergic respiratory disease (COPD)
Lungworm
Foals
Rhodococcus equi infections
Adenovirus (Arabians)
Viral respiratory disease
Bacterial bronchitis/pneumonia
Parasites (roundworm infestations)
Sex
No significant effect

---

*Denotes most likely diagnosis.

History
How long has the horse been coughing?
Has the horse been dewormed recently?
Has there been a nasal discharge at any stage?
Is more than one horse in the stable affected?
Is the cough related to feeding?
Is the cough related to exercise?
Is the cough related to stabling?
Is the horse eating and drinking normally?
Has the horse lost weight?
Are there signs of systemic disease (e.g., fever)?
Has the horse been in contact with any donkeys?
How would the cough be described?
Has the horse been vaccinated?
Physical Examination
General Inspection
Presence of nasal discharge
Lymph node enlargement
Odor of breath
Character of respiration
General body condition
Detailed Examination
Sinus percussion
Retropharyngeal lymph node palpation
Palpation of larynx (muscular process)
Auscultation of the chest, including rebreathing
Respiratory frequency
Diagnostic Procedures
Transtracheal Aspiration
Cytologic examination
Bacteriologic examination
Endoscopic Examination
Rhinolaryngoscopy
Examination of the trachea to level of tracheal bifurcation
Radiography
Head, sinuses, and larynx, if upper airway problem
Chest
Ultrasound
Examination of chest for presence of fluid
Arterial Blood Gas Analysis
PaO_2 determination
Hematology
Total and differential white cell count
Plasma fibrinogen
Differential Diagnoses
Viral upper respiratory tract infection*
Pharyngitis/tracheitis*
Allergic bronchiolitis (COPD)*
Pneumonia/pleuritis, bacterial
Exercise-induced pulmonary hemorrhage
Rhodococcus equi infection—foals
Lungworm
Epiglottic entrapment
Previous laryngoplasty surgery
Parasitic infestation (e.g., roundworms in foals)
Strangles

DIARRHEA

Signalment
  Age of the Horse
    Parasites—young horses
    "Foal heat" diarrhea—foals 7 to 14 days old
    Gastrointestinal ulcers—young horses
    Intussusception—young horses
    Salmonellosis—young horses
    Clostridial diarrhea—young horses
    Inflammatory bowel disease—older horses
    Neoplasia—older horses
    Nutritional—foals
    Colitis X—older horses
    Equine monocytic erhlichiosis ("Potomac fever")—older horses
  Breed and Use
    Thoroughbred and Quarter Horse Racehorse
      Idiopathic
      Drug-induced diarrhea (e.g., phenylbutazone, antibiotics)
      Stress-induced diarrhea
      Salmonellosis
      Gastroduodenal ulcers
      Colitis X
      Equine monocytic erhlichiosis ("Potomac fever")
      Intestinal clostridiosis
      Chronic liver disease
      Strongylosis
      Toxemia
      Peritonitis
    Standardbred Trotter and Pacer
      Idiopathic
      Drug-induced diarrhea (e.g., phenylbutazone, antibiotics)
      Stress-induced diarrhea
      Salmonellosis
      Gastroduodenal ulcers
      Colitis X
      Equine monocytic erhlichiosis ("Potomac fever")
      Intestinal clostridiosis
      Chronic liver disease
      Strongylosis
      Toxemia
      Peritonitis
    Working Quarter Horse
      Idiopathic
      Drug-induced diarrhea (e.g., phenylbutazone, antibiotics)
      Stress-induced diarrhea
      Salmonellosis
      Gastroduodenal ulcers
      Colitis X
      Equine monocytic erhlichiosis ("Potomac fever")
      Intestinal clostridiosis
      Chronic liver disease
      Strongylosis
      Toxemia
      Peritonitis

    Pleasure Horses
      Idiopathic
      Drug-induced diarrhea (e.g., phenylbutazone)
      Stress-induced diarrhea
      Salmonellosis
      Gastroduodenal ulcers
      Colitis X
      Equine monocytic erhlichiosis ("Potomac fever")
      Intestinal clostridiosis
      Chronic liver disease
      Strongylosis
      Heavy-metal intoxication
      "Blister beetle" intoxication
      Fungal diarrhea
      Peritonitis
    Foals
      "Foal heat" diarrhea
      Rotavirus
      Gastroduodenal ulcers
      Small intestine intussusception
      Strongyloides westeri infestation
      Parascaris equorum (roundworm) infestation
      Bacterial septicemia
      Bacterial GIT infection: *Salmonella, E. coli, Clostridium, R. equi*
      Failure of passive transfer of immunity
      Nutritional diarrhea
  Sex
    No significant effect

History
  How long has the diarrhea been present?
  Is the horse drinking, and if it is, how much?
  Have there been dramatic changes in fecal consistency?
  Is the horse regularly dewormed?
  Are there other horses in contact that are affected with diarrhea?
  Have there been any stressful events (e.g., transport) associated with diarrhea onset?
  Has the horse been undergoing any drug treatment, particularly antibiotics?
  Has the horse had any change in its diet recently?

Physical Examination
  General Inspection
    Attitude—depressed or bright
    Frequency and volume of diarrhea
    Consistency and composition of feces
    Signs of pain
  Detailed Inspection
    Vitals: HR, RR, temperature, pulse quality
    Gut sounds
    Capillary refill time
    Mucous membrane color
    Skin turgor
    Temperature of extremities

Diagnostic Procedures
  Clinical Pathology
    Hematocrit and total serum/plasma protein

White cell count and differential
Venous or arterial acid–base status
Serum/plasma electrolytes, osmolality
Plasma/serum fibrinogen
Liver enzymes: GGT, SDH, AP
Abdominal fluid analysis: total protein, WCC,
   cytology, bacteriology
Urinary cantharadine concentration
Fluid Balance
Weight of horse
Estimation of fluid loss: TPP, PCV, osmolality,
   skin turgor, capillary refill
Fecal Examination
Fecal volume estimation
Fecal occult blood
Fecal bacteriology: cultures over several days
   necessary for *Salmonella* (results improved
   if combined with culture of rectal mucosal
   biopsy)
Parasite ova
Fecal mycology
Examination for sand
Nutritional Examination
Heavy-metal measurement in feed samples
History of eating off sandy soil
Blister beetles
Rectal Examination
Abnormal masses
Distended bowel
Areas of localized pain
Abdominocentesis
Fluid color
Fluid turbidity
Presence of blood
Small Intestinal Absorption Tests
D-Glucose
D-Xylose
Differential Diagnoses
Adult Horses
Idiopathic*
Cyathostome infestations*
Stress-induced diarrhea*
Gastroduodenal ulcers
Salmonellosis
Drug-induced diarrhea (e.g., phenylbutazone,
   antibiotics)
Colitis X
Equine monocytic erhlichiosis ("Potomac fe-
   ver")
Intestinal clostridiosis
Chronic liver disease
Strongylosis
Toxemia
Heavy-metal intoxication
"Blister beetle" intoxication
Fungal diarrhea
Nutritional diarrhea
Postimpaction diarrhea
Peritonitis

Foals
Idiopathic*
Cyathostome infestations*
"Foal heat" diarrhea*
Rotavirus
Small intestine intussusception
Strongyloides westeri infestation
Parascaris equorum (roundworm) infestation
Bacterial septicemia
Salmonellosis
Failure of passive transfer of immunity
Nutritional diarrhea
Drug-induced diarrhea (e.g., phenylbutazone,
   antibiotics)

DYSPHAGIA

Signalment
Age of the Horse
Cleft palate—foals
Guttural pouch tympany—foals
Botulism—older horses
Choke—older horses
Encephalomyelitis—older horses
Guttural pouch mycosis—older horses
Strangles—young horses
Rabies—older horses
Toxoinfectious botulism—foals (Shaker
   foals)
Septicemia—foals
Breed and Use
Thoroughbred and Quarter Horse Racehorse
Choke
Strangles
Pharyngeal paralysis
After laryngoplasty/laryngeal surgery
Teeth problems
Esophageal stricture
Head trauma
Guttural pouch disease
Equine protozoal myeloencephalitis
Viral encephalomyelitis (EEE and WEE)
Standardbred Trotter and Pacer
Choke
Strangles
Pharyngeal paralysis
Teeth problems
Esophageal stricture
Head trauma
Guttural pouch disease
Equine protozoal myeloencephalitis
Viral encephalomyelitis (EEE and WEE)
Working Quarter Horse
Choke
Strangles
Pharyngeal paralysis
Teeth problems
Esophageal stricture
Head trauma
Rabies
Guttural pouch disease

---

*Denotes most likely diagnosis.

Equine protozoal myeloencephalitis
Viral encephalomyelitis (EEE and WEE)
Pleasure Horses
   Choke
   Strangles
   Pharyngeal paralysis
   Teeth problems
   Esophageal stricture
   Head trauma
   Rabies
   Lead poisoning
   Guttural pouch disease
   Hepatoencephalopathy
   Equine protozoal myeloencephalitis
   Viral encephalomyelitis (EEE and WEE)
Foals, All Breeds
   Cleft palate
   Guttural pouch tympany
   Head trauma
   Septicemia with CNS signs
   Liver failure/hepatoencephalopathy
   Toxoinfectious botulism (Shaker foals)
   Haloxon toxicity

Sex
No significant effect

History
How long have the signs been present?
Is there a known history of trauma?
Are any other horses affected?
Is there a recent change in diet?
Is the horse attempting to eat?
Are the signs progressive?
Does the horse have access to yellow star thistle or Russian knapweed at pasture?
Have the horses been vaccinated against viral encephalomyelitides?
Are there other signs of neurologic dysfunction?
Is there saliva, pus, or blood coming from the mouth or nose?
Has the horse received any medication or other treatment?

Physical Examination
General Inspection
Vitals: HR, RR, temperature, capillary refill, gut sounds
Evidence of salivation
Demeanor
Skin turgor
Presence of feed, pus, or blood at the nose
Detailed Examination
Palpation of the throat and esophagus
Cranial nerve examination
General neurologic examination
Chest auscultation for evidence of aspiration pneumonia

Diagnostic Procedures
Nasogastric Intubation
Determination of any obstruction sites
Radiography of the Head and Neck
Plain radiographs
Contrast radiography (e.g., barium)

Clinical Pathology
PCV and total plasma or serum protein
Fibrinogen
Electrolytes and osmolality
Plasma urea and creatinine
Liver enzymes/biochemistry: GGT, SDH, AP (bile acids)
Endoscopic Examination
Examination of pharynx and larynx
Examination of soft palate
Examination of guttural pouch openings
Examination of nasopharynx during attempted swallowing
Examination of the esophagus
CSF Examination
Color
Cytology
Protein
Serology
Titers for EEE and WEE
Fluorescent Antibody Detection for Rabies
Skin, brain (consult laboratory)
Differential Diagnoses
Choke*
Teeth problems*
Strangles
Pharyngeal paralysis
Hepatoencephalopathy
Esophageal stricture
After laryngoplasty/laryngeal surgery
Head trauma
Botulism
Guttural pouch disease
Nigropallidal encephalomalacia (e.g., yellow star thistle, Russian knapweed poisoning)
Equine protozoal myeloencephalitis
Viral encephalomyelitis (EEE and WEE)
Rabies
Lead poisoning

DYSPNEA (RESTING)

Signalment
Age of the Horse
Viral respiratory disease—young horses
Bacterial respiratory disease—young horses
Nasal and thoracic tumors—older horses
Breed and Use
Thoroughbred and Quarter Horse Racehorse
   Viral respiratory disease
   Strangles
   Bacterial pneumonia/pleuritis/bronchitis
   Chronic obstructive pulmonary disease (COPD)
   Nasal tumors
Standardbred Trotter and Pacer
   Viral respiratory disease

---

*Denotes most likely diagnosis.

Strangles
Bacterial pneumonia/pleuritis/bronchitis
Nasal/thoracic tumors
COPD
Working Quarter Horse
Viral respiratory disease
Strangles
Bacterial pneumonia/pleuritis/bronchitis
Nasal tumors
Progressive hematoma of the ethmoid
Thoracic tumors
Pleasure Horse
Viral respiratory disease
Strangles
Bacterial pneumonia/pleuritis/bronchitis
Chronic allergic bronchitis (COPD)
Nasal tumors
Progressive hematoma of the ethmoid
Thoracic tumors
Foals
Bacterial pneumonia
Guttural pouch tympany
Congenital malformations of the upper airway
Sex
No significant effect
History
Is the horse normal at rest?
If the dyspnea is apparent only during exercise, at what speed does it occur?
Is there a history of nasal discharge?
Does the horse have a cough?
If the dyspnea is apparent at rest, is it related to the horse being housed?
Is the dyspnea seasonal?
Is the dyspnea worsened by feeding?
Physical Examination
General Inspection
Examination of the nares for discharge (uni/bilateral)
Evidence of systemic disease (e.g., weight loss)
Examination of the head and upper respiratory tract for swellings
Detailed Examination
Percussion of the sinuses
Look in the nose
Oral examination to determine presence of tooth problems
Auscultation of the thorax
Smell the horse's breath
Palpation over the guttural pouches
Palpation of the trachea
Examination of the lymph nodes
Diagnostic Procedures
Rhinolaryngoscopy
Examination of nasal conchae (turbinates)
Guttural pouch openings
Examination of guttural pouches
Ethmoid region
Pharynx
Larynx and trachea

Radiography
Sinuses
Guttural pouches
Nasal conchae
Ethmoid
Tooth roots
Chest
Ultrasound
Chest
Bacteriology
Transtracheal aspirate
Guttural pouch aspirate
Bronchoalveolar lavage
Hematology and Biochemistry
White cell count and differential
Fibrinogen
Red cell count
Protein electrophoresis
General biochemical profile
Differential Diagnoses
Viral or bacterial lower respiratory tract disease*
Chronic allergic bronchitis (COPD)*
Pleural effusion*
Interstitial pneumonia
Tooth-root tumors
Nasal tumors
Endotoxemia
Partial upper airway obstructions
Guttural pouch tympany
Progressive hematoma of the ethmoid
Heart failure
Liver failure
Anaphylaxis
Bronchospasm

EDEMA, PERIPHERAL

Signalment
Age of the Horse
Septicemia—young horses
Congestive heart failure—older horses
Vasculitis—older horses
Pleuropneumonia—older horses
Rhodococcus equi infection—young horses
Breed and Use
No significant effect
Sex
No significant effect
History
When was the swelling/edema first noticed?
Is the edema increasing in size?
Is the horse demonstrating evidence of pain associated with the edema?
Are there other systemic signs associated with the edema (e.g., petechial hemorrhages)?
Is the edema associated with the recent administration of any medications?

*Denotes most likely diagnosis.

Has the horse received any treatment for the edema, and if so, what effect has it produced?

Is the edema initiated or exacerbated when the horse is confined?

Is the appetite normal?

Is the horse losing weight?

Has there been a recent change in the diet?

Does the horse have normal feces?

Does the horse drink and urinate normal volumes?

Physical Examination

General Inspection

Note the distribution of the edema

Is there evidence of systemic disease (e.g., weight loss, diarrhea, or nasal discharge)?

Determine whether the edema is pitting

General body condition

Attitude—depressed or bright

Detailed Inspection

Vitals: HR, RR, temperature, capillary refill time, presence or absence of icterus

Is the edema hot, painful, or pitting on palpation?

Is the horse lame?

Check mucous membranes for petechiae

Detailed auscultation of the chest

Rectal examination

Diagnostic Procedures

Clinical Pathology

CBC and differential WBC, fibrinogen, electrolytes

Total plasma protein and protein electrophoresis

Fecal egg count

Liver enzymes, serum bile acid concentration

Creatinine and urea

Urinalysis

Fractional electrolyte excretions

Coombs' test

Coggins' test

Abdominocentesis (if indicated)

Acid–base status

Bacteriology

Fecal culture for *Salmonella*

Culture of thoracic or abdominal fluid (if indicated)

Blood culture (septicemic foals)

Thoracocentesis (if indicated)

Transtracheal aspirate

Ultrasound and Radiology

Echocardiography

Thoracic examination for presence of fluid

Radiography of the chest

Gastrointestinal Studies

Oral D-glucose absorption test

Oral D-xylose absorption test

Liver biopsy

Differential Diagnoses

Lymphatic obstructions*

Trauma*

Cellulitis*

Parasitism

Drug reaction (eruption)

Primary hypersensitivity (e.g., urticaria)

Secondary hypersensitivity (e.g., neoplasia)

Erythema multiforme

Vasculitis

Protein-losing enteropathy

Liver failure

Phenylbutazone toxicity

Heart failure

Glomerulonephritis

Pleuropneumonia

Confinement

Chronic abscessation

Rhodocoocus equi infection (foals)

Angioedema

EXERCISE INTOLERANCE

Signalment

Age of the Horse

Congenital cardiovascular anomalies—foals

Neonatal isoerythrolysis—foals

Vitamin E/selenium deficiency—foals

COPD—mature horses

Breed and Use

Thoroughbred and Quarter Horse Racehorse

Lameness

Infectious respiratory disease

Subclinical respiratory disease

Exercise induced pulmonary hemorrhage (EIPH)

Laryngeal hemiplegia

Recurrent rhabdomyolysis

Upper airway disorders

Cardiovascular disease

Paroxysmal atrial fibrillation

Anemia

Cervical vertebral malformation

Standardbred Trotter and Pacer

Atrial fibrillation

Lameness

Infectious respiratory disease

Subclinical respiratory disease

EIPH

Recurrent rhabdomyolysis

Upper airway disorders

Cardiovascular disease

Anemia

Neurologic disease

Working Quarter Horse

Lameness

Infectious respiratory disease

COPD

Cardiovascular disease

Recurrent rhabdomyolysis

Hyperkalemic periodic paralysis

Anemia

Neurologic disease

*Denotes most likely diagnosis.

Pleasure Horses
 Lameness
 Infectious respiratory disease
 COPD
 Cardiovascular disease
 Recurrent rhabdomyolysis
 Parasitic infections
 Anemia
 Malnutrition
 Liver or renal disease
Foals, All Breeds
 Vitamin E/selenium deficiency
 Congenital heart disease
 Infectious respiratory disease
 Septicemia
Sex
 No significant effect

History
 Is there evidence of intercurrent disease?
 Does the horse make a respiratory noise?
 Is the horse distressed after exercise?
 Does the horse have a cough?
 Is there a history of exercise-induced pulmonary hemorrhage?
 Is there a nasal discharge?
 Has any lameness been noted?
 If a racehorse, is there a decrease in performance on previous form or has the horse never performed up to expectation?
 Is there a history of trauma?
 If the horse is racehorse, is the decrease in performance abrupt during a race?

Physical Examination
 General Inspection
  Note general condition of horse
  Mental status of the horse
  Presence of jugular pulse
  Presence of cough
  Respiratory stridor
 Detailed Examination
  Vitals: HR, RR, temperature
  Auscultation of thorax, including rebreathing
  Percussion of the thorax
  Evidence of arrhythmia
  Lameness examination
  Neurologic examination
  Palpation of regional lymph nodes
  Palpation of muscular process of arytenoid cartilage
  Laryngeal adductor ("slap") test

Diagnostic Procedures
 Clinical Pathology
  CBC and fibrinogen
  Plasma or serum biochemistry: AST, GGT, CPK, electrolytes, urea, creatinine
  Glutathione peroxidase activity, serum vitamin E concentration
 Endoscopy
  Examination of upper airway
  Examination of trachea, presence of mucopus and blood

Bronchoalveolar Lavage and/or Transtracheal Aspiration
 Cytology
 Bacteriology
Electrocardiography
 Atrial fibrillation
 Major conduction disturbances
 Presence of ventricular premature contractions
Arterial Blood Gas Analysis
 Evidence of hypoxemia during exercise
Radiography
 As indicated by lameness and/or neurologic examinations
Serology
 Respiratory viruses
 Coggins' test
Treadmill Exercise Testing
 Telemetry electrocardiography
 Blood lactate measurements
 Oxygen uptake measurements
 Blood volume determination
 Arterial blood gas measurements during exercise

Differential Diagnoses
 Lameness (clinical and subclinical) and back disorders*
 Infectious respiratory disease (clinical and subclinical)*
 Inadequate fitness*
 Laryngeal hemiplegia and other upper airway disorders
 Recurrent rhabdomyolysis
 Acquired cardiovascular disease (e.g., paroxysmal atrial fibrillation)
 Infectious disease with systemic manifestations
 EIPH
 Anemia
 Neurologic disease (e.g., cervical vertebral malformation)
 Parasitic infections
 Malnutrition
 Vitamin E/selenium deficiency
 Congenital heart disease
 Liver disease
 Renal disease

INFERTILITY, MARE

Signalment
 Age of the Horse
  Ovarian atrophy—older mares
  Conception rate decreases linearly with age of the mare.
 Breed and Use
  No significant effect

---

*Denotes most likely diagnosis.

History
　Has the mare had a foal previously?
　Is the mare cycling regularly?
　How long does the mare remain in season?
　Has there been any discharge noted from the vulva?
　Has the behavior of the mare changed?
　How many times was the mare bred?
　When was the last time the mare was bred?
　Has the mare conceived but the pregnancy has not continued?
　Are other mares pregnant that have been bred to the same stallion?
Physical Examination
　General Inspection
　　General body condition
　　Attitude—depressed or bright
　　Evidence of systemic disease
　　Evidence of chronic musculoskeletal problems
　Detailed Inspection
　　Examination of perineal conformation (note vulval angle)
　　Examination for evidence of discharge from the reproductive tract
　　Vitals: HR, RR, temperature, mucous membranes, capillary refill time
　　Examination of the udder
Diagnostic Procedures
　Speculum Examination
　　Examination of the vagina for scars, lacerations
　　Examination of the cervix.
　Rectal Examination
　　Palpation of any abnormal abdominal masses
　　Palpation of the uterus
　　Palpation of the ovaries
　　Palpation of the cervix
　Clinical Pathology
　　Cervical or uterine bacteriologic swab
　　Endometrial biopsy: histologic examination
　　Endometrial or cervical cytology
　Ultrasound Examination
　　Ultrasound examination of uterus
　　Ultrasound examination of the ovaries
　Endoscopic Examination
　　Examination of the uterus
　Endocrinologic Examination
　　Plasma progesterone concentration
Differential Diagnoses
　Endometritis*
　Urine pooling*
　Pneumovagina*
　Cervical abnormalities (e.g., adhesions, cervicitis)*
　Uterine hypoplasia
　Transitional estrus, particularly if early in breeding season

*Denotes most likely diagnosis.

Ovarian problems (e.g., follicular atresia, ovulation failure, tumor, persistent corpus luteum)
Fallopian tube abnormalities
Poor mare management (e.g., breeding at wrong time, poor estrus detection, etc.)
Perineal lacerations or rectovaginal fistula
Subfertile or infertile stallion
Chromosomal abnormalities
General physical problem (e.g., malnutrition, chronic laminitis, severe degenerative joint disease, etc.)

INFERTILITY, STALLION

Signalment
　Age of the Horse
　　Testicular degeneration—older stallions
　Breed and Use
　　No significant effect
History
　Has the stallion had systemic disease in the past few months?
　Has the stallion been in race training prior to the breeding season?
　Has the stallion received anabolic steroids?
　Is there any discharge from the penis or prepuce?
　Is the stallion reluctant to mate?
　Are mares failing to conceive, or is there early embryonic loss?
　What percentage of mares have become pregnant in the current and previous breeding seasons?
　Has the stallion had any injuries?
Physical Examination
　General inspection
　　General body condition
　　Attitude—depressed or bright
　　Evidence of systemic disease
　　Evidence of chronic musculoskeletal problems
　Detailed Inspection
　　Examination of penis and prepuce
　　Examination of testicles for size, resilience, signs of pain
　　Examination for evidence of discharge from prepuce
　　Vitals: HR, RR, temperature, mucous membranes, capillary refill time
Diagnostic Procedures
　Rectal Examination
　　Examination of accessory sex glands
　　Examination of inguinal rings
　Semen Examination
　　Motility
　　Abnormalities of sperm
　　Total sperm count
　　Urea concentrations

Bacteriology
    Semen culture, including microaerophilic techniques
    Cytologic examination
Histopathology
    Testicular biopsy (only if indicated)
Differential Diagnoses
    Systemic disease*
    Trauma*
    Testicular degeneration*
    Venereal infections
    Infectious orchitis
    Balanoposthitis
    Urethritis
    Phimosis
    Paraphimosis
    Tumors of the penis, prepuce, or testicle
    Urospermia
    Hemospermia
    Habronemiasis
    Cryptorchidism
    Torsion of the spermatic cord
    Varicocele
    Epididymitis
    Seminal vesiculitis
    Lack of libido

LACRIMATION, EXCESSIVE AND/OR PHOTOPHOBIA

Signalment
  Age of the Horse
    Entropion—young foals
    Periodic ophthalmia—older horses
    Eye cancer—older horses
    Habronemiasis—older horses
    Nasolacrimal duct obstruction—older horses
    Atresia of the lacrimal puncta—foals
  Breed and Use
    No significant effect
  Sex
    No significant effect
History
    Is there a history of trauma?
    How long has the problem been present?
    Is the horse reluctant to go out in the daylight?
    Does the eye remain closed at all times or only in the light?
    Does the horse show any systemic signs (e.g., depression, inappetence)?
    Is the discharge from the eye clear or purulent?
    Is the cornea cloudy?
    Does the eye appear inflamed?

*Denotes most likely diagnosis.

Physical Examination
  General Inspection
    Note whether one or both eyes affected
    Attitude and mental status of the horse
  Detailed Inspection
    Vitals: HR, RR, temperature, capillary refill time
    Globe size: increased or decreased
    Presence of swelling or other abnormalities of the eyelids
    Inspection of nasal opening of nasolacrimal duct
    Examination of the conjunctiva and sclera
    Pupillary light reflexes
    Menace response
    Examination of the third eyelid
    Examination of corneal surface using direct light source
Diagnostic Procedures
  Nerve Blocks
    Auriculopalpebral block to remove motor function of upper eyelid
    Supraorbital block to desensitize the eye
    Topical anesthesia using proparacaine 0.5% to desensitize conjunctiva and cornea
  Fluorescein Test
    Fluorescein strip to demonstrate corneal imperfections
  Bacteriology and Cytology
    Scraping and culture for establishing cause of corneal ulcer
  Ophthalmoscopy
    Examination of the anterior chamber and lens
    Examination of the retina
Differential Diagnoses
    Corneal ulcers*
    Trauma*
    Conjunctivitis*
    Periodic ophthalmia (e.g., recurrent uveitis, immune-mediated uveitis)*
    Blepharitis
    Retrobulbar abscess
    Squamous cell carcinoma of the third eyelid
    Orbital cellulitis
    Entropion
    Habronemiasis
    Ectopic cilia
    Distichiasis
    Sarcoid
    Absence of distal nasolacrimal duct punctum

LAMENESS, ACUTE

Signalment
  Age of the Horse
    Metabolic bone disease—young horses
    Degenerative conditions—mature horses
    Septic conditions—foals
    "Bucked" shins—2-year-old racehorses

Breed and Use
Thoroughbred and Quarter Horse Racehorse
  "Bucked" shins
  Chip fractures, fetlock, carpus
  Bowed tendons (tendon strain)
  Suspensory desmitis
  Nail prick
  Tying up
  Sesamoid fractures
  Joint disease
  Long bone fractures, proximal phalanx, condylar fractures McIII
  Fissure fracture, McIII, proximal phalanx
  Laminitis
Standardbred Trotter and Pacer
  Bowed tendons (tendon strains)
  Suspensory desmitis
  Check ligament injuries
  Fractures of distal phalanx
  Sesamoid bone fractures
  Nail prick
  Fractures of McII
  Joint disease
  Curb
  Tying up
  Long bone fractures
  Laminitis
Working Quarter Horse
  Acute joint conditions
  Bowed tendons (tendon strains)
  Nail prick
  Suspensory desmitis
  Muscle injuries
  Long bone fractures
  Laminitis
  Tying up
Pleasure Horses
  Foot abscess
  Nail prick
  Long bone fractures
  Direct trauma
  Laminitis
  Tying up
Foals, All Breeds
  Septic arthritis, polyarticular
  Trauma, fractures of long bones

Sex
  No significant effect

History
  Was the lameness related to a specific exercise episode?
  Did the lameness worsen in the period immediately after exercise?
  Did the lameness worsen in the days following the episode?
  Did the lameness improve with rest?
  Did the lameness improve with "bute"?
  Was the horse shod recently?
  Has the horse rested the leg, and if so, what position does it adopt?

Has the horse been injected in a joint in the affected leg recently?
Physical Examination
General Inspection
  Presence of swelling: joints, tendons, dorsal metacarpus
  Symmetry of the limbs
  Weight bearing of limbs
  Examination of gait at the walk and trot (hard, even surface)
Detailed Examination
  Digital pulse, prominence
  Temperature (subjective), foot to carpus/tarsus (comparison with normal leg)
  Pain on palpation or flexion
  Hoof testers
  Hoof hammer
  Flexion test response
Diagnostic Procedures
Nerve Blocks
  If a fracture is suspected, nerve blocks should be avoided.
  Palmar digital
  Palmar (abaxial)
  It is essential to exclude the foot before proceeding to other possible sites.
  Palmar metacarpal
Intraarticular Local Analgesia
  Distal interphalangeal (coffin) joint
  Fetlock joint
  Intercarpal (mid-carpal)
  Radiocarpal (proximal carpal)
  Elbow
  Shoulder
  Hock, tarsometatarsal and tarsocrural joints
  Stifle
Radiography
  Additional oblique views of the foot, fetlock, carpus, and tarsus.
  Also, the use of skyline views of the carpal bones.
  Fractures of the third carpal bone can sometimes be missed without inclusion of a skyline view.
  Air arthrograms can be considered to delineate soft-tissue swellings in the dorsal fetlock.
Ultrasound
  Use to better define tendon and ligament injuries for prognosis.
Differential Diagnoses
  Subsolar (foot) abscess*
  Acute joint sprains*
  Osteochondral (chip) fractures in fetlock or carpus*
  Nail prick*
  "Bucked" shins
  Tendon strains and suspensory desmitis
  Tying up (rhabdomyolysis)

---

*Denotes most likely diagnosis.

Muscle injuries
Fractures of a long bone
Laminitis
Fissure fracture, proximal phalanx, McIII
Septic arthritis
Infection of tendon sheath
Infection of navicular bursa
Fractures of sesamoid bones

KEY POINT ► If a fissure fracture is suspected, although no radiographic changes are found, it is essential to immobilize the leg with a cast and check the radiographic appearance after 7 days.

LAMENESS, CHRONIC

Signalment
  Age of the Horse
    Metabolic bone disease—young horses
    Degenerative conditions—mature horses
    Congenital deformities—young horses
    Navicular disease—mature horses
  Breed and Use
    Thoroughbred and Quarter Horse Racehorse
      Degenerative joint disease
      Pedal osteitis
      Navicular disease
      Bone spavin
      Osteochondrosis dissecans (OCD)
      Bowed (strained) tendons and suspensory desmitis
    Standardbred Trotter and Pacer
      Degenerative joint disease
      Pedal osteitis
      Nonunion of pedal bone fractures
      Sacroiliac pain
      Bone spavin
      OCD
      Back injuries
      Stifle problems
      Bowed tendons and suspensory desmitis
    Working Quarter Horse
      Navicular disease
      Degenerative joint disease
      Fibrotic myopathy
      Chronic laminitis
    Pleasure Horses
      Navicular disease
      Degenerative joint disease
      Chronic laminitis
      Back injuries
      Pedal osteitis
    Foals
      OCD
      Bone cysts
      Angular limb deformities
  Sex
    Chronic lameness is more likely to be presented in geldings.

History
  What is duration of the lameness?
  Has the lameness gradually been worsening?
  Does the lameness improve with exercise?
  Is the lameness more apparent immediately after exercise?
  Is the lameness more apparent after the horse has "cooled down"?
  Does the lameness improve with rest?
  Is there an improvement with "bute"?
  Has the horse been shod recently?
  Does the horse rest the affected leg?
  If the leg is rested, how does the horse hold the affected leg?
  Have there been any temperament changes noted?
Physical Examination
  General Inspection
    Presence of swelling: joints, tendons
    Atrophy of muscles, particularly gluteal
    Hoof wear
    Hoof cracks
    Old scars
  Detailed Examination
    Temperature (subjective), foot to carpus/tarsus (comparison with normal leg)
    Pain on palpation or flexion, particularly distal joints
    Hoof testers (middle third of frog)
    Flexion test response*
Diagnostic Procedures
  Nerve Blocks
    Palmar digital
    Palmar (abaxial)
    It is essential to exclude the foot before proceeding to other possible sites.
    Palmar metacarpal
    Subcarpal (check ligament) block
  Intraarticular Local Analgesia
    Distal interphalangeal (coffin) joint
    Fetlock joint
    Intercarpal (mid-carpal)
    Radiocarpal (proximal carpal)
    Elbow
    Shoulder
    Hock, tarsometatarsal and tarsocrural joints
    Stifle
  Radiography
    Additional oblique views in the foot, fetlock, carpus, tarsus.
    Also, the use of skyline views of the carpal bones.
    Fractures of the third carpal bone can sometimes be missed without inclusion of a skyline view.
    Air arthrograms can be considered to delineate soft-tissue swellings in the dorsal fetlock.

---

*Flexion tests of the fetlock and carpus are essential in aiding localization of pain. Spavin test in the hindleg will aid localization of pain to the hock and stifle.

Ultrasound
Use to better define tendon and ligament injuries for prognosis.

Differential Diagnoses
Chronic degenerative joint disease*
Navicular disease*
Pedal osteitis*
Bone spavin*
Articular ringbone
Tendon and ligament strain/sprain
Back injuries/sacroiliac pain
"Wobblers"
OCD and bone cysts
Chronic proliferative synovitis
Nonunion fractures of pedal bone

KEY POINT ▶ In some chronic lamenesses, several conditions may be contributing to the problem.

LIMB SWELLING

Signalment
Age of the Horse
Septic arthritis—foals
Osteomyelitis—foals
Epiphysitis—yearlings
"Bucked shins"—2-year-old racehorses
Tendon/ligament injuries—young horses
Joint disease—young horses
Breed and Use
Thoroughbred and Quarter Horse Racehorse
"Bucked shins"
Joint disease, fetlock and carpus
Tendon/ligament injuries
Fractures, chip fractures involving fetlock and carpus
Soft-tissue injuries/trauma
Splints
Monarticular septic arthritis
OCD
Abscess
Palmar annular ligament constriction
Hematoma
Bog spavin
Standardbred Trotter and Pacer
Joint disease, fetlock and carpus
Tendon/ligament injuries
Fractures, chip fractures involving fetlock and carpus
Soft-tissue injuries/trauma
Splint bone (McII) fractures
Monarticular septic arthritis
OCD
Interference, knee knocking

*Denotes most likely diagnosis.

Hobble chafing
Abscess
Palmar annular ligament constriction
Curb
Hematoma
Working Quarter Horse
Trauma/soft-tissue injuries
Hygroma
Tendon/ligament injuries
Fractures
Joint disease
Ringbone
Periosteal new bone reaction
Abscess
Muscle injuries
Hematoma
Pleasure Horses
Trauma/soft-tissue injuries
Hygroma
Splints
Fractures
Joint disease
Ringbone
Localized osteomyelitis
Abscess
Periosteal new bone reaction
Muscle injuries
Hematoma
Foals
Septic arthritis (joint ill)
Osteomyelitis
Trauma/soft-tissue injuries
Tumoral calcinosis
Abscess
Sex
No significant effect
History
Is the horse lame?
How long has the swelling been present?
Has the swelling changed in size?
Is the horse showing signs of systemic illness?
Is there heat and pain associated with the swelling?
Is the swelling related to a joint?
Is the swelling related to a tendon or tendon sheath?
Is the swelling hard or soft?
Is there a draining sinus related to the swelling?
Physical Examination
General Inspection
Symmetry of the swelling
Location of the swelling
Examination at walk and trot to detect lameness
Relationship of swelling to a joint
Detailed Inspection
Palpation of the swelling
Aspiration, if indicated
If related to a joint, determination of pain on flexion

Diagnostic Procedures
  Radiography
    Oblique views are important.
    Use low kVp and slight underexposure to high-light soft tissues.
    Contrast radiography, if indicated.
  Ultrasound
    Essential in tendon and ligament injuries
    May be useful in other swellings to determine soft tissue changes
  Joint Fluid Analysis
    Only indicated if there is suspicion of septic ar-thritis
  Nerve Blocks
    To confirm relationship between swelling and lameness
    Intraarticular anesthesia is important if swell-ing is joint effusion
Differential Diagnoses
    Localized trauma*
    Degenerative joint disease/joint effusion*
    Splints*
    Tendon/ligament injuries*
    Abscess
    Hematoma
    "Bucked" shins
    Bog spavin
    Splint bone fractures
    OCD
    Septic arthritis
    Tenosynovitis
    Ringbone
    Bone spavin

NASAL DISCHARGE

Signalment
  Age of the Horse
      Viral respiratory disease—young horses
      Bacterial respiratory disease—young horses
      Cleft palate—young horses
      Nasal tumors—older horses
      Guttural pouch infections—all ages
      Progressive hematoma of the ethmoid—older horses
  Breed and Use
    Thoroughbred and Quarter Horse Racehorse
      Viral respiratory disease
      Strangles
      Bacterial pneumonia/pleuritis/bronchitis
      Pharyngitis
      Exercise-induced pulmonary hemorrhage
      Guttural pouch infection
      Sinusitis
      After laryngoplasty surgery
      Tooth-root infections
      Nasal conchal (turbinate) necrosis

    Standardbred Trotter and Pacer
      Viral respiratory disease
      Strangles
      Bacterial pneumonia/pleuritis/bronchitis
      Pharyngitis
      Guttural pouch infection
      Sinusitis
      After laryngoplasty surgery
      Nasal conchal (turbinate) necrosis
    Working Quarter Horse
      Viral respiratory disease
      Strangles
      Bacterial pneumonia/pleuritis/bronchitis
      Guttural pouch infection
      Sinusitis
      Nasal conchal (turbinate) necrosis
      Nasal tumors
      Tooth-root infections
      Progressive hematoma of the ethmoid
    Pleasure Horse
      Viral respiratory disease
      Strangles
      Bacterial pneumonia/pleuritis/bronchitis
      Guttural pouch infection
      Sinusitis
      Nasal conchal (turbinate) necrosis
      Nasal tumors
      Tooth-root infections
      Progressive hematoma of the ethmoid
    Foals
      Cleft palate
      Congenital pharyngeal abnormalities
      Bacterial pneumonia
  Sex
    No significant effect
History
    Is the discharge unilateral or bilateral?
    Is the discharge clear, mucoid, purulent, or bloody?
    Is the discharge related to feeding or head pos-ture?
    How long has the discharge been present?
    Is the quantity of the discharge increasing?
    Is there an associated cough?
    Are other animals in the barn/pasture affected?
    Is there evidence of systemic disease (e.g., depression, inappetence, fever, etc.)?
    Has the horse been vaccinated?
    Is the discharge malodorous?
    Has there been any change in facial contours?
Physical Examination
  General Inspection
    Examination of the nares for discharge (uni/bi-lateral)
    Evidence of systemic disease (e.g., weight loss)
    Examination of the head and upper respiratory tract for swellings
  Detailed Examination
    Percussion of the sinuses
    Look in the nose

*Denotes most likely diagnosis.

Oral examination to determine presence of tooth problems

Auscultation of the thorax

Smell the horse's breath

Palpation over the guttural pouches

Diagnostic Procedures

Rhinolaryngoscopy

Examination of nasal conchae (turbinates)

Guttural pouch openings

Examination of guttural pouches

Ethmoid region

Pharynx

Larynx and trachea

Radiography

Sinuses

Guttural pouches

Nasal conchae

Ethmoid

Tooth roots

Chest

Bacteriology

Sinus centesis

Transtracheal aspirate

Guttural pouch aspirate

Bronchoalveolar lavage

Anaerobic culture

Hematology and Biochemistry

White cell count and differential

Fibrinogen

Red cell count

Protein electrophoresis

Thoracocentesis

Cytologic examination

Bacteriologic examination

Glucose measurements

Differential Diagnoses

Viral or bacterial respiratory disease*

Pharyngitis*

Pneumonia*

Sinusitis*

Strangles

Exercise-induced pulmonary hemorrhage

Dysphagia

Guttural pouch infections

Progressive hematoma of the ethmoid

Tooth-root infections

Nasal tumors

Nasal conchal (turbinate) necrosis

Heart failure

Cleft palate

Congenital pharyngeal abnormalities

PRURITUS

Signalment

Age of the Horse

Culicoides hypersensitivity—older horses

---

*Denotes most likely diagnosis.

Dermatophytosis—younger horses

Urticaria—older horses

Breed and Use

No significant effect

Sex

No significant effect

History

Does the problem occur in a certain season?

Is more than one horse affected?

How long has the problem been present?

How severe is the pruritus?

Does the condition adversely affect the horse's behavior?

Has the horse been treated?

What was the response to treatment?

How long since the horse has been treated?

Is the horse eating normally?

Is the horse losing weight?

Physical Examination

General Inspection

General body condition

Attitude—depressed or bright

Detailed Inspection

Vitals: HR, RR, temperature, gut sounds, capillary refill time

Determine whether the lesions are localized or generalized

Is there alopecia associated with the pruritus

Is there evidence of self-trauma

Clipping of hair in a pruritic region and examination of skin with a hand lens

Clinical Pathology

CBC, differential

Total plasma protein

Examination of the Skin

Skin scrapings

Impression smears

Intradermal skin testing

Acetate tape preparations

Bacterial/fungal cultures

Skin biopsies (histopathology, fluorescent antibody testing)

Differential Diagnoses

Culicoides hypersensitivity (Queensland itch)*

Dermatophytosis*

Ectoparasites (e.g., biting flies, lice, ticks, harvest mites or "chiggers," mosquitoes)*

Cutaneous onchocerciasis

Pinworm infestation, *Oxyuris equi*

Folliculitis/furunculosis

Urticaria due to inhaled allergens or drug administration

Contact dermatitis

Eosinophilic dermatitis

Photosensitization, primary and secondary

Dermatophilosis

Seborrheic dermatosis

Pemphigus foliaceus

Scratches ("grease heel")

Phycomycosis

Habronemiasis

Neurologic diseases (e.g., rabies, polyneuritis equi, self-mutilation syndrome)

RESPIRATORY NOISE

Signalment
  Age of the Horse
    Congenital airway disorder—newborn foal
    Laryngeal hemiplegia—young racehorse
    Epiglottic problems—young horse
    Soft palate dislocation—young horse
    Strangles—young horse
    Nasal tumor—older horse
    Guttural pouch tympany—foal
  Breed and Use
    Thoroughbred and Quarter Horse Racehorse
      Laryngeal hemiplegia
      Epiglottic entrapment
      Subepiglottic cysts
      Soft palate dislocation
      Pharyngitis
      Rostral displacement of the palatopharyngeal arch
      Atheroma of the false nostril
      Tooth-root abnormalities impinging on ventral meatus
      Nasal tumors
    Standardbred Trotter and Pacer
      Epiglottic entrapment
      Subepiglottic cysts
      Soft palate dislocation
      Pharyngitis
      Nasal tumors
    Working Quarter Horse
      Pharyngitis
      Atheroma of the false nostril
      Nasal tumors
      Retropharyngeal abscess
    Pleasure Horses
      Tooth-root abnormalities
      Nasal tumors
      Retropharyngeal abscess
      Tracheal stenosis
    Foals, All Breeds
      Guttural pouch tympany
      Retropharyngeal abscess
      Bilateral laryngeal paralysis
  Sex
    Males are more likely to be affected by laryngeal hemiplegia than females.
History
  Can you describe the type of noise (e.g., roaring, whistling, gurgling)?
  Is the noise apparent when the horse is at rest?
  If the noise occurs during exercise, is it present at all speeds?
  Is the noise getting worse with time?
  Has the horse had a nasal discharge?
  Has the horse been coughing?
  Is the noise related to inspiration or expiration? (During cantering or galloping, as the leading leg hits the ground, the horse expires, whereas inspiration occurs when the forelegs are protracted.)
  Is there any noticeable swelling associated with the nose or face?
  Has the horse been vaccinated?
Physical Examination
  General Inspection
    Presence of any nasal/facial swelling
    Inspection of the external nares
  Detailed Examination
    Percussion of the paranasal sinuses
    Palpation of muscular process for prominence (atrophy of dorsal cricoarytenoid muscle)
    Auscultation of upper airway and thorax
    Palpation for soft-tissue mass in pharyngeal region
    Postexercise arytenoid depression maneuver (pushing on muscular process to worsen the respiratory noise)
    "Slap test" to assess adductor function
Diagnostic Procedures
  Rhinolaryngoscopy
    Appearance of upper airway
    Symmetry of the larynx
    Evidence of inflammation
    "Slap test" of adductor function
    Appearance immediately after exercise
    Endoscopic appearance of trachea
    Appearance of upper airway during treadmill exercise
  Radiography
    Radiography of the larynx
    Radiography of the nose and sinuses
  Arterial Blood Gas Analysis
    Resting values for PaO_2
    Arterial blood samples during exercise (requires a treadmill)
Differential Diagnoses
  Laryngeal hemiplegia*
  Soft palate dislocation (dorsal displacement)*
  Epiglottic entrapment
  Subepiglottic cysts
  Atheroma of the false nostril
  Pharyngitis
  Rostral displacement of the palatopharyngeal arch
  Tracheal stenosis
  Tooth-root tumors
  Nasal tumors
  Retropharyngeal abscess
  Guttural pouch tympany
  Hypoplasia of the epiglottis

SUDDEN DEATH

Signalment
  Age of the Horse
    No significant effect

---

*Denotes most likely diagnosis.

Breed and Use
No significant effect
Sex
No significant effect
History
Was the horse observed at the time of death?
Have there been any recent changes in management?
Has the horse received any medication recently?
Was the death related to exercise?
Was there evidence of struggling?
Have there been any other recent horse deaths?
Has the horse been ill recently?
Was the horse at pasture or in a box stall?
If a mare, has it recently foaled?
Physical Examination
General Inspection
Note the position of the horse
Note any signs of struggling
Detailed Inspection
Age of horse
Presence of blood from any of the body orifices
Evidence of trauma
Evidence of diarrhea or blood in the feces
Note evidence of abdominal distension
Evidence of skin abrasions
Diagnostic Procedures
Necropsy
Note distension or torsion of intestine or severe enteritis
Presence of hemorrhage (thoracic or abdominal)
Trauma (fractures of vertebrae, ribs, etc.)
Samples of blood, gut contents, liver, kidney or heart for toxicologic profile
Sampling of pasture and/or feed for toxins
Differential Diagnoses
Rupture of the aorta
Acute respiratory distress following adverse drug reaction
Mare—rupture of the uterine artery at parturition
Electrocution/lightning strike
Acute fulminant colitis
Trauma (e.g., gunshot)
Snakebite
Pneumothorax
Skull fractures
Toxic plants (e.g., yew)
Cantharidin toxicosis
Endotoxemia
Monensin toxicity
Organic/chemical toxins

URINE OUTPUT CHANGES

Signalment
Age of the Horse
Ruptured urinary bladder—foals

Chronic renal failure—older horses
Urolithiasis—older horses
Cystitis—older horses
Paralytic bladder—older horses
Psychogenic polydipsia—older horses
Breed and Use
No significant effect
Sex
No significant effect
History
When was the change in urine output first noticed?
Has the horse had a change in water consumption?
Does the horse strain to urinate?
Is the urine discolored?
Is there blood in the urine, and if so, at what stage of urination does it occur?
Is the horse losing weight?
Is the change in urine output related to exercise?
Has the horse received any medication, particularly phenylbutazone?
Physical Examination
General Inspection
General body condition
Attitude—depressed or bright
Detailed Inspection
Vitals: HR, RR, temperature, gut sounds, capillary refill time
Rectal examination, particularly for examination of urinary tract
Clinical Pathology
Urinalysis
Serum/plasma urea and creatinine
Fractional electrolyte excretions
Total serum/plasma protein
Urinary gamma-glutamyl transpeptidase
CBC
Abdominocentesis
Peritoneal fluid/serum creatinine ratio (foals)
Water Deprivation Test
Check urinary concentrating ability in selected cases
Bacteriology
Bacterial culture of urine
Endoscopic Examination/Cystoscopy
Lower urinary tract and bladder
Ultrasound
Renal
Abdominal (foals, suspected ruptured bladder)
Abdominal Radiography
Plain and contrast (foals, suspected ruptured bladder)
Injection of Nontoxic Dye (Methylene Blue, Fluoroscein)
Via urethral catheter (foals, suspected ruptured bladder)
Renal Biopsy
For prognosis/diagnosis, ultrasound guided (if possible)

Differential Diagnoses
  Oliguria
    Acute renal failure*
    Chronic renal failure*
    Severe dehydration*
    Shock
    Urolithiasis
    Equine herpesvirus myelitis
    Ruptured urinary bladder (foals)
  Polyuria
    Chronic renal failure*
    Psychogenic polydipsia*
    Cushing's syndrome
    Fluid administration
    Steroid administration
    Tumors of the pars intermedia of the pituitary
      gland
    Diabetes mellitus
    Cantharadin toxicosis

WEIGHT LOSS OR FAILURE TO THRIVE

Signalment
  Age of the Horse
        Parasites—young horses
        Gastrointestinal ulcers—young horses
        Chronic diarrhea—young horses
        Tooth problems—older horses
        Inflammatory bowel disease—older horses
        Neoplasia—older horses
        Liver disease—older horses
        Renal disease—older horses
  Breed and Use
    Thoroughbred and Quarter Horse Racehorse
      Chronic infections
      Chronic diarrhea
      Gastrointestinal ulcers
      Abdominal abscesses
      Peritonitis
      Inflammatory bowel disease
      Neoplasia (e.g., lymphosarcoma)
    Standardbred Trotter and Pacer
      Chronic infections
      Chronic diarrhea
      Gastrointestinal ulcers
      Abdominal abscesses
      Peritonitis
      Inflammatory bowel disease
      Neoplasia (e.g., lymphosarcoma)
    Working Quarter Horse
      Chronic infections
      Chronic diarrhea
      Gastrointestinal ulcers
      Abdominal abscesses
      Peritonitis
      Inflammatory bowel disease
      Neoplasia (e.g., lymphosarcoma)

---

*Denotes most likely diagnosis.

        Liver disease
        Renal disease
    Pleasure Horses
      Malnutrition
      Teeth problems
      Chronic infections (e.g., pleuritis)
      Chronic diarrhea
      Gastrointestinal ulcers
      Abdominal abscesses
      Peritonitis
      Inflammatory bowel disease
      Neoplasia (e.g., lymphosarcoma)
      Liver disease
      Chronic colic (e.g., sand, enterolith)
      Renal disease
      Heart failure
    Foals
      Chronic infections
      Congenital gastrointestinal abnormalities
      Malnutrition/maldigestion
      Chronic intussusception
      Internal abscessation
  Sex
    No significant effect
History
    Is the horse eating normally?
    How long has the horse been losing weight?
    Is the appetite increased or decreased?
    Is the appetite capricious?
    What is the composition of the diet?
    Are there any behavioral changes?
    How frequently is the horse wormed?
    Are there any signs of abdominal pain?
    Are there signs of systemic disease?
    Has there been a disease outbreak in the herd
      (e.g., "strangles")?
    Are the feces normal in color, volume, and
      consistency?
    Have any medications been given, and what is
      the response?
    Where is the horse housed?
    Is the horse low on the social structure within
      the herd?
Physical Examination
  General Inspection
    Estimation of weight loss: mild/moderate/se-
      vere
    Attitude—depressed or bright
    Consistency and composition of feces
    Signs of pain
    Evidence of systemic disease
    Evidence of dysphagia or problems with pre-
      hension
  Detailed Inspection
    Vitals: HR, RR, temperature
    Examination of teeth and tongue
    Body weight
    Capillary refill time—mucous membrane color
    Skin turgor
    Gut sounds
    Auscultation of heart and thorax
    Palpation of superficial lymph nodes

Diagnostic Procedures

Clinical Pathology

Hematocrit and total serum/plasma protein
White cell count and differential
Plasma/serum fibrinogen
Liver enzymes/biochemistry: GGT, SDH, AP, bilirubin, bile acids
Renal function tests: BUN, creatinine, urinalysis
Abdominal fluid analysis: total protein, nucleated cell count, cytology, bacteriology
Serum protein electrophoresis

Serology

Coggins' test

Fecal Examination

Fecal consistency
Parasite ova
Fecal occult blood
Fecal bacteriology, e.g., *Salmonella* (cultures over several days necessary; results improved if combined with culture of rectal mucosal biopsy)
Fecal/rectal mucosal mycology
Examination for sand

Nutritional Examination

History of eating off sandy soil
Quality and volume of feed

Rectal Examination

Abnormal masses
Distended/thickened bowel
Areas of localized pain

Abdominocentesis

Fluid color
Fluid turbidity
Presence of blood

Small Intestinal Absorption Tests

D-Glucose
D-Xylose

Other Procedures (If Indicated)

Rectal mucosal biopsy
Liver biopsy
Renal biopsy
Exploratory laparotomy

Differential Diagnoses

Adults

Malnutrition*
Teeth problems*
Parasitism (e.g., strongylosis)
Chronic infections
    Chronic pleuritis
    Abdominal abscesses
    Peritonitis
Chronic diarrhea
Gastrointestinal ulcers
Liver disease
Chronic colic (e.g., sand, enterolith)
Renal disease
Inflammatory bowel disease
Neoplasia (e.g., lymphosarcoma)
Heart failure
Heavy-metal intoxication (e.g., lead)
Idiopathic

Foals

Malnutrition*
Bacterial septicemia*
Failure of passive transfer of immunity*
Strongyloides westeri infestation
Parascaris equorum (roundworm) infestation
Rhodococcus equi infection
Small intestine intussusception
Chronic diarrhea
Bacterial GIT infection: *Salmonella, E. coli, Clostridium, R. equi*
Idiopathic
Liver disease
White muscle disease

---

*Denotes most likely diagnosis.

3

Musculoskeletal System

Problems involving the musculoskeletal system are common reasons for veterinary attention to all breeds and types of horses. In racehorses, surveys in all countries have indicated that musculoskeletal problems are the most common reason for interruptions to training programs. In evaluation of horses prior to sale, considerable attention should be paid to the musculoskeletal system because this is likely to be the major cause of future disputes between the seller, purchaser, and veterinarian.

Most horses are presented because of lameness, with or without some degree of swelling in one or more of the limbs.

KEY POINT ► A systematic examination procedure should be adhered to in all cases of lameness because, on occasions, the most spectacular swellings of the limbs may be of little functional significance.

Before a detailed examination commences, a rapid evaluation of the conformation and symmetry of the musculoskeletal system should be undertaken. Particular note should be made of any swellings or muscle atrophy for later detailed investigation. Clinical significance can be attached to swellings involving one of the joints, particularly if there is evidence of synovial effusion.

GENERAL CONSIDERATIONS

The examination should commence after obtaining a precise history that should indicate whether the onset was sudden or insidious, the relationship of the presenting signs to exercise, and details of medications received. It is important to remember that the history may not be reliable because many owners or trainers will provide a history that is consistent with their view of the problem.

The horse should be walked, initially, on a hard surface, and note should be taken of limb coordination and any indications of lameness. *Forelimb lameness* is most easily diagnosed by watching the horse walk and trot on a firm, even surface both toward and away from the observer. When the horse is walked, special note should be made of any signs of incoordination indicating a possible neurologic problem. These signs may be less apparent at the trot.

As weight is borne on the affected forelimb, the head is lifted, and the head is dropped when weight is placed on the unaffected forelimb.

KEY POINT ► For the inexperienced observer, it is easier to watch for the forelimb on which the head drops because this allows concentration on one phase of the gait.

In the case of bilateral forelimb lameness (such as cases of navicular disease), it may be difficult to detect any head movement. However, affected horses will usually show a reluctance to stretch forward and will have a stilted or shuffling gait. Many owners and trainers will describe such horses as being "tied up in the shoulders." While some books emphasize classification of the lameness into a "swinging leg" or "supporting leg" lameness, we have found that such a classification is seldom helpful. It is impossible to determine from the gait of the horse whether the problem is in the upper or lower limb. Only a detailed physical examination together with nerve blocks will definitively localize the lameness to a particular site.

Hindlimb lameness is more subtle, and an affected horse will usually show no signs of head movement during trotting. Many owners or trainers will be unaware that their horse is lame, and the horse may be presented because of reduced performance or for having a "rough" or "choppy" gait. In the case of standardbred trotters and pacers, the trainers sometimes describe the horse as "jumping out of its gear." Diagnosis is best undertaken by watching the horse walk and trot on firm, even ground away from the observer.

KEY POINT ▶ As weight is placed on the affected hindleg, the tuber coxa on that side is raised, together with the hindquarters.

Conversely, as weight is taken on the sound hindlimb, the tuber coxa on the affected side and the hindquarters appear to drop. Additionally, it can be noted that the fetlock joint on the sound limb will descend further than on the affected leg. This occurs because the unaffected limb bears more weight than the affected limb.

In this section of the handbook, particular emphasis will be placed on diagnosis, prognosis, and treatment. One of the important early lessons learned by all clinicians is that often it is extremely difficult to provide an accurate prognosis for the client. We have all suffered damage to our egos when the racehorse with multiple limb problems, degenerative joint disease in several joints, and a strained tendon, which we have told the owner or trainer will never race again, ends up winning a major race. The important lesson from this is that forecasting likely outcomes is always a matter of probabilities, with some injuries carrying a better prognosis than others.

KEY POINT ▶ However, never tell the owner or trainer of a horse that it will never win another race or compete successfully, unless you know the horse is dead! This is the only way you can be sure that you will be correct.

EXAMINATION PROCEDURE

When examining a horse for either a forelimb or hindlimb lameness, the examination always should commence at the foot and progress proximally.

KEY POINT ▶ It is important to remember that the majority of conditions causing lameness occur in the carpus or distally in the forelimb and in the tarsus or distally in the hindlimb.

Therefore, the examination should concentrate on the distal limb. There is an old saying that "the foot is the cause of lameness until proven otherwise," and this saying has considerable truth.

KEY POINT ▶ In any lameness investigation, the foot should always be inspected and

eliminated as a potential source for the lameness before any further examination.

With the busy schedule of practice, most of us ignore this sooner or later—to our cost. A typical story is as follows: A horse is presented with obvious carpal swelling, and radiographs are taken that show soft-tissue swelling. Advice is to treat with phenylbutazone for 7 days and rest the horse. The swelling disappears, but the horse is still quite lame. An examination performed by another practice shows that the horse has considerable pain on application of hoof testers and there is a fracture involving the wing of the distal phalanx (pedal bone). If the veterinarian performing the initial examination failed to examine the foot, he or she can appear incompetent. Clients always remember your mistakes more than your successes.

Forelimb

Foot

Inspection and Assessment of Shoeing. The foot is inspected for signs of cracks, discharge, uneven wear, and improper shoeing. Particular note should be made as to how the shoe lies on the foot.

KEY POINT ▶ The most common shoeing fault is where the shoe has excessive contact with the sole, resulting in extra pressure on an area that was not designed for weight bearing.

The shoe normally should maintain contact with the hoof wall and a small amount of sole around the area of the white line. Uneven trimming of the foot may be evident when one stands behind the horse and evaluates the symmetry of the heels. If ground contact is not even, the heels may assume a "sheared" appearance, one of the bulbs of the heel being pushed higher than the other. A common shoeing fault in thoroughbred horses occurs when the toe of the foot is left too long and the heel is cut too short. This may be one of the conformational contributors to navicular disease.

Detailed Examination. Signs of increased heat around the coronary band and hoof wall should be determined by comparing with the opposite foot. This may be most easily assessed by using the back of the hand rather than the palm. With weight off the foot, the palmar region is examined to determine if there has been any loss of elasticity of the lateral cartilages, indicating the development of sidebone. Hoof testers can then be used to attempt to determine if pain is present in any part of the foot (Fig. 3-1).

KEY POINT ▶ If a painful response is found, it should always be rechecked and compared with the opposite foot.

Some horses with a unilateral forelimb lameness will show evidence of pain with hoof testers on the

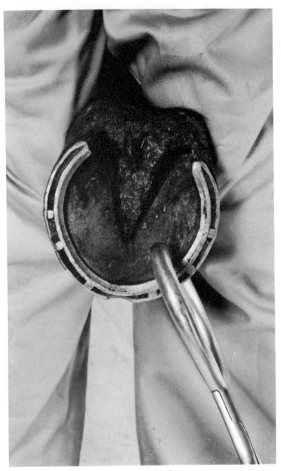

Figure 3–1. Examination of the foot using hoof testers. The hoof testers are applied between the hoof wall and the sole to find whether pain is present.

affected hoof, which initially can be thought to be the site of the problem. However, examination of the unaffected foot may disclose a similar painful response to hoof testers. Careful use of hoof testers applied around the hoof wall and periphery of the sole may localize the pain to a particular region of the foot, which is especially useful in dealing with problems such as foot abscesses. The hoof testers also should be applied across the frog (Fig. 3-2) and across the heels (Fig. 3-3) to determine if there are signs of pain. With the foot on the ground, the hoof wall is then tapped with a hoof hammer (Fig. 3-4) or closed hoof testers to determine if any painful areas are present, which may have been inapparent with the hoof testers.

Pastern

Most problems in the pastern are due to direct trauma or concussion. Injuries to the proximal or middle phalanges usually result in swelling and pain, evident on various degrees of flexion or palpation of this region.

KEY POINT ▶ Many normal horses will have swellings on the medial and lateral aspects of the distal part of the proximal phalanx, which are of little clinical significance.

However, in degenerative joint disease involving the proximal interphalangeal joint (ringbone), there can be severe changes present but little or no pain on flexion or palpation. Therefore, great care should be taken in assessment of pastern swelling and should include radiography of the pastern region if there is suspicion of joint involvement.

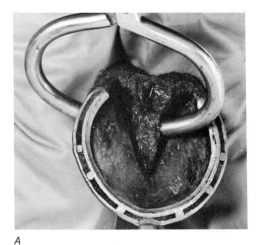

A

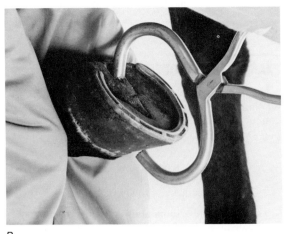

B

Figure 3–2. Examination of the foot using hoof testers. (*A*) The hoof testers are applied over the middle third of the frog. Horses with pain in the navicular region may show pain on application over this area. (*B*) The hoof testers are applied between the frog and the dorsal surface of the hoof wall. This will sometimes reveal pain in the navicular region.

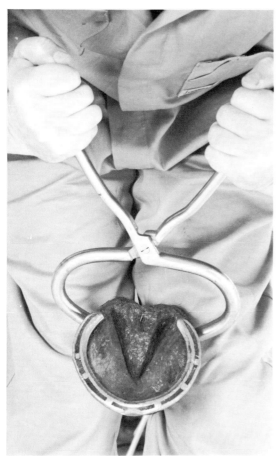

Figure 3–3. Examination of the foot using hoof testers. The hoof testers are being applied across the heels of the foot to localize pain to the palmar aspect of the foot.

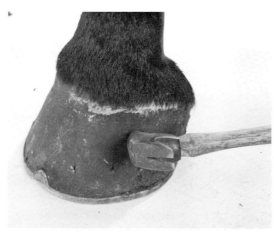

Figure 3–4. Tapping of the hoof wall with a hoof hammer, with the foot on the ground. Sometimes this will reveal pain when the use of hoof testers does not.

Fetlock

Inspection of the fetlock should be undertaken to detect swelling over the dorsal region of the joint and the palmar pouches. The palmar pouches are located between the interosseous (suspensory) ligament and the palmar aspect of the third metacarpal bone. In the normal fetlock this area will appear indented, but in joint disorders this will become distended with synovial fluid (Fig. 3-5). The fetlock joint should then be flexed as much as possible (Fig. 3-6) to determine the normal range of movement (usually 90 degrees) and to evaluate any pain that may be present in the joint. [Note that the range of fetlock flexion will decrease as the horse's age increases.] After this, the sesamoid bones are palpated over the abaxial surface of the fetlock to ascertain if pain is present.

KEY POINT ► If pain is found in the joint, a flexion test should be performed to determine if the degree of lameness can be aggravated.

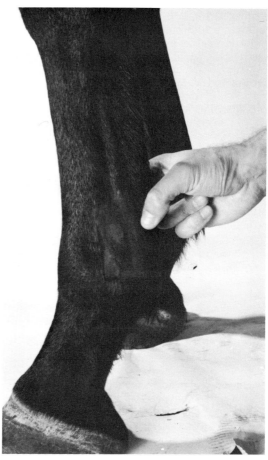

Figure 3–5. Lateral view of the palmar pouch of the left fetlock showing distension of the pouch. The pouch is located between the suspensory ligament and the palmar aspect of the third metacarpal bone in the distal metacarpus.

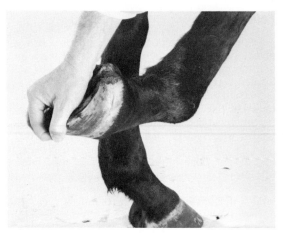

Figure 3–6. Flexion of the right fetlock to determine if there is a painful reaction.

This is performed by holding the fetlock flexed for 1 minute and trotting the horse off (Fig. 3-7). Fetlock and phalangeal flexion tests are nonspecific and will accentuate lameness due to a variety of problems ranging from the foot to the fetlock. Note that the test should be performed with the carpus extended as much as possible so that lameness proximal to the fetlock is not emphasized.

Metacarpus

The structures of importance to the examination are the superficial and deep flexor tendons, inferior check ligament, interosseous (suspensory) ligament, and second, third, and fourth metacarpal bones. The tendons and suspensory ligament should all be palpated individually with the weight off the affected leg (Figs. 3-8 and 3-9). The superficial flexor tendon is flat, whereas the deep flexor tendon is round. Particular note should be paid to any signs of swelling or pain on palpation.

KEY POINT ▶ It must be kept in mind that all horses will show some pain on firm palpation of the interosseous (suspensory) ligament.

Pain should be evaluated against the findings on palpation, where a thickened main body of the ligament or its branches indicates a probable desmitis. The inferior check ligament, situated in the proximal metacarpal region, should be palpated for signs of pain and swelling. The second, third, and fourth metacarpal bones should be palpated for signs of pain and swelling. While the fourth metacarpal bone is rarely a source of lameness, the second metacarpal bone is quite frequently injured in pleasure horses and standardbred racehorses.

KEY POINT ▶ The dorsal aspect of the third metacarpal bone should be palpated carefully in 2- and 3-year old

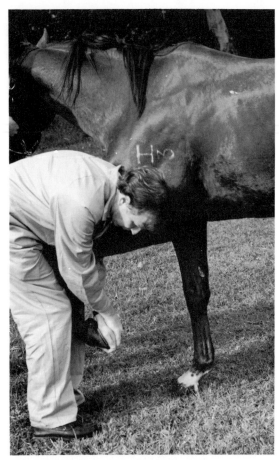

Figure 3–7. Flexion test demonstrating flexion of the fetlock and phalanges. Note that the carpus should be kept as extended as possible so that lameness can be localized to the distal limb. After 1 min the horse is trotted off to determine if the extent of lameness is aggravated.

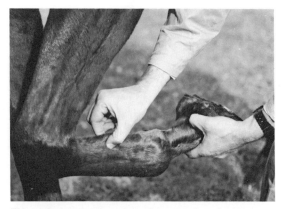

Figure 3–8. Palpation of the flexor tendons in the metacarpal region of the left foreleg. Note should be taken of heat and swelling as well as pain.

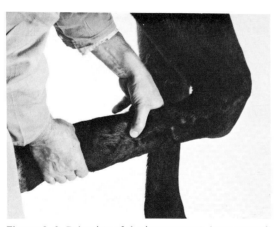

Figure 3–9. Palpation of the interosseous (suspensory) ligament of the right foreleg to determine swelling and pain.

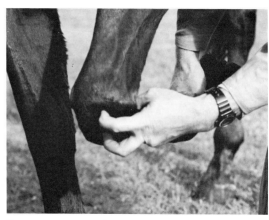

Figure 3–10. Palpation of the dorsal aspect of the left carpus for joint capsule distension and thickening over the proximal (radiocarpal) and middle (intercarpal) carpal joints.

racehorses because "bucked shins" is a very common cause of lameness.

Carpus

Most horses with carpal injuries will show some degree of distension of the joint capsules of the middle (intercarpal) and/or proximal (radiocarpal) carpal joints. The dorsal aspect of the carpus should be palpated over the appropriate joint to check for signs of synovial effusion and joint capsule swelling (Fig. 3-10), followed by extreme flexion of the carpus to determine whether there is resistance to flexion, reduced flexion, or pain.

KEY POINT ▶ Many horses only will show signs of pain during the last few degrees of flexion.

Therefore, the foot should be pulled up past the elbow joint to determine the response to severe flexion (Fig. 3-11). If there are doubts about the response to static flexion, a carpal flexion test should be carried out, where the carpus is held flexed for 1 minute and the horse is trotted off. An increase in the degree of lameness indicates the probability of a carpal problem.

Upper Forelimb (Radius, Elbow, Humerus, and Shoulder)

KEY POINT ▶ Horses with lameness arising from the upper forelimb will seldom reveal any signs of pain on examination.

However, these areas of the leg are palpated, flexed, abducted, and extended to determine if any localizing signs can be found (Figs. 3-12 to 3-14). Attention also should be paid to careful inspection and palpation of the musculature to determine whether muscle injuries contribute to the lameness.

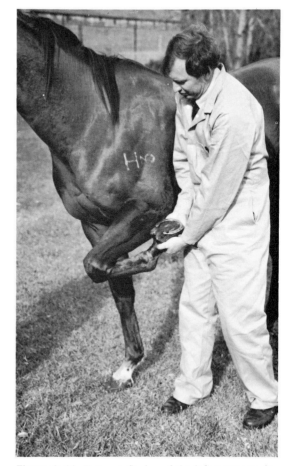

Figure 3–11. Extreme flexion of the left carpus to determine signs of pain localized to the carpus.

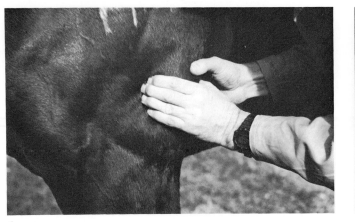
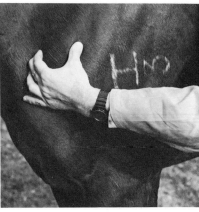

A   B

Figure 3–12. Palpation of the musculature in the upper forelimb to localize pain. (*A*) Palpation over the triceps muscles. (*B*) Palpation over the supraspinatus muscle.

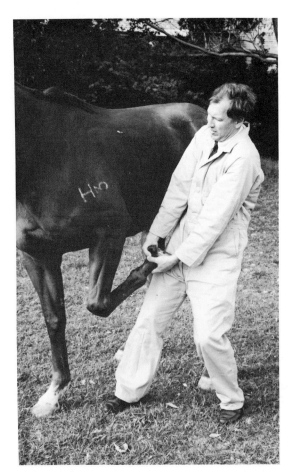
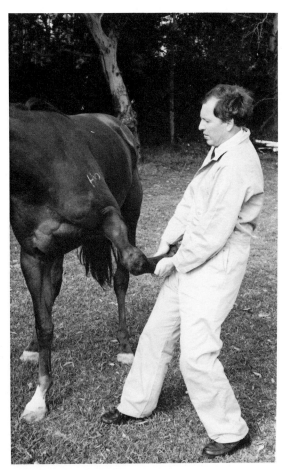

Figure 3–13. Flexion of the upper foreleg to determine whether pain is present.

Figure 3–14. Abduction of the upper foreleg to determine whether pain is present.

Hindlimb

The initial part of the examination (foot, pastern, fetlock, and metatarsus) is similar to that for the forelimb. However, chronic lamenesses are usually in the upper hindleg and may be caused by injuries to the hock (most common), stifle, or hip (least common).

KEY POINT ▶ It is particularly important in chronic hindleg lamenesses to evaluate the symmetry of the left and right gluteal region because atrophy of the gluteal muscles is a feature of such lamenesses.

This is best done by standing the horse square on level ground and examining the appearance of the hindquarters from behind the horse (but not too close).

Tarsus (Hock)

The hock should be inspected for signs of swelling, particularly the tibiotarsal joint capsule, which is prominent on the dorsomedial aspect of the joint. The hock should be flexed and extended; however, this seldom produces any signs of pain, even in severe hock disorders.

KEY POINT ▶ After the initial examination, a spavin test should be carried out (Fig. 3-15).

This test will aggravate chronic lamenesses involving the hock and stifle joints. The hock is held flexed for 2 minutes (timed by watch) by holding the leg at the midmetatarsus and parallel to the ground. The horse is then trotted off, and if there is an intraarticular problem, the lameness may be aggravated for the first six to eight steps. The spavin test will aggravate lameness due to problems in the stifle and occasionally the hip. However, in most cases where there is a dramatic positive response to the spavin test, the hock is the site of the problem.

Stifle

In most stifle problems there is distension of the joint capsule of the femoropatellar pouches just distal to the patella and between the patellar ligaments.

KEY POINT ▶ The femoropatellar pouches should be examined by palpating either side of the middle patellar ligament to detect distension (Fig. 3-16).

Even minor degrees of distension are of significance, and abnormal findings should be compared with those of the opposite stifle joint. However, it should be remembered that in young horses where there is distension of the femoropatellar pouches due to osteochondritis dissecans in one stifle joint,

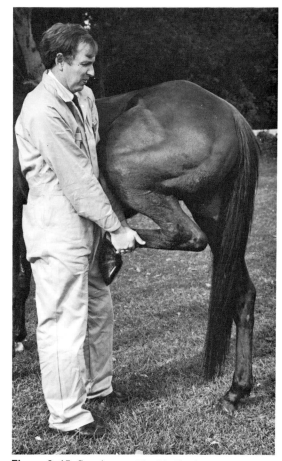

Figure 3–15. Spavin test. The hindleg is held in flexion for 2 min, after which the horse is trotted off to determine whether the lameness is aggravated.

the opposite stifle is frequently affected and may be equally distended.

Hip

The hip can only be palpated indirectly by placing the palm of the hand over the greater trochanter of the femur (Fig. 3-17). In some cases of damage to the hip joint, crepitus can be detected in this fashion as the horse walks. Soft-tissue injuries around the hip joint are much more common than damage to the hip joint itself. Examination of this region should include palpation of the gluteal muscle mass bilaterally, since pain in this region is not uncommon and may contribute to reduced performance.

Back

The clinical signs of back injuries may be quite varied and range from changes in temperament to reduced performance. Temperament problems as a

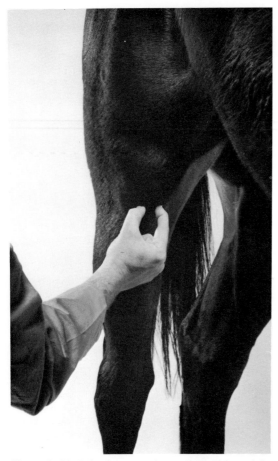

Figure 3–16. Palpation over the medial and lateral femoropatellar pouches to determine whether there is synovial effusion.

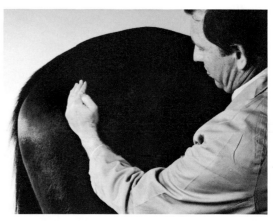

Figure 3–17. Palpation over the greater trochanter of the femur to detect signs of pain and crepitus involving the hip joint.

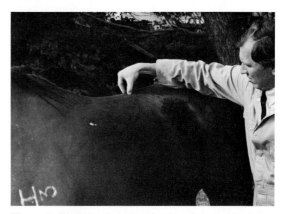

Figure 3–18. Palpation over the dorsal thoracic spinous processes for signs of pain or hypersensitivity.

clinical sign are quite common in dressage horses. The majority of problems arise from the thoracolumbar region, although sacroiliac pain is a common problem, particularly in standardbreds.

The examination should begin with palpation over the dorsal thoracic spinous processes (Fig. 3-18) to detect any pain and should proceed caudally to the sacral region. Normal horses will "dip" their backs on stroking with a blunt object such as a pen over the thoracolumbar region (Fig. 3-19) and arch their backs on stroking over the caudal sacral region (Fig. 3-20). A back problem may be suspected in horses that do not show these responses, since the horse may be attempting to protect itself from back pain by holding its back rigid. Because a number of back problems involve soft-tissue injuries, the longissimus dorsi muscles on either side of the dorsal spinous processes also should be palpated and may be stroked with a firm object such as the blunt end of a ballpoint pen to check lateral flexibility of the back.

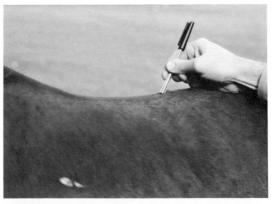

Figure 3–19. Examination of the thoracolumbar region by stroking with a pen. The horse will normally dip its back.

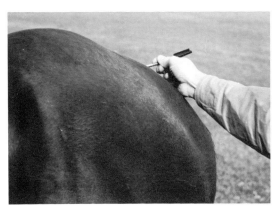

Figure 3–20. Examination of the caudal sacral region of the back. The horse will normally arch its back on firm stroking.

If sacroiliac pain exists, palpation over the tuber sacrale (point of the croup; Fig. 3-21) will result in the horse crouching toward the ground. Sacroiliac problems are common in standardbred horses and may be manifested as gait disorders of a nonspecific nature. Trainers often complain about horses "jumping out of their gear" or "breaking on turns."

DIAGNOSTIC AIDS
Local Anesthesia–Nerve Blocks

In many cases it may be impossible to localize the site of lameness from the clinical examination or there may be more than one contributing cause. In such cases, diagnostic nerve blocks should be undertaken, either to localize the source of the problem or to confirm the suspected site. This may be done either by blocking sensory nerves innervating specific regions or by injecting local anesthetic intraarticularly. Prior to all injections, a strict

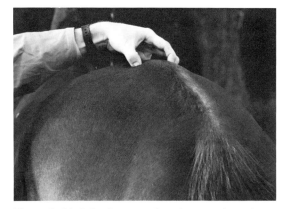

Figure 3–21. Palpation over the tuber sacrale to determine if there is pain in the sacroiliac region.

surgical disinfection of the site should be performed. For intraarticular injections, correct placement of the needle in the joint can be confirmed in most joints by the presence of synovial fluid that drips from the needle or may be found on aspiration. It is important to use sterile gloves for intraarticular injections, and clipping or shaving the surgical site is preferred.

KEY POINT ► In some performance horses, clients object to the hair being removed over the site, and in these cases it is acceptable not to remove the hair.

However, the site should be well prepared by scrubbing two to three times for at least 1 minute with povidone-iodine scrub, followed by application of 70% alcohol. A final skin preparation utilizes an iodine-based product, which can either be tincture of iodine mitis or povidone-iodine (see Disinfectants, Chap. 17). It is important to use a new needle to enter the joint rather than the needle used for aspiration of local anesthetic into the syringe.

Choice of Local Anesthetic

While a variety of local anesthetics may be used, lidocaine (Treatment No. 67) is somewhat more irritating to the tissues than such drugs as prilocaine and mepivacaine (Treatment Nos. 72 and 93). For this reason, and because the latter local anesthetics diffuse better and have a more rapid onset of action than lidocaine, prilocaine and mepivacaine are the local anesthetic drugs of choice.

KEY POINT ► If the local anesthetic is to be administered intraarticularly, a new bottle should be used rather than one from which samples have already been taken.

Onset of Analgesia

With the use of prilocaine or mepivacaine, blocking regional nerves usually results in analgesia within 3 to 5 minutes. A positive result can be assessed quickly, but if there is no improvement, a period of 10 to 15 minutes should elapse before a negative response is assumed. With intraarticular blocks we have often found immediate improvement in gait, but it may require as long as 20 to 30 minutes for a complete effect. This is an important point because if a subsequent nerve block is performed too quickly, the improvement in the lameness may be the result of the previous block rather than the current one.

Problems in Interpretation of Nerve Blocks

While the failure of a horse's gait to improve after a nerve block usually indicates that the problem is elsewhere in the leg, there are occasions where nerve blocks may provide incorrect information. In cases where the lameness is of neurologic origin or where there are fractures, lameness may not be abolished by the nerve block. Therefore, this possibility should be considered when a horse's gait fails to improve despite considerable certainty that the region of the leg blocked is the site of the problem. A common example of this failure to respond to nerve blocks occurs in a horse with a fracture of the distal phalanx involving the distal interphalangeal joint. An abaxial nerve block, which should abolish the lameness, will result in only partial improvement in the gait.

The following sequence, commencing with the foot and proceeding proximally, is used in investigating a lameness problem where no localizing signs can be found during examination. If a specific area of the limb is thought to be involved, that region can be blocked to determine if the lameness originates from that area.

Forelimb

Desensitizing the Palmar Aspect of the Foot: Palmar Digital Nerve Block

With the affected limb held up, the foot is extended and the ergot on the palmar aspect of the fetlock is pulled proximally. This tenses the ligaments of the ergot, which run palmaromedial and palmarolateral in the pastern (Fig. 3-22). The medial and lateral palmar digital nerves run just deep to these ligaments, and the nerves may be desensitized by inserting a 23-gauge, 12-mm (0.5-in) needle to a depth of approximately 6 mm (0.25 in) as shown in Figure 3-23. Local anesthetic (1.5–2.0 ml of 2% prilocaine or a similar local anesthetic) is in-

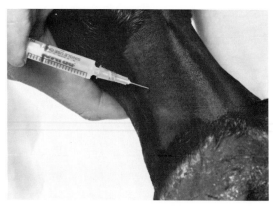

Figure 3–23. Palmar digital nerve block. A 23-gauge, 15-mm (⅝″) needle is inserted just underneath the ligament of the ergot. The photograph shows the position for desensitizing the right lateral palmar digital nerve. A volume of 1.5 ml of 2% local anesthetic is injected.

jected into each site, and the block can be assessed by pricking the palmar aspect of the heel with a pen about 5 minutes after injection. The horse is then trotted, and if the lameness is not abolished, the next site more proximal is assessed. However, in some cases, the effect of the block may not be complete for up to 15 minutes. Therefore, this period of time should elapse before a negative response to the nerve block is considered.

Desensitizing the Distal Interphalangeal (Coffin) Joint

To localize lameness to the coffin joint, a 21-gauge, 25-mm (1-in) needle is inserted almost vertically, about 12 mm (0.5 in) above the coronary band and 18 mm (0.75 in) medial or lateral to the dorsal midline (Fig. 3-24). Then 5 ml of 2% local anesthetic is injected, and a period of 15 minutes should elapse before the gait is reevaluated.

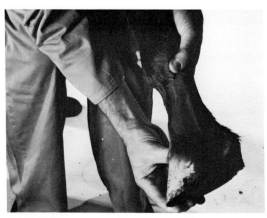

Figure 3–22. With the right front fetlock extended and the ergot pulled proximally, the ligament of the ergot can be seen as the taut structure just distal to the left thumb of the person holding the foot. This is the landmark for insertion of the needle for the palmar digital nerve block. The photograph shows the lateral ligament of the ergot.

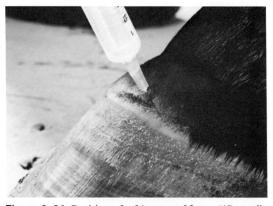

Figure 3–24. Position of a 21-gauge, 25-mm (1″) needle in the coffin (distal interphalangeal) joint to desensitize the joint. A volume of 5 ml of 2% local anesthetic is injected.

Desensitizing the Proximal Interphalangeal (Pastern) Joint

Localization of lameness to the proximal interphalangeal joint is seldom necessary. However, the joint can be desensitized in the distal third of the pastern by insertion of a 21-gauge, 25-mm (1-in) needle on the dorsum of the pastern, about 10 to 15 mm (0.5 in) lateral or medial to the dorsal midline (Fig. 3-25). Then 5 ml of 2% local anesthetic is injected into the joint.

Desensitizing the Foot, Pastern, and Sesamoids: Abaxial Block

The abaxial block desensitizes structures distal to the fetlock joint as well as the sesamoid bones. With the limb held up, the palmar vessels can be palpated over the palmar aspect of the sesamoid bones. The palmar nerves run palmar to these vessels and can be desensitized by inserting a 23-gauge, 25-mm (1-in) needle subcutaneously as shown in Figure 3-26. The needle is inserted at the

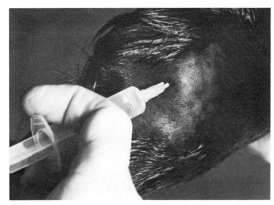

Figure 3–26. Palmar (abaxial) nerve block. The 23-gauge, 25-mm (1″) needle is inserted just palmar to the vessels over the abaxial surface of the sesamoid bones. The photograph shows the needle position for the lateral abaxial block in the right foreleg. A volume of 3 ml of 2% local anesthetic is injected.

base of the sesamoid bones. Approximately 3 to 4 ml of 2% local anesthetic is injected. This nerve block will not desensitize the dorsal aspect of the fetlock. The block can be assessed by using a ball-point pen or similar object to prick the dorsal aspect of the pastern. While this block is probably the easiest to perform of all the nerve blocks, its nonspecific nature often makes it difficult to localize the problem when there is improvement in gait.

Desensitizing the Dorsal Aspect of the Fetlock: Palmar Metacarpal Nerve Block

If the dorsal aspect of the fetlock requires desensitization following a negative response to the abaxial block, the palmar metacarpal nerves can be blocked. These nerves emerge from under the distal ends of the second and fourth metacarpal bones (splint bones) and can be desensitized by injecting 2 to 3 ml of 2% local anesthetic under the distal ends or "buttons" of the second and fourth metacarpal bones (Fig. 3-27).

Desensitizing the Fetlock Joint Intraarticularly

If primary fetlock joint pathology is thought to be the cause of lameness, the fetlock joint can be desensitized by injection of 8 to 10 ml of 2% local anesthetic directly into the joint. A 21-gauge 25-mm (1-in) needle is used for this block, which can be performed through one of three sites. The principal site used by most veterinarians is the palmar pouch (Fig. 3-28), particularly if it is distended with synovial fluid. It is easier to gain access to this site if the leg is held off the ground. An alternative site is

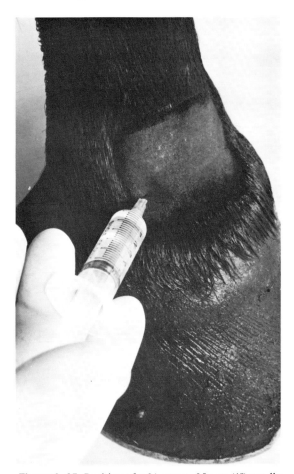

Figure 3–25. Position of a 21-gauge, 25-mm (1″) needle in the pastern (proximal interphalangeal) joint to desensitize the joint. A volume of 5 ml of 2% local anesthetic is injected.

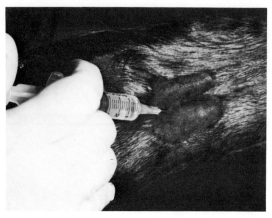

Figure 3–27. Palmar metacarpal nerve block. A 23-gauge, 15-mm (⅝″) needle is positioned underneath the distal end ("button") of the 4th metacarpal bone in the right foreleg. A volume of 2 to 3 ml of 2% local anesthetic is injected.

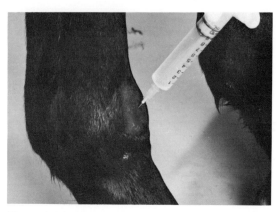

Figure 3–29. Position of a 21-gauge, 25-mm (1″) needle in the dorsal aspect of the right fetlock joint to desensitize the joint. To desensitize the joint a total of 10 ml of 2% local anesthetic is injected.

the dorsal aspect of the fetlock joint, between the common and lateral extensor tendons (Fig. 3-29). This site provides more certain access, but there is potential for the point of the needle to traumatize the articular cartilage. Recently, a more distal site on the lateral aspect of the fetlock joint with the needle inserted through the lateral collateral sesamoidean ligament has been advocated as a superior location for fetlock arthrocentesis (Fig. 3-30). The technique should be carried out with the horse's leg in flexion. Advantages include less hemorrhage into the joint and more definite appearance of synovial fluid after needle insertion.

Desensitizing from Subcarpal Area Distally: High Palmar Nerve Block

This site may be useful to desensitize the entire limb distal to the carpus via a single needle site. With the affected leg on the ground and the opposite forelimb held up, a small amount (0.5–1 ml) of 2% local anesthetic is injected under the skin at the dorsal aspect of the deep flexor tendon on the lateral side of the proximal palmar metacarpus. A 21-gauge, 36-mm (1.5-in) needle is inserted through the bleb at right angle to the long axis of the leg (Fig. 3-31) so that the point of the needle lies 2 to 3 mm

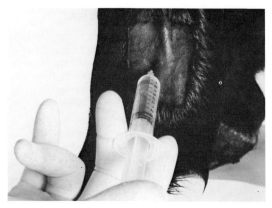

Figure 3–28. Position of a 21-gauge, 25-mm (1″) needle in the palmar pouch, between the third metacarpal bone and suspensory ligament of the left foreleg, to desensitize the fetlock joint. It is sometimes easier to obtain synovial fluid when the needle is inserted with the joint flexed. To desensitize the joint, a total of 10 ml of 2% local anesthetic is injected.

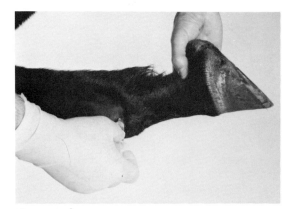

Figure 3–30. Position of a 21-gauge, 25-mm (1″) needle through the lateral collateral sesamoidean ligament to desensitize the left fetlock joint. This site is the most reliable for obtaining joint fluid and causes the least hemorrhage. The landmarks are most easily located with the joint held in slight flexion. The needle has to be placed more deeply than the other two sites for fetlock joint arthrocentesis. To desensitize the joint a total of 10 ml of 2% local anesthetic is injected.

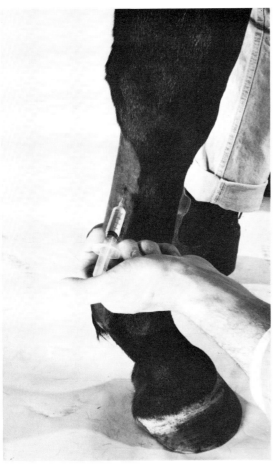

Figure 3–31. High palmar nerve block showing the position of a 21-gauge, 36-mm (1.5″) needle underneath the deep flexor tendon to block the lateral palmar nerve of the right foreleg. Note that the needle is located just beneath the skin over the dorsal edge of the deep flexor tendon. A volume of 3 ml of 2% local anesthetic is injected.

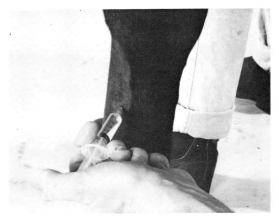

Figure 3–32. High palmar nerve block showing the position of a 21-gauge, 36-mm (1.5″) needle for blocking the medial palmar nerve of the right foreleg. The needle has been pushed along the dorsal margin of the deep flexor tendon so that its point can be palpated on the medial side of the leg. Care must be taken that the needle does not penetrate the medial palmar artery. A volume of 3 ml of 2% local anesthetic is injected.

(0.1-in) under the skin, immediately dorsal to the deep flexor tendon. Then 2 ml of 2% local anesthetic is injected at this point, following which the needle is pushed through medially so that its point can be palpated beneath the skin on the medial side of the leg (Fig. 3-32). Aspiration should then be performed to check that the needle has not entered the palmar artery, after which a further 2 ml of 2% local anesthetic is injected to desensitize the medial palmar nerve.

Desensitization of the Proximal Metacarpus

In some horses, inferior check ligament injury may result in a low-grade lameness that is not readily diagnosed. In these cases, deposition of 5 to 6

ml of 2% local anesthetic will be useful to aid in diagnosis (Fig. 3-33).

Desensitization of the Carpus

The most common carpal joint involved in injury is the middle carpal (intercarpal) joint. This does not communicate with the proximal carpal (radiocarpal) joint, which must be desensitized separately. However, the middle carpal joint does communicate with the distal carpal (carpometacarpal) joint, and this should be taken into account when evaluating a positive response to a nerve block.

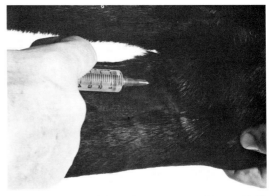

Figure 3–33. Position of a 21-gauge, 36-mm (1.5″) needle in the proximal metacarpus, deep to the deep flexor tendon to desensitize the region of the inferior check ligament. A volume of 5 to 6 ml of 2% local anesthetic is injected.

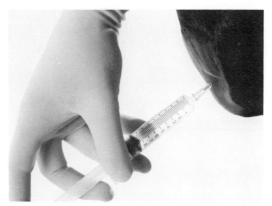

Figure 3–34. Position of a 21-gauge, 25-mm (1″) needle in the left middle carpal (intercarpal) joint to desensitize the joint. A volume of 10 ml of 2% local anesthetic is injected.

Both the proximal and middle carpal joints are easily blocked by holding the affected leg off the ground so that the carpus is well flexed. A 21-gauge, 25-mm (1-in) needle is placed into the middle or proximal carpal joints, either medial or lateral to the extensor carpi radialis tendon (Figs. 3-34 and 3-35) in the depressions formed by the openings of the joints. Then 10 ml of 2% local anesthetic is injected into the affected joint. At least 10 minutes should elapse before reevaluating the horse's gait.

Desensitizing from the Distal Radius to the Foot

To desensitize the distal radius (and all structures distally), it is possible to block the median, ulnar, and musculocutaneous nerves. While these nerve

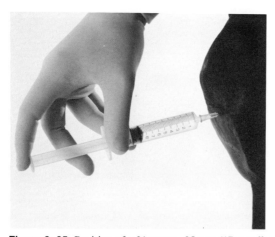

Figure 3–35. Position of a 21-gauge, 25-mm (1″) needle in the left proximal carpal (radiocarpal) joint to desensitize the joint. A volume of 10 ml of 2% local anesthetic is injected.

blocks are seldom necessary in practice, they are sometimes useful if the veterinarian wants to ensure that the problem is proximal to the carpus by allowing complete desensitization of the distal limb. The nerve blocks are illustrated in Figures 3-36 to 3-38. Between 10 and 20 ml of local anesthetic is injected at each of the sites.

Desensitizing the Elbow Joint

Lameness arising from the elbow joint is uncommon, but when it does occur, it is almost impossible to diagnose by physical examination because there is seldom pain on palpation and synovial effusion may not be detectable. Arthrocentesis of the elbow joint is achieved by palpating the lateral collateral ligament and determining its point of insertion on the lateral radius. A notch can then be felt imme-

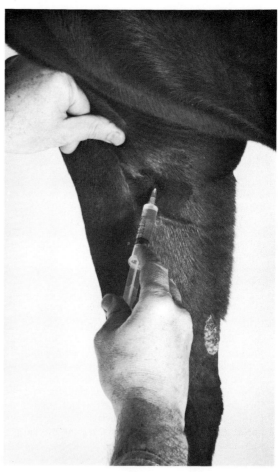

Figure 3–36. Median nerve block. A 19-gauge, 36-mm (1.5″) needle is inserted underneath the belly of the pectoralis descendens muscle, in a proximal direction and just caudal to the radius. Because the median artery lies close to this site, it is possible to penetrate the vessel. Therefore, if blood drips from the needle, it should be directed more caudally. A volume of 10 ml of 2% local anesthetic is injected.

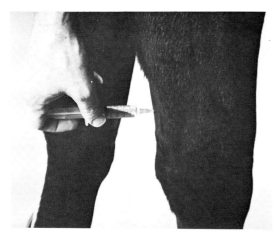

Figure 3–37. Ulnar nerve block. A 21-gauge, 25-mm (1″) needle is inserted 8 to 10 cm above the acessory carpal bone in the groove between the ulnaris lateralis and the flexor carpi ulnaris muscles. A volume of 10 ml of 2% local anesthetic is injected.

diately caudal to the ligament, and a 21-gauge, 25-mm (1-in) needle is placed into this notch to a depth of approximately 12 mm (0.5 in) (Fig. 3-39). A total of 15 to 20 ml of 2% local anesthetic is injected.

Desensitizing the Shoulder Joint

As for the elbow joint, horses with lameness arising from the shoulder joint seldom show pain on palpation or flexion. The site for needle insertion for intraarticular local anesthesia is determined by palpating the lateral tuberosities of the humerus with the thumb and forefinger (Fig. 3-40). After desensitizing the skin with a bleb of local anesthetic, an 18-gauge, 7.5-cm (3-in) spinal needle is passed in the groove between the tuberosities, along the humeral head (Fig. 3-41). When the point of the needle enters the joint, a slight sucking sound is usually heard, and aspiration with a 10-ml syringe produces synovial fluid. Approximately 20 ml of 2% local anesthetic is injected to desensitize the joint.

Hindlimb

The regimen for local anesthesia in the hindlimb is similar to that for the forelimb, from the foot proximally to below the hock. However, the nerve distribution is slightly more variable than that of the forelimb, particularly that of the plantar digital nerves. Additionally, the deep peroneal nerve has branches that can innervate the distal structures. Distal limb nerve blocks are also more difficult in the hindlimb because the leg must be held off the

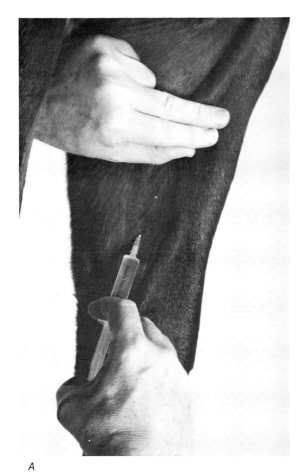

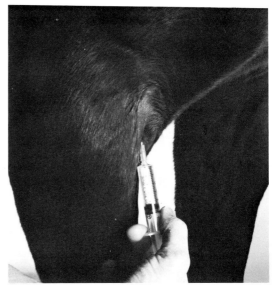

A   *B*

Figure 3–38. Musculocutaneous nerve block. Two injection sites are necessary to desensitize the musculocutaneous nerve. (*A*) One site is on the medial aspect of the mid radius, close to the cephalic vein. The nerve can be palpated and a 21-gauge, 25-mm needle used to inject 5 ml of local anesthetic. (*B*) The more proximal site is over the lacertus fibrosis. A 21-gauge, 25-mm needle is inserted where the nerve can be palpated, and 5 ml of 2% local anesthetic is injected.

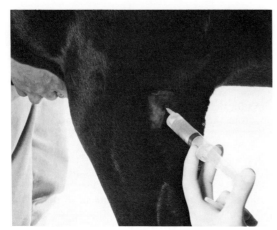

Figure 3–39. Position of a 19-gauge, 36-mm (1.5″) needle in the left elbow joint to desensitize the joint.

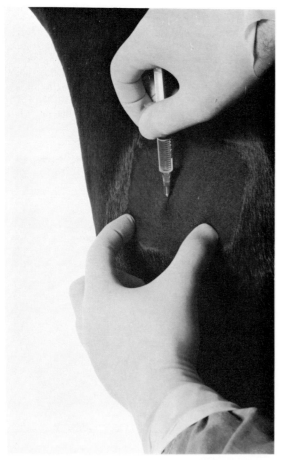

Figure 3–40. Palpation of the lateral tuberosities of the left humerus and deposition of local anesthetic to desensitize the skin prior to insertion of the spinal needle.

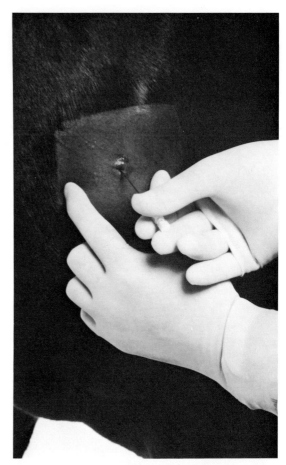

Figure 3–41. An 18-gauge, 12.5-cm (5″) spinal needle inserted along the humeral head into the left shoulder joint.

ground by the veterinarian while carrying out the blocks and the risk of injury to the operator is potentially greater. Most chronic hindleg lamenesses arise from the hock and (less commonly) the stifle. Intraarticular local anesthesia is particularly helpful in positively localizing the site of chronic hindlimb lameness.

Tarsus (Hock)

The hock is a complex joint, with four possible sites for intraarticular pathology: tarsocrural (tibiotarsal), proximal intertarsal, distal intertarsal and tarsometatarsal joints. The tarsocrural and proximal intertarsal joints communicate, whereas the distal intertarsal and tarsometatarsal joints communicate in only 20% to 30% of cases. Arthritis of the hock (bone spavin) is usually confined to the tarsometatarsal and distal intertarsal joints, and therefore, these joints are blocked first.

Desensitizing the Tarsometatarsal Joint

Arthrocentesis of the tarsometatarsal joint is undertaken over the head of the fourth metatarsal bone on the plantarolateral surface of the distal hock. A 21-gauge, 25-mm (1-in) needle is inserted to a depth of 12 to 18 mm (0.5–0.75 in) (Fig. 3-42). In a difficult horse, it may be helpful to insert a bleb of local anesthetic in the skin prior to the needle being inserted into the joint. If synovial fluid does not appear in the hub of the needle, it should be rotated, after which synovial fluid should emerge. Despite the small volume of this joint (1.5–2.0 ml), approximately 5 ml of 2% local anesthetic should be injected because such volume will disrupt the joint capsule, separating the tarsometatarsal and distal intertarsal joints thus leading to communication between the two joints. Therefore both joints may be blocked from the same site. However, it should be noted that horses with intraarticular problems involving the distal intertarsal and tarsometatarsal joints will seldom become completely sound after desensitization of the latter joint.

Desensitizing the Distal Intertarsal Joint

The distal intertarsal joint can be desensitized on the medial aspect of the hock, 10 to 12 mm (0.5 in) above the head of the second metatarsal bone and slightly farther dorsally. It is usually difficult to palpate the joint space, whereas the space of the proximal intertarsal joint above it is more readily discernible. A 23-gauge, 25-mm (1-in) needle is introduced at a right angle to the long axis of the leg (Fig. 3-43), and 2 ml of 2% local anesthetic is injected.

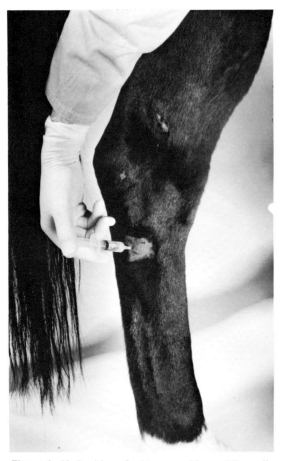

Figure 3–42. Position of a 21-gauge, 25-mm (1″) needle in the right tarsometatarsal joint to desensitize the joint. The needle is inserted at an angle over the head of the fourth metatarsal bone. A volume of 5 ml of 2% local anesthetic is injected.

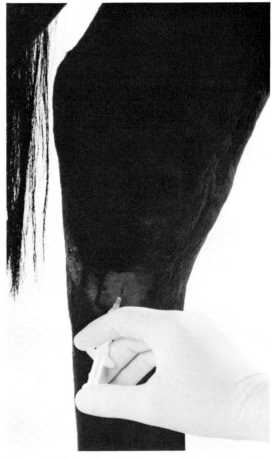

Figure 3–43. Position of a 23-gauge, 15-mm (⅝″) needle on the medial aspect of the left distal intertarsal joint on the medial aspect of the hock. A volume of 2 to 3 ml of 2% local anesthetic is injected.

Desensitizing the Tarsocrural (Tibiotarsal) and Proximal Intertarsal Joints

The tarsocrural joint and proximal intertarsal joint can both be desensitized by introducing local anesthetic into the tarsocrural joint, on the medial aspect of the hock. After palpation of the medial malleolus of the distal tibia, a 21-gauge, 25-mm (1-in) needle is inserted just distal to it and either dorsal or plantar to the saphenous vein to a depth of 12 mm (0.5 in) (Fig. 3-44). A total of 8 to 10 ml of 2% local anesthetic is injected to achieve desensitization.

Desensitizing from the Distal Tibia to the Foot

As with the median, ulnar, and musculocutaneous nerve blocks in the foreleg, desensitization of the peroneal and tibial nerves is seldom neces-sary. We use these blocks to exclude the hock and structures distally as the possible sites of lameness. The tibial nerve is blocked on the medial aspect of the hindleg, approximately 8 cm (3 in) above the point of the hock, on the caudal border of the deep flexor tendon (Fig. 3-45). To block the left tibial nerve, the operator should stand on the lateral side of the right hindleg and have an assistant hold up the left foreleg. After a bleb of local anesthetic has been placed in the skin, a 19-gauge, 25-mm (1-in) needle is inserted under and along the edge of the deep flexor tendon. A total of 20 ml of 2% local anesthetic is deposited in several locations by moving the needle.

The peroneal nerves are located in the groove between the lateral and long digital extensor muscles on the lateral aspect of the tibia approximately 10 to 12 cm (4–5 in) above the point of the hock (Fig. 3-46). Both deep and superficial peroneal nerves should be blocked using 15 to 20 ml of 2% local anesthetic.

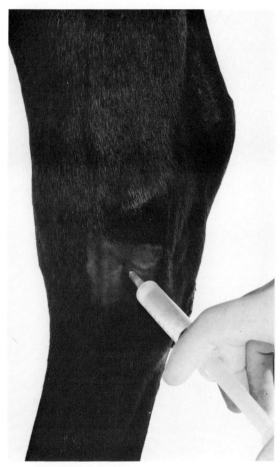

Figure 3–44. Position of a 21-gauge, 25-mm (1″) needle in the right tarsocrural (tibiotarsal) joint just distal to the medial malleolus of the tibia. Note the position of the needle on the medial aspect of the leg, just plantar to the saphenous vein.

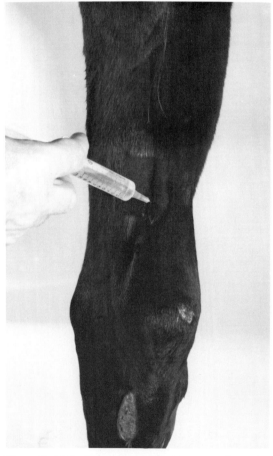

Figure 3–45. Position of 19-gauge, 25-mm needle on the medial aspect of the hock to block the tibial nerve, just caudal to the deep flexor tendon. Approximately 20 ml of 2% local anesthetic is deposited in several sites.

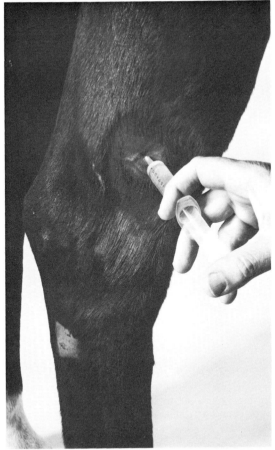

Figure 3–46. Position of 19-gauge, 3.75-cm needle on the lateral aspect of the distal tibia to block the peroneal nerves. The needle is located about 10 cm above the point of the hock, in the groove formed between the lateral and long extensor muscles. Local anesthetic is injected at a depth of 3 cm to block the deep peroneal and withdrawn superficially to block the superficial peroneal.

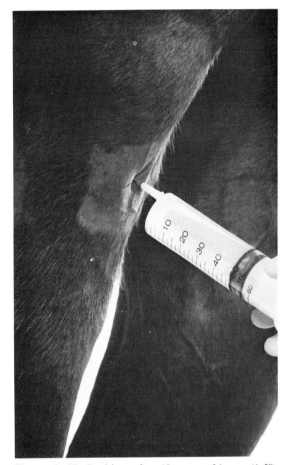

Figure 3–47. Position of a 19-gauge, 36-mm (1.5″) needle in the medial femoropatellar pouch to desensitize the medial side of the stifle joint.

Desensitizing the Stifle

The stifle joint is most easily desensitized by injecting local anesthetic into the medial or lateral femoropatellar pouch. The medial femoropatellar pouch always communicates with the medial aspect of the femorotibial joint, whereas the lateral femoropatellar pouch only communicates with the lateral part of the femorotibial joint in about 20% of cases. To desensitize the medial part of the joint, a 19-gauge, 36-mm (1.5-in) needle is introduced into the medial femoropatellar pouch approximately 25 mm (1 in) above the tibial crest (Fig. 3-47). Where the joint capsule is distended, synovial fluid will be obtained, after which 50 ml of 2% local anesthetic is injected. To desensitize the lateral aspect of the joint, a 19-gauge, 36-mm (1.5-in) needle is introduced on the lateral aspect of the stifle after palpating the joint space (Fig. 3-48). The location for needle insertion is between the lateral patellar ligament and the lateral collateral ligament of the femorotibial joint. Then 50 ml of 2% local anesthetic is injected.

Desensitizing the Hip

Due to its depth and muscle covering, the hip is probably the most difficult joint to access. Fortunately, hip problems in horses are extremely rare, and the hip joint seldom requires desensitization. The joint is desensitized by using an 18-gauge, 15-cm (6-in) spinal needle. After locating the greater trochanter of the femur, the needle is passed cranial to this, along the femoral neck and head (Fig. 3-49). Aspiration with a 10-ml syringe will indicate entry to the joint, which is 10 to 13 cm (4–5 in) deep, and 20 ml of 2% local anesthetic is injected.

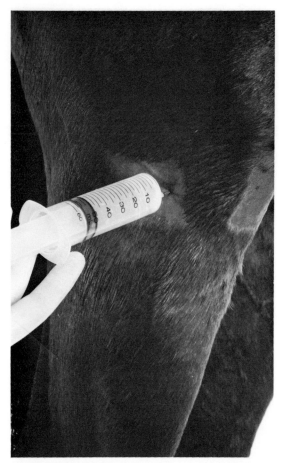

Figure 3–48. Position of a 19-gauge, 36-mm (1.5″) needle between the lateral patellar ligament and the lateral collateral ligament to desensitize the lateral side of the stifle joint.

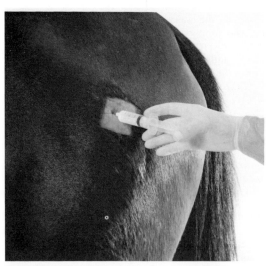

Figure 3–49. Desensitization of the hip joint. Position of an 18-gauge, 15-cm (6″) spinal needle in the hip joint.

Synovial Fluid Analysis

Synovial fluid analysis is useful in distinguishing septic from nonseptic forms of joint disease. While cytologic analyses have been advocated by some veterinarians to assist in determining the stage of degenerative joint disease, we have not found such analyses useful.

KEY POINT ► There is no correlation between synovial fluid cytologic findings and the severity of degenerative joint disease.

Rather, clinical and radiographic findings are of more use in establishing prognosis and treatment of joint disorders. If synovial fluid is to be collected, it should be obtained as previously described, and portions should be placed in a tube containing EDTA as well as in a sterile plain tube. If samples are to be submitted for bacteriology because of suspected septic arthritis, great care should be taken to ensure that the fluid does not become contaminated during collection. It may be necessary to collect the samples with the horse under general anesthesia, particularly if there is severe pain associated with manipulation of the joint. The fluid sample in the sterile tube can be submitted for bacteriology (see Chap. 15). Worthwhile analyses include total and differential white cell count, total protein, and alkaline phosphatase. Normal values for most joints are as shown in Table 3-1.

In septic arthritis, total protein is increased to more than 30 g/L (3 g/dL), and the total white cell count increases to a value usually in excess of $10,000 \times 10^6$/L (10,000/μL), with neutrophils usually contributing more than 90% of the leukocytes.

Radiology

Once the site of the lameness has been localized with nerve blocks or intraarticular local anesthesia, radiographs can be taken. While it has become common for clients to request radiographs of all four limbs, from the foot to the carpus or tarsus, interpretation of the changes found is often difficult. For this reason, it is best to perform a thorough clinical examination followed by radiography only of areas that are of concern. Several radiographic views are usually required, with lateral to medial and oblique views being the most rewarding. While there are a number of excellent books indi-

TABLE 3–1. Normal Values for Synovial Fluid Analyses

Total protein (g/L)	10–20 (1–2 g/dL)
White cell count ($\times 10^6$/L)	100–800 (100–800/μL)
Differential count	
Neutrophils	<20%
Mononuclear cells	80–95%
Alkaline phosphatase (U/L)	20–40

cating radiographic positioning and interpretation, we will provide some perspective and practical tips for each of the areas that are commonly radiographed.

Foot

While many veterinarians will attempt to examine the navicular bone and distal phalanx (pedal bone) on the same radiograph, the exposure necessary to properly examine the navicular bone will result in overexposure of the pedal bone on the dorsopalmar view.

KEY POINT ▶ Separate exposures must be made of the pedal and navicular bones depending on the suspected site of the problem.

The sulci of the frog should be cleaned and packed with Play-Doh to eliminate the possibility of radiolucent lines over the distal phalanx and navicular bone. The dorsopalmar view can be taken in either of two ways: The first is the *upright pedal view,* where the foot is positioned in a block so that the sole is at right angles to the ground and the foot rests on the toe. To radiograph the navicular bone using this view, the x-ray beam should be centered about 12 mm (0.5 in) above the coronary band. The second is the *high coronary view,* where the foot is positioned in a normal weight-bearing stance on a reinforced cassette. This view provides a satisfactory view of the pedal bone but causes magnification of the navicular bone, making assessment of minor changes difficult. *Oblique views* are of particular use when evaluating horses with fractures of the pedal bone. The normal lines of the frog sulci, together with the direction of the fracture line, often result in a fracture being inapparent. The appropriate oblique view enables a fracture line to be seen more easily and potential involvement of the articular surface to be evaluated. The *special navicular or palmar (skyline) view* enables the wings of the pedal bone and the flexor surface of the navicular bone to be assessed. This view is particularly useful in cases of suspected fracture of the navicular bone. The *lateral view* of the foot enables the orientation of the pedal bone in the foot to be evaluated, which is essential when assessing possible pedal bone rotation in cases of laminitis. It is useful to stick a short piece of wire longitudinally on the middorsal hoof wall to aid this evaluation. This view should be taken with the foot on a wooden block around 25 to 50 mm (1–2 in) high so that the solar aspect of the pedal bone can be assessed.

Pastern and Fetlock

The four standard views (dorsopalmar, lateral, dorsomedial to palmarolateral, dorsolateral to palmaromedial) should be used when assessing problems involving the pastern or fetlock.

KEY POINT ▶ A lateral view of the fetlock is particularly important to evaluate the dorsal aspect of the distal third metacarpal bone.

This site is important when determining changes to the dorsal contour of the distal metacarpus, which occur when there is chronic proliferative synovitis (villonodular synovitis). If this condition is suspected, an air arthrogram of the fetlock, where 15 ml air is injected into the fetlock joint, is useful in defining the extent of the soft-tissue proliferation in the dorsal fetlock when combined with a lateral view.

Metacarpus and Metatarsus

Oblique views are very important to evaluate the second and fourth metacarpal bones if fractures are suspected. Lateral views of the metacarpus or metatarsus with good detail are important if fissure fractures of the dorsal cortex are suspected.

Carpus

KEY POINT ▶ The view that can be eliminated from a routine radiographic screening of the carpus is the dorsopalmar view.

Because most carpal problems occur on the dorsomedial side of the joint, the dorsolateral to palmaromedial oblique view (45 degrees) is the most useful view for showing lesions, in combination with the lateral to medial view.

KEY POINT ▶ Some undisplaced chip and slab fractures of the third carpal bone may be difficult to detect using standard views, and a skyline view can be valuable.

The *flexed lateral view* is useful for assessment of the articular surfaces of the distal radial carpal and proximal third carpal bones.

Elbow and Shoulder

For adequate radiographs of both these areas, the horse is best anesthetized, although standing shots are possible. While x-ray machines with capacities for high (about 300 mA) output are optimal for radiographing the elbow and shoulder, it is possible to obtain adequate exposures with portable x-ray machines. This is achieved by using repeated exposures with the same plate in position.

Hock

Four views, dorsoplantar, lateral, and two obliques, are necessary for full evaluation of hock disorders.

KEY POINT ▶ Because the majority of hock problems involve the distal joints, the primary beam should be centered at the level of the chestnut.

Although many horses with bone spavin have lesions on the dorsomedial aspects of the tarsometatarsal and intertarsal joints, we have found that the dorsomedial to plantarolateral oblique view, which highlights lesions on the dorsolateral aspect of the hock, often demonstrates significant changes that may not be apparent on the other views. Therefore, this view should always be included when radiographing the hock for suspected bone spavin. Note that some standardbred horses have radiographic changes involving the hock without signs of lameness.

Stifle

KEY POINT ▶ Radiographs of the stifle are difficult to take with the portable x-ray machines that are used to radiograph the distal limbs.

This is particularly so for the craniocaudal view of the stifle. However, because one of the most common lesions involving the stifle is osteochondrosis dissecans of the lateral trochlear ridge of the femur, a lateral radiographic view, often possible with a portable machine, may be useful.

Hip

By positioning the x-ray machine under the horse's hindleg, standing radiographs of the hip and pelvis are possible. The x-ray tube is positioned underneath the abdomen and just cranial to the hindleg. The head of the x-ray machine is angled (35 degrees from the vertical) so that the beam is directed slightly caudally and dorsally. The cassette and grid are positioned above the gluteal muscle mass and angled to the natural slope of the croup.

To obtain a radiograph of the ilium, the same technique is used, with a less acute angle of the tube.

Ultrasound

Ultrasound has become an important aid for assessing the prognosis of tendon and ligament injuries. A number of portable machines are now available and provide the resolution necessary to evaluate the extent of lesions and whether the core of the tendon or ligament is involved. Hypoechoic areas show up as black holes, indicating disruption of fibers and local edema and hemorrhage. Monitoring the progress of tendon and ligament lesions via repeated ultrasound examinations allows determination of the rate of healing of the injury and the time at which the horse can be returned to training.

References

Blevins, W. E., and Widmer, W. R.: Radiology in racetrack practice. *Vet. Clin. North Am. (Equine Pract.)* 6:31, 1990.

Dik, K. J., and Gunsser, I.: *Atlas of Diagnostic Radiology of the Horse,* Part 1: *Diseases of the Front Limb.* London: Wolfe Publishing, 1988.

Dyson, S.: Problems associated with the interpretation of regional and intraarticular anaesthesia in the horse. *Vet. Rec.* 118:419, 1986.

May, S. A., Wyn-Jones, G., and Peremans, K. Y.: Importance of oblique views in radiography of the equine limb. *Equine Vet. J.* 18:7, 1986.

May, S. A., Patterson, L. J., Peacock, P. J., and Edwards, G. B.: Radiographic technique for the pelvis in the standing horse. *Equine Vet. J.* 23:312, 1991.

Rantanen, N. W. (ed): Diagnostic ultrasound. *Vet. Clin. North Am. (Equine Pract.)* 2:1986.

Rose, R. J., and Frauenfelder, H. C.: Arthrocentesis in the horse. *Equine Vet. J.* 14:173, 1982.

Forelimb Abnormalities

FOOT PROBLEMS

Corns (Subsolar Hematoma)

The term *corns* is really a misnomer because it refers to a hematoma between the sensitive and insensitive layers of the hoof rather than the condition described in people. The usual site is at the heel, between the bars and the wall. The condition often results from an ill-fitting shoe, with the heel of the shoe resting on the sole between the bar and wall of the foot. This produces excessive pressure in a region that was not designed to bear weight directly. The diagnosis of corns is a favorite one of farriers, and many chronic forelimb lamenesses are ascribed to corns. However, great care should be taken in making this diagnosis, and all other possibilities must be excluded.

History and Presenting Signs

- Chronic, low-grade forelimb lameness
- Reluctance to stretch out during exercise

Clinical Findings and Diagnosis

- Horses may or may not show signs of lameness depending on the extent of the hematoma.
- Examination of the foot seldom reveals any abnormalities. However, application of hoof testers across the heel(s) produces a painful response.

KEY POINT ▶ Although corns are a frequent finding in lame horses, they are seldom the cause of lameness. Therefore, a careful examination of the rest of the leg is important before the lameness can be attributed to the corns.

- If the corns involve only one side of the foot and are causing lameness, a unilateral palmar digital nerve block of the medial or lateral nerve should result in the horse becoming sound.

Differential Diagnosis

- Foot abscesses
- Navicular disease
- Nonarticular fractures of the pedal bone
- Pedal osteitis

Treatment

KEY POINT ▶ Improper shoeing, with the heel of the shoe bearing weight in the angle of the bars, is often the cause, so correct placement of the shoe should be ensured.

- The shoe should normally have little contact inside the white line and be evenly placed on the foot.
- A heart bar shoe may be useful in more severe cases. This shoe distributes weight evenly over the foot and prevents the concentration of force and pressure over the angle of the bars of the foot.
- If there is intense pain in the heel region, the sole should be pared away over the site to release the pressure. However, it is possible for bacteria to colonize the exposed area and an abscess to form.
- Alternative or coincident therapy is to administer anti-inflammatory drugs such as phenylbutazone (Treatment No. 88) for 5 to 7 days. A dose rate of 4.4 mg/kg should be used for 24 hours, followed by 2.2 mg/kg q12h thereafter.

Coronitis

Coronitis is an inflammation of the coronary band and usually results from systemic disease. It is a rare condition in clinical practice but may be seen in febrile illnesses or in horses with laminitis.

History and Presenting Signs

- Sudden onset of lameness with reluctance to bear weight
- Swelling around the dorsal coronary band of the foot
- Systemic illness

Clinical Findings and Diagnosis

- Two or more feet are usually involved, and there is initial swelling of the coronary band, followed by exudate development and severe pain.
- Over a period of 7 to 14 days, there may be complete separation of the hoof wall from the coronary band.
- The end result may be complete loss of the protective hoof horn from the affected foot.

Differential Diagnosis

- Foot abscesses
- Laminitis
- Fractures of the pedal bone
- Septic arthritis of the coffin joint

Treatment

- There appears to be little effective treatment for this condition. The nonsteroidal anti-inflammatory drugs such as phenylbutazone (Treatment No. 88), meclofenamic acid (Treatment No. 69), or flunixin meglumine (Treatment No. 52) should be used, but the prognosis is very poor.
- In many cases that do resolve, the coronary band is permanently affected so that abnormal hoof growth results.

Foot Abscesses (Subsolar Abscesses, Nail Prick)

KEY POINT ► Foot abscesses are probably the most common cause of acute lameness encountered in equine practice.

An abscess usually results from nails or other foreign bodies entering the sensitive structures of the foot, usually via the sole, and depositing bacteria. Due to the anaerobic conditions, bacteria such as *Clostridium* species may be found, and therefore, tetanus prophylaxis should always be given.

History and Presenting Signs

- Horse recently shod with suspicion that the sensitive structures were "pricked"
- Horse kept at pasture in wet conditions following a dry period
- Chronic laminitis with secondary abscessation
- Known history of foreign-body penetration of the sole

Clinical Findings and Diagnosis

- Acute, severe lameness unassociated with exercise, with the horse reluctant to bear weight on the affected leg.
- Early stages of infection—increased heat in the affected foot and coronary band, increased rate and amplitude of the pulse in the palmar or plantar digital arteries. After several days there may be little or no heat in the affected foot.
- After 24 to 48 hours there may be swelling in the pastern and fetlock.
- If untreated, the infection may underrun the hoof wall and ultimately form a sinus with a discharging point at the coronary band.
- The use of hoof testers demonstrates severe generalized pain (acute cases) or localized pain (chronic cases) over the sole. With care, even in acute, severe cases, the use of hoof testers around the sole should localize one site where

there is more pain. Then this site can be investigated with a hoof knife.
- Paring of the sole with a hoof knife may indicate the site of penetration of the sole.
- Abaxial nerve block should abolish or substantially relieve the pain and lameness.
- In cases where the history of a penetrating injury is not clear, radiographs of the foot may be necessary to eliminate the possibility of a fracture of the distal phalanx.

Differential Diagnosis

- Fractures of the distal phalanx (pedal bone)
- Infection of the navicular bursa or deep flexor tendon sheath
- Laminitis
- Severe subsolar hematoma (corn)
- Fractures of the navicular bone

Treatment

- Determine the most painful site over the sole, since this is the point to begin paring with the hoof knife. It may be necessary to perform an abaxial block (Fig. 3-26) to desensitize the foot in cases where there is severe pain. Once pus is located, the paring should continue until the origin of the abscess is opened.
- Establish effective drainage of the infected area.
- Soak the entire foot for 10 minutes in a bucket of warm to hot water containing a suitable disinfectant (see Chap. 17), followed by application of a poultice dressing to the foot to encourage further drainage.
- In most cases, antibiotic therapy is not necessary and will be ineffective because the infection is localized. In a more generalized infection, the antibiotic of choice will be procaine penicillin (Treatment No. 83) (see Chap. 17) administered for 4 to 5 days at a dose rate of 15 mg/kg q12h.
- Effective drainage is the key to successful treatment. Local irrigation and soaking of the foot are repeated daily for the next 3 to 5 days depending on the extent of the infection.
- A protective boot can be applied until provisional keratinization protects the sensitive structures of the foot (5–7 days).
- Where there is extensive infection with underrunning of the sole and/or wall of the hoof, stripping of the sole and hoof wall may be necessary.

KEY POINT ► It is essential to administer tetanus prophylaxis, and the usual regimen is to give 3000 IU of tetanus antitoxin (Treatment No. 115) subcutaneously, plus intramuscular tetanus toxoid (Treatment No. 116) administered in a site remote from the antitoxin injection. The tetanus toxoid injection should be repeated 4 weeks later in a horse with no previous vaccination history.

Foot Cracks (Sand Cracks)

Foot cracks usually result from the hoof becoming dehydrated and brittle. Most cracks are longitudinal and extend proximally up the hoof wall from the solar aspect. However, some hoof cracks arise from previous trauma to the coronary band with subsequent failure of horn growth at the injured site. In these cases the crack will extend from proximal to distal as the hoof grows.

History and Presenting Signs

- Previous trauma to the coronary band
- Poor hoof care
- Wet followed by prolonged dry pasture conditions

Clinical Findings and Diagnosis

- In most cases, the cracks, which are self-evident, will not cause any lameness. If, however, they extend into the deeper sensitive structures of the foot, infection may ensue, with signs of a foot abscess.
- It is important to determine the depth of the cracks to determine whether infection is likely.

KEY POINT ► Foot conformation should be evaluated carefully together with assessment of shoe placement. Some cracks, particularly those toward the quarters and heels, may be due to abnormal conformation or poor shoe placement.

Differential Diagnosis

- If no lameness is present, the cracks are self-evident and probably do not involve sensitive structures in the deeper part of the foot.
- If lameness is present, infection of the sensitive structures should be suspected.

Treatment

- Rehydrating the hoof is important, and a hoof dressing made up of a combination of ⅓ stockholm tar and ⅔ neatsfoot oil is appropriate. A number of other commercial hoof dressings are available.
- The proximal extent of the crack may be limited by making a deep groove with a hoof rasp at right angles to the crack. In severe cracks, it may be necessary to deepen the crack with a hand drill or grinder such as a Moto-Tool so that wire and hoof acrylic can be used to strengthen the wall and prevent the crack from widening.
- If the crack occurs toward the heel, it may be necessary to cut away the wall behind the crack so that it does not bear weight. Combining this with a heart bar or straight bar shoe is important to ensure that the surface area of contact is evenly distributed and the crack is not enlarged.

Fracture of the Distal Phalanx (Pedal Bone, Third Phalanx)

Fracture of the pedal bone is a condition that occurs in all athletic horses and is more common in standardbred trotters and pacers than thoroughbred racehorses. Most fractures occur through the lateral wing of the pedal bone, and horses will show the most pain if the fracture extends intraarticularly.

History and Presenting Signs

- The most common history is that a horse shows acute lameness immediately after a race and within 30 to 60 minutes will be reluctant to bear weight on the affected leg.
- In cases where there is an intraarticular fracture, the lameness will gradually improve over 2 to 3 days with box rest, whereas in the case of nonarticular fractures, the degree of improvement is usually more pronounced.

Clinical Findings and Diagnosis

KEY POINT ► An acute non-weight-bearing lameness is a feature of the presenting signs in horses with pedal bone fractures.

- Severe pain is evident on application of the hoof testers. This is usually concentrated on the lateral side of the sole and wall of the affected foot.
- Occasionally, horses will not show marked pain with hoof testers but will react to tapping around the affected side of the hoof wall with a hoof hammer or closed hoof testers.
- An abaxial block (see Fig. 3-26) will resolve the lameness, but most horses do not become completely sound.
- In many cases, horses will show considerable improvement after 48 hours rest in a stall and, if the fracture does not extend into the joint, will walk almost sound.
- Radiography should include dorsopalmar, lateral to medial, dorsolateral to palmaromedial, and dorsomedial to palmarolateral oblique views. It is essential to establish whether or not the fracture extends into the coffin joint. In some cases, the fracture may be difficult to visualize on the dorsopalmar view. However, one of the oblique views will usually show the fracture more clearly.

Differential Diagnosis

- Fractures of the other phalanges
- Foot abscess
- Infection of the navicular bursa
- Fractures of the navicular bone

Treatment

- If the fracture does not extend into the coffin joint, conservative treatment with the application of a bar shoe (i.e., a bar of steel welded across the heels of an ordinary shoe) is sufficient. The use of quarter clips to limit hoof expansion is also useful and will help to immobilize the fracture. Good results also have been reported recently with the use of a continuous-rim bar shoe.

- The bar shoe requires changing every 6 weeks or so, and the fracture will usually heal following 6 to 7 months rest. In some cases, healing may be delayed for up to 12 months. During the first 2 to 3 months of rest, the horse should be confined to a box stall, after which a small yard or pasture is adequate.
- If the fracture is intraarticular, the application of a bar shoe for 6 months together with rest for 9 to 12 months may result in the fracture healing if the horse is less than 3 years of age.

KEY POINT ► In horses over 3 years of age, conservative treatment using a bar shoe will result in fracture healing in less than 20% of horses with intraarticular fractures. The most successful treatment is insertion of a cortical bone screw in the distal phalanx, using the technique of interfragmentary bone compression (lag-screw fixation). Most fractures will heal in 6 to 9 months.

- A disadvantage of internal fixation of pedal bone fractures is the possibility of osteomyelitis owing to the difficulty in disinfecting the hoof prior to surgery. Although anabolic steroids have been advocated, there is no evidence that they hasten fracture healing.
- If internal fixation is used, a bar or rim shoe also should be applied. Some horses subsequently require screw removal because the screw loosens and irritates the sensitive laminae.

Canker

Canker is a rare condition resulting in chronic hypertrophy of the horn-producing tissues of the foot. Although the hindfeet are more commonly affected, any one of or all the feet may be involved. It is usually found in hot, humid conditions, such as those found in the southern part of the United States.

History and Presenting Signs

- Usually no lameness until well advanced
- Often there is neglect of the feet or poor hoof care
- Persistent, foul-smelling exudate from the frog region, with little tendency to resolve spontaneously

Clinical Findings and Diagnosis

- The foot has a distinct odor, and the frog, which may have a frayed appearance, loosens easily to reveal a foul-smelling, localized necrotic horn covered with a caseous cream-colored exudate.
- The condition often goes unrecognized until well advanced, when the corium shows chronic proliferation and the sole and wall may be involved.
- The appearance of the foot together with the characteristic odor is diagnostic of canker.

Differential Diagnosis

- Thrush
- Foot abscess

Treatment

- Thorough debridement with removal of all affected tissue is essential. The foot should then be soaked in a bucket of hot water containing a suitable disinfectant (see Chap. 17) and a bandage applied. Astringent agents such as a mixture of 30 g zinc sulfate and 20 g lead acetate in 500 ml water (White lotion) may be used.
- We have found the use of topical chloramphenicol useful, when applied by soaking a pad of cotton wool and bandaging this to the foot, repeating the treatment daily for 5 to 7 days. However, the use of chloramphenicol is banned in some countries owing to the classification of the horse as a food-producing animal.
- Systemic penicillin therapy (see Chap. 17) has been advocated for the treatment of canker but in our experience is not useful.
- The foot should be dressed until the condition has resolved, and the horse should be kept in a clean, dry environment. The prognosis is guarded, and improvement, when it occurs, is slow.
- It is common for the hoof to require extensive debridement on a number of occasions.

Fracture of the Extensor Process of the Distal Phalanx (Pedal Bone)

Fracture of the extensor process of the pedal bone is usually an avulsion fracture at the site of insertion of a part of the common extensor tendon.

KEY POINT ► While this type of fracture can cause a significant lameness, small fractures can occur that are not responsible for lameness.

Therefore, care needs to be taken in ascribing lameness (particularly chronic lameness) to extensor process fractures. Many older horses without lameness can be found to have small extensor fractures when radiographs are taken as part of a prepurchase examination. In these cases it may be difficult to provide clear advice to the client.

History and Presenting Signs

- Acute onset of a moderate forelimb lameness after exercise
- Low-grade, chronic forelimb lameness

Clinical Findings and Diagnosis

- Some horses with small fractures will show no clinical signs, and the extensor process fracture only may be found on a routine radiograph of the foot.
- In other cases, where larger portions of the extensor process have been fractured, there is lameness with swelling of the coronary band in the dorsal midline.
- Diagnosis should be made by a confirmatory nerve block to localize the lameness to the dorsal region of the foot (abaxial block or coffin joint block), together with a lateral radiograph of the foot to demonstrate the presence of a fracture.

Differential Diagnosis

- Trauma to soft tissues of the dorsal midline
- Low ringbone
- Pyramidal disease

Treatment

- Long-standing fractures that may not be causing lameness should be left untreated.
- Small fractures of the extensor process can be removed surgically, using an approach through the common extensor tendon, the incision commencing just above the coronary band in the dorsal midline.
- Small fragments also can be removed arthroscopically.
- Larger fragments may have to be reaffixed using a lag screw to achieve stability. However, secondary arthritis is common, and a change in shape of the hoof wall (see Pyramidal Disease) may occur.

Grease Heel (Pastern Dermatitis, Scratches)

Grease heel is a condition that may result from improper foot care. It is a seborrheic dermatitis involving the skin at the palmar aspect of the pastern and occasionally the fetlock. It is quite common in horses stabled in moist conditions and is well known to all horse owners. While the condition obviously causes irritation to the horse, it is seldom the cause of lameness.

History and Presenting Signs

- Stabling in moist conditions
- Evidence of poor foot care and stable hygiene

Clinical Findings and Diagnosis

- In the early stages there may be a mild dermatitis with swelling in the palmar region of the pastern.
- This is usually followed by secretion and exudate formation. In the chronic stages, the skin is thickened, and there may be excoriation.

Differential Diagnosis

Other skin disorders, including contact dermatitis and allergic dermatitis, should be considered.

Treatment

- Cleaning the area is important, and it may be necessary to clip the hair. It is essential that the affected area be kept dry.
- An astringent preparation such as White lotion (see Treatment under Canker) can be applied topically to the affected area until the condition resolves. This treatment is quite effective and is economical.
- In severe cases, a systemic course of an antibiotic such as procaine penicillin (Treatment No. 83) at a dose rate of 15 mg/kg (15,000 IU/kg) q12h may be necessary.

Infection of the Navicular Bursa

Penetrating injuries of the sole of the foot that occur in the middle of the frog may lead to penetration of the navicular bursa, which lies between the deep flexor tendon and the navicular bone on the palmar aspect of the pedal bone. Infection in this location leads to a severe non-weight-bearing lameness of the affected leg that is very difficult to treat successfully.

History and Presenting Signs

- Nail or wire penetration to the foot
- Sudden onset of an acute foreleg lameness with the horse reluctant to take weight on the affected leg.

Clinical Findings and Diagnosis

- Severe non-weight-bearing unilateral foreleg lameness.
- If any weight is taken on the leg, it is usually only on the toe, with heel held off the ground.
- Increased heat in the foot and increased digital pulse are found.
- Pain is evident on application of hoof testers, particularly over the frog.
- Improvement in gait is found after palmar digital nerve block (see Fig. 3-23), and further improvement usually occurs after abaxial nerve block (see Fig. 3-26). However, usually horses will not become sound.
- Radiographs may not show any abnormalities in the early stages of the condition unless some of the penetrating object (if radiopaque) has lodged at the site.
- If the lameness has been present for several days, radiographs may show radiolucency on the palmar aspect of the navicular bone, indicating the presence of infection. These changes are often most obvious on the lateral and skyline views of the navicular bone.

- In some cases it is possible to confirm the presence of infection by inserting a needle into the navicular bursa to aspirate purulent material. This is done following an abaxial nerve block to desensitize the distal limb. An 18-gauge, 8.5-cm (3.5-in) needle is inserted in the axial plane in the palmar midline between the bulbs of the heels.

Differential Diagnosis

- Foot abscess
- Fracture of pedal bone
- Septic tenosynovitis
- Fracture of the navicular bone

Treatment

KEY POINT ▶ It is important to make an early diagnosis of navicular bursa infection because response to treatment is dependent on early intervention.

Surgical exposure of the navicular bursa should be performed using the "street nail operation." This is undertaken by resecting the middle third of the frog down to the depth of the deep flexor tendon with an oscillating saw. A window can then be cut in the deep flexor tendon that permits drainage. Once drainage and exposure to air can occur, there is usually rapid improvement of the lameness. However, in cases where the infection has been present for more than 1 week, the degree of improvement may be limited. Many horses will be left with a chronic lameness even if there is initial improvement in gait.

Laminitis

Laminitis is an avascular necrosis involving the sensitive laminae, which intermesh with the hoof wall. The hoof (particularly the capillary blood supply) appears to be a target organ for endotoxins, which can be released as a result of a variety of causes. While the blood supply to the feet is the main area apparently affected, it seems likely that other vascular beds are also involved. However, the unique housing of the blood supply to the foot in a nonexpandable structure (the hoof) may accentuate the impact of blood flow changes. Systemic hypertension is found in the early stages of the disease. The end mediators of the endotoxins are prostaglandins that affect blood supply to the feet, leading to opening of arteriovenous anastomoses. The outcome is a loss of blood supply to the laminae, despite an increase in blood flow to the foot. The most common causes are grain engorgement, grazing in lush pastures, postfoaling metritis, and systemic gram-negative bacterial infections. In fat ponies, it is common to find laminitis during the spring months, when the soluble carbohydrate content increases in grasses and clovers.

History and Presenting Signs

- Overfeeding of grain
- Gastrointestinal problems, particularly after colic surgery
- Mare recently foaled having had retained fetal membranes
- Fat pony grazing pasture rich in legumes
- Recent pleuritis or pneumonia due to gram-negative infection

Clinical Findings and Diagnosis

- Although all four feet can be involved in laminitis, the forelimbs are more frequently affected than the hindlimbs.
- Affected horses show reluctance to move and a typical "sawhorse" stance with the forelimbs placed well out in front of the body. It will be difficult to pick up one of the forelegs.
- Examination will usually reveal increased heat in the feet and around the coronary band, with intense pain on application of the hoof testers.
- Palpation of the palmar arteries over the abaxial surface of the sesamoid bones will disclose an increase in both rate and amplitude of the pulse.
- An abaxial nerve block (see Fig. 3-26) will improve the signs of lameness.
- In more chronic cases, or where there is a severe acute condition, rotation of the pedal bone may occur owing to the pull of the deep flexor tendon. In these cases, the dorsal part of the pedal bone may protrude through the sole of the foot, or there will be evidence of distortion of the sole as a result of the rotated bone.

KEY POINT ▶ If rotation of the pedal bone is suspected, lateral radiographs should be taken of the feet to reveal the extent of rotation. It may be helpful to put a radiopaque marker, such as a strip of metal, on the dorsal midline of the foot so that the degree of rotation can be measured accurately.

Differential Diagnosis

- Pedal osteitis
- Foot abscess
- Fractures of the pedal bone

Treatment

KEY POINT ▶ It is important to establish the cause of the laminitis prior to treatment. While endotoxins are the end product, it is important to treat the originating cause of endotoxin release.

- In cases of grain engorgement, 3 to 4 liters of paraffin should be administered by stomach tube to prevent further endotoxin absorption and help eliminate the grain from the gastrointestinal tract.

- Where metritis is the initiating cause, bacteriologic swabs should be taken so that appropriate intrauterine and systemic antimicrobial therapy can be commenced (see Endometritis, Chap. 7).
- If there are signs of shock (prolonged capillary refill time, injected mucous membranes, etc.), intravenous fluid therapy may be required (20–40 ml/kg of a polyionic, isotonic fluid). For further details, see Fluid Therapy (in Chap. 17).

KEY POINT ► Formerly it was thought that walking exercise was helpful to prevent vascular stasis. Now it has been found that walking often worsens the condition and may cause separation of the hoof wall from the coronary band. In all but the mildest cases, it is best that the horse not be forced to walk.

- Prostaglandin synthetase inhibitors such as phenylbutazone (Treatment No. 88), flunixin meglumine (Treatment No. 52), or meclofenamic acid (Treatment No. 69) are essential. Maximal dose rates are used for the first 2 to 4 days, and continuation of therapy for between 7 and 21 days may be necessary depending on the response. Of the nonsteroidal anti-inflammatory drugs, phenylbutazone appears to be the drug of choice for effective pain relief. If endotoxemia is suspected, flunixin appears to be more efficacious as an antiendotoxic agent.
- Intravenous heparin at a dose rate of 40 IU/kg has been found to be useful in some cases, particularly where there are indications of disseminated intravascular coagulation.
- The use of a support shoe with elevation of the heel may be helpful in some acute cases where there is no initial response to medical therapy. Heart bar shoes are very useful, applied so that the V provides support to the frog. However, if this shoe is incorrectly applied, it can produce excessive pressure and necrosis at the tip of the frog.
- In severe acute laminitis, nailing a shoe may be contraindicated because of the concussion. In such cases, supporting the frog with a bandage may be useful or a glue on shoe may be required.
- In severe cases where there is no response to the usual therapy, dorsal resection of the hoof wall and/or section of the deep flexor tendon has been used. We have not found these treatments to be helpful as "last ditch" measures. Recent information suggests that earlier resection of the dorsal hoof wall may be indicated in acute, severe cases of laminitis.
- In chronic laminitis, corrective trimming of the feet is essential. The idea is to trim back the excessively long heel to maintain normal heel height and to square the toe to facilitate breakover. Progress can be assessed from lateral radiographs.

- Some horses with low-grade lameness from chronic laminitis have shown a response to a 2- to 3-week course of isoxsuprine hydrochloride (Treatment No. 61) administered orally at a dose rate of 1 mg/kg twice daily before feeding.

Navicular Disease

KEY POINT ► Navicular disease is the most common cause of chronic forelimb lameness in pleasure horses.

The disease was originally believed to be an arthritis resulting from irritation to the navicular bursa and progression to involve the coffin joint, but this is now debated. The condition is surrounded by considerable controversy as to the pathogenesis, with some investigators proposing a vascular origin and others favoring a degenerative process. It seems clear that a spectrum of conditions may be lurking under the general heading of *navicular disease* and that there is no simple single entity involved. For this reason, some research workers have labeled the condition *navicular syndrome*. It is widely held that conformational abnormalities of the foot can predispose to the disease. However, no one has unequivocally demonstrated all the factors involved. While it is overdiagnosed by some and referred to as the "last refuge of the diagnostically destitute" by others, definitive diagnosis is possible in all cases by progressing through a series of diagnostic steps outlined below.

KEY POINT ► It is important to note that navicular disease is a clinical rather than a radiologic diagnosis.

History and Presenting Signs

- An older (6- to 8-year-old) horse is the most common candidate with a chronic, low-grade forelimb lameness.
- Intermittent, progressive lameness with exacerbations and remissions in the early stages.
- Thoroughbreds, quarter horses, and warmbloods are affected more commonly than standardbreds and other riding breeds.
- Horses are often presented with a history of being "tied up in the shoulders."

Clinical Findings and Diagnosis

- A unilateral or bilateral chronic forelimb lameness that is gradually progressive in a horse with no obvious swelling in the leg(s) or abnormal findings on clinical examination are the main clues to the possibility of navicular disease.
- The average age of horses involved is 6 to 7 years, but navicular disease has been found in horses as young as 2 years of age.

KEY POINT ► It is important to note that the majority of horses with navicular disease will not show a positive response to hoof testers.

■ Examination of the foot will reveal pain on application of hoof testers across the middle third of the frog in approximately 30% to 50% of cases. While some authors have indicated that a lack of hoof-tester response indicates that navicular disease cannot be present, we have not found this to be the case.

KEY POINT ▶ A phalangeal and fetlock flexion test is one of the most useful diagnostic tests for horses with suspected navicular disease.

■ The test should be performed by flexion of the fetlock and phalanges, pulling up on the toe of the foot. After 1 to 2 minutes the horse is trotted off, and lameness is aggravated in approximately 80% of cases. This test is not diagnostic because a range of other distal limb disorders will show worsening of lameness after fetlock flexion. However, in most of these conditions there will be evidence of pain during flexion, which is seldom the case in horses with navicular disease.

KEY POINT ▶ A positive diagnosis can be made by performing a palmar digital nerve block (see Fig. 3-23).

■ Horses that fail to become completely sound after this block should be followed up with a coffin joint block (see Fig. 3-24) to determine whether secondary involvement of the joint has occurred. It should be noted that a palmar digital nerve block will desensitize other structures in the palmar area of the foot apart from the navicular bone.

■ Radiographs (upright pedal or high coronary views) will reveal a change in shape of the distal foramina. The normal triangular shape changes to an inverted flask or "lollipop" shape, and a grading system has been suggested as a prognostic aid. The more foramina that are visible and the greater the change in shape from a normal triangular appearance, the less is the likelihood for a response to medical therapy. The presence of radiographic changes without clinical signs is not consistent with a diagnosis of navicular disease. Some of the important factors in obtaining good-quality radiographs of the navicular bone are discussed in the section on radiology (p. 69).

Differential Diagnosis

■ Pedal osteitis
■ Corns
■ Low ringbone
■ Shoulder problems
■ Arthritis involving the distal joints of the forelimbs
■ Fetlock degenerative joint disease

Treatment

KEY POINT ▶ There is no treatment that is invariably successful for navicular disease.

■ Since many horses with navicular disease have bad foot conformation, it is important to assess this and trim the foot correctly. The most common fault is the toe being left too long with the heels cut excessively short.

■ Corrective shoeing, involving a rolled-toe, raised-heel shoe may be useful, particularly in pleasure horses. An egg-bar shoe also has been suggested and found useful in horses other than those used for racing.

■ Analgesic drugs such as phenylbutazone (Treatment No. 88) will give temporary relief of lameness, but signs will usually return on withdrawal of therapy.

■ Palmar digital neurectomy has been advised, but there are many complications that may result from this surgery. However, in severe cases of navicular disease that no longer respond to medical therapy, we have been pleased with the results of neurectomy.

■ Surgery to section the navicular suspensory ligament has been reported to be successful in the treatment of navicular disease. However, we have not had good results in a limited number of cases treated in this way.

■ The oral use of warfarin to produce an increase in clotting time has been successful in improving more than 70% of horses with navicular disease. An initial dose rate of 0.05 mg/kg is used, and the one-stage prothrombin time of blood is monitored so that an increase of 2 to 4 seconds is maintained. It is, however, difficult to maintain a stable one-stage prothrombin time, and some horses on warfarin therapy have been reported to have had fatal hemorrhage. Horses should not receive phenylbutazone and warfarin therapy concurrently because differential plasma protein binding of the two drugs may result in fatal hemorrhage.

KEY POINT ▶ We find that the most effective therapy is the oral use of isoxsuprine hydrochloride in a paste form (Treatment No. 61).

■ Horses that respond best are those which have few major radiographic changes or that have been lame for a period less than 6 months. The use of isoxsuprine in capsule form is also effective, but it must be given on an empty stomach to ensure complete absorption. An initial dose rate of 1.0 mg/kg q12h for 3 weeks is used. If there is complete relief of lameness, then an additional 3 weeks at the same dose rate is given, followed by 3 weeks of treatment once daily. If complete relief of lameness does not occur in the first 3-week period, the dose of isoxsuprine is increased by 50%, and therapy is maintained for a further 6 weeks. If the horse is sound at the end of this period, the treatment can be decreased to once daily. We have found that there is a better long-term response to therapy if the drug dosage is not acutely discontinued but rather goes to an every-other-day schedule following the once-daily treatment. Many horses will have up to 6 to 12 months free of lameness after withdrawal of isoxsuprine therapy, particularly in milder cases of navicular disease.

- Isoxsuprine has been successful in 60% to 80% of horses with navicular disease, with horses becoming sound on treatment. In longer-term follow-up we have found more than 60% of horses remaining sound for 3 months or more after ceasing therapy. In pleasure horses, we have found that the use of an egg-bar shoe as well as isoxsuprine treatment gives better longer-term results than using isoxsuprine alone.

Navicular Bone Fracture

Fracture of the navicular bone is a rare condition that can cause an acute forelimb or hindlimb lameness. Although causing an acute lameness, the fracture may not be diagnosed initially, so it is possible to have horses presented with a chronic lameness, particularly if the fracture is undisplaced.

KEY POINT ▶ A misdiagnosis of fracture of the navicular bone can be made because radiolucent lines associated with the sulci of the frog can appear to overlie the navicular bone in radiographs taken of the foot.

History and Presenting Signs

- The most common presentation is that of an acute unilateral forelimb lameness following exercise, with reluctance of the horse to bear weight on the foot.
- If the fracture is displaced, the toe of the foot is rested on the ground, there being hesitation of the horse to bear weight on the heel of the foot.
- The condition is found more commonly in pleasure horses than in horses used for athletic pursuits.

Clinical Findings and Diagnosis

- Acute, severe non-weight-bearing unilateral foreleg lameness is most common.
- Occasionally, a more chronic unilateral forelimb lameness may be found.
- Pain on application of hoof testers across both heels and also over the middle third of the frog is typically found.

KEY POINT ▶ Dramatic improvement of the lameness occurs following a palmar digital nerve block. However, many horses with navicular fractures do not

become completely sound after this block.

- Good-quality radiographs are essential for an accurate diagnosis. Because the lines of the sulci of the frog appear radiolucent on radiographs, it is easy to mistake these lines for fractures. Packing of the foot with a material such as Play-Doh will eliminate lines of the frog sulci.

KEY POINT ▶ The radiographic views that are most useful to enable a diagnosis are the dorsopalmar (high coronary or upright pedal) and skyline (special) navicular views.

- The skyline navicular view is taken with the foot on an x-ray plate and the direction of the beam coming down at an angle of 60 to 75 degrees vertical and from behind the leg. This demonstrates the flexor surface of the navicular bone and often permits a definitive diagnosis that may not be possible using the other views. If the fracture has been present for more than 2 to 3 weeks, considerable rarefaction will be found.

Differential Diagnosis

- Fracture of the pedal bone
- Infection of the navicular bursa
- Subsolar (foot) abscess
- Navicular disease

Treatment

- The prognosis is poor for athletic soundness in horses that have sustained fractures of the navicular bone.
- Rest will sometimes result in healing of the fracture, particularly if it is undisplaced. However, in many cases the union is incomplete, and the fracture line can often be demonstrated several years after the fracture was sustained.
- A surgical technique for insertion of a screw into the fractured navicular bone has been described and may be worth considering if you like a surgical challenge. Because the screw has to be placed "blind," practice on cadaver specimens is essential.

Pedal Osteitis

Pedal osteitis is an inflammatory disorder associated with the sensitive structures of the solar aspect of the front feet, usually resulting from concussion. It is a common condition in athletic horses, usually associated with exercise on hard tracks, and is usually bilateral.

KEY POINT ▶ In many cases the problem arises from improper shoeing or hoof trimming so that excessive weight is taken on the sole of the foot.

History and Presenting Signs

- Often found in thoroughbred racehorses
- Horse not stretching out during exercise
- Decreased performance
- The gait may be described as "looking like the horse is stepping on hot bricks."

Clinical Findings and Diagnosis

- The horse may have a shuffling forelimb gait and may be reluctant to stretch forward when trotting so that there is a reduced anterior phase of the stride.

KEY POINT ▶ Examination reveals pain over the entire sole on application of hoof testers. It is common for there to be more sensitivity at the toe and the heels of the foot.

- Pedal osteitis usually occurs bilaterally in the front feet. However, one foot may be affected more severely than the other.
- There is a great improvement in gait following an abaxial nerve block. There also may be some improvement following a palmar digital nerve block.
- Radiographs of the feet may show areas of roughening around the margins of the pedal bone, indicating periosteal new bone formation. Additionally, there is often rarefaction around the wings and toe of the pedal bone. Changes are usually visible on dorsopalmar (upright pedal or high coronary) and lateral to medial views.

Differential Diagnosis

- Corns
- Navicular disease
- Fracture of the wing of the pedal bone (nonarticular)
- Chronic, low-grade laminitis

Treatment

- The shoes should be checked to ensure that the soles are not bearing excessive pressure from the shoes.

KEY POINT ▶ If there is excessive contact of the shoe with the sole, the inside margin of the solar aspect of the shoe should be ground down using an electric grinder to relieve sole pressure so that the shoe only maintains contact with the wall up to the region of the white line.

- A heart-bar shoe, which has a V-shaped section extending from the heel of the shoe (with the tip of the V toward the apex of the frog), may help by extending the surface area of contact of the shoe with the foot.
- Various types of pads are available for use under the shoe, and some farriers favor rubber under the rim of the shoe to reduce the concussion. However, such padding reduces the solar surface area for ground contact, and padding should be used only in extreme situations.
- A course of phenylbutazone (Treatment No. 88) for 10 to 14 days (4.4 mg/kg q12h for 1 day, 2.2 mg/kg q12h for 5 days, followed by 2.2 mg/kg q24h) in conjunction with stall rest usually assists in resolution of the condition.

Club Foot

Club foot is the term given to a condition where one or more of the feet is abnormally shaped, with upright conformation and a foot axis of 60 degrees or more.

KEY POINT ▶ The condition apparently results from initial flexure deformity of the deep digital flexor tendon.

The superficial digital flexor tendon and suspensory ligament also may be involved. In young horses it may be congenital or a result of nutritional deficiencies during growth. However, club foot may develop in horses of any age as a result of prolonged disuse of the foot and contraction of the flexor tendons resulting from injury.

History and Presenting Signs

- May be an incidental finding on clinical examination
- Abnormal foot conformation usually concerns breeders at the time of weaning or prior to the sale of yearlings.

Clinical Findings and Diagnosis

- The affected hoof (hooves) appears smaller and more upright than unaffected feet. Measurement may indicate a hoof axis of 60 degrees or greater; however, this criterion alone is not diagnostic.
- The appearance of the foot is diagnostic, and the gait may or may not be affected.

KEY POINT ▶ Radiographs are essential to discern whether the pedal bone has moved relative to the dorsal aspect of the hoof wall. In many cases, the pedal bone will appear misshapen, and there is periosteal new bone formation at the tip of the bone on a lateral-projection radiograph.

Differential Diagnosis

- Contracted heels
- Chronic laminitis

Treatment

- Club foot is a malformation that is permanent once it develops. Immature horses that are affected should have their diet assessed for possible deficiencies or imbalances. However, dietary manipulations will not cure the problem.

- Although there is some controversy, careful and regular trimming of affected feet may render the horse suitable for athletic use.

KEY POINT ► Care should be taken when inspecting the feet during clinical examinations, since corrective trimming, as described above, may disguise a club foot, and although the gait may appear normal, this condition is regarded as an unsoundness in a horse for sale.

- Inferior check ligament desmotomy can be of value in some early cases.
- Many horses with milder forms of club foot may have no lameness and can have a normal athletic career.

Pyramidal Disease

Pyramidal disease is a condition that results in abnormal growth of the hoof wall in the dorsal midline so that the hoof wall at this point projects forward from the surrounding horn. It is usually the result of a chronic injury such as low ringbone or fracture of a large part of the extensor process of the pedal bone.

History and Presenting Signs

- Long-standing injury to the distal limb
- Gradual change in the shape of the dorsal hoof wall
- Low-grade lameness

Clinical Findings and Diagnosis

- The change in shape of the hoof wall is diagnostic, with the appearance of a ridge in the hoof wall gradually extending from the coronary band to the sole.
- This change probably takes place from the local increase in blood supply. The horse usually will show lameness due to coffin joint arthritis.
- Radiographs should be taken of the foot. A lateral radiograph will demonstrate the extent of any bony changes involving the coffin joint.
- If lameness is present, a coffin joint block should be performed to determine if this joint is the site of the problem.

Differential Diagnosis

- Chronic laminitis
- Extensor process fracture
- Trauma to coronary band

Treatment

- The change in shape of the hoof wall is only a clinical sign of underlying pathology, which may or may not cause lameness.

- If radiographs indicate arthritis of the coffin joint, intraarticular medication may be useful. The best response is from long-acting corticosteroids. (For further details, see section on arthritis, page 125.)

Quittor

Quittor is infection of the lateral cartilage, usually following trauma around the heels. This is an uncommon injury these days, but it can be difficult to treat because of the avascular nature of cartilage and the failure of antibiotics to penetrate the area. The condition was most commonly found in draught horses following local cuts and trauma to the heel region of the foot.

History and Presenting Signs

- Lacerations around the heel of the foot
- Chronic purulent discharge in the palmar area of the distal pastern

Clinical Findings and Diagnosis

- Purulent discharge from the palmar/plantar aspect of the foot is usually found.
- Lameness is not usually a feature of the condition, particularly when the problem has been present for some period of time.
- Radiographs should be taken to determine whether there is any involvement of the pedal bone. If there is infection, there may be a radiolucency in one of the wings of the pedal bone.

Differential Diagnosis

- Osteomyelitis of the pedal bone
- Foot abscess
- Trauma to the heel
- Foreign-body (wood, wire) localization near the lateral cartilages

Treatment

- Infection in the lateral cartilage does not respond to conservative treatment (antibiotics, irrigations).

KEY POINT ► Radical surgery is necessary to resect any infected cartilage.

- Because the cartilage is distal to the coronary band at the heel, an incision should be made in the skin above the coronary band. Any discolored cartilage should be removed by sharp dissection, and the area should be packed with gauze soaked in povidone-iodine (Treatment No. 91).

Seedy Toe

Seedy toe is a condition that results from separation between the hoof wall and the sensitive laminae, usually taking place at the toe of the foot. The space resulting is usually filled with crumbly horn.

It is often a sequel to laminitis, particularly in ponies. The condition predisposes to infection underrunning the hoof wall.

KEY POINT ▶ Horses frequently have a chronic lameness associated with infection that gains access to the sensitive structures under the horn.

History and Presenting Signs

- Previous history of laminitis
- Lameness, which may be low grade or acute and severe depending on the presence of infection.

Clinical Findings and Diagnosis

In most cases there is no associated lameness. However, when the separation becomes filled with dirt or small stones so that there is pressure on the sensitive laminae, lameness ensues. It is also possible for infection to gain entrance to this site, causing lameness because of infection being trapped between the hoof wall and laminae.

Differential Diagnosis

- Foot abscess
- Chronic laminitis

Treatment

KEY POINT ▶ Seedy toe is an unrewarding condition to treat, with recurrence quite common. Once separation has occurred between the laminae and the hoof wall, it is difficult to reestablish the connection.

The cavity can be cleaned out with a hoof knife, and in extensive cases, a complete wall strip can be performed in the hope that new horn growth will occur without separation. Even with this radical treatment, results are poor, and up to 12 months is needed for regrowth of the hoof wall.

Sidebone (Calcification of the Lateral Cartilages)

Sidebone is a calcification of the lateral cartilages that usually occurs in the front feet of older horses. While it seldom causes lameness, and mild forms of the condition may be an incidental finding on foot radiographs, it is considered an unsoundness in a horse for sale.

History and Presenting Signs

- Older horses are usually affected.
- Lameness is seldom found, except if there is a fracture of the calcified cartilage.

Clinical Findings and Diagnosis

KEY POINT ▶ Most horses with sidebone formation will have normal gaits, and there are few clinical signs indicating the presence of sidebone. Sidebone may therefore be an incidental finding in the examination of a limb.

- The lateral cartilages are normally quite resilient and can be easily palpated above the coronary band at the heels. When sidebone occurs, the calcified cartilage can be palpated above the coronary band, the structure losing its resiliency. Palpation of the lateral cartilages should be part of every lameness examination so that an impression can be gained of normal findings.
- When calcification occurs, the lateral cartilages are prone to fracture, and the horse may be presented acutely lame following fracture of the calcified cartilage.
- Dorsopalmar (upright pedal or high coronary) and lateral radiographs will reveal the extent of the sidebone formation.

Differential Diagnosis

- Trauma to the heel of the foot
- Fracture (nonarticular) of the wing of pedal bone

Treatment

- Because lameness is seldom found in cases of sidebone, no treatment is required.
- If the calcified cartilage is fractured, rest for 6 months with the horse shod with a bar shoe will usually result in healing.

Thrush

Thrush is a bacterial infection of the sulci of the frog resulting from prolonged exposure to excessively moist conditions where the horse is stabled. It results from improper foot care, where the sulci of the frog are not cleaned out daily.

KEY POINT ▶ Thrush is seldom the cause of lameness unless the condition has been present for a prolonged period with deep erosion of the sulci.

History and Presenting Signs

- Usually found in stabled horses
- No lameness unless the condition is severe
- Owners may notice a foul smell associated with the feet

Clinical Findings and Diagnosis

KEY POINT ▶ There is a characteristic foul-smelling discharge associated with the affected frog sulci.

- The discharge is usually black in color, and there is a deep erosion of the medial and lateral sulci in severely affected cases.
- Most horses will not show any signs of lameness. However, when deep erosion and extension of infection occurs, the sensitive structures of the caudal foot may be involved, and the horse will become lame.
- Diagnosis is made by observation of the black discharge associated with the sulci of the frog.

Differential Diagnosis

- Foot abscess
- Canker
- Greasy heel

Treatment

- It is important that the sulci of the frog are cleaned out and all necrotic horn is removed with a hoof knife.
- Steps should be taken to ensure that the frog is bearing weight (e.g., by lowering the heels of the foot) if there is inadequate frog pressure.
- Once the sulci of the frog have been cleaned out, various disinfectants (see Chap. 17) may be used.
- Antibiotics are not usually necessary. However, if there is chronic infection with deep erosion of the sulci and lameness, it may be necessary to give a 5- to 7-day course of procaine penicillin (Treatment No. 83) at a dose rate of 15 mg/kg (15,000 IU/kg) q12h.
- Astringent preparations such as White lotion (see Treatment under Canker) can be applied to the affected areas to help dry the sites and therefore prevent further infection.
- The client must be asked to clean the horse's feet out on a daily or twice-daily basis, and if the horse is being stabled in moist conditions, an attempt should be made to relocate it to a dry surface until the condition is controlled.

References

Honnas, C. M., O'Brien, T. R., and Linford, R. L.: Distal phalanx fractures in horses: A survey of 274 horses with radiographic assessment of healing in 36 horses. *Vet. Radiol.* 29:98, 1988.
Stashak, T. S.: Lameness. In T. S. Stashak (ed.), *Adams' Lameness in Horses,* 4th Ed. Philadelphia: Lea & Febiger, 1987, p. 486.
Turner, T. A.: Proper shoeing and shoeing principles for the management of navicular syndrome. *Proc. Am. Assoc. Equine Pract.,* 1988, p. 299.
Yovich, J. V. (ed.): The equine foot. *Vet. Clin. North Am. (Equine Pract.)* 5, 1989.

PASTERN PROBLEMS

Longitudinal Fractures of the Proximal (First) Phalanx (Split Pastern)

Fracture of the proximal phalanx is a common injury in performance horses. Fractures are usually longitudinal, extending from the fetlock joint distally, and may or may not involve the pastern joint.

KEY POINT ► Fractures of the proximal phalanx are frequently undisplaced and may not be easily visible on radiographs.

Because of this, it is important to cast any suspected case of proximal phalanx fracture so that displacement of the fracture does not occur.

History and Presenting Signs

- Acute lameness following work or a race
- Lameness usually worsens dramatically in the first 30 minutes after stopping exercise.
- The horse is usually presented unable to bear weight on the leg.

Clinical Findings and Diagnosis

- Reluctance to place any weight on the affected leg
- If examined immediately after the injury, there will be little or no swelling.
- Intense pain is found on palpation, particularly over the dorsal aspect of the pastern and fetlock.
- Pain on fetlock flexion
- Lameness improves after abaxial block, but the horse does not become sound. Lameness may improve further with a four-point block (abaxial together with palmar metacarpal nerve blocks). If a fracture is suspected, it is best to avoid nerve blocks because the horse is able to bear weight on the affected leg, which may cause fracture displacement.
- Radiography of the pastern region may demonstrate fracture line(s), but in some cases the fractures may be difficult to detect. The most useful radiographic view is the dorsopalmar projection. If a fracture is suspected but cannot be seen on the radiographs, oblique views (10 degrees from the dorsal midline) should be taken.
- Most fractures are in the sagittal plane and extend from the fetlock to the proximal interphalangeal (pastern) joint. However, a number of the fractures may be oblique, extending from the proximal articular surface of the proximal phalanx to the lateral or medial cortex, proximal to the proximal interphalangeal joint.
- The fractures with the best prognosis are those which involve only one (usually the fetlock) joint.

Differential Diagnosis

- Foot abscess
- Fractures of other phalanges
- Condylar fractures of McIII
- Acute joint sprain
- Fractures of other long bones
- Tenosynovitis
- Fracture of the navicular bone

Treatment

KEY POINT ► If radiographs do not reveal any fracture lines but the clinical signs indicate a fracture, the leg should be immobilized in a cast extending from the foot to just below the carpus (see Casting, Chap. 17).

- Radiographs taken 7 to 10 days later will then reveal the presence of fracture line(s), if a fracture has occurred.
- If a fracture line can be clearly demonstrated, the treatment of choice is internal fixation using two or more cortical bone screws with the technique of interfragmentary compression. Screws can be inserted using stab incisions after careful measurements are made on a dorsopalmar radiographic view to assess the degree of overdrilling necessary for the proximal drill hole. If this is to be done, allowance must be made for magnification. In most cases, the screws do not have to be removed subsequently, and healing is usually complete in 12 to 16 weeks. The horse should be reradiographed before returning to training.
- While immobilization of the leg in a cast will result in healing in 10 to 12 weeks, imperfect alignment of the fracture sites at the joint surface(s) usually results in secondary arthritis. Therefore, if it is uneconomic to treat the case surgically, cast immobilization will result in healing but is unlikely to allow return of the horse to athletic competition when the fracture is undisplaced.
- If there are multiple fracture lines with involvement of the proximal interphalangeal (pastern) joint, it may be necessary to arthrodese this joint at the same time as fracture reduction and fixation.

Fracture of the Middle (Second) Phalanx

Fractures of the middle phalanx are most common in pleasure horses performing cutting, roping, barrel racing, etc.

KEY POINT ► Fractures are usually comminuted and may be difficult to treat successfully in terms of athletic function.

History and Presenting Signs

- Acute lameness following exercise or a race
- Inability to bear weight on the affected leg

Clinical Findings and Diagnosis

- As with proximal phalanx fractures, horses with fractures of the middle phalanx will show acute lameness immediately after work.
- There will be severe pain on flexion or palpation of the distal pastern region, and the horse will be reluctant to bear weight. Nerve blocks should not be performed because of the possibility of worsening the fracture displacement.

KEY POINT ► At least four radiographic views (dorsopalmar, lateral, and obliques) should be taken to ensure that the complete extent of the fracture lines can be seen, which may not be apparent if only dorsopalmar and lateral views are taken. Because of the comminution of these fractures, it is important to detect all fracture lines so that reduction and internal fixation can be undertaken.

Differential Diagnosis

- Foot abscess
- Fractures of other phalanges
- Acute joint sprain
- Fractures of other long bones

Treatment

- If a horse requires transport to a referral center, immobilization of the leg to below the carpus should be undertaken using a Robert Jones bandage (see Chap. 17) or a temporary cast.
- The prognosis for complete soundness following healing of these fractures is very poor because of the difficulty in achieving perfect anatomic reduction. Usually both the proximal and distal interphalangeal joints (pastern and coffin joints, respectively) are involved in fractures of the middle phalanx.
- Because the fractures are usually comminuted, internal fixation is difficult. It is important to evaluate the three-dimensional aspects of the fractures prior to undertaking surgery. Unlike fractures of the proximal phalanx, where internal fixation is possible via several stab incisions, fractures of the middle phalanx usually require open reduction because of the large number of fragments. Cortical bone screws are then inserted using the technique of interfragmentary bone compression.
- Immobilization in a cast (see Casting, Chap. 17) extending from the foot to below the carpus is an alternative treatment, although secondary arthritis will usually result. Reduction of a comminuted

fracture of the middle phalanx is possible under general anesthesia using a block and tackle system. After drilling wires through the medial and lateral sides of the hoof wall, in a similar plane to that in which shoe nails are placed, the block and tackle system is attached and tension is applied until radiographs show reasonable reduction. The cast can then be applied. This usually will result in fracture healing so that the horse is paddock sound, but it is unlikely to result in athletic soundness.

Ringbone (Phalangeal Exostosis)

Ringbone is the name given to a periostitis and osteitis with new bone growth involving the pastern region. Although it can affect both forelimbs and hindlimbs, it is most common in the forelimbs. It is classified in two ways:

Articular or nonarticular—Depending on whether or not the proximal (pastern) or distal (coffin) interphalangeal joints are involved.

High or low—*High ringbone* is that which involves the distal aspect of the proximal phalanx and the proximal part of the middle phalanx. *Low ringbone* is the term used to describe an osteitis and periostitis of the distal part of the middle phalanx and the proximal part of the distal phalanx (pedal bone). Ringbone is usually the result of direct or indirect trauma to the pastern and may be associated with an upright pastern conformation.

History and Presenting Signs

- Chronic unilateral or bilateral forelimb lameness
- Swelling around the phalanges
- Usually older horses are affected.

Clinical Findings and Diagnosis

- There is a variable degree of swelling involving the dorsal and medial and/or lateral aspects of the pastern, usually around the middle to distal pastern region.

KEY POINT ▶ If the ringbone is nonarticular, the horse may not be lame. However, if the ringbone is articular, then there will usually be a chronic lameness that varies in severity with the extent of the joint involvement.

- There may be no pain on palpation or flexion of the pastern, particularly if the problem is chronic.
- If there is lameness, there should be an improvement in gait following an abaxial nerve block.
- Radiographs (a minimum of dorsopalmar and lateral views) should be taken to assess the extent of joint involvement. Changes usually will be most apparent on the lateral view. Typical findings include variable periosteal new bone production and narrowing of the joint space.

Differential Diagnosis

- Osteochrondritis dissecans (OCD) of the distal first phalanx
- Phalangeal fractures
- Trauma (e.g., wire cuts to the phalangeal region), resulting in periosteal new bone growth
- Collateral ligament damage

Treatment

- Once the problem is chronic, with extensive new bone growth and articular involvement, there is little that can be done apart from surgical arthrodesis of the pastern joint.
- Arthodesis of the pastern joint can be accomplished using three screws inserted through the distal dorsal aspect of the proximal phalanx. The prognosis for athletic function is good after this surgery, with some thoroughbred and standardbred horses even returning to racing.
- Arthrodesis of the coffin joint is not possible. It may be useful to inject 80 mg of a long-acting corticosteroid such as methylprednisolone acetate (Treatment No. 74) into the coffin joint. However, this is usually only a short-term solution.
- In the early stages of the condition, before new bone growth has occurred, it may be possible to limit the extent of the new bone growth. This can be done by giving a 2- to 3-week course of phenylbutazone (Treatment No. 88) at a dose rate of 4.4 mg/kg q12h for 1 day, 2.2 mg/kg q12h for 5 days, and 2.2 mg/kg q24h for 5–10 days. This medication is combined with restriction of movement and perhaps immobilization using a Robert Jones bandage (see Chap. 17).
- We have also had a good response, in some cases of early, nonarticular ringbone, to the injection of 1 to 2 ml of a long-acting corticosteroid such as methylprednisolone acetate (Treatment No. 74) subperiosteally along the area of the bone where the reaction is present.
- Radiation therapy has been found to be helpful in some cases if applied in the early stages of the condition to limit the extent of the periosteal reaction. Cobalt-60 packs are usually used, and doses of 500 to 1000 rads are given. This treatment has to be undertaken by a veterinarian who has a radiation therapy license.

References

McIlwraith, C. W., and Goodman, N. L.: Conditions of the interphalangeal joints. *Vet. Clin. North Am. (Equine Pract.)* 5:161, 1989.

McIlwraith, C. W., and Turner, A. S.: Arthrodesis of the Proximal Interphalangeal Joint. In *Equine Surgery: Advanced Techniques.* Philadelphia: Lea & Febiger, 1987, p. 179.

Rick, M. C., Herthel, D., and Boles, C.: Surgical management of middle phalangeal fractures and high ringbone in the horse: A review of 16 cases. *Proc. Am. Assoc. Equine Pract.,* 1986, p. 315.

Stashak, T. S.: Management of lacerations and avulsion injuries of the foot and pastern regions, and hoof wall cracks. *Vet. Clin. North Am. (Equine Pract.)* 5:195, 1989.

Stashak, T. S.: Lameness. In T. S. Stashak (ed.), *Adams' Lameness in Horses*, 4th Ed. Philadelphia: Lea & Febiger, 1987, p. 551.

Swanson, T. D.: Degenerative disease of the proximal interphalangeal (pastern) joint in performance horses. *Proc. Am. Assoc. Equine Pract.*, 1988, p. 393.

Trotter, G. W.: Degenerative joint disease with osteochondrosis of the proximal interphalangeal joint in young horses. *J. Am. Vet. Med. Assoc.* 180:1312, 1982.

FETLOCK PROBLEMS

Arthritis of the Fetlock Joint (Osselets, Fetlock Joint Sprain)

Arthritis of the fetlock is a relatively common condition in athletic horses and is thought to be a wear-and-tear injury.

KEY POINT ▶ In the early stages, there may be only a serous arthritis, with joint effusion, soft-tissue swelling, and little articular damage.

It is essential not only that horses are treated effectively at this stage but also that they have a period of rest. If this is not done, a vicious cycle of trauma and cartilage degeneration evolves, eventually leading to narrowing of the joint space and the formation of periarticular new bone.

History and Presenting Signs

- Variable degrees of forelimb lameness
- Swelling around the fetlock joint
- Usually found in horses used for racing or other high-speed athletic events

Clinical Findings and Diagnosis

- In the early stages, there may only be swelling around the dorsal aspect of the fetlock and/or the palmar pouches.

KEY POINT ▶ The most consistent clinical finding in horses with fetlock joint pathology is distension of the palmar pouches of the fetlock joint. The palmar pouch is located between the suspensory ligament and the palmar aspect of the distal third metacarpal bone.

- Even in the early stages of the condition there is pain on flexion of the joint, with more severe pain in the acute stage.
- If the horse continues in work, lameness will become evident.

KEY POINT ▶ The lameness can be aggravated by holding the fetlock flexed for 1 minute, after which the horse is trotted off.

- Radiographs are essential to establish the extent of joint involvement. Four views (dorsopalmar, lateral to medial, and two oblique views) are necessary. It is important that the x-ray beam be aligned with the joint space so that any narrowing can be assessed on the dorsopalmar and lateral views.
- If the horse is lame, soundness should result from a combination of abaxial and palmar metacarpal nerve blocks (see Figs. 3-26 and 3-27), or alternatively, local anesthetic can be introduced directly into the joint (see Figs. 3-28, 3-29, and 3-30).

Differential Diagnosis

- Chip fracture of dorsal aspect of proximal articular margin of the proximal phalanx
- Chronic proliferative synovitis (villonodular synovitis)
- Tearing of the insertion of the common and/or lateral extensor tendons on the proximal dorsal area of the proximal phalanx

Treatment

- There are a variety of treatments for arthritis of the fetlock. However, it is important that the horse have at least 6 to 8 weeks rest after treatment. Most fetlock pain appears to center on the soft tissue of the fetlock joint, particularly the dorsal joint capsule. This appears to be inflammatory in nature and often responds well to rest and topical anti-inflammatory drugs such as dimethylsulfoxide (DMSO) (Treatment No. 34).
- The most effective therapy is that given intraarticularly. Full details of intraarticular medications are given in the section on arthritis (p. 125). In the early stages of fetlock arthritis when there is no radiographic evidence of degenerative joint disease, we have noted an excellent response to intraarticular sodium hyaluronate (Treatment No. 60). In the later stage of arthritis or where there has been little response to hyaluronate or polysulfated glycosaminoglycans (Treatment No. 90), intraarticular long-acting corticosteroids (Treatment Nos. 12 and 74) should be considered.

Chip Fracture of the Proximal Phalanx

Chip fractures in the fetlock joint usually occur at the dorsal aspect of the proximal articular margin of the proximal phalanx and appear to arise from overextension of the fetlock joint during fast exercise. The chips occur either medial or lateral to the common extensor tendon. Chip fractures are common injuries in racehorses and other athletic horses.

History and Presenting Signs

- Standardbred, thoroughbred, and quarter horse racehorses most commonly
- Low-grade forelimb lameness after initial acute episode
- Swelling around fetlock joint, particularly dorsal aspect

Clinical Findings and Diagnosis

KEY POINT ► In many cases there will be little or no lameness resulting from these fractures, and the presence of a chip fracture on a radiograph may be an incidental finding.

- Because these fractures may not be the cause of the current lameness, an intraarticular block should be performed (see Figs. 3-28, 3-29, and 3-30) to demonstrate an improvement in gait before it can be concluded that the fracture is causing a problem.
- There will be swelling over the dorsal aspect of the fetlock joint, distension of the palmar pouches of the joint capsule, and perhaps slight pain on flexion of the fetlock.

KEY POINT ► The chip fracture is most easily seen on a lateral radiograph of the fetlock.

- Oblique views (dorsolateral to palmaromedial and dorsomedial to palmarolateral) should be used to determine whether the fracture involves the dorsolateral or dorsomedial aspect of the proximal articular margin of the proximal phalanx.

Differential Diagnosis

- Arthritis of the fetlock joint
- Chronic proliferative synovitis (villonodular synovitis)
- Tearing of the insertion of the common and/or lateral extensor tendons on the proximal dorsal area of the proximal phalanx
- Synovitis of the dorsal fetlock joint capsule

Treatment

- If these chip fractures are causing lameness, they can be removed. Arthrotomy of the fetlock is still performed by some veterinarians to remove such fractures.

KEY POINT ► Arthroscopic surgical removal is the technique of choice, and the procedure results in less trauma to the joint and faster return to athletic function.

- Most horses with small fractures can resume training 4 to 6 weeks after surgery. However, this is dependent on the status of the articular cartilage of the dorsal fetlock as visualized during arthroscopy. If there are extensive areas of cartilage erosion, a 3- to 6-month rest period should be given together with the possible use of intraarticular medication.
- Intraarticular medications of choice are sodium hyaluronate (Treatment No. 60) and polysulfated glycosaminoglycans (Treatment No. 90).

Palmar Annular Ligament Constriction

The palmar annular ligament is the tough, fibrous band of material present at the palmar aspect of the fetlock and encompasses such contents as the flexor tendons, sesamoid bones, nerves, and vessels. If there is inflammation of the contents at the level of the palmar fetlock, the palmar annular ligament is inelastic and can constrict the contents of this region.

KEY POINT ► The most consistent aspect of palmar annular ligament constriction is the characteristic fluid-filled swelling on the palmar aspect of the fetlock involving the tendon sheaths.

History and Presenting Signs

- Racehorses and other athletic horses usually affected
- Chronic, progressive, but low-grade forelimb lameness
- Swelling noted above and below the palmar aspect of the fetlock joint, there being a characteristic "notched" appearance

Clinical Findings and Diagnosis

- Because of the constriction, there is usually notching at the palmar aspect of the fetlock, with distension of the flexor tendon sheaths above and below the annular ligament. The notching is a result of the inability of the inelastic ligament to swell in response to inflammation, and therefore, the swelling occurs above and below the joint.
- It is essential to radiograph the fetlock joint (dorsopalmar, lateral to medial, and two oblique views) to determine whether there is any bone damage.

KEY POINT ► Ultrasound examination is useful to establish whether there are tendon lesions, particularly involving the deep flexor tendon.

- The horse will show various degrees of lameness depending on the initiating cause of the swelling and its severity.
- A high palmar nerve block will usually result in improvement of the lameness.

Differential Diagnosis

- Sesamoid bone injuries
- Flexor tendon injuries
- Sesamoidean ligament injuries

Treatment

■ Sectioning of the palmar annular ligament (desmotomy), to relieve the constriction, is effective. This surgery can be undertaken via a small stab incision just above the annular ligament, followed by section of the ligament with scissors underneath the skin. While most horses show improvement after surgery, the underlying cause of the problem should be established—in particular, whether there is any tendon damage.

KEY POINT ► The majority of horses show an excellent response to surgery. However, we have noted that in a small percentage of horses there may be recurrence of the fluid distension and lameness. In some of these cases, the lameness and effusion have improved following administration of 80 to 120 mg of a long-acting corticosteroid such as methylprednisolone acetate (Treatment No. 74) into the flexor tendon sheath. However, in some cases, the effusion and lameness have persisted despite further medication.

■ If surgery is uneconomic, some horses may show short-term (1–3 months) response following injection of 80 to 120 mg methylprednisolone (Treatment No. 74) into the distended area of the flexor tendon sheaths.

Proximal Sesamoid Fracture

The sesamoid bones are part of the suspensory apparatus and receive reflections to their abaxial surfaces from the suspensory ligament. With overextension of the fetlock joint, which occurs during fast exercise, fracture of the sesamoid bone(s) may occur as a result of the distracting forces.

History and Presenting Signs

■ Acute forelimb lameness with variable degrees of swelling
■ Athletic horses (racehorse, polo horse, eventing horse, etc.)

Clinical Findings and Diagnosis

■ Acute, severe lameness is apparent following sesamoid fracture(s).
■ The horse is usually reluctant to bear weight on the affected leg for 3 to 5 days after the injury. However, in small chip fractures involving the proximal articular margin of the sesamoid, the lameness may be less severe. The forelimbs are more frequently involved than the hindlimbs.
■ Examination reveals severe pain on flexion of the fetlock joint or palpation over the affected sesamoid bone(s). Within 12 to 24 hours there is swelling around the palmar fetlock that will vary

in degree depending on the extent of the sesamoid fracture(s). If both sesamoid bones in the one leg are fractured, there will be complete loss of support for the fetlock joint, with the result that the joint becomes overextended and the fetlock sinks toward the ground.
■ Radiographs will establish the extent of the fracture(s), and it is important that the relevant oblique view be included in addition to the dorsopalmar and lateral views. A dorsolateral to palmaromedial oblique projection will demonstrate the lateral sesamoid bone, whereas the opposite oblique projection will show up the medial sesamoid. With some basal fractures, it may not be clear whether the fracture arises from the distal articular margin of the sesamoid bone or the proximal palmar aspect of the proximal phalanx. In such cases, a flexed lateral view may be helpful.

Differential Diagnosis

■ Sesamoiditis
■ Injury to the sesamoidean ligaments
■ Palmar annular ligament constriction
■ Flexor tendon and suspensory ligament injuries

Treatment

KEY POINT ► The time that the fracture has been present is vital to the prognosis. Fractures that have been present for less than 1 month have a favorable prognosis with surgery, whereas fractures present for greater than 1 month should not be operated on.

■ The course of treatment will depend on the extent and type of fracture found on radiographs. With apical fractures, where less than one-third of the bone is involved, surgical removal is the treatment of choice, and the prognosis is quite good. If more than one-third of the bone is involved, removal of the fractured piece of bone should not be undertaken because there will be too much damage and loss of support for the suspensory apparatus. Surgery is performed via a vertical incision in the lateral or medial palmar pouch of the fetlock joint.
■ In fractures involving more than one-third of the bone or basilar fractures, initial immobilization in a cast (see Casting, Chap. 17) followed by a rest of 9 to 12 months may result in healing. Better results can be obtained by harvesting a cancellous bone graft from the tuber coxa and inserting it into the fracture site via an incision on the palmar aspect of the fetlock. Internal fixation, using cortical bone screws, can be performed, but the technique is difficult and the results poor. Internal fixation of sesamoid bone fractures is seldom performed these days.
■ Small basilar chip fractures seem to have a better prognosis when the chips are removed, although

this can be difficult, than when such fractures are left undisturbed and treated by rest.

Sesamoiditis

The sesamoid bones are maintained in position via the reflection of the suspensory ligament to their abaxial surfaces and by a number of sesamoidean ligaments. Because of the great stress placed on the fetlock during fast exercise, tearing of some of these ligaments can take place, resulting in sesamoiditis. Sesamoiditis is found most commonly in racehorses, and despite treatment, recurrence is common.

History and Presenting Signs

- Low-grade, unilateral or bilateral foreleg lameness
- Usually found in racehorses (thoroughbred or quarter horse)
- History of gait restriction during exercise

Clinical Findings and Diagnosis

- The clinical signs of sesamoiditis are similar to but less severe than those resulting from sesamoid fractures.
- Depending on the extent of the damage, there will be varying degrees of lameness and swelling. In most cases, lameness will be substantially improved following an abaxial nerve block (see Fig. 3-26).
- Pain on flexion of the fetlock joint and on palpation of the sesamoid bone(s) usually is found. Some cases of severe sesamoiditis may be difficult to distinguish from sesamoid bone fracture, and therefore, good radiographs are required.

KEY POINT ▶ The most useful views for examining the sesamoids are dorsolateral to palmaromedial oblique (shows the lateral sesamoid bone), dorsomedial to palmarolateral oblique (shows the medial sesamoid bone), and lateral to medial views.

- The radiographic features of sesamoiditis include periosteal new bone growth, particularly on the abaxial surface of the affected sesamoid, and radiolucent lines (looking similar to fracture lines except that there is no fragment distraction) running obliquely lateromedially across the bone. These changes are most easily seen on oblique views.

KEY POINT ▶ Many horses with sesamoiditis also will have suspensory ligament damage.

- It is important to palpate both medial and lateral branches of the suspensory ligament and to compare the findings with those of the opposite foreleg. If there are suspected abnormalities, ultrasound examination should be undertaken.

Differential Diagnosis

- Sesamoid bone fracture
- Navicular disease
- Pedal osteitis
- Suspensory ligament injury
- Palmar annular ligament constriction

Treatment

- Despite a variety of treatment regimens, the prognosis for horses with sesamoiditis is not good. A high percentage of horses that have had prolonged rest will become lame 6 to 8 weeks after recommencing training.

KEY POINT ▶ We have found that the best response is gained from the oral administration of isoxsuprine hydrochloride (Treatment No. 61).

- A minimum dose rate of 0.9 mg/kg q12h should be given for a period of 3 weeks. During this time the horse can be kept in light exercise. A further course of the drug may be required depending on the initial response.
- In cases where there is local swelling and evidence of inflammation, a 7- to 10-day course of oral phenylbutazone (Treatment No. 88) may be useful. The dosage regimen is 4.4 mg/kg q12h for 1 day, followed by 2.2 mg/kg q12h for 3 to 5 days and then 2.2 mg/kg q24h.
- Depending on the severity of the problem and the response to initial therapy, a rest period may be necessary. In mild cases, a 3- to 4-week rest period is required, but in more severe sesamoiditis, 3 to 6 months of rest may be needed.

Chronic Proliferative Synovitis (Villonodular Synovitis)

Chronic proliferative synovitis is a condition that causes a low-grade foreleg lameness in racehorses and other athletic horses. Hypertrophy of tissue on the dorsal aspect of the third metacarpal bone, just distal to the attachment of the joint capsule, results in a space-occupying lesion and pressure on the dorsal aspect of the joint capsule.

History and Presenting Signs

- Low-grade chronic forelimb lameness
- Swelling of dorsal fetlock region

Clinical Findings and Diagnosis

- Unilateral forelimb lameness
- Distension of fetlock joint capsule, including the palmar pouches
- Pain on flexion and marked worsening of lameness following 1 minute of flexion
- Improvement in gait following intraarticular anesthesia of the fetlock (see Figs. 3-28 to 3-30)
- Radiography of the fetlock should be done, using

four radiographic views (dorsopalmar, lateral, dorsolateral to palmaromedial oblique, and dorsomedial to palmarolateral oblique).

KEY POINT ▶ On the lateral view, there is a characteristic indentation on the dorsal distal aspect of the third metacarpal bone, just above the articular surface.

- The space-occupying lesion in the dorsal fetlock can be demonstrated by an air arthrogram (see p. 69), which is simpler, cheaper, and causes less joint reaction than iodine-based contrast agents.

Differential Diagnosis

- Fetlock arthritis
- Chip fracture of dorsal aspect of proximal articular surface of the proximal phalanx
- Fetlock joint sprain

Treatment

- Surgery should be performed to remove the synovial proliferation. This can be done by an open technique to expose the mass via a longitudinal incision medial or lateral to the common extensor tendon on the dorsal midline.

KEY POINT ▶ With smaller masses, removal is possible using arthroscopy; however, even small masses are very tough, and small bites can only be taken with sharp rongeurs.

- The prognosis for return to full athletic function after surgery is excellent in horses with small masses. With larger masses, recurrence of the problem is possible, and there may be subsequent development of degenerative joint disease. Horses should be rested for approximately 3 months after the surgery.

References

Bukowiecki, C. V., Bramlage, L. R., and Gabel, A. A.: Proximal sesamoid bone fractures in horses: Current treatment and prognoses. *Compend. Contin. Educ. Pract. Vet.* 7:684, 1985.

Ferraro, G. L.: Lameness diagnosis and treatment in the thoroughbred racehorse. *Vet. Clin. North Am. (Equine Pract.)* 6:63, 1990.

McIlwraith, C. W.: *Diagnostic and Surgical Arthroscopy in the Horse,* 2d Ed. Philadelphia: Lea & Febiger, 1990, p. 85.

Poulos, P. W.: Radiographic and histologic assessment of proximal sesamoid bone changes in young and working horses. *Proc. Am. Assoc. Equine Pract.,* 1988, p. 347.

Stashak, T. S.: Lameness. In T. S. Stashak (ed.), Adams' Lameness in Horses, 4th Ed. Philadelphia: Lea & Febiger, 1987, p. 568.

Swanson, T. D.: Degenerative disease of the metacarpophalangeal (fetlock) joint in performance horses. *Proc. Am. Assoc. Equine Pract.,* 1988, p. 399.

Yovich, J. V., and McIlwraith, C. W.: Arthroscopic surgery for osteochondral fractures of the proximal phalanx of the metacarpophalangeal and metatarsophalangeal (fetlock) joints in horses. *J. Am. Vet. Med. Assoc.* 188:273, 1986.

Yovich, J. V., Turner, A. S., Stashak, T. S., and McIlwraith, C. W.: Luxation of the metacarpophalangeal and metatarsophalangeal joints in horses. *Equine Vet. J.* 19:295, 1987.

METACARPAL PROBLEMS
Bucked Shins (Dorsal Metacarpal Disease)

"Bucked shins" is the lay term for a periostitis and osteitis affecting the dorsal aspect of the middle third of the third metacarpal bone.

KEY POINT ▶ Bucked shins is by far the most common lameness affecting 2-year-old racehorses in their first training season.

The reason for this is unclear, but it may be associated with immaturity, excessive forces on the dorsal aspect of the immature third metacarpal bone, and dietary imbalances. Of particular concern are diets that have a too low calcium–phosphorus ratio.

History and Presenting Signs

- Two-year-old racehorse
- Bilateral forelimb lameness (more common than unilateral)
- Shuffling forelimb gait with reluctance of horse to stretch out

Clinical Findings and Diagnosis

- Both forelegs usually are affected, and the horse may show a range of signs from reluctance to stretch out to severe lameness.
- There is usually some swelling in the dorsal midmetacarpus with severe pain on mild palpation of this region.
- In cases that have resolved, there may be periosteal new bone production in the dorsal midmetacarpal region, but there will be no pain on palpation.
- Radiographs may be necessary in cases with recurrent or severe lameness because some horses have fissure or saucer fractures of the dorsal cortex of the third metacarpal bone. Such fractures cause a more severe lameness that tends not to respond to the usual treatments of anti-inflammatory drugs and rest. If a horse fails to respond to rest and has a recurrence of lameness, fissure fractures should be suspected.

Differential Diagnosis

- Fissure fracture of the dorsal cortex of the third metacarpal bone
- Condylar fracture of third metacarpal bone

- Soft-tissue swelling of tissues over the dorsal metacarpus
- Saucer fracture of the dorsal cortex of the third metacarpal bone

Treatment

- Whatever treatment is used, it is important for the horse to have a period of rest. However, experiments have shown considerable loss in bone strength, as measured with ultrasound, at the time of onset of bucked shins, and with rest the bone strength will continue to decrease.
- Once shin soreness occurs, it is very difficult to keep the horse in training because the condition will be aggravated by exercise. Unfortunately, the condition usually occurs in thoroughbred racehorses at a time when the important 2-year-old races take place. Therefore, there is a lot of pressure on the veterinarian to try to keep the horse in work.

KEY POINT ▶ It is important to return the horse to training as soon as the acute pain from the bucked shins has resolved. This usually requires between 10 and 14 days of rest. After this, periods of training that are slow to moderate in intensity can be commenced.

- Treatment can involve local anti-inflammatory measures, including cold hosing and bandaging with cold gel packs. Anti-inflammatory drugs such as phenylbutazone (Treatment No. 88) are useful, and a 2-week course is usually sufficient. An initial dose rate of 4.4 mg/kg q12h is given orally for 1 day, followed by 2.2 mg/kg q12h for 5 days and 2.2 mg/kg q24h for 5 days.
- Topical treatment with dimethylsulfoxide (DMSO, Treatment No. 34) is useful in reducing the inflammation. The DMSO is painted on the area once or twice daily for 5 to 10 days.
- Studies have shown that the type of track surface that the horse trains on has a bearing on the incidence of bucked shins. Horses trained on dirt have a higher incidence of this problem than those trained on a wood-fiber track. One would also anticipate that the incidence of this problem would be lower in horses trained on turf tracks. This is borne out to some extent by the lower incidence of bucked shins reported in the United Kingdom, where horses are trained on grass, than in the United States.

Fractures of the Third Metacarpal (Cannon) Bone

Fractures of the third metacarpal bone (McIII) may be the result of direct trauma (e.g., kicks), in which case they are usually *transverse fractures* in the midmetacarpus, or a racing injury, in which fractures are usually longitudinal oblique fractures (*condylar fractures*) extending proximally from the distal articular surface of the McIII. The other types of fractures are *fissure fractures and saucer fractures* involving the middle third of the dorsal cortex of the McIII.

History and Presenting Signs

- Direct trauma, usually a kick from another horse, particularly in foals
- Acute lameness following fast exercise (racehorses)

Clinical Findings and Diagnosis

Transverse midmetacarpal fractures provide no difficulty in diagnosis because the leg is obviously fractured. It is important to establish whether the fracture is open or not, because compound fractures have a very poor prognosis. Radiographs (a minimum of lateral to medial and dorsopalmar views) are necessary to determine the extent of the fractures. *Condylar fractures* usually occur following racing or fast work and result in a severe, acute lameness. Examination reveals some pain on flexion of the fetlock joint together with pain on palpation over either the medial or lateral surface of the dorsal metacarpus.

KEY POINT ▶ Most commonly, the fractures are of the lateral condyle, and thoroughbred racehorses are most frequently affected.

A dorsopalmar view is usually the best radiographic view to demonstrate the presence of a fracture line(s). However, in some cases there may only be a fissure fracture, and radiographs may fail to reveal any fracture lines. If the clinical signs indicate the likelihood of a condylar fracture despite negative radiographic findings, a number of oblique radiographic views should be taken at 10-degree intervals from the vertical midline. Such views may show small fissure fractures that may not be apparent on routine views.

Fissure and saucer fractures of the dorsal cortex are sometimes found in thoroughbred racehorses. Clinical signs include variable lameness that is mild to moderate. Usually horses will show some lameness at the trot, and there is pain over the middorsal metacarpal region on palpation. Lateral radiographs with good detail show the presence of a very fine fracture line, usually in the middle of the dorsal cortex and/or a saucer-shaped fragment. These fractures can sometimes be difficult to see, and fine-detail film may be necessary. Scintigraphy or xeroradiography, if available, will be useful in these situations.

Differential Diagnosis

- Fracture of the proximal phalanx (condylar fracture)
- Fracture of the sesamoid bones (condylar fracture)

- Fracture of the pedal bone
- "Bucked shins" (dorsal metacarpal periostitis and cortical fractures)

Treatment

Transverse Midmetacarpal Fractures

- With transverse fractures of the midmetacarpus, the most important aspect of treatment is the effective immobilization of the leg prior to transport to a surgical facility. This is best done using a Robert Jones bandage together with some form of splinting. Inflatable splints are also available commercially and are useful for short-term immobilization of the limb.
- Some midmetacarpal fractures may heal with a cast (see Chap. 17) applied from the foot up to just below the elbow. However, prolonged immobilization (3–6 months) is often required, and nonunion or delayed union often occurs.

KEY POINT ▶ The treatment of choice is internal fixation using compression plates and screws, and this is most successful in foals.

- In very young foals, one plate is sufficient, but in weanlings, yearlings, and older horses, two plates usually are necessary. Surgery needs to be combined with external fixation using a cast for 4 to 6 weeks. After the cast is removed, a Robert Jones supporting bandage is necessary for a further period, until there is some radiographic evidence of fracture healing. The plates and screws may require removal if a discharging sinus or lameness develops from screw movement.

Condylar Fractures

- Condylar fractures that are undisplaced can be treated with a cast applied to just below the carpus (see Chap. 17). However, if there is some displacement of the fractured piece, arthritis may result because of the difficulty in achieving perfect anatomic reduction with external coaptation alone.

KEY POINT ▶ The treatment of choice is the insertion of two or three cortical bone screws starting just above the fetlock joint using the technique of interfragmentary compression (lag-screw fixation).

- With good preoperative radiographs, it is possible to measure the distance required for overdrilling the proximal fragment so that surgery can be performed via stab incisions on the lateral or medial aspect of the metacarpus using a C clamp. A cast (see Chap. 17) or a heavy Robert Jones bandage (see Chap. 17) is applied for the immediate postoperative period, but after 7 to 10 days, a lighter bandage is all that is required. The horse should be kept in a box stall for 4 to 6 weeks, and healing

should be complete in 4 to 6 months. In most cases, the screws need not be removed. However, if lameness develops as a result of the screws loosening (radiography shows lysis around screw heads), then the screws should be removed.

Fissure and Saucer Fractures of the Dorsal Cortex.

- Dorsal cortical fractures often do not heal satisfactorily with rest alone.

KEY POINT ▶ The treatment of choice is forage around the site of the fracture.

This is usually performed with a 2-mm drill bit, with several holes being drilled into the dorsal cortex of the third metacarpal bone. This results in stimulation of osteogenesis and subsequent fracture healing. Some larger saucer fractures are treated by the placement of a lag screw in the dorsal cortex. A 3-month rest period after surgery is usually adequate.

Fracture of the Second or Fourth Metacarpal (Splint) Bones

The small metacarpal bones are prone to trauma.

KEY POINT ▶ Fracture of the second metacarpal bone is more common than fracture of the fourth and is most commonly found in standardbred trotters and pacers.

Horses with fracture of the second metacarpal bone often have an associated suspensory ligament desmitis.

History and Presenting Signs

- Low-grade forelimb lameness
- Swelling around medial aspect of midmetacarpus

Clinical Findings and Diagnosis

- There is usually a mild lameness and a variable degree of swelling depending on the extent of the fracture.

KEY POINT ▶ In both acute and more long-standing cases, there is pain on palpation over the fracture site.

- When the second metacarpal bone is fractured, it usually occurs in the middle to lower third of the bone. Dorsomedial to palmarolateral oblique radiographs are necessary to evaluate the extent of the fracture. Usually there is little displacement of the fracture line, but depending on the time since the fracture, there may be periosteal new bone growth around the fracture site.
- It is difficult to block out the lameness with standard nerve blocks, but infusion of 2 to 3 ml of 2% prilocaine (Treatment No. 93) subcutaneously

around the site of the fracture usually results in improvement in the gait.

■ If the fracture has been present for several weeks, there will be new bone production around the fracture site. The main differential diagnosis is "splints." However, there is seldom lameness from splint formation.

Differential Diagnosis

■ Splints
■ Suspensory ligament sprain
■ Condylar fracture of the third metacarpal bone
■ Osteomyelitis of the splint bones

Treatment

■ Most fractures of the splint bones will heal spontaneously in 3 to 6 months. However, there is usually quite a lot of callus formation around the fracture site, which may be unsightly, particularly in a show horse.

KEY POINT ▶ An alternative that results in a shorter rest period is surgical removal of the fractured portion of bone. This reduces the rest time, and horses are usually able to return to work 6 to 8 weeks after surgery.

■ The splint bone is removed just above the fracture site using a chisel, with the chisel positioned so that the proximal part of the splint bone is tapered at the removal site. Care should be taken to disturb the periosteum at the level of the third metacarpal bone as little as possible. If more than two-thirds of the bone is removed, the proximal portion should be stabilized using a cortical bone screw to attach the proximal portion of the splint bone to the third metacarpal bone.

KEY POINT ▶ The best cosmetic results are obtained by attempting to reduce the swelling following surgery.

■ This is done using pressure bandaging for the first 2 weeks after surgery together with oral phenylbutazone administration (Treatment No. 88). The dose rate of phenylbutazone is 4.4 mg/kg q12h for the first 24 hours, followed by 2.2 mg/kg q12h for 5 days and then 2.2 mg/kg q24h for 4 days. A total of 8 weeks of rest usually is required following surgery before the horse returns to exercise.

Rupture of the Suspensory Apparatus

Traumatic rupture of the suspensory apparatus may occur with or without fractures of both the proximal sesamoid bones and results in a loss of support for the fetlock. It usually occurs as a racing injury and needs immediate and appropriate attention. Treatment should be regarded as a salvage measure, however, because affected horses will not return to athletic competition.

History and Presenting Signs

■ Acute, severe lameness, usually of the foreleg
■ Lameness usually occurs after racing or after fast training exercise.
■ Sometimes found in foals as a result of jumping off a ridge in the pasture

Clinical Findings and Diagnosis

■ Severe overextension of the fetlock is the characteristic feature of rupture of the suspensory apparatus.
■ With a loss of support for the fetlock, the palmar aspect of the fetlock sinks toward the ground when the horse attempts to put weight on the leg.
■ Radiographs, a minimum of four views (dorsopalmar, lateral to medial, and two obliques), should be taken to determine if the sesamoid bones have been fractured. In some cases, luxation of the fetlock joint occurs.
■ Diagnosis is not difficult because of the extreme nature of the fetlock appearance when the horse attempts to bear weight on the affected leg.

Differential Diagnosis

■ Fetlock luxation
■ Weak flexor tendons (following casting or in newborn foals)

Treatment

KEY POINT ▶ It is vital to stabilize the limb to prevent further trauma and damage of the blood supply to the affected leg.

■ Stabilization is best achieved by casting the leg (see Chap. 17) with the fetlock in flexion. If this cannot be done, it may be possible to immobilize the fetlock by nailing the sole of the foot to a plank of wood, following appropriate padding of the pastern, fetlock, and metacarpus with cotton wool. The plank is then taken up the palmar aspect of the leg so that weight is taken only on the toe of the affected foot. The plank is then secured in position over the top of the bandages. This allows the fetlock to be stabilized until surgery can be done.
■ There is no athletic future for a horse with rupture of the suspensory apparatus. However, such horses can be made paddock sound by arthrodesis of the fetlock joint. This surgery is very complex and should only be undertaken at a specialist referral center.

Splints

"Splint" is a lay term used to describe an osteitis and periostitis usually involving the proximal part of the second metacarpal bone. This results in localized swelling and new bone production. The cause in many cases is abnormal conformation, with the metacarpal bones being set too far to the lateral side of the carpus. This results in excessive weight being placed on the second metacarpal bone, which causes movement and local periostitis. Other cases may be the result of direct trauma to the metacarpus, in which case other anatomic sites may be involved.

History and Presenting Signs

- Swelling, usually over the medial aspect of the metacarpus
- Little or no lameness
- May affect any breed of horse
- Most commonly found in younger horses (2 to 5 years old)

Clinical Findings and Diagnosis

KEY POINT ► Usually, there is little or no lameness resulting from splints.

- Occasionally, during the early stages, involving inflammation, there may be a mild lameness. If there is marked or persistent lameness associated with the swelling, it is more likely to be a fracture of the second metacarpal bone.
- The most obvious clinical sign is swelling over the proximal third of the medial aspect of the second metacarpal bone. During the acute stages of the reaction, this swelling may be diffuse, whereas later the swelling will be localized and will vary in size from a marble to a golf ball. Care should be taken in excluding other areas of the leg before lameness is ascribed to a splint.
- Radiographs may be necessary to exclude a fracture of the second metacarpal bone. The most important radiographic view is usually the 45-degree dorsomedial to palmarolateral oblique view. This view shows the outline of the second metacarpal bone, and the extent of soft tissue versus new bone growth can be assessed accurately. Because the junction between the second and the third metacarpal bones can appear as an oblique radiolucent line through the body of the second metacarpal bone, a fracture may be diagnosed mistakenly.

Differential Diagnosis

- Fracture of the small metacarpal bones
- Suspensory ligament strain
- Soft-tissue trauma to the metacarpus

Treatment

- During the very early stages, before new bone growth has occurred, local anti-inflammatory measures (cold hosing, bandaging) together with injection of 20 to 40 mg of a long-acting corticosteroid such as methylprednisolone acetate (Treatment No. 74) subperiosteally will reduce the swelling and limit the extent of new bone growth.

- Anti-inflammatory drugs such as phenylbutazone (Treatment No. 88) also may be used orally for 10 to 14 days. The initial dose rate is 4.4 mg/kg q12h for 1 to 2 days, followed by 2.2 mg/kg q12h for 3 to 5 days.
- Radiation therapy also has been used with some success. However, because of stimulation of local blood supply, if further trauma occurs, there may be more profuse new periosteal bone growth.
- A variety of iodine-based blistering agents and firing have been used as counterirritants in attempts to resolve the swelling associated with the splint. These procedures do not improve the end result and have no place in therapy.

KEY POINT ► Once new bone formation has occurred, the splint will seldom cause the horse any problem, apart from being a cosmetic blemish.

- At this stage, only surgical removal of the new bone growth will resolve the problem. However, there is a high chance of recurrence of the bone formation. The best cosmetic result is achieved by taking great care in avoiding disruption to the periosteum around the area of new bone growth. Pressure bandaging for at least 2 weeks after surgery is important, after which a lighter bandage should be applied for a further 2 weeks. During the first 2 weeks after surgery, phenylbutazone (Treatment No. 88) should be given orally at a dose rate of 4.4 mg/kg q12h for 1 day, followed by 2.2 mg/kg q12h for 5 days and then 2.2 mg/kg daily for 5 days. This helps to reduce swelling and prevent new periosteal bone formation following surgery.

Suspensory (Interosseous) Ligament Sprain

The suspensory (interosseous) ligament is part of the suspensory apparatus and has its origin in the proximal palmar metacarpus or metatarsus. It divides approximately 5 to 7.5 cm (3 in) above the fetlock joint, and the medial and lateral branches attach to the abaxial surfaces of the sesamoid bones before joining the extensor tendon in the dorsal midpastern region.

KEY POINT ► Sprain of the suspensory ligament usually occurs after the site of division of the ligament in one or other of the branches, and the medial branch of the ligament appears to be injured more commonly than the lateral.

History and Presenting Signs

- Swelling in the middle to distal metacarpus
- Most common in racehorses, particularly standardbred pacers and trotters, and other athletic horses
- Mild or no lameness

Clinical Findings and Diagnosis

- There may or may not be signs of lameness, depending on the severity of the sprain. The lameness is usually low grade, and horses are usually presented because of swelling rather than lameness.
- There is usually swelling in the distal metacarpus, associated with the affected branch of the suspensory ligament. There is also pain on gentle palpation of the affected area of the suspensory ligament. (Note that firm palpation will result in a painful response in most normal horses.) In long-standing cases, there may be gross enlargement of the ligament due to scar-tissue formation at the site of injury.

KEY POINT ▶ Note that the sesamoid bones are often involved secondarily, owing to tearing of the insertion of the ligament.

- Additionally, it is relatively common to find fractures of the second metacarpal bone in many standardbred horses wih suspensory ligament desmitis. It is essential, therefore, to obtain radiographs (particularly oblique views of the fetlock and metacarpus) before deciding on the eventual treatment.
- Ultrasound examination is useful to determine the extent of damage to the suspensory ligament. Repeated examinations assist in indicating the course of healing, which helps in deciding when the horse should be returned to work.

Differential Diagnosis

- Fracture of the small metacarpal bones
- Splints
- Deep flexor tendon strain
- Sesamoiditis

Treatment

- Rest is a major factor in successful treatment, and up to 9 to 12 months may be required. Repeated ultrasound examinations at regular intervals will indicate the course of healing of the lesion in the ligament.
- If there is a fracture of the distal part of the second metacarpal bone, this results in continued irritation to the ligament, and therefore, the fractured portion of bone should be surgically removed.
- In the acute phase of the injury, local anti-inflammatory measures (cold hosing, cold packs, pressure bandaging), together with anti-inflammatory drugs such as phenylbutazone (Treatment No. 88) for 10 to 14 days, will help reduce the swelling and pain. Oral administration at a dose rate of 4.4 mg/kg q12h for 1 day, followed by 2.2 mg/kg q12h for 5 days and then 2.2 mg/kg daily for up to 5 days, is usual.
- A number of different surgical treatments have been tried, none of which has proved very successful. Rest is the key, followed by a graded exercise program to increase the strength of the soft tissues when returning the horse to training. We have found treadmill training to be particularly useful for this purpose. The consistent surface for exercise and the control of the speed of training are the most useful aspects of treadmill exercise.
- If there is associated sesamoiditis, a course of isoxsuprine hydrochloride (see Sesamoiditis) may be helpful.

Tendon Strain ("Bowed Tendon")

The deep and superficial flexor tendons are both prone to injury because of the forces placed on them by galloping horses.

KEY POINT ▶ The superficial flexor tendon is far more commonly injured than the deep flexor tendon, and the most frequent site for injury is the midmetacarpal region.

The reason for the injuries being largely confined to the midmetacarpal region may be because the cross-sectional area is the smallest in this part of the tendon. Tendon strains are uncommon in the hindlegs. The expression "bowed tendon" is used by owners and trainers because of the characteristic swelling at the palmar aspect of the midmetacarpus.

History and Presenting Signs

- Variable degrees of swelling in the palmar aspect of the midmetacarpus
- Lameness is uncommon but, when it does occur, is usually mild.
- Most commonly found in racehorses (quarter horses, standardbreds, and thoroughbreds) and other horses used for high-intensity exercise

Clinical Findings and Diagnosis

- The first sign of injury is swelling in the affected area of the tendon, together with heat and pain on palpation. Initially, the degree of swelling may be quite mild and may be ignored by the owner or trainer because the horse is not lame.
- In mild injuries there is usually no lameness, but in severe tendon strains there may be a mild to moderate foreleg lameness.
- Examination of the tendons should be performed with the weight off the affected leg, because the horse may show no signs of pain on palpation if examined when bearing weight. With weight off the leg, each of the tendons can be palpated, progressing 1 cm (0.5 in) at a time, to localize the area where swelling and pain are present.
- In chronic cases, there is usually considerable thickening of the tendon, with an increase of up to four to five times in area, due to scar-tissue formation. Even in long-standing cases, it is pos-

sible to detect pain on palpation. A useful guide to tendon healing is gained from palpation of the affected site to determine if pain is still present in the area. If there is pain on palpation, exercise should be restricted to slow training only.

■ Ultrasound examination is important to assess the extent of the tendon injury and will distinguish swelling in the peritendinous tissue from that within the tendon fibers. It is also useful to document the rate of healing, giving a guide as to when the horse can return to training. The most severe ultrasound lesions are those showing up as anechoic areas in the central region of the tendon when examined in cross section. These so-called core lesions indicate major tendon fiber disruption and local hemorrhage. The proximal to distal extent of the tendon lesion should be quantified, and a hard copy should be made of the ultrasound results so that reexamination will allow determination of the rate and extent of tendon healing.

Differential Diagnosis

■ Suspensory ligament desmitis
■ Soft-tissue trauma around flexor tendons
■ Palmar annular ligament constriction
■ Tendon sheath infection

Treatment

There have probably been more treatments advocated for tendon strain than for any other musculoskeletal problem. This indicates that few of the treatments are efficacious.

KEY POINT ▶ The limiting factor to any form of treatment is that when a tendon is injured, healing is very slow, and the normal type I collagen, which is very strong, is replaced by type III collagen, which has poor tensile strength. Additionally, the normal longitudinal orientation of the tendon fibers is lost, so some of the mechanical properties of the tendon are altered.

Treatments still in current use include:

Firing—Application of a hot firing iron to the skin over the damaged area of tendon has *absolutely no merit* and should not be done. Studies in England in experimental tendon injuries have demonstrated that firing has no beneficial effects and most probably some adverse effects on tendon healing. Most equine practitioner professional bodies recommend that it should not be used.

Tendon Stab or Tendon Splitting—This surgical procedure originated in Sweden and consists of a number of stabs being made into the tendon or the tendon being split longitudinally. The aim of this surgery was to promote vascularity to the damaged area of tendon. Older experimental evidence in normal tendons suggests that the procedure is of lim-

ited value and may actually delay tendon healing. More recently, there has been some ultrasound evidence that in horses with severe core tendon lesions, stabs into the area of the damaged tendon may lead to more rapid healing, particularly when combined with superior check ligament desmotomy.

Injection of Sodium Hyaluronate in or Around the Tendon Lesion—Some studies have shown that sodium hyaluronate (Treatment No. 60) injected around a damaged tendon may result in fewer adhesions and more rapid return to function. However, the efficacy of this treatment is still uncertain.

Carbon Fibers—Carbon fibers were originally thought to be the ideal treatment because when they were surgically implanted, they imparted strength and encouraged longitudinal orientation of collagen. While this treatment appears to have some merit, reinjury is common, and few studies have shown any improvement in tendon function. Most practitioners that advocate carbon fiber implantation undertake the implant by insertion of the fibers, via a large-gauge needle, longitudinally down the body of the affected tendon. Horses are then given a 6- to 12-month rest period before returning to exercise.

Conservative Treatment—The idea of conservative treatment is to limit the inflammatory reaction with local anti-inflammatory measures plus 10 to 14 days of oral phenylbutazone (Treatment No. 88) at a dose rate of 4.4 mg/kg q12h for 1 day, followed by 2.2 mg/kg q12h for 3 to 5 days and then 2.2 mg/kg daily for up to 7 days. Approximately 21 days after injury, passive mobilization of the flexor tendon is begun by swimming the horse, thus preventing restrictive adhesions. A rest period should be given, depending on the ultrasound appearance of the tendon lesion and the change in appearance upon reexamination. If the proximodistal extent of the lesion and the cross-sectional area of involvement are not excessive, early mobilization of the tendon (swimming), followed by graded light exercise, appears to be useful for returning normal tendon function. Slow, long-distance training is useful to strengthen tendon fibers, with the speed of exercise not to exceed 600 m/min. Treadmill exercise is extremely useful for rehabilitation of horses with tendon strain.

Superior Check Ligament Desmotomy

KEY POINT ▶ Section of the superior check ligament is acknowledged by most equine practitioners to be the treatment that gives the most successful results in terms of return to athletic function in horses with superficial flexor tendonitis.

The theory behind this surgery is that by cutting one of the points of attachment to the superficial flexor tendon, there is more flexibility and elasticity in the tendon. The surgery is difficult because in some horses the check ligament is hard to find and there are frequently some large vessels that may be inapparent when cutting the fibers of the ligament. Retraction of these vessels, once cut, makes ligation extremely difficult because the origin of the bleeding cannot be found. There appears to be quite a degree of individual variation in the appearance of the check ligament, and while the diagrams in surgical books make the technique appear simple, it is not a procedure that is easy to perform. Exactly when the surgery should be performed in relation to the tendon injury has not been absolutely clarified. Recent evidence has indicated that with large core lesions in the superficial flexor tendon, a combination of a tendon stab operation and a check ligament desmotomy may be more effective than desmotomy alone. Following surgery, the horse should be given a minimum of 6 months of rest, after which time the lesion can be evaluated using ultrasound examination. If the ultrasound appearance has improved, consideration can be given to returning the horse to training, with an emphasis on low-speed exercise for the first 8 to 10 weeks. Swimming also appears to be beneficial in these circumstances and may be useful in the first few weeks after injury to reduce adhesions.

Conclusions. Despite the various treatments used, there is a high rate of recurrence of the tendon injuries. This is so because in the region of tendon injury, the type III collagen formed is much weaker than the type I collagen in normal tendon. The most effective treatment for superficial tendon strain appears to be superior check ligament desmotomy, together with a graded exercise program in the convalescent period. There are some differences in prognosis between various classes of performance horses. Tendon reinjury is far less common in standardbred pacers and trotters than in thoroughbred racehorses.

Tendon Transection

Complete rupture of tendons is very rare in the horse. However, transection of tendons is quite common as a result of trauma to the metacarpal region. This can occur as a result of having limbs caught in fences, trauma from exposed areas of sharp iron around barns or box stalls, wire cuts, and other similar traumas. The flexor tendons are more commonly involved than the extensor tendons, but the prognosis is better for extensor tendon transection.

History and Presenting Signs

- Trauma to the limb
- Hyperextension of the fetlock
- Severe, non-weight-bearing lameness

Clinical Findings and Diagnosis

- If both superficial and deep flexor tendons are transected, the fetlock joint will drop as a result of the lack of support, so hyperextension of the fetlock occurs.
- In some cases, the transection will be obvious, particularly if there is extensive skin laceration. However, sometimes there is transection with minimal skin trauma, particularly if the transection is due to tin on barns. In such cases, the presenting signs may be similar to those in horses with rupture of the suspensory apparatus.

Differential Diagnosis

- Rupture of the suspensory apparatus
- Fracture of the proximal sesamoid bones
- Fracture of the metacarpus

Treatment

- Often the wound and the tendon ends are contaminated by the time the horse is examined. In this case, lavage of the area using saline should be performed, preferably using a pulsating lavage system such as a Water-Pik. The leg can be wrapped in a Robert-Jones bandage (see Chap. 17) or immobilized with a cast (see Chap. 17) for 7 to 10 days.
- If the horse is examined within 6 to 12 hours of the injury and there is no evidence of wound contamination, primary surgical repair of the tendon can be performed; otherwise, repair should be delayed until infection is under control. Any foreign material lodged in the tendon may cause a chronic infection, and if there is also infection of the tendon sheath, infection is difficult to control (see Tendon Sheath Infections, p. 99).
- Tendon repair can be performed with monofilament nylon inserted between the tendon ends. It does not seem to be necessary to completely appose the tendon ends. The fetlock is set in flexion and is cast (see Chap. 17) to just below the carpus for 6 to 8 weeks. After this time, a trailer shoe is applied to prevent overextension of the foot.

KEY POINT ► A trailer shoe is easily made by welding a heavy metal strip (such as an old rasp) from the toe of the shoe to extend about 5 cm (2 in) behind the heels of the shoe.

- If there is evidence of local infection, the leg can be cast to the subcarpal region without any attempt to surgically approximate the tendon ends. It is important to cast the limb in flexion so that the tendon ends are apposed. Casting for a total of 8 to 12 weeks is required, after which a trailer shoe (see above) should be applied. This type of injury will always heal, although it may be insufficient for athletic function in racehorses. Healing is accompanied by a large amount of scar tissue with residual swelling at the site.

Inferior Check Ligament Desmitis

The inferior check ligament is approximately the same width as the deep flexor tendon and runs from its origin on the palmar surface of the proximal metacarpus to join the deep flexor tendon in the mid-metacarpal region. Inferior check ligament desmitis is an uncommon cause of lameness and can be easily overlooked.

KEY POINT ▶ Inferior check ligament desmitis is usually found in standardbred trotters and pacers and causes a low-grade lameness.

Diagnostic nerve blocks are essential to establish a definitive diagnosis. This is a condition used by some clinicians as a last-resort diagnosis when no other cause for lameness can be found.

History and Presenting Signs

- Usually a standardbred pacer or trotter
- Mild, chronic foreleg lameness
- No swelling reported by the trainer or owner

Clinical Findings and Diagnosis

- Mild to moderate foreleg lameness
- Clinical examination of the leg usually reveals no areas of pain or swelling. In some cases there is pain on deep palpation in the area palmar to the third metacarpal bone in the proximal metacarpal region.

KEY POINT ▶ Infusion of 6 to 8 ml of 2% prilocaine or mepivacaine (Treatment No. 72) into the region around the check ligament will result in relief of the lameness.

- Ultrasound examination is useful to demonstrate an anechoic area within the substance of the check ligament.
- In some chronic cases, there is sclerosis of the trabeculae and enthesopathic formations visible on dorsopalmar and oblique radiographs of the proximal metacarpus.

Differential Diagnosis

- Deep flexor tendon strain
- Stress fractures of the third metacarpal bone
- Suspensory ligament desmitis
- Fractures and osteitis of the small metacarpal (splint) bones

Treatment

- Rest is the only treatment that is worthwhile. If there are signs of local inflammation, the use of oral phenylbutazone (see Treatment No. 88) for 5 to 7 days, together with topical application of dimethylsulfoxide (DMSO) (Treatment No. 34), is useful therapy. The dose rate of phenylbutazone should be 4.4 mg/kg q12h for 1 day, followed by 2.2 mg/kg q12h for 5 to 6 days.
- Most cases of inferior check ligament desmitis will resolve with a period of 2 to 3 months of rest.

Tendon Problems in Foals

Two types of tendon problems occur in newborn foals. The first is *weak flexor tendons,* mainly found in the hindlegs and common in premature foals. The second is *flexure deformity,* which also can be found in weanlings and yearlings, particularly if on a high plane of nutrition. In such cases, it is usually an excessive amount of energy in the diet that is the problem. Therefore, in combination with other treatment, it is important to reduce the amount of energy in the diet.

History and Presenting Signs

- Most commonly found in newborn foals, although flexure deformities may develop in weanlings and yearlings, particularly those on high energy diets.
- Obvious change in the contour of the legs. *Weak flexor tendons* are usually found in the hindlegs of newborn foals, with overextension of the limbs. *Flexure deformities* result in the foal or weanling standing very upright, usually in the forelegs, and in severe cases there may be knuckling over on the dorsal surface owing to the degree of flexion.

Clinical Findings and Diagnosis

- *Weak flexor tendons* are easily diagnosed because when the foal stands, the palmar aspect of the fetlock will descend toward the ground as a result of overextension.
- With *flexure deformity,* the pastern and fetlock will be very upright, and in severely affected cases, the foal may actually knuckle over on the dorsal fetlock owing to overflexion. The foal will be unable to place the affected feet flat on the ground and usually bears weight on the toe.
- A neurologic examination is important because in some foals with tendon problems the cause may be related to problems during development or hypoxic damage at birth. If neurologic function is normal, the prognosis for recovery is good.
- With the foal in lateral recumbency, the distal joints should be flexed and extended to ensure that a normal range of movement exists.

Differential Diagnosis

- Arthrogryposis
- Neurologic disorders

Treatment

KEY POINT ▶ *Weak flexor tendons* will self-correct if the foal is confined to a box stall with its mother for 3 to 4 days. During this period, support may have to be provided to ensure that trauma does not occur to the palmar or plantar aspect of the affected fetlocks.

- To prevent overextension from occurring, application of one or several wooden tongue depressors to the sole of the affected foot so that they project 3 to 5 cm (1.5 to 2 in) behind the heels, in a similar fashion to a trailer shoe, should be done.
- In larger foals, several tongue depressors or other suitable wood may need to be used to provide sufficient strength. These usually can be fixed in place with elastic adhesive bandage.

KEY POINT ► Many cases of young foals with *flexure deformity* also will respond well to stall rest, and the foot will assume a normal position over a period of several days. However, in some foals, and especially in weanlings and yearlings, this condition may not correct despite lowering the plane of nutrition.

- In newborn foals, it is worthwhile to consider splinting the leg using inflatable splints. Such splints were designed principally for temporary immobilization of human limbs, but they are effective for splinting foal limbs and have the advantage over other splinting techniques of lessening the risk of pressure sores. The inflatable splint is applied after bandaging the limb from the pastern to the upper forearm with cotton wool to reduce the possibility of pressure sores. With the foal in lateral recumbency, an inflatable splint is applied from the fetlock to the midforearm and inflated so that no flexion of the carpus is possible. If both limbs are affected, only one leg is splinted at a time, alternating every 4 to 6 hours, until correction occurs.
- In older foals or in more severe cases, surgery should be performed to section the inferior check ligament. If the flexure deformity principally involves the phalanges, a better response to surgery is found by cutting the superior check ligament. However, the surgery is more difficult than inferior check ligament desmotomy.

Tendon Sheath Infections

The flexor tendons have sheaths in areas immediately distal to the carpus and around the fetlock. The middle third of the tendons in the metacarpal region have no tendon sheaths. Infection of the tendon sheath is extremely difficult to treat successfully. This difficulty results from the infection being in a contained synovial space where it is hard to establish drainage, together with variable penetration of antibiotics into the affected sheath.

History and Presenting Signs

An acute traumatic incident is usual, there being a cut or penetrating injury in the area of one of the tendon sheaths.

KEY POINT ► Acute severe lameness, with the horse reluctant to bear weight on the affected leg, together with gross swelling of the affected area, is usual.

Clinical Findings and Diagnosis

- Heat and swelling around the affected area of the leg, with distension of the tendon sheath
- In the early stages of a tendon sheath infection, there may be an increase in rectal temperature and an elevation of heart and respiratory rates.
- Aspiration of the swollen tendon sheaths should be performed aseptically, following surgical preparation of the area. Fluid should be collected into tubes containing EDTA for cytologic examination and measurement of total protein. In normal tendon sheath fluid, there are few cells (<1000 $\times$ 10^6/L or 1000/μL), and total protein values are less than 25 g/L or 2.5 g/dL. Fluid also should be collected into sterile tubes for bacteriologic examination using similar techniques to those for joint fluid (see Chap. 16).

Differential Diagnosis

- Septic arthritis
- Infection of navicular bursa
- Fracture of the phalanges

Treatment

- Appropriate systemic bactericidal antibiotic therapy should be commenced as soon as samples have been obtained for culture and sensitivity. Once the results of bacteriology are known, the antibiotic therapy can be amended appropriately.
- Irrigation of the tendon sheath with an isotonic polyionic solution should be performed under general anesthesia. Approximately 1 to 2 L should be flushed through the tendon sheath using large-gauge (12 or 14 gauge) catheters. It may be worthwhile to include a nonirritant antibiotic, such as sodium or potassium penicillin, with the fluid solution. The concentration should never exceed 1 million units (0.6 g) per liter of polyionic fluid. Flushing the sheath with 3–4L of a 20% solution of DMSO (Treatment No. 34) may also be useful.
- In many cases it is difficult to culture bacteria, particularly if antibiotic therapy has been instituted prior to samples being taken for bacteriology. The prognosis is poor for successful resolution of the problem, even with aggressive therapy. Horses tend to remain chronically lame, despite receiving prolonged antibiotic courses.

References

Allen, D., and White, N. A.: Management of fractures and exostosis of the metacarpals and metatarsals II and IV in 25 horses. *Equine Vet. J.* 19:326, 1987.

Dyson, S.: Proximal suspensory desmitis: Clinical, ultrasonographic and radiographic features. *Equine Vet. J.* 23:25, 1991.

Ferraro, G. L.: Lameness diagnosis and treatment in the thoroughbred racehorse. *Vet. Clin. North Am. (Equine Pract.)* 6:63, 1990.

Moyer, W., Ford, T. S., and Ross, M. W.: Proximal suspensory desmitis. *Proc. Am. Assoc. Equine Pract.*, 1988, p. 409.

Reef, V. B., Martin, B. B., and Elser, A.: Types of tendon and ligament injuries detected with diagnostic ultrasound: Description and follow-up. *Proc. Am. Assoc. Equine Pract.*, 1988, p. 245.

Rick, M. C., O'Brien, T. R., Pool, R. R., et al.: Condylar fractures of the third metacarpal bone and third metatarsal bone in 75 horses: Radiographic features, treatment and outcome. *J. Am. Vet. Med. Assoc.* 183:287, 1983.

Turner, A. S., and McIlwraith, C. W.: *Techniques in Large Animal Surgery,* 2d Ed. Philadelphia: Lea & Febiger, 1989, p. 147.

PROBLEMS OF THE CARPUS AND DISTAL RADIUS

Carpitis

Carpitis is an osteitis and periostitis affecting various carpal bones and may include an arthritis of the proximal or middle carpal joints. Usually it is from overextension of the carpus and is found most frequently in thoroughbred racehorses. However, carpitis can be a cause of lameness in any type of athletic horse and may be the result of direct trauma in the jumping horse. The most common sites affected are the dorsal aspects of the radial, third, and intermediate carpal bones as well as the distal radius. In some cases, there may be only soft-tissue damage to the dorsal carpus.

History and Presenting Signs

- Lameness and/or swelling involving the dorsal aspect of the carpus
- History may be either of acute or chronic lameness depending on the stage of the condition
- In some cases with trauma to the soft tissues overlying the carpal bones, the horse may be presented with swelling over the dorsal carpus but no significant lameness.

Clinical Findings and Diagnosis

- The most obvious clinical sign is swelling of the dorsal aspect of the carpus and, perhaps, distension of the involved joint capsules.
- Most horses in the acute stage are lame, but in chronic cases without joint involvement there may be localized swelling without any signs of lameness.
- On examination of the carpus, there may be pain on palpation over the affected carpal bones (particularly in the acute stage), and pain on flexion of the carpus is a consistent finding.
- If lameness is present, intraarticular nerve blocks should be performed to determine whether the lameness can be localized to the proximal or middle carpal joints. Although the distal (carpometacarpal) joint communicates with the middle (intercarpal) joint, primary disease of the distal carpal joint is unusual.
- A radiographic survey of the carpus is essential, and at least two oblique views (lateral and a flexed lateral) are required. Because the clinical signs are similar to those in horses with chip fractures of the carpal bones, it is important to exclude such fractures. If there is any doubt from the initial radiographs, additional oblique and skyline views should be taken.

Differential Diagnosis

- Chip fractures of the carpal bones
- Soft-tissue trauma to dorsal aspect of the carpus
- Extensor tendon sheath synovitis
- Carpal arthritis
- Hygroma of the carpus

Treatment

- It is important that an accurate diagnosis be made prior to treatment and, in particular, that no chip fractures are present. If radiographs reveal only soft-tissue swelling and no periosteal reaction, local anti-inflammatory measures (cold hosing, application of cold packs and pressure bandages, and/or topical application of dimethylsulfoxide Treatment No. 34), together with a 7- to 10-day course of phenylbutazone (Treatment No. 88), will reduce the swelling and prevent new periosteal bone growth. Local radiation therapy can be beneficial in preventing the new bone growth if it is applied before new bone formation occurs.
- If degenerative joint disease involving the proximal intercarpal (radiocarpal) or middle carpal (intercarpal) joints is evident, intraarticular therapy is required (see Treatment under Degenerative Joint Disease, p. 126). Good long-term results may be obtained with the use of intraarticular medication: sodium hyaluronate (Treatment No. 60) or polysulfated glycosaminoglycans (Treatment No. 90) in the affected joint. In some cases, intraarticular corticosteroids (Treatment Nos. 12 and 74) can be useful.

Carpal Canal Syndrome (Carpal Tunnel Syndrome)

Carpal canal syndrome is a lameness resulting from inflammation and pressure on the contents of the carpal canal. Because of the tough, fibrous palmar annular ligament, no expansion of the carpal canal contents is possible when there is trauma. This syndrome is unusual as a cause of lameness and is found most commonly in jumping horses. It also may be found following fracture of the accessory carpal bone.

History and Presenting Signs

- Low-grade to moderate forelimb lameness
- Swelling on the caudal aspect of the distal radius

Clinical Findings and Diagnosis

- There is lameness of the affected limb with pain on extreme flexion of the carpus and an absence of lesions on the dorsal aspect of the carpal bones.
- The most consistent finding is fluid distension of the sheaths of the flexor carpi ulnaris and ulnaris lateralis proximal to the annular ligament of the carpus.
- Radiographs should include lateral and flexed lateral, oblique, and skyline views. In some cases, carpal canal syndrome is secondary to fracture of the accessory carpal bone.

Differential Diagnosis

- Fracture of the accessory carpal bone
- Synovitis or desmitis of the flexor tendons proximally at the palmar aspect of the carpus

Treatment

Resection of an elliptical strip of the annular ligament on the medial side of the carpus results in relief of pressure on the contents of the carpal canal. The concept of the operation is similar to section of the palmar annular ligament of the fetlock in cases of constriction.

Carpal Fractures ("Knee Chips")

Fractures of various carpal bones are common injuries in racehorses and are thought to result from a combination of conformation problems (particularly calf knees) and overextension of the carpus during fast exercise.

KEY POINT ▶ The majority of the fractures are small chip fractures on the dorsal aspect of the carpus, but slab fractures (particularly of the third carpal bone) are also found.

The most common sites for carpal fractures are the dorsal distal articular margin of the radial carpal bone, the dorsomedial proximal articular margin of the third carpal bone, and the dorsolateral aspect of the distal articular margin of the radius. The intermediate carpal, ulnar carpal, and accessory carpal bones are sometimes fractured. However, fractures of the second and fourth carpal bones are extremely unusual.

History and Presenting Signs

- Most carpal fractures occur in thoroughbred racehorses
- The left carpus is usually affected in horses racing in a clockwise direction, whereas the right carpus is usually affected in horses racing in a counterclockwise direction.
- Fractures involving the middle carpal joint are mostly on the dorsomedial aspect, whereas those involving the proximal carpal joint are usually on the dorsolateral aspect.

Clinical Findings and Diagnosis

- There is acute lameness immediately after the fracture that will vary in severity depending on the extent of the fracture.
- Distension of the joint capsule is apparent over the dorsal aspect of the affected carpus within 3 to 6 hours after the injury. This distension often appears like a small bubble that is localized to the dorsal joint capsule over the affected joint. This localized joint capsule swelling is an important clinical sign of intraarticular pathology of the carpus, and therefore, the joint capsules of the proximal and middle carpal joints should always be palpated carefully when performing a lameness examination.
- If there is a slab fracture of the third carpal bone, the horse will be reluctant to bear any weight on the leg, and the carpus will be considerably swollen. Pain on flexion of the carpus is found, but if the fracture is long-standing, pain may be difficult to demonstrate. In these cases, extreme flexion of the carpus will be necessary to demonstrate a painful response. In long-standing cases, intraarticular local anesthesia may be required to confirm that the carpus is the site of lameness. This is particularly the case in chip fractures of the distal radius, because many horses with these fractures will show no lameness. Good radiographs are essential to diagnosis and should include at least a lateral, flexed lateral, and two oblique views.
- Sagittal fractures of the third carpal bone are uncommon but will not be seen on the standard radiographic views. This type of fracture can only be diagnosed using a skyline view, where a radiolucent line is seen running in a dorsopalmar direction.

Differential Diagnosis

- Extensor tendon sheath synovitis
- Carpitis
- Soft-tissue trauma to the carpus
- Nonspecific carpal lameness

Treatment

- Although surgery to remove the chip fracture is the most logical treatment, this may not always carry with it a good prognosis for further racing. Careful assessment of radiographs to determine if any arthritis is present, the size of the chip, and the extent of articular involvement is important. These factors allow advice to be given to the client regarding the prognosis for future athletic function.
- If only a small chip fracture is present and the fracture is undisplaced, there is the possibility that 6 months of rest will enable successful healing and return to racing. However, because of continued irritation to the joint from the presence of the chip, it is best in most cases to remove the fracture via arthroscopy.
- Arthroscopic surgery provides the possibility of fracture removal with little disturbance to the joint capsule.

KEY POINT ▶ While most horses with chip fractures of the carpal bones will benefit from arthroscopy, it must be remembered that horses with coexistent degenerative joint disease may not respond to the extent of allowing a return to successful athletic function.

- The best results are obtained with small fragments, where there is little cartilage erosion. In some cases, this is clear prior to surgery, because there are radiographic signs of degenerative joint disease. However, in other cases, the radiographs appear to indicate a good prognosis, but once the arthroscope is placed, there may be quite extensive cartilage erosion involving a number of the carpal bones. Because surgeons like doing arthroscopic surgery, there has been a tendency for horses to be operated on without due regard for the prognosis.
- Fractures of the ulnar carpal bone are quite rare, but when they occur, they have a very poor prognosis. Joint instability is often the result, and horses are left with chronic lameness.
- Postoperatively, the horse's carpus remains bandaged for 7 to 10 days. Usually only a light bandage is required, with one bandage change in the week after surgery. The horse should be confined to a box stall for the first 2 to 3 weeks after surgery, followed by a larger yard for 2 to 3 weeks, before being turned out to pasture. The degree of rest required after surgery will show great variation. In horses with small chips and little cartilage erosion, a return to training is possible within 2 weeks of surgery. However, the latter situation cannot be regarded as good practice and has generally been used when the horse has an important race scheduled soon after surgery. Generally, a minimum rest period of 3 months is given, but with more severe cartilage erosion, rest of at least 6 months is required.

- Where extensive cartilage erosion has been found at the time of surgery, it is worthwhile to consider the intraarticular administration of polysulfated glycosaminoglycans (Treatment No. 90). Three treatments are given at weekly intervals, and the first injection usually is left until 2 weeks after surgery because problems have been encountered with isolated cases of septic arthritis following intraarticular use of polysulfated glycosaminoglycans administered in the first 5 to 10 days after surgery. The reason for the infection is not clear, but experimental studies have shown that when a subclinical number of bacteria are placed in the joint together with polysulfated glycosaminoglycans, clinical septic arthritis is more likely than with other medications. For this reason, it would appear to be prudent to delay this intraarticular medication for at least 2 weeks after surgery.
- If there is a slab fracture of the third carpal bone, internal fixation with a cortical bone screw is required. In many cases, this can be accomplished using a stab incision over the dorsal aspect of the third carpal bone and visualization of the fracture line using the arthroscope. A cortical bone screw, usually 4.5 mm in diameter, is inserted using the principle of lag-screw fixation.
- Fractures of the accessory carpal bone are usually longitudinal and are best treated conservatively with 6 to 9 months of rest. However, some cases may require internal fixation. This is quite difficult because the bone is curved.
- Sagittal fracture of the third carpal bone is rare and difficult to treat. It is not possible with these fractures to use internal fixation. However, with rest periods of up to 6 months, the fracture may heal. If the horse is kept in training because the fracture fails to be diagnosed initially, the prognosis for successful healing is poor. Rarefaction often is found on subsequent radiographs, and the fracture never shows satisfactory signs of healing.

Epiphysitis

Epiphysitis is a condition involving the growth plates of various bones of young horses. It mainly affects the distal radial growth plate in weanlings and yearlings. In most cases it is a result of feeding a high-grain diet with a low ratio of calcium to phosphorus and too high an energy content.

History and Presenting Signs

- Commonly seen in foals and weanlings from 4 to 5 months of age
- Some cases are found in thoroughbred yearlings during early phases of training.
- Swellings around the distal radial growth plate and the distal metacarpal growth plates are the most common presenting sign.
- In some cases, horses may be presented because of lameness. However, this is uncommon.

Clinical Findings and Diagnosis

- Swelling at the site of the growth plate in the distal radius is the most obvious sign. This swelling is usually bilateral.
- There may be pain on palpation over the affected growth plates.
- Radiographs will show a variety of changes in the region of the epiphysis and metaphysis. Most common findings include flaring of the metaphysis, sclerosis of bone immediately adjacent to the epiphysis, and in some cases an irregular and lytic appearance of the physis.

Differential Diagnosis

- Carpitis
- Carpal chip fractures
- Extensor tendon sheath synovitis
- Trauma to the distal radius
- Carpal valgus deformity (may coexist with epiphysitis)

Treatment

- Analysis of the diet is important and may reveal inadequate calcium or a calcium–phosphorus ratio that is too low. Computer programs such as the *Equine Nutritionist* (Nsquared, Silverton, Oregon) are available and allow comprehensive dietary analyses, comparing results with recommended National Research Council (NRC) values.
- Correction of this relative calcium deficiency using calcium carbonate or decreasing the amount of grain in the diet may be useful.
- Excessive energy intake appears to contribute to epiphysitis, particularly in yearlings. Therefore, decreasing the energy intake is of use in treatment.

Hygroma of the Carpus and Extensor Tendon Sheath Synovitis

Hygroma of the carpus is a large, fluid-filled subcutaneous swelling on the dorsal aspect of the carpus, usually resulting from direct trauma. Although unsightly, it rarely causes lameness. Extensor tendon sheath synovitis causes a similar swelling, although it is confined to the tendon sheath of the extensor carpi radialis.

KEY POINT ► Usually, neither of these problems causes significant lameness.

History and Presenting Signs

- Usually found in showjumping and eventing horses
- History of trauma to the dorsal carpus and distal radius
- Considerable swelling of the carpal region without significant lameness

Clinical Findings and Diagnosis

- A gross swelling, from the size of a golf ball up to that of a tennis ball or larger, is the most obvious sign.
- Palpation of the swelling indicates that it is fluid-filled. In cases of hygroma of the carpus, the swelling is diffuse and usually localized to the dorsal carpus. However, in cases of extensor tendon sheath synovitis, the extensor carpi radialis sheath is affected, with obvious fluid distension evident over the distal part of the tendon, which inserts on the proximal aspect of the third metacarpal bone.
- Usually there is no pain on palpation or flexion of the carpus, although invariably there is some restriction to the degree of flexion.
- Radiographs should be taken to ensure that there is no involvement of the carpal bones. In some cases there may be a coexisting carpitis with evidence of new periosteal bone formation.
- If there is any doubt, a needle can be inserted at the lowest point of the swelling to aspirate some fluid.

Differential Diagnosis

- Extensor tendon sheath synovitis
- Carpitis
- Carpal fractures
- Trauma to the medial tuberosity of the distal radius

Treatment

KEY POINT ► The only worthwhile treatment is surgical drainage of the fluid, insertion of a Penrose drain, and application of a pressure bandage.

- The Penrose drain is inserted via two stab incisions at the most proximal and distal aspects of the fluid swelling. The drains are fixed in place with a single suture in the skin, and a sterile dressing is applied.
- This treatment is indicated both in hygroma of the carpus and extensor tendon sheath synovitis. While the extensor carpi radialis is the most common tendon sheath involved in extensor tendon sheath synovitis, the common extensor tendon is occasionally involved.
- The Penrose drain should remain in place for 5 to 7 days, being removed when there is no evidence of fluid discharge from the distal drainage site. Initially, a daily bandage change is required, but after 2 to 3 days, this can be every other day if the amount of fluid discharge has reduced.
- Drainage of the fluid and injection of various corticosteroids are used by some practitioners but are generally not useful because the fluid will recur.

Nonspecific Carpal Lameness

A small proportion of horses presented with lameness will have no localizing signs on examination, but with sequential nerve blocks, the problem is localized to the carpus. The majority of horses in this group will become sound after intraarticular local anesthesia of the middle carpal joint.

KEY POINT ► Horses with nonspecific carpal lameness are difficult to manage, particularly because radiography may reveal few, if any, abnormalities.

History and Presenting Signs

■ Unilateral forelimb lameness
■ No obvious swelling in the affected leg

Clinical Findings and Diagnosis

■ Lameness may vary from moderate to severe.
■ In some cases, there may be signs of effusion involving the middle or proximal carpal joints, although our experience is that it is more common to have no or minimal abnormalities on clinical examination.
■ In the majority, but far from all cases, there is pain on extreme flexion of the carpus and a positive response to a carpal flexion test.
■ Often a detailed examination will reveal no localizing signs, despite the horse showing signs of lameness at the trot.

KEY POINT ► Intraarticular local anesthesia results in the horse becoming sound. Most commonly this occurs after introducing local anesthetic into the middle carpal joint.

■ Radiographs of the carpus (including skyline views) usually do not show anything of consequence.
■ In some cases, diagnostic arthroscopy is helpful to define whether or not there is gross evidence of intraarticular pathology, which may not be apparent on radiographic examination.
■ Because intraarticular local anesthesia of the middle carpal joint also blocks pain in the distal carpal (carpometacarpal) joint, it is important to evaluate this joint carefully on radiographs.

Differential Diagnosis

■ Chip, slab, or sagittal fractures of one of the carpal bones
■ Lesions involving the distal carpal joint, including possible soft-tissue lesions at the palmar aspect of the proximal metacarpus.

Treatment

■ Because a precise diagnosis is seldom possible, it is difficult to provide effective therapy. Because of this, if further diagnostic tests (bone scans, arthroscopy) are not performed, symptomatic treatment involving intraarticular medication is the only possibility for therapy, apart from resting the horse.
■ If the radiographs reveal no fracture lines or indication of joint disease, the treatment of choice is the use of intraarticular sodium hyaluronate (Treatment No. 60) and/or intraarticular corticosteroids. The intraarticular corticosteroids that are most effective are betamethasone acetate (Treatment No. 12) and methylprednisolone acetate (Treatment No. 74).

KEY POINT ► To ensure that there are no intraarticular lesions, diagnostic arthroscopy is worthwhile.

■ Occasionally, a fracture will be found on arthroscopy despite no abnormal radiographic findings. Other findings may include localized, severe cartilage erosion, and tearing of the palmar carpal ligament, which can be demonstrated at the palmar aspect of the third carpal bone. This ligament attaches from the palmar aspect of the third carpal bone to the radial and intermediate carpal bones. We have noted that many horses with carpal lameness have no other lesions on arthroscopy apart from tearing of this ligament. We presume that the ligament tearing leads to instability of the joint.
■ In many horses with nonspecific carpal lameness, we have found nothing significant on arthroscopic examination, and horses have remained lame despite intraarticular medication and prolonged rest periods.
■ Nonspecific carpal lameness is a frustrating condition with which to deal.

Trauma to the Medial Tuberosity of the Distal Radius

This is a condition, most commonly found in standardbred pacers, in which one forefoot traumatizes the skin and soft tissue over the medial tuberosity of the distal radius. Most trainers describe this as the horse "getting on the knee." Horses with this problem will usually have a "toe out" or "penguin-toed" conformation. For this reason, many pacers will wear "knee boots."

History and Presenting Signs

■ Swelling noted by trainer or owner over the medial aspect of the distal radius
■ Lameness is unusual in this disorder.
■ Horses are occasionally presented with a "big knee."

Clinical Findings and Diagnosis

■ Swelling over the medial aspect of the distal radius is quite apparent, and there will be pain on palpation.

KEY POINT ► In most cases the horse is not lame. If the condition is chronic, there may be extensive soft-tissue swelling over the medial tuberosity of the distal radius.

- Radiographs are not usually necessary and reveal only soft-tissue swelling. However, if there is any lameness or significant pain on palpation or flexion of the carpus, a full series of radiographs should be taken.

Differential Diagnosis

- Distal radial fractures
- Hygroma of the carpus
- Chip fractures of the proximal carpal joint

Treatment

- Local anti-inflammatory measures are usually all that is required to resolve some of the swelling. These measures include cold hosing, cold packs, and locally applied dimethylsulfoxide (DMSO, Treatment No. 34).
- If extensive swelling is present, a 7-day course of phenylbutazone (Treatment No. 88) may be necessary.
- To prevent further trauma, the use of a "knee boot" during training should be advised.

KEY POINT ► Corrective shoeing, with the application of square-toe shoes on the front feet, will help by enforcing breakover at the toe. Pacers and trotters should be exercised wearing "knee boots."

Valgus or Varus Deformity of the Carpus

KEY POINT ► Valgus deviation of the carpus is the most common limb deformity in growing foals and results in deviation of the third metacarpal bone away from an imaginary line drawn through the midline of the limb viewed from in front of the foal.

The opposite of this (carpus varus) is less common, although it more frequently affects the fetlock. One of the main etiologic factors is uneven forces on the growth plate of the distal radius. In the case of carpus valgus, there is faster growth on the medial aspect of the growth plate than on the lateral aspect and hence an apparent medial deviation of the carpus with resultant lateral deviation of the limb distal to the carpus. The condition is usually found in young, rapidly growing foals. Where the condition is apparent immediately after birth, the limb deviation may be due to abnormal limb position in utero.

History and Presenting Signs

- Owner or studfarm manager notices that the foal's forelimb(s) show progressive deviation with the foal appearing more "knock kneed."

- Usually first noticed when the foal is around 1 month of age but in some cases (particularly premature foals) may be apparent shortly after birth.
- In cases that are obvious soon after the foal stands, the appearance of the limbs will often improve considerably over the first week of life as the foal develops better muscle tone.

Clinical Findings and Diagnosis

- The deviation of the limb is apparent, although in some cases it initially may be quite mild.
- Radiographs are essential to enable an accurate diagnosis. The most important radiographic view is the dorsopalmar. This allows determination of whether the deviation is occurring as a result of malformation of the carpal bones (common in premature foals) or is due to abnormalities in the distal radial growth plate. The latter problem has a much better prognosis than the former. The source of the deviation can be determined by drawing lines down the long axes of the radius and third metacarpal bones. The lines intersect at the major source of the limb deviation.

Differential Diagnosis

- Carpal bone hypoplasia
- Mild conformation faults

Treatment

- If the deformity is mild, restriction of movement together with corrective trimming of the hoof may be all that is required. The medial aspect of the hoof wall is usually worn, and therefore, the lateral side may be trimmed, but not excessively.
- In more severe cases, slowing of growth of the medial side or increasing the growth on the lateral side of the distal radial growth plate is necessary. This should be performed before the foal is 4 months of age in order for sufficient "catch-up" growth to occur on the lateral aspect of the limb.
- Slowing of growth of the medial aspect of the radial growth plate may be achieved in several ways. Internal fixation with cortical bone screws inserted either side of the growth plate and a figure of eight wire to exert compression is effective. Because growth is slowed on the medial aspect of the distal radial growth plate, the lateral side can catch up, and the limb straightens. It is essential to remove the implants prior to limb straightening. If the implants are left in until the limb straightens, there can be overcorrection of the problem so that a varus carpal deformity results. The screw and wire technique was commonly used, or staples, but is now reserved for cases that do not respond to periosteal stripping.

KEY POINT ► Periosteal "stripping," i.e., elevation of a T-shaped portion of periosteum over the lateral aspect of the distal radial growth plate, has been shown to be effective in increasing growth on the lateral side of the forelimb, where the deviation is the result of growth problems originating in the distal radial growth plate.

■ Periosteal stripping is ineffective if the deviation is due to malformation of the carpal bones. The best results with periosteal stripping occur when the surgery is performed before the foal is 3 months of age because the most rapid growth rate occurs up to this time, and this provides an opportunity for the limb to return to a normal conformation. There are few risks with surgery for periosteal stripping, and it is interesting that the limb will correct but not overcorrect, such as when using the screw and wire technique. The periosteal stripping technique also gives better cosmetic results than the staple or screw and wire technique.

Carpal Collapse or Carpal Bone Hypoplasia

Carpal collapse is a problem noted most frequently in premature foals and results from the foals placing abnormal stresses on the carpal bones before the bones are properly developed. Similar problems can be encountered in the tarsus. The foal usually presents with a carpus valgus or carpus varus deformity.

History and Presenting Signs

■ Foal born prematurely
■ Limb deviation apparent shortly after birth
■ If the expected birth date is not known, there is usually a history of excessive laxity of the flexor tendons for several days after birth.

Clinical Findings and Diagnosis

■ Deviation of the forelimbs is common.
■ The most common deviation in foals with carpal bone hypoplasia is carpus valgus (see p. 105).
■ Dorsopalmar radiographs should be taken of both carpi to evaluate the shape of the carpal bones.
■ Longitudinal lines drawn through the long axes of the third metacarpal bone and the radius will indicate that the site of the deviation is the carpus.

Differential Diagnosis

■ Angular limb deformities arising primarily from the distal radial growth plate
■ Malformation of the second or fourth metacarpal bones

Treatment

■ Because of the asymmetrical loading of the distal radial growth plate, there is usually compression of one side of the growth plate. Because the defect originates within the carpus, the prognosis with any form of treatment is poor.

■ The medial side of the distal radial growth plate grows comparatively more quickly than the lateral side, resulting in a carpus valgus deformity, which requires treatment.
■ The treatment of choice is transphyseal bridging using a screw and wire technique.

References

Bertone, A. L., Schneiter, H. L., Turner, A. S., and Shoemaker, R. S.: Pancarpal arthrodesis for treatment of carpal collapse in the adult horse: A report of two cases. Vet. Surg. 18:353, 1989.
French, D. A., Barber, S. M., Leach, D. H., and Doige, C. E.: The effect of exercise on the healing of articular cartilage defects in the equine carpus. Vet. Surg. 18:312, 1989.
Goodman, N. L., and Baker, B. K.: Lameness diagnosis and treatment in the quarter horse racehorse. Vet. Clin. North Am. (Equine Pract.) 6:85, 1990.
Martin, G. S., Haynes, P. F., and McClure, J. R.: Effect of third carpal slab fracture and repair on racing performance in thoroughbred horses: 31 cases (1977–1984). J. Am. Vet. Med. Assoc. 193:107, 1988.
McIlwraith, C. W., Yovich, J. V., and Martin, G. S.: Arthroscopic surgery for the treatment of osteochondral chip fractures in the equine carpus. J. Am. Vet. Med. Assoc. 191:531, 1987.

FOREARM AND ELBOW PROBLEMS
Fractures of the Radius

Radial fractures are most commonly found in foals and yearlings. Such fractures are due to direct trauma such as kicks and usually occur when horses are run in herds. The long-term prognosis for athletic function in horses with radial fractures is very poor, and owners should be advised of this before treatment is commenced. Most fractures are midshaft and require referral to a specialist center for application of one or two bone plates. There is a prolonged hospitalization time, up to several months, and the attempted internal fixation of these fractures should only be undertaken in valuable animals that have some breeding future.

History and Presenting Signs

■ Most horses are usually unable to bear weight on the affected leg.
■ It is uncommon for the traumatic event to be seen by anyone on the stud farm, and there may be no external signs of trauma.

Differential Diagnosis

■ Fracture of the humerus or ulna
■ Fracture of carpal bones

Diagnosis and Treatment

- Non-weight-bearing lameness indicates the likelihood of a long bone fracture.
- There may be some degree of swelling over the midradius, but this is not always the case.
- Close examination of the forearm reveals crepitus to be present on palpation and manipulation of the limb.
- Because penetration of part of the fractured bone through the skin will result in a much worse prognosis, it is important to establish early if the fracture is compound.

KEY POINT ► If the horse requires transport to a facility to take radiographs for further evaluation, the limb should be immobilized as effectively as possible.

- In general, the use of splints is contraindicated because these usually slip and may result in the fracture becoming compound by acting as a fulcrum. A Robert Jones bandage (see Chap. 17), using three to four rolls of cotton wool, provides the best immobilization. This bandage should be applied as far proximally on the forearm as possible.
- Anteroposterior and lateral radiographs are essential to determine the type of fracture present.
- In horses of low economic value, more distal fractures of the radius may be successfully treated by external immobilization alone.

KEY POINT ► However, the treatment of choice is internal fixation using two bone plates placed on the craniomedial and craniolateral aspects of the radius.

- Following internal fixation, a cast (see Casting, Chap. 17) is applied during the initial convalescent period.
- In adult horses, the prognosis for successful healing of radial fractures is very poor, and surgery is best attempted in foals and weanlings.

Fractures of the Ulna

Fractures of the ulna are usually the result of kicks and therefore are more commonly found in horses running in herds. While the fractures cause dramatic clinical signs, the prognosis for full athletic recovery is excellent, particularly if the fracture does not involve the elbow joint. In foals, physeal fractures of the olecranon tuberosity are quite common.

History and Presenting Signs

- Acute history of non-weight-bearing lameness
- Presented with a "dropped elbow" appearance

Clinical Findings and Diagnosis

- Limited or no weight bearing on the affected leg is a typical sign.

- There is a "dropped elbow" appearance to the leg, with the horse unable to extend the elbow.
- Fractures involving the elbow joint usually result in signs of more pain and reluctance to bear weight compared with fractures not involving the joint.
- Examination of the elbow region usually will show limited swelling and pain on palpation. In some cases, crepitus may be detected.
- A lateral radiographic view is most important for diagnosis. Because there may be considerable distraction of the proximal fragment, it is important to ensure that the radiographic field includes the area up to 15 cm (6 in) proximal to the elbow joint.

Differential Diagnosis

- Fracture of the proximal radius
- Fracture of the distal humerus
- Radial nerve paralysis

Treatment

- Horses that can bear some weight on the affected limb may have undistracted fractures of the ulna not involving the elbow joint. These fractures often heal with stall rest alone, and activity needs to be restricted for 2 to 3 months.
- If the fracture is distracted or involves the joint, internal fixation provides the best results. Using the tension-band principle, a bone plate is placed along the caudal border of the olecranon and ulna. If the proximal fragment is displaced some distance proximally, reduction of the fracture can be difficult.
- The prognosis for ulnar fractures is quite good, even in cases where there is severe distraction of the proximal fragment. However, where there has been involvement of the elbow joint in the fracture, there may be secondary degenerative joint disease that may result in a chronic, low-grade lameness.
- Physeal fractures in foals have a good prognosis, unless there is a Salter II type fracture with involvement of the elbow joint.

Hygroma of the Elbow ("Shoe Boil")

Hygroma of the elbow is a fluid-filled subcutaneous swelling at the point of the elbow. It results from trauma and may be due to the shoe hitting the elbow when the horse is lying down. Hence the lay term for the condition is "shoe boil." It is also referred to as "capped elbow." If the condition is chronic, there may be extensive fibrous tissue formation rather than simple fluid accumulation.

History and Presenting Signs

- Usually found in horses kept in stables
- Obvious swelling over the point of the elbow noted by owner or trainer

Clinical Findings and Diagnosis

- A fluid-filled, nonpainful swelling on the point of the elbow is pathognomic.
- This condition does not cause the horse any problems and is merely a cosmetic blemish.

KEY POINT ▶ Lameness is not a feature of this condition, and if lameness is found, it is likely to be due to problems at an additional site.

- Radiographs are not necessary unless the area is painful on palpation.

Differential Diagnosis

- Fractures of the ulna
- Soft-tissue trauma/foreign-body penetration
- Damage to tendon of triceps brachii muscle

Treatment

- Surgical drainage and insertion of a Penrose drain are the only effective treatments (see Hygroma of the Carpus, p. 103).
- In chronic cases there may be extensive scar-tissue formation. Surgical resection of the entire mass is the only possibility if a cosmetic result is desired. However, because of the location of the surgical site, wound breakdown is common. Tension sutures, using buttons, are helpful, and a Robert Jones bandage (see Chap. 17), applied from the foot up to the proximal part of the forearm, prevents elbow flexion.

Intraarticular Elbow Lameness

Lameness arising from the elbow joint is very uncommon. A survey of our records at the University of Sydney Equine Clinic showed that over a 16-year period, only three horses were confirmed as having an intraarticular problem of the elbow resulting in lameness. However, in lamenesses that do not block out in the distal limb, the possibility of an elbow joint problem should not be discounted. Fortunately, intraarticular anesthesia of the elbow joint is very simple, allowing a definitive diagnosis to be made.

History and Presenting Signs

- Usually a chronic forelimb lameness
- Lameness thought to be in the shoulder or foot because no swelling is present anywhere in the affected limb

Clinical Findings and Diagnosis

- Chronic, low-grade unilateral forelimb lameness is typically found.
- A careful clinical examination of the affected leg may not reveal any swelling, heat, or pain.
- Regional anesthesia commencing at the foot and ascending proximally to the carpus does not result in improvement in gait.
- Lameness is abolished after desensitizing the elbow joint (see p. 62).
- Radiographs may not reveal any abnormalities in the joint. In some cases, there are changes involving the anconeal process of the ulna, with joint irregularity and spur formation. These changes may only be found on a flexed lateral view of the elbow joint.

Differential Diagnosis

- Problems involving the shoulder joint
- Rupture of the medial collateral ligament of the elbow joint

Treatment

- Intraarticular medications (see Degenerative Joint Disease) may result in temporary alleviation of the clinical signs. However, the prognosis for athletic soundness in horses with intraarticular elbow lameness is very poor.
- Arthroscopy of the elbow joint is possible and may be helpful in establishing a diagnosis if no radiographic changes are evident.

References

Denny, H. R., Barr, A. R. S., and Waterman, A.: Surgical treatment of fractures of the olecranon in the horse: A comparative review of 25 cases. *Equine Vet. J.* 19:319, 1987.

Nixon, A.: Arthroscopic approaches and intraarticular anatomy of the equine elbow. *Vet. Surg.* 19:93, 1990.

Sanders, S. M., Bramlage, S. R., and Gable, A. A.: Radius fractures in the horse: A retrospective study of 47 cases. *Equine Vet. J.* 18:432, 1986.

Wilson, D. G., and Riedesel, E.: Nonsurgical management of ulnar fractures in the horse: A retrospective study of 43 cases. *Vet. Surg.* 14:283, 1985.

SHOULDER PROBLEMS

Shoulder lameness is quite uncommon in horses. However, it is a favorite diagnosis of horse trainers and owners as well as those involved in chiropractic manipulation of horses. The difficulty often lies in convincing the client that the problem does not originate in the shoulder but is elsewhere in the leg. This is particularly so in horses with navicular disease. Soft-tissue injuries may occur in the muscles around the shoulder, and we have seen such problems most commonly in endurance horses that have been ridden over difficult and slippery terrain.

KEY POINT ▶ In many shoulder problems, there are no localizing signs on clinical examination, and unless the problem is intraarticular, it may be difficult to establish a definitive diagnosis.

Intraarticular problems are easily diagnosed by depositing local anesthetic into the shoulder joint. The technique for intraarticular anesthesia of the shoulder is not difficult and in the majority of horses is well tolerated.

In cases where there is a suspicion of a shoulder problem, a careful examination of the shoulder should be carried out. Flexion, extension, and abduction of the shoulder should be performed to determine whether there is any restriction of movement or pain. Particular note should be paid to the muscles around the shoulder for signs of atrophy and pain on palpation. In some conditions, applying flexion to the shoulder joint for 1 minute and trotting the horse off may accentuate the lameness.

Bicipital Bursitis

The bicipital bursa is interposed between the tendon of the biceps brachii and the head of the humerus. Because the bursa is situated over the point of the shoulder, it is subjected to trauma, resulting in a bursitis. Occasionally, the same injury may result in damage to the suprascapular nerve. On rare occasions, the bicipital bursa may become infected with *Brucella abortus* via a similar mechanism to that for fistulous withers.

History and Presenting Signs

- Low-grade lameness found after a history of trauma to the shoulder
- Lameness without any evidence of swelling or heat in the leg

Clinical Findings and Diagnosis

- An acute forelimb lameness with evidence of marked lifting of the head is a good indicator of shoulder lameness.
- Circumduction of the leg also may be seen as the limb is advanced. In most cases, pain can be elicited by palpation over the bicipital bursa.
- Attempts are made to restrict the movement of the shoulder joint. This is quite noticeable during walking.

Differential Diagnosis

- Sweeney
- Fractures of the scapula
- Fractures of the humerus
- Osteochrondritis dissecans (OCD) of the shoulder

Treatment

- Rest for 3 to 4 weeks is most important to allow the inflammatory response to resolve. A course of phenylbutazone (Treatment No. 88) for 7 to 10 days is also useful in aiding resolution.
- Topical treatment with dimethylsulfoxide (DMSO, Treatment No. 34) is useful.

Fractures of the Humerus

Fractures of the humerus are not as common as other long bone fractures and have a slightly better prognosis because of the success of conservative treatment. Humeral fractures are most commonly associated with falling but may be due to direct trauma such as a kick from another horse. Because the course of the radial nerve is intimately associated with the humerus, any possible damage must be assessed before treatment is commenced.

History and Presenting Signs

- Non-weight-bearing lameness of the affected leg
- "Dropped elbow" appearance of the leg

Clinical Findings and Diagnosis

- In many cases there is swelling over the fracture site and abrasion of the skin.
- The degree of "dropped elbow" appearance will depend on the extent of the fracture displacement and overriding of the major fracture fragments.
- Crepitus may be difficult to detect in many humeral fractures.
- If a fracture is suspected, excessive manipulation of the leg should be avoided because trauma to the radial nerve is a possibility.
- Radiographs should be taken, and these may require general anesthesia. This could be difficult because the fracture may be worsened during recovery. Therefore, if adequate radiographs cannot be taken with the horse conscious, it may be better to postpone radiographs until the time of surgery.

Differential Diagnosis

- Fracture of the olecranon
- Fracture of the scapula
- Radial nerve paralysis

Treatment

- In some humeral fractures, confining the horse to a box stall is sufficient to result in fracture healing. This is so because many fractures of the humerus are spiral and will heal satisfactorily because of the support of the large muscle mass when the horse does not bear weight on the leg. The healing that results may not produce a horse that is athletically sound, but it may be sound for breeding purposes.
- If there is fracture displacement, the horse should be immobilized in a sling. An alternative is partial immobilization in a tank of warm saline to reduce the weight on the affected and unaffected legs. The problem with this technique is that there is substantial loss of calcium because of the reduced weight on the skeleton.
- In foals, it may be possible to partially immobilize the humerus by bandaging the upper part of

the forearm to the thorax. The main complication in foals is the development of various angular limb deformities. For this reason, fracture repair can be attempted and successful repair has been reported using two bone plates.

■ Because of the increased weight borne by the un-affected forelimb, there are many cases where rotation of the distal phalanx occurs due to a mechanical laminitis. It is important to support the unaffected limb using a Robert Jones bandage (see Chap. 17) and to apply corrective shoeing if signs of distal phalanx rotation occur.

Fractures of the Scapula

The majority of fractures of the scapula that we have seen have been due to falls. However, direct blows to the shoulder also may produce scapular fractures. Fractures are mostly simple and usually involve the supraglenoid tubercle and the glenoid cavity. Occasionally, the spine of the scapula will fracture, and in rare cases, there will be comminution, usually involving the neck of the scapula.

History and Presenting Signs

■ History of direct trauma is usual.
■ Horses may present with mild lameness or, in severe comminuted fractures, may present unable to bear weight on the affected leg.

Clinical Findings and Diagnosis

■ Fractures of the scapular spine may result in mild lameness. However, fractures involving the glenoid cavity that result in a nonunion usually produce a more severe lameness.
■ Palpation around the shoulder joint usually reveals pain, and there may be pain on flexion of the shoulder.
■ Because the suprascapular nerve may be involved in scapular fractures, there may be signs of atrophy of the supraspinatus and infraspinatus muscles.
■ Fracture of the scapula is confirmed by radiography, which must be performed under general anesthesia.

Differential Diagnosis

■ Suprascapular nerve paralysis
■ Fractures of the proximal humerus

Treatment

KEY POINT ▶ Many fractures of the scapula will heal sufficiently well with box stall rest to permit pasture soundness. We have seen one Standardbred horse with a fracture of the glenoid cavity return to successful racing, despite a nonunion, muscle atrophy, and moderate lameness.

■ Comminuted fractures with a lot of displacement have a poor prognosis, and it may be necessary to attempt to place horses with these fractures in a sling.
■ Some fractures involving the neck of the scapula in foals can be repaired by internal fixation using bone plates.
■ Fractures of the supraglenoid tubercle are difficult to repair successfully. While these fractures often will heal, the pull of the biceps brachii results in displacement of the fragment and, therefore, long-term mechanical restriction of limb movement. However, horses with this fracture have a good prognosis for pasture soundness.

Osteochondrosis Dissecans of the Shoulder Joint

Osteochondrosis dissecans (OCD) of the shoulder is a condition that causes a severe lameness in yearling or 2-year-old horses. It generally involves the head of the humerus toward the caudal limit of the scapulohumeral joint. More details on OCD are given in the section on general musculoskeletal problems (p. 129). Shoulder joint OCD is the most common form of shoulder lameness in young thoroughbred horses.

History and Presenting Signs

■ Yearling or 2-year-old horse with moderate lameness
■ Lameness usually noted at the walk as well as at the trot

Clinical Findings and Diagnosis

■ The clinical signs are very similar to those for bicipital bursitis except that in most cases there is no pain on palpation of the shoulder.
■ Some horses with OCD become severely lame and in severe cases may be such that a long bone fracture could be considered. In the majority of cases, lameness can be seen at the walk.
■ Some horses with localized OCD lesions, particularly involving the caudal region of the humeral head, may have a history of low-grade, intermittent lameness.
■ Diagnosis is aided by intraarticular local anesthesia (see p. 63) because all horses with OCD of the shoulder will show dramatic improvement of lameness afterwards.
■ Radiographs are necessary to determine the extent of the lesion(s) and the prognosis. These should be performed under general anesthesia. Contrast arthrography of the shoulder joint can be useful to delineate smaller lesions involving the articular surface.
■ Because the opposite shoulder joint also may be affected, radiographic examination of the unaffected shoulder also should be performed.

Differential Diagnosis

- Bicipital bursitis
- Fractures of the scapula
- Fractures of the humerus
- Shoulder muscle injuries

Treatment

- Rest is often a worthwhile treatment, and in cases where there are small lesions, healing may be complete in 9 to 12 months.
- In cases where the lesions are extensive, severe arthritis may be a secondary result and cause chronic lameness.
- Arthroscopic surgery of the shoulder joint enables visualization of the joint surface and permits removal of loose fragments and curettage of the damaged articular surface.
- Where the lesions are quite localized, the prognosis following arthroscopic surgery is very good, and horses will return to successful athletic endeavors after 6 to 12 months of rest.
- The use of intra-articular polysulfated glycosaminoglycans (Treatment No. 90) at weekly intervals for 3 weeks may be helpful where there is evidence of cartilage erosion.

Sweeney (Suprascapular Nerve Damage)

Sweeney is the term used to describe atrophy of the supraspinatus and infraspinatus muscles due to paralysis of the suprascapular nerve. Most cases result from trauma to the point of the shoulder, although it is possible that damage to the nerve can arise because of the nerve being stretched. This could occur if the shoulder joint were suddenly thrust caudally.

History and Presenting Signs

- In the chronic cases, atrophy is clearly visible.
- The shoulder can "pop" outward when the horse places weight on the affected leg.

Clinical Findings and Diagnosis

- In early cases, prior to visible atrophy of the affected muscles, outward movement of the shoulder joint can be seen when the horse takes weight on the leg.

KEY POINT ► Atrophy of the supraspinatus and infraspinatus muscles is readily apparent after several weeks, and the spine of the scapula becomes more prominent. This is the classical clinical sign of suprascapular nerve damage.

- With sweeney, there may be acute lameness immediately after the injury that improves after 7 to 10 days.
- Radiographs may be taken to ensure that there are no bony lesions.

Differential Diagnosis

- Myopathies
- Disuse atrophy

Treatment

- Most cases of sweeney do not improve even with prolonged rest.
- The use of intraarticular corticosteroids (Treatment Nos. 12 and 74) has been reported to yield good results in some cases of chronic sweeney.

KEY POINT ► Surgery to free the suprascapular nerve is the treatment of choice, and while a large case series has not been reported in the veterinary literature, complete recoveries have been noted in individual cases.

- After the nerve has been dissected free of any scar tissue, a wedge of bone is removed from underneath the nerve. The bone removed should be no more than 1.5 cm² (0.5 in²), because fractures of the scapula have occurred during recovery when larger sections were removed.
- Immediate improvement and return of function to the suprascapular nerve do not take place. However, improvement usually occurs over a period of 4 to 6 months.

References

Adams, S. B., and Blevins, W. E.: Shoulder lameness in horses, part I. *Compend. Contin. Educ. Pract. Vet.* 11:64, 1989.
Adams, S. B., and Blevins, W. E.: Shoulder lameness in horses, part II. *Compend. Contin. Educ. Pract. Vet.* 11:191, 1989.
Bertone, A. L., and McIlwraith, C. W.: Arthroscopic surgical approaches and intraarticular anatomy of the equine shoulder joint. *Vet. Surg.* 16:312, 1987.
Bertone, A. L., and McIlwraith, C. W.: Osteochondrosis of the equine shoulder: Treatment with arthroscopic surgery. *Proc. 33rd Conv. Am. Assoc. Equine Pract.*, p. 683, 1987.
Dyson, S.: Shoulder lameness in horses: An analysis of 58 suspected cases. *Equine Vet. J.* 18:29, 1986.
Miller, R. M., and Dresher, L. K.: Treatment of equine shoulder sweeny with intraarticular corticosteroids. *Vet. Med. Small Anim. Clin.* 72:1077, 1977.

Hindlimb Abnormalities

Injuries to the foot, pastern, fetlock, and metatarsus are similar to those found at equivalent sites in the forelimb. Hindlimb injuries are less common than those in the forelimb and account for approximately 20% of musculoskeletal problems in thoroughbreds and 40% in standardbreds. Acute hindleg problems are generally due to problems in the distal limb, such as subsolar (hoof) abscesses, phalangeal fractures, and fractures of the sesamoid bones. Unlike foreleg lameness, which many owners and trainers are aware of, hindleg lameness may remain undetected. Horses with chronic, low-grade hindleg lameness may be presented for performance problems rather than specific lameness.

Details of the examination procedure are outlined in the introductory section (p. 000). However, there are a few additional points about examining horses for hindleg lameness.

1. In chronic lameness, gluteal muscle atrophy is common and can be viewed standing directly behind the horse. This is an important sign of chronic upper (hock or above) hindleg problems.

2. The nerve distribution in the distal hindleg appears to be more variable than in the foreleg. This results in some nerve blocks (particularly the plantar digital) being less reliable and more difficult than in the foreleg.

3. Unless there is a distal limb problem, there may be few localizing signs (e.g., heat, swelling, pain) to indicate where the problem is located. For this reason, intraarticular local anesthesia of the hock and stifle is very important to enable a diagnosis to be established.

4. In a chronic, low-grade hindleg lameness, the hock is likely to be the site of the problem in more than 80% of cases.

HOCK AND TIBIA PROBLEMS

Bog Spavin (Tarsal Hydrarthrosis)

"Bog spavin" is the common name given to distension of the tarsocrural (tibiotarsal) joint with synovial fluid. The tarsocrural joint capsule extends from the dorsomedial aspect of the joint, where the saphenous vein overlies it, to the lateral aspect of the hock. In cases of distension, the joint can contain more than 100 ml of synovial fluid. Bog spavin is chiefly a cosmetic problem, but because osteochondritis dissecans also can present with similar features, radiographs of the hock should always be taken. The cause of the condition is unknown.

History and Presenting Signs

- Usually found in young horses
- Horses are usually presented because of gross swelling over the dorsomedial aspect of the hock.

Clinical Findings and Diagnosis

- Despite the degree of distension of the joint capsule, horses with bog spavin do not show signs of lameness.
- The fluid can be demonstrated to move from the medial to lateral aspects of the joint by palpation over the distended dorsomedial joint capsule.
- There is no heat or pain on palpation.
- Radiographs (lateral and oblique views) should be taken to ensure that there are no chip fractures from the talus or OCD lesions. It is particularly important to examine the area of the intermediate ridge on the radiographs because small OCD lesions in this location can easily be missed.
- Synovial fluid examination is not necessary, but if a sample is taken, it will reveal low protein content (<20 g/L or 2.0 g/dL) and low cell count (<400 × 10^6/L or 400/μL).

Differential Diagnosis

- Tarsal chip fractures
- Thoroughpin
- Osteochondrosis dissecans (OCD)

Treatment

- Bog spavin requires no treatment, because the condition does not interfere with function.
- Because it is cosmetically undesirable, many clients request treatment.
- Although a variety of treatments have been tried, none has been successful.

KEY POINT ▶ The most useful treatment consists of draining the excess synovial fluid from the tarsocrural joint (see Fig. 3-44) and injecting 200 to 250 mg of medroxyprogesterone acetate (Treatment No. 70) intraarticularly.

- The treatment has an antisecretory effect on synovia and will be successful in some but by no means all cases. A pressure bandage similar to a Robert-Jones bandage (see Chap. 17) is then applied to the leg to attempt to prevent the recurrence of fluid accumulation.

Bone Spavin

"Bone spavin" is an osteoarthritis and osteitis usually involving the tarsometatarsal and distal intertarsal joints. In some cases, the proximal intertarsal joint may be involved.

KEY POINT ▶ Bone spavin is the most common cause of chronic hindlimb lameness in horses.

While all breeds of horses may be affected, bone spavin is a common problem in standardbred pacers or trotters. The condition is progressive and results in a lameness that gradually worsens with time.

History and Presenting Signs

- Poor racing performance
- Standardbreds may have history of "jumping out of their harness" or a "stabbing" hindleg action.
- Standardbreds also may have a history of not running straight in the cart, with the hindquarters moving toward the shaft of the sulky on the affected side.

Clinical Findings and Diagnosis

- Bone spavin causes a chronic progressive hindlimb lameness and is usually unilateral.
- Many owners or trainers may complain of the horse being "tied up," reluctant to stretch out, or having a jerky or stabbing hindleg gait.
- In the early stages of the disease, horses will "warm out" of the lameness as they exercise. However, as the condition progresses, the lameness worsens, and the horses no longer improve as they exercise.
- Examination of the hindleg will usually reveal nothing significant, and there is no pain on flexion or palpation of the hock.
- Careful examination of the gait at the trot may show a lower arc of flight of the foot, in an attempt to limit the degree of hock flexion, when the horse trots.
- Application of the spavin test will usually accentuate the lameness when the horse is trotted off after 2 minutes of hindleg flexion.
- A positive diagnosis can be made by intraarticular local anesthesia of the tarsometatarsal and distal intertarsal joints (see p. 65). In most cases, the lameness will not be abolished, but there will be a definite improvement in the gait.
- Radiographs should be taken with the x-ray beam centered about 10 cm (4 in) distal to the point of the hock. Changes are found most commonly on the lateral and plantarodorsal oblique views.

- Radiographic changes are found most commonly in and around the tarsometatarsal joint. Periarticular new bone growth is often found around the dorsal margins of the proximal aspect of the third metatarsal bone. There also may be narrowing of the joint space and bone sclerosis and lysis, most easily visible on the dorsomedial aspect of the joint. If there are radiographic changes involving the proximal intertarsal joint, the prognosis is poor for future athletic function. In milder cases of bone spavin, we have found that changes may be more common on the dorsolateral aspect of the hock, involving the tarsometatarsal and distal intertarsal joints. These changes may not be apparent on the plantarodorsal or lateral views.

KEY POINT ▶ For this reason, it is important to take oblique radiographic views when examining the hock. The least useful radiographic view is the plantarodorsal view.

Differential Diagnosis

- Cunean tendon bursitis
- Stifle joint problems

Treatment

- Bone spavin is a progressive disease that may eventually result in ankylosis of the affected joints. Once ankylosis has occurred, the signs of lameness will abate.

KEY POINT ▶ In the early stages of joint disease, intraarticular medications such as sodium hyaluronate (Treatment No. 60) and/or long-acting corticosteroids (Treatment Nos. 12 and 74) can be injected into the affected joints.

- We have had good results with 1 ml (20 mg) of sodium hyaluronate and 2 ml (80 mg) of methylprednisolone acetate (Treatment No. 74). Relief of the clinical signs has persisted for up to 6 months after a single treatment, although the time period is usually much shorter. This treatment can be repeated if surgery is not an option because of the expense.

KEY POINT ▶ Hastening of the naturally occurring ankylosis is probably the treatment of choice, because once ankylosis is complete, the horse will not be lame.

- One way of hastening ankylosis is to continue to work the horse while it receives analgesic drugs such as phenylbutazone (Treatment No. 88) at dose rates of 1 to 2 g daily. A more radical (and quicker) method of hastening ankylosis is surgical arthrodesis of the affected joint(s) using a drill to remove some of the articular cartilage. Because both hocks are usually affected with bone spavin, it is usual to drill the tarsometatarsal and distal intertarsal joints in both hindlegs. Originally, a 4.5-mm drill bit was advocated for drilling the joints, but horses were often in severe pain for some time after surgery. We have found that use of a 3.2-mm drill bit provides adequate subchondral bone removal to result in subsequent ankylosis.

■ More recently, the use of a chemical agent, sodium iodoacetate, has been advocated as a non-surgical method for arthrodesis of the small hock joints. Injection of 100 mg diluted in 2 ml saline into the tarsometatarsal and distal intertarsal joints at 3 weekly intervals for a total of three injections has been advocated in experimental studies. This treatment has not been evaluated in clinical cases but appears to be a promising alternative to surgical fusion of the joints. To control the pain associated with the injection, horses should receive phenylbutazone for 5 days, with the first treatment administered prior to injection of the iodoacetate. Exercise should be commenced about 1 week after treatment to hasten the process of ankylosis.

■ Corrective shoeing has been suggested by some veterinarians but is seldom effective in relieving lameness.

Capped Hock

Capped hock is a subcutaneous swelling that develops at the point of the hock as a result of trauma. It is a hygroma or traumatic bursitis and in some acute cases may be filled with a large amount of fluid.

History and Presenting Signs

■ Swelling over the point of the hock
■ No lameness

Clinical Findings and Diagnosis

■ Swelling over the point of the hock without any lameness is a consistent finding.
■ If the injury is acute, there will be pain on palpation over the swollen area, but in long-standing cases there will be no pain and only fibrous enlargement.
■ Radiography is not necessary, unless there are signs of lameness.

Differential Diagnosis

■ Thoroughpin
■ Curb (plantar ligament sprain)
■ Luxation of the superficial digital flexor tendon

Treatment

■ If the swelling is long-standing, with only fibrous tissue present, no treatment will be successful. Surgery to improve the cosmetic appearance of the leg should only be attempted by the brave surgeon who has access to a good attorney.
■ In acute cases, cold hosing and a topical anti-inflammatory preparation such as dimethylsulfoxide (DMSO, Treatment No. 34) can be useful, followed by a Robert-Jones type of dressing (see Chap. 17).
■ If a large amount of fluid is present, drainage of the fluid and a pressure bandage may be successful.

Cunean Tendon Bursitis

The cunean tendon is the medial tendon of the cranial tibial muscle that runs obliquely and in a medial direction to insert in the region of the head of the second metatarsal bone. Lying underneath the tendon is a bursa, which can occasionally become inflamed and lead to lameness.

KEY POINT ▶ Cunean tendon bursitis is a condition found most commonly in standardbred trotters and pacers but is probably overdiagnosed.

History and Clinical Signs

■ Low-grade hindleg lameness
■ History of performance problems

Clinical Findings and Diagnosis

■ A typical hindleg lameness, usually low-grade, is seen, and the trainer may complain that the horse is not running straight in the cart and moves its hindquarters so that they come to lie up against one of the shafts.
■ Some clinicians think that the condition may be contributed to by the use of abnormal shoes with calks and trailers, which are prevalent in the standardbred industry.
■ Little will be found on clinical examination, and the only way a positive diagnosis can be made is to inject 5 ml of 2% mepivacaine (Treatment No. 72) under the cunean tendon to determine if the lameness is relieved. This is most easily done with the hock flexed, because the cunean tendon can then be palpated easily, running across the dorsal aspect of the hock. It may take up to 20 to 30 minutes after injection of the local anesthetic for the gait to improve.
■ Care must be taken with the mepivacaine infusion because it is possible for this local anesthetic to diffuse into the small hock joints and confuse the diagnosis.
■ Radiographs should be taken to ensure that no bony changes are present, indicative of bone spavin.

Differential Diagnosis

■ Bone spavin
■ Tarsal chip fractures

Treatment

- Injection of 3 to 4 ml of a long-acting corticosteroid such as methylprednisolone acetate (Treatment No. 74) into the cunean bursa may result in temporary relief of the condition.
- The only permanent solution is surgical resection of a portion of the cunean tendon. This surgery can be performed with the horse standing.

Curb (Plantar Ligament Sprain)

"Curb" is the common name given to sprain of the plantar ligament. The plantar ligament runs down the plantar aspect of the hock along the calcaneus. Curb is a condition most commonly found in standardbred trotters or pacers. While excessive hock angulation (so-called sickle hock) may contribute to the condition, it is not clear what produces the condition. Most cases of curb cause only mild lameness and resolve quickly with rest.

Clinical Findings and Diagnosis

- The first sign of curb is swelling at the plantar aspect of the hock and about 8 to 10 cm (3.5–4 in) distal to the point of the hock.
- In the acute stage there will be heat, swelling, and pain, and there may be a mild hindleg lameness.
- In chronic cases, swelling will be the only residual sign.
- Ultrasonography will differentiate effusion alone from ligament or tendon damage, and serial examinations will give a guide to progress.
- Radiographs reveal only soft-tissue swelling on the plantar aspect of the calcaneus. However, in severe cases of trauma to the plantar ligament, there may be subsequent new periosteal bone growth along the plantar border of the calcaneus.
- If an apparent curb is seen in a foal or yearling, radiographs should be taken. Most such cases suffer tarsal collapse, where the central or third tarsal bones collapse, and the third tarsal bone may be fractured. Surprisingly, in horses such as these that are not in active training, there may be little or no lameness, despite marked radiographic changes involving the small hock joints. The cause of tarsal collapse is not known, although there have been reports incriminating hypothyroidism.

Differential Diagnosis

- Periligamentous or peritendinous effusion
- Tendinitis/tenosynovitis of the proximal superficial digital flexor tendon
- Thoroughpin
- Tarsal collapse

Treatment

- In the acute stage, local anti-inflammatory measures such as cold water hosing, application of cold packs, and bandaging will help reduce the swelling.
- Anti-inflammatory drugs such as phenylbutazone (Treatment No. 88), given for 7 days, also can help to reduce the swelling.
- Topical preparations such as dimethylsulfoxide (DMSO, Treatment No. 34) are useful in reducing the swelling and inflammation.
- Some practitioners advocate injection of corticosteroids locally into the area of the swelling. This results in immediate reduction in swelling but may encourage the trainer to put the horse back into full training before the damage has healed.
- Most cases of curb will resolve with 2 to 4 weeks of rest or light exercise. Horses in which there is structural damage to the superficial flexor tendon require a long period of rest and carry a poorer prognosis.
- Where there is recurrence of the injury, injection of sclerosing agents (sodium iodide, ethanolamine oleate) into the plantar ligament has been found to be useful. However, it may be that the rest after the injection of a sclerosing agent is more effective than the sclerosing agent itself.

Fracture of the Talus (Tibial Tarsal Bone)

The talus articulates with the tibia, calcaneus, and central tarsal bone. It has medial and lateral trochlear ridges, and chip fractures may occur at these sites. Such fractures are uncommon, and it is more usual to find lesions on the trochlear ridges associated with osteochondrosis dissecans (OCD).

History and Clinical Signs

- Variable degrees of lameness
- Distension of the tarsocrural joint

Clinical Findings and Diagnosis

- Lameness may or may not be present.
- Occasionally, small chip fractures of the talus will be found on radiography of the hock and may be of no consequence.
- It is important to use local anesthesia in the tarsocrural joint to positively localize the site of lameness.
- There is usually some distension of the tarsocrural joint capsule, and the condition must be differentiated from bog spavin and OCD.
- When radiographs are taken, the fracture is usually most visible on the lateral view. Oblique views assist in determining whether the fracture is off the medial or lateral trochlear ridge.

Differential Diagnosis

- Bog spavin
- Fractures of other tarsal bones
- Osteochondrosis dissecans (OCD)

Treatment

- Some horses with very small chip fractures will return to successful work with a rest period of 3 to 6 months.
- However, with most chip fractures and especially larger chips, surgical removal is necessary, and this may be done arthroscopically. Cases where there is significant cartilage damage at surgery may benefit from the administration of intraarticular medications such as polysulfated glycosaminoglycans (Treatment No. 90) postoperatively. However, if degenerative joint disease is severe, the prognosis for long-term resolution of the lameness is less favorable.

Osteochondrosis Dissecans of the Hock

Osteochondrosis dissecans (OCD) may affect the hock in yearling and 2-year-old horses and usually involves the talus and/or the dorsal edge of the sagittal ridge of the tibia. Hock OCD is especially common in standardbreds.

History and Presenting Signs

- Distension of the tarsocrural (tibiotarsal) joint
- Little or no lameness

Clinical Findings and Diagnosis

- There is distension of the tarsocrural joint capsule with fluid and varying degrees of lameness depending on the extent of the lesion.
- The opposite hock also may be affected and therefore needs to be examined carefully.
- Intraarticular local anesthesia of the tarsocrural joint (see p. 66) will result in improvement of the gait, although we have found that the majority of horses do not become sound.
- Radiographs will indicate the exact site and extent of the lesion(s). Important views are the lateral and two oblique views. Lesions involving the dorsal sagittal ridge may only be seen on the dorsolateral aspect of the hock. The view of importance is therefore the plantarolateral to dorsomedial oblique projection.

Differential Diagnosis

- Fracture of the talus
- Bog spavin

Treatment

- If a small fragment is present, no treatment may be required apart from rest, although intraarticular medications such as sodium hyaluronate (Treatment No. 60) or polysulfated glycosaminoglycans (Treatment No. 90) have been found to be useful.

KEY POINT ▶ The treatment of choice is arthroscopic surgery to remove the osteochondral fragments, curette the damaged articular surface, and lavage the joint.

- Following surgery, there is usually a dramatic reduction in the degree of joint effusion. A period of 3 to 6 months of rest is usually advocated, depending on the extent of the cartilage damage. Polysulfated glycosaminoglycans (Treatment No. 90) can be used 2 to 3 weeks after surgery if there was extensive cartilage erosion visible at the time of surgery.

Rupture of the Peroneus Tertius

The peroneus tertius is part of the stay apparatus of the hindlimb. Its origin is on the dorsal aspect of the distal part of the femur, and it inserts on the dorsal aspect of the proximal third metatarsal bone. Rupture of the peroneus tertius is an uncommon injury, but it produces typical clinical signs and is therefore easily diagnosed.

History and Presenting Signs

- Abnormal hindleg carriage
- Extension of the hock with stifle flexion

Clinical Findings and Diagnosis

- The horse usually bears weight without trouble but shows reduced flexion of the hock as the limb is advanced.
- The typical sign of rupture is that it is possible to flex the stifle while extending the hock. This is most easily seen by moving the hindleg backward.
- The limb also may appear to tremble as it is advanced and has a loose or slack appearance.

Differential Diagnosis

The ability to extend the hock while the stifle is flexed is pathognomonic.

Treatment

- Rest is the only treatment that is feasible, and most cases will resolve with time. In most cases, 3 to 4 months of rest will give resolution of the problem. The early part of the rest period should take place in a box stall so that movement is restricted.
- Because cases are uncommon, there have been no reports of the follow-up of a large series of cases of rupture of the peroneus tertius.

Stringhalt

Stringhalt is a condition that results in involuntary flexion of one or (usually) both hindlimbs. Where the condition is bilateral, it is found in horses that depend on pasture for nutrition (so-called Australian stringhalt). Therefore, it has been suggested that a pasture-derived neurotoxin may be important in the pathogenesis. In the United States, lathyrism (sweetpea toxicity) has been reported to result in a stringhalt-like syndrome, and in Australia, flatweed-dominated unimproved pastures have been incriminated in some cases. A common history in outbreaks of the disease in Australia is that horses are affected following a period of drought followed by substantial rain with fresh pasture growth. Most commonly this occurs in spring, and substantial numbers of horses have been affected within the same geographic area.

History and Presenting Signs

Involuntary flexion involving one or both hindlegs

Clinical Findings and Diagnosis

- A typical goose-stepping gait with hyperflexion of the hindlegs is characteristic.
- This gait is more evident when the horse is first walked off and improves as the horse "warms up."
- The severity of the gait abnormality varies and may be accompanied by atrophy of the hindlimb muscles and left laryngeal hemiplegia. If the condition has been present for weeks to months, atrophy of the muscles on the lateral aspect of the tibia is a consistent finding.
- Because the condition appears to be a long nerve problem and, therefore, the left recurrent laryngeal nerve may be affected, endoscopic examination of the larynx should be considered. If an endoscope is not available, the "slap test" may be applied to assess laryngeal function. The left and right muscular processes of the larynx are palpated while an assistant slaps the midthorax. Movement of the muscular process on the contralateral side to the thorax can be felt if there is normal recurrent laryngeal nerve function.
- In severe cases, flexion of the limb may be so severe that the dorsal fetlock makes contact with the ventral abdomen.

Differential Diagnosis

- Upward fixation of the patella
- Adhesions as a result of damage to the extensor tendons in the proximal metatarsus

Treatment

- While many cases will resolve spontaneously, this may take months to years. If the condition is thought to arise from plant toxins, removal of the horse to another paddock may give resolution. However, this may take several months.
- In cases that do not resolve, surgical resection of the lateral extensor tendons is a popular treatment, and success rates of approximately 80% have been reported. It is interesting, however,

that where horses do improve with surgery, the improvement is never immediate and takes up to 7 to 10 days.
- Recent studies have demonstrated the widespread axonopathy and neurogenic muscle atrophy in this condition. The validity of surgical treatment, therefore, may be open to question.
- The use of phenytoin (Treatment No. 89) has been reported to result in improvement in clinical signs while horses were on treatment. The dose rate recommended is 15 mg/kg given in capsule or powder form twice daily.
- Recently, there has been some success at our clinic with the use of a GABA inhibitor, baclofen, given orally at a dose rate of 1 mg/kg three times daily (Malik and Kannegieter, personal communication). Some cases have shown a dramatic response within days of treatment, while others have continued to improve after ceasing therapy, despite the presence of clinical signs for more than 12 months. In other cases, there has been no significant improvement. Because baclofen is a centrally acting drug, it may be that there is a central as well as a peripheral component to stringhalt.

Thoroughpin

Thoroughpin is the term used to describe a tenosynovitis of the deep flexor tendon sheath. It may occur in yearlings or older horses, and in many cases there is no apparent cause. In the majority of cases, the condition is found in young horses and there is no lameness.

History and Presenting Signs

- Fluid-filled swelling on the plantar aspect of the hock
- Young horses usually affected

Clinical Findings and Diagnosis

- A nonpainful, fluid-filled swelling just proximal to the point of the hock, on both medial and lateral sides, is typical. Horses will not show any lameness with simple thoroughpin.
- Radiography is recommended to rule out the possibility of bony lesions. A special radiographic view that is often useful is the skyline view of the hock. This is undertaken by flexing the hindlimb and placing the x-ray plate along the plantar aspect of the proximal metacarpus so that the calcaneus is outlined in relief.
- Ultrasonography, while not generally required, will demonstrate effusion in the deep flexor tendon sheath.

Differential Diagnosis

- Bog spavin
- Curb

Treatment

- Drainage of the fluid and injections of corticosteroids are seldom successful.
- While cold hosing and anti-inflammatory drugs such as phenylbutazone (Treatment No. 88) may be given in the acute stages, these are seldom of benefit.
- In most horses, thoroughpin is purely a cosmetic fault and will not interfere with limb function. The degree of effusion may decrease with time.

Tibial Fractures

Fractures of the tibia are usually oblique or spiral ones and often result from direct trauma. In adult horses, fractures of the tibia represent a considerable challenge to the surgeon. Our experience with these fractures suggests that even in a valuable horse, surgery may not be worthwhile because the success rates are so low. This is particularly so if the fracture is compound or open, with the certainty of osteomyelitis developing. In younger horses, the outcome is more likely to be successful.

History and Presenting Signs

- Non-weight-bearing lameness
- Visible alteration in the tibial contour

Clinical Findings and Diagnosis

- There is inability to bear weight on the affected leg when the fracture is complete.
- Extensive soft-tissue swelling is found, and the skin should be examined carefully for the presence of trauma indicating that bone has penetrated.
- Fractures of the growth plates can occur in foals, and these have a slightly better prognosis for pasture soundness.
- Crepitus is usually found on palpation over the affected site.
- Suitable radiographs can be taken even with smaller mobile x-ray machines. The radiographs should include caudocranial and lateral views.

Differential Diagnosis

- Fractures of the tibial growth plates
- Femoral fractures

Treatment

- Surgery, using internal fixation with two bone plates, is necessary if salvage of the horse is to be attempted.
- In most tibial fractures it is difficult to effectively immobilize the leg for transport to a surgical facility. Care should be taken to ensure that if a Robert Jones bandage (see Chap. 17) is used, it does not worsen the fracture or result in a compound or open fracture.

- Some spiral fractures are nondisplaced, and if these occur in the middle to distal part of the tibia, they may be treated successfully using external fixation. More proximal fractures should be treated using internal fixation followed by external fixation.

References

Bohanon, T. C., Schneider, R. K., and Weisbrode, S. E.: Fusion of the distal intertarsal and tarsometatarsal joints in the horse using intraarticular sodium monoiodoacetate. *Equine Vet. J.* 23:289, 1991.

Huntington, P. J., Jeffcott, L. B., Friend, S. C. E., et al: Australian stringhalt: Epidemiological, clinical and neurological investigations. *Equine Vet. J.* 21:266, 1989.

MacDonald, M. H., Honnas, C. M., and Meagher, D. M.: Osteomyelitis of the calcaneus in horses: 28 cases (1972–1987). *J. Am. Vet. Med. Assoc.* 194:1317, 1989.

Wyn-Jones, G., and May, S. A.: Surgical arthrodesis for the treatment of osteoarthrosis of the proximal intertarsal, distal intertarsal and tarsometatarsal joints in 30 horses: A comparison of four different techniques. *Equine Vet. J.* 18:59, 1986.

STIFLE AND HIP PROBLEMS

Fibrotic and/or Ossifying Myopathy

Injuries to the semimembranosus and semitendinosus muscles can occur from horses slipping during rodeo events or during restraint with sidelines or breeding hobbles. The localized muscle trauma results in fibrosis, and occasionally, this develops into a local ossified area. The end result of this injury is to interfere with muscle function so that the horse has a restricted anterior phase of the stride.

History and Presenting Signs

- Unusual hindleg gait
- Leg jerks backward on advancing affected hindleg

Clinical Findings and Diagnosis

- Unilateral gait abnormality so that as the foot is advanced, the adhesions and scarring in the semimembranosus and semitendinosus muscles result in the leg being suddenly jerked caudally.
- Palpation of the affected muscles reveals a firm to hard area, usually in the middle to distal regions of the semimembranosus and semitendinosus muscles. Usually there is no pain found on palpation of these areas.

Differential Diagnosis

- Neurologic problems
- Gonitis

Treatment

- Surgical treatment is necessary to resolve the gait abnormality.
- Myectomy of the affected muscles was the treatment of choice, but the surgery is rather traumatic.
- Simple transection of the tendon of the semitendinosus muscle near its insertion on the caudomedial region of the proximal tibia has given good results, and this is now the technique of choice.

Femoral Subchondral Bone Cysts

Subchondral bone cysts are a common cause of hindleg lameness in yearling and 2-year-old horses. The cysts invariably occur on the medial femoral condyle. There is some controversy about the etiology, with some authors certain that subchondral bone cysts are part of the OCD complex. Others are of the opinion that subchondral bone cysts have a separate etiology. These cysts are often difficult to diagnose because there are few localizing signs.

History and Presenting Signs

- Young horse, usually yearling or 2-year-old
- Most common in thoroughbreds

Clinical Findings and Diagnosis

- Most commonly the hindleg lameness is unilateral. The degree of lameness can be quite variable, with some horses showing very mild degrees of lameness.
- Lameness is often gradual in onset and slowly worsens with time.

KEY POINT ▶ Unlike OCD lesions affecting the lateral trochlear ridge of the femur, bone cysts seldom cause effusion, and therefore, there may be few abnormalities on clinical examination.

- In most cases there is a definite worsening of lameness following a spavin test.
- Good-quality radiographs are essential, particularly a caudocranial view of the stifle. If the films are slightly underexposed, it is possible to miss the presence of a bone cyst. Close examination of the articular surface of the medial femoral condyle will usually reveal some degree of flattening, and a radiolucent area, often up to 2 to 3 cm (1 in) in diameter, can be seen extending within the medial condyle.
- Although it is usual to have the condition presenting as a unilateral hindleg lameness, it is common to have lesions in both stifle joints. Therefore, it is essential that radiographs be taken of the apparently unaffected stifle.

Differential Diagnosis

- OCD of the stifle
- Hock lamenesses
- Ligament and meniscal injuries to the stifle

Treatment

- In small bone cysts causing little or no lameness, conservative therapy involving pasture rest for 6 to 12 months will often result in a horse that is sound for athletic endeavors.
- Even where the cysts do cause significant lameness, we have seen horses race successfully despite the hindleg lameness.
- Larger cysts, where there is significant lameness, require surgical treatment because conservative treatment has been disappointing in our experience.
- Surgical treatment involves visualization of the medial femoral condyle with an arthroscope and curettage of the cavity of the cyst. This should be followed by forage of the cavity of the cyst using a 2- to 3.2-mm-diameter drill bit. The latter technique permits ingrowth of vessels and accelerates bone deposition within the cystic cavity.
- Horses require up to 12 months of rest following surgery.

Gonitis: Stifle Lameness

Gonitis is the term used to describe inflammation of the stifle joint owing to a variety of disorders. It is a general term indicating the region of pathology only and may reflect soft-tissue or bony lesions, although the latter are more common.

History and Presenting Signs

- Hindleg lameness
- Distension of the femoropatellar pouches

Clinical Findings and Diagnosis

- Distension of the femoropatellar pouches is characteristic.
- If there is any suggestion of a septic arthritis, a synovial fluid sample should be taken for a white cell count and total protein determination.
- Affected horses will show varying degrees of lameness, depending on the specific problem.
- Various techniques for manipulation of the stifle can be undertaken, but these give the investigator a great chance of being injured and seldom reveal worthwhile information.
- Intra-articular local anesthesia (see Figs. 3-47 and 3-48) should be used to confirm the site.
- Radiography of the stifle is essential and should include a minimum of caudocranial and lateral views. In some cases, extra information may be gained from flexed lateral views.

■ Arthroscopic examination of both the femorotibial and femoropatellar joints is often useful in defining the pathology and for removing any osteochondral fragments.

Differential Diagnosis

■ Damage to medial or lateral collateral ligaments
■ Meniscal damage
■ Cruciate ligament damage
■ OCD
■ Subchondral bone cysts
■ Septic arthritis
■ Fractures of the patella
■ Osteoarthritis

Treatment

■ For most of the causes of gonitis, rest is the only treatment possible.
■ Rest periods of up to 12 months may give resolution of osteochondritis, bone cysts, meniscal damage, and ligament rupture.
■ Depending on the etiology of the gonitis, it may be possible to remove osteochondral fragments or gain access to the joint for other surgical treatments using arthroscopy.

Osteochondrosis Dissecans of the Stifle Joint

Osteochondrosis dissecans affecting the stifle is a common condition, particularly in young thoroughbred horses. The most common site affected is the lateral trochlear ridge of the femur.

History and Presenting Signs

■ Hindleg lameness
■ Effusion of the femoropatellar pouches
■ Horses 2 years old or less are usually presented.

Clinical Findings and Diagnosis

■ Variable hindleg lameness that is usually unilateral
■ Obvious effusion involving the femoropatellar pouches
■ Effusion is usually bilateral, with lesions involving both stifle joints.
■ Standard radiographic views should be taken. Lesions are most easily seen on the lateral view, and the lateral trochlear ridge and patella are most commonly affected.

Differential Diagnosis

■ Meniscal injuries
■ Collateral ligament injuries
■ Cruciate ligament injuries
■ Bone cysts

Treatment

■ Unless the lesion is very small, the treatment of choice is arthroscopic surgery to remove the osteochondral fragments.
■ We have had excellent results where the extent of damage is limited to localized areas of the lateral trochlear ridge. Removal of the osteochondral fragments and curettage of the damaged cartilage are performed easily using arthroscopic visualization.
■ A prolonged rest period of up to 6 months is usually required after surgery.

Tumoral Calcinosis (Calcinosis Circumscripta)

Tumoral calcinosis is a condition in which one or sometimes more circumscribed, hard swellings are found. It is characterized by the formation of amorphous, calcified, granular deposits in the subcutaneous tissues that induce a granulomatous reaction. In most cases these are located over the lateral aspect of the proximal tibia, just distal to the stifle joint. Other sites are occasionally involved, and sometimes the lesions occur bilaterally. They are usually first noticed in weanlings or yearlings. There is a low incidence of lameness associated with this condition.

History and Presenting Signs

Large, firm swelling on the lateral aspect of the proximal tibia

Clinical Findings and Diagnosis

KEY POINT ► The typical appearance of a round, hard swelling over the lateral aspect of the proximal tibia is very characteristic of tumoral calcinosis.

■ The diameter of the swellings is approximately 3 to 12 cm (1–5 in), and they are immobile.
■ There is usually no lameness.
■ If radiographs are taken, there will be a circumscribed radiopaque mass that has a somewhat granular appearance.
■ If fine-needle aspiration is attempted, this will indicate that the mass is extremely hard and calcified, and it will not be possible to obtain a sample.

Differential Diagnosis

■ Soft-tissue abscess
■ Foreign body
■ Neoplasia

Treatment

■ Surgery is the only feasible treatment, and while many are easily dissected, in some cases they will attach to the joint capsule of the stifle and are impossible to remove without entering the joint.

- Therefore, since this condition often causes only a cosmetic blemish, it is probably best left untreated except in cases in which lameness can be attributed directly to the lesion.

Upward Fixation of the Patella ("Locking Stifle")

Upward fixation of the patella is a condition that is found commonly in shetland ponies and standardbreds. It is usually the result of a conformational fault, whereby the stifle is excessively straight, giving rise to the medial patellar ligament "locking" over the medial trochlea of the femur. In most cases, it affects young horses, and many will recover spontaneously. Because surgical section of the medial patellar ligament is simple to perform, many horses with obscure hindleg lamenesses are operated on by equine practitioners in the hope that a partially "locked stifle" may be the problem. Recently, it has been found that such surgery may have some ill effects.

History and Presenting Signs

- Inability of the horse to flex the limb
- Dragging of toe when the limb is advanced, with sudden hyperflexion

Clinical Findings and Diagnosis

- The typical gait of a horse with upward fixation of the patella is that the limb locks in extension and cannot be moved forward. The result of this is that the toe is dragged as the horse tries to move forward.
- This may occur in one or both hindlimbs.
- If the patella then unlocks, the hindlimb may suddenly hyperflex, so confusion with stringhalt is possible by horse trainers and owners.
- In most cases, upward fixation of the patella is seen when the horse is first taken out of its stall or perhaps unloaded from a trailer.
- In milder cases it may not be possible to positively demonstrate the condition, which is intermittent, and reliance may have to be placed on the history.
- Some clinicians have advocated manipulation of the patella to produce upward fixation. In our experience this is not only very difficult but also has a high chance of injury to the operator.

Differential Diagnosis

- Stringhalt
- Damage to the proximal portion of the extensor tendons with adhesion formation
- Fibrotic myopathy

Treatment

- In young horses (yearlings and 2-year-olds), if the condition is not severe, many horses will grow out of it. Exercise up hills, which develops the quadriceps muscle group, may aid resolution.
- However, where the upward fixation occurs very frequently or in older horses, surgical treatment (medial patellar ligament desmotomy) is indicated. This is best performed under sedation using xylazine (Treatment No. 108) or detomidine (Treatment No. 28) and butorphanol (Treatment No. 15) (see Chap. 17) and local infiltration with 3 to 5 ml of mepivacaine (Treatment No. 72). A 2.5-cm (1-in) incision is made between the middle and medial patellar ligaments, just proximal to the tibial crest. After a sharp stab incision is made in the fascia, a pair of blunt-pointed scissors is pushed through the fascia between the ligaments. This enables a blunt-nosed teat bistoury to be used to sever all fibers of the medial patellar ligament. Only one or two skin sutures are necessary, and the subcutaneous tissue is left unsutured. Following surgery, horses should be rested for 1 month before resuming training.
- Recent studies reporting bone pathology, including patellar chip fractures, following medial patellar desmotomy suggest that conservative treatment should always be tried, with surgery reserved for severe, nonresponsive cases.
- Some clinicians favor the injection of sclerosing agents into the medial patellar ligament to "tighten" it. We have used sodium iodide injected into the ligament. An 18-gauge needle is pushed into the body of the ligament, and 0.5 ml of the irritant agent is injected into the ligament. While some clinicians report good results with this technique, we have not had consistent improvement and favor desmotomy if treatment is necessary.

References

Gibson, K. T., and McIlwraith, C. W.: Identifying and managing stifle disorders that cause hindlimb lameness. *Vet. Med.* 85:188, 1990.

McIlwraith, C. W.: Fragmentation of the distal patella in horses: A complication of medial patellar desmotomy. *Proc. 34th Conv. Am. Assoc. Equine Pract.*, 1988, p. 660.

Sanders, S. M., Bukowiecki, C. F., and Biller, D. S.: Cruciate and collateral ligament failure in the equine stifle: Seven cases (1975–1985). *J. Am. Vet. Med. Assoc.* 193:573, 1988.

HIP AND PELVIS PROBLEMS

Femoral Fractures

While femoral fractures are less common than fractures of the radius and tibia, they are nonetheless a relatively common long bone fracture. While direct trauma is a possible cause, particularly in young horses, our experience is that by far the majority of fractures of the femur in mature horses have been the result of bad inductions and recoveries from anesthesia. In such cases, the fracture usually involves the diaphysis, and there is considerable comminution. Younger horses sometimes have fractures that involve the growth plates.

History and Presenting Signs

- History of severe trauma or anesthesia
- Non-weight-bearing lameness
- In some cases, a history of a loud crack or bang, like a gun going off

Clinical Findings and Diagnosis

- Non-weight-bearing lameness on affected hindleg
- The affected hindleg may appear shorter than the unaffected hindleg because of the overriding of the proximal and distal fragments and the comminution.
- Crepitus may or may not be felt on manipulation of the leg, but if the area is auscultated with a stethoscope, crepitus can be heard.
- The fracture can usually be diagnosed from the clinical examination. Radiographs are indicated in a valuable horse, where attempts at surgical repair may be considered. However, in the majority of cases, the prognosis is so poor that it is not worthwhile considering surgery. Therefore, radiographs may not be of economic benefit because general anesthesia is necessary.

Differential Diagnosis

- Fracture of the tibia
- Fracture of the patella
- Dislocation of the hip

Treatment

- In mature horses, femoral fractures are remarkably difficult to treat successfully. At this stage there have been isolated cases that have been treated successfully, but the majority of cases have failed. It may be that the development of an implant such as the Huckstep nail, which is inserted into the medullary cavity and cross-fixed through the pin with transverse screws, may be a surgical approach with merit for the future.
- There have been reports in young foals of successful treatment of femoral fractures using multiple intramedullary pins. The use of bone plates provides more secure stabilization of the fracture and may carry a better prognosis for healing in young foals than the pinning technique.
- Some femoral fractures in young horses, particularly those through the growth plate that are not completely distracted, may heal for pasture soundness with box-stall confinement.

Dislocation of the Hip Joint

The hip joint is maintained by a round and an accessory ligament. If these ligaments are ruptured, dislocation of the hip joint will occur. This type of injury occurs secondary to trauma but is quite uncommon. In some cases of dislocation of the hip joint in ponies, it may be accompanied by upward fixation of the patella. Rarely, the round ligament is ruptured but the hip joint does not dislocate. The result of the instability is degenerative arthritis of the hip joint. Lameness associated with hip problems is very rare, although we have seen occasional cases in standardbred pacers and trotters.

History and Clinical Signs

- History of trauma or slipping on the leg
- Hindleg lameness
- Turning outward of the toe and stifle of the affected leg
- Inability to advance the hindleg

Clinical Findings and Diagnosis

- Rupture of the round ligament of the hip joint is associated with a typical appearance of the hindleg, with the stifle and toe rotated outward.
- Complete dislocation of the hip joint may not occur. When it does, there is a marked effect on gait, with the horse being reluctant to bear weight.
- The femur is rotated outward, and the greater trochanter is more prominent than usual.
- Radiographs can be used to confirm the diagnosis, but it can be difficult to obtain views that demonstrate the dislocation. Standing films can be obtained (see Radiography, p. 70).

Differential Diagnosis

- Fractures of the femur
- Fractures of the pelvis
- Upward fixation of the patella

Treatment

- Relocation of the hip joint may be attempted under general anesthesia, but this is difficult, and the long-term results are usually poor.
- Surgical transposition of the greater trochanter of the femur has been reported to be useful but is still an experimental procedure at this stage.

Pelvic Lameness and Fractures

Pelvic lameness nearly always results from trauma. For accurate diagnosis, radiography under general anesthesia is necessary. Rectal examination also may be useful in some cases. There is invariably a history of trauma, and fractures are common after heavy falls. Most pelvic problems will resolve with time, but some fractures will produce a long-standing lameness.

History and Presenting Signs

- History of the horse having fallen
- Hindleg lameness
- Change in contour of the pelvic region

Clinical Findings and Diagnosis

- If there is a fracture of the pelvis, there will usually be a chronic unilateral hindlimb lameness with atrophy of the gluteal muscles if the fracture involves one side of the pelvis.
- Where soft-tissue injuries occur, there may be only a vague history of lameness or reduced performance. If fracture of the pelvis has occurred, it may be possible to detect crepitus on a rectal examination in acute cases, but this is not present in chronic cases.
- The most common injury to the pelvis is a "knocked down hip," or fracture of the tuber coxae. This injury is reasonably common, with horses sometimes sustaining the fracture when they suddenly rush through box-stall doors and traumatize the tuber coxa on the door entrance.
- If a pelvic injury is suspected, good-quality radiographs are important to determine the prognosis. Such radiographs must be taken under general anesthesia, and the horse should be referred to an institution that has a powerful x-ray machine.

Standing radiographs of the hip and pelvis are possible (see p. 70).
- If the acetabulum is not involved, most pelvic fractures will heal satisfactorily in a period of 12 months. However, we have had a few horses that were left with a chronic hindleg lameness even 12 months after a pelvic fracture that did not appear to involve a vital area of the pelvis. For this reason, a guarded prognosis should be given.

Differential Diagnosis

- Fractures of the pelvis
- Thrombosis of the caudal aorta or iliac arteries

Treatment

- Rest is the only treatment possible, and periods of up to 12 months may be necessary.

References

Little, C., and Hilbert, B.: Pelvic fractures in horses: 19 cases (1974–1984). *J. Am. Vet. Med. Assoc.* 190:1203, 1987.

May, S. A., Patterson, L. J., Peacock, P. J., and Edwards, G. B.: Radiographic technique for the pelvis in the standing horse. *Equine Vet. J.* 23:312, 1991.

Rutkowski, J. A., and Richardson, D. W.: A retrospective study of 100 pelvic fractures in horses. *Equine Vet. J.* 21:256, 1989.

Back Abnormalities

Back problems make up only a small proportion of musculoskeletal problems in horses, accounting for less than 1% of cases in most veterinary practices. However, in practices where there is a large proportion of pleasure, dressage, eventing, and hunting horses, back injuries are more common. Back problems are also more common in standardbred trotters and pacers than in thoroughbred gallopers. Many veterinarians have difficulty in the diagnosis of back disorders. Because of this, horse owners and trainers have tended to use chiropractors and horse manipulators who have little or no training. One of the major difficulties in establishing a diagnosis in horses with suspected back problems is achieving adequate radiographs of the region. Apart from radiographing the thoracic dorsal spinous processes, which can be achieved with most x-ray machines, those with a capability of more than 120 kVp and 500 mA are needed for radiographs to be taken of other areas of the back.

In some dressage horses, the rider may complain of various temperament problems, but the veterinarian may find nothing wrong. There may be subclinical back problems, but in some cases it may simply be that the horse is not responding well to the schooling or is being given conflicting signals by the rider. Such horses often present as "head shakers."

History and Presenting Signs

- History of fall or trauma
- Temperment changes
- Poor performance
- Resentment of saddling
- Adverse reactions to being groomed
- Hindleg lameness
- Adverse reactions to a heavy rider

Clinical Findings and Diagnosis

- The most consistent history is of a change in the temperment of the horse, with or without a loss of performance.
- The horse also may resent weight on its back and show signs of hindlimb lameness or reluctance to "stretch out."
- Examination should concentrate on evaluating the flexibility of the back together with assessment of any areas of asymmetry. Particular note should be taken of any excessively prominent spinous processes, deformities of the spinal column such as lordosis (sway back), kyphosis (roach back), or scoliosis (lateral deviation), and areas of hypersensitivity.
- Firm pressure should be applied over the dorsal midline, palpating over each spinous process to determine if there is a localized area of pain. After this, the area over the longissimus dorsi muscles should be palpated at intervals of 2 to 3 cm (1 in). Hypersensitivity may be found, or the horse may attempt to kick, indicating pain.
- Stroking over the dorsal midline with the blunt end of a pen will result in the horse crouching away (ventroflexion) from the pen, particularly over the thoracolumbar region. Over the caudal sacral region, firm stroking with a pen will result in the horse arching (dorsiflexion) its back. Stroking over the longissimus dorsi muscles normally results in lateral flexion of the thoracic spine away from the side being stroked. These responses may be abolished or modified when there are back problems, because movement of the back causes pain.
- In standardbreds in particular, palpation over the tuber sacrale should be performed to determine if any hypersensitivity is present, since sacroiliac pain is a common problem. Pain in this area is manifested as the horse flexing its hindlegs and crouching toward the ground when the region over the tuber sacrale has firm pressure applied. In some horses, there may be evidence of shifting of the sacrum, with the tuber sacrale being higher on one side than the other.
- If a localized area of pain is found, particularly over the thoracic spinous processes, it may be helpful to deposit 5 ml of a local anesthetic such as 2% prilocaine (Treatment No. 93) or mepivacaine (Treatment No. 72) to determine if there is an improvement in gait or in temperament.
- Radiographs may be indicated in some cases. The thoracic dorsal spinous processes are relatively easily radiographed. However, for radiographs of the vertebral bodies or the sacrum, general anesthesia is required together with a large-capacity x-ray machine.
- Rectal examination should be performed as a routine, although in most cases there are negative findings.

Differential Diagnosis

- Rhabdomyolysis ("tying up")
- Hindlimb lameness
- Temperament problems
- Rider/horse incompatibility

Treatment

- Checking on the equipment used, particularly the fitting of the saddle, is important because an ill-fitting saddle may result in a chronic back problem.
- Manipulation under general anesthesia has been advocated by some veterinarians, whereas others favor techniques such as acupuncture. Unfortunately, the results of a large number of cases treated by these techniques have not been published, so assessment is impossible. While we remain unconvinced about some of the methods used for treatment of back problems, we have seen horses improve greatly after manipulation and acupuncture. A common form of manipulation in the conscious horse involves pulling one hindleg at a time quickly backward as far as possible. This is followed by abduction and flexion of each hindleg. Some horses will show a reduction in pain after such manipulation. However, the improvement is usually transient.
- Some veterinarians have reported good results from acupuncture in the treatment of back injuries. Our experience is limited, but we have not seen dramatic results in horses with chronic back pain that we have referred for acupuncture therapy.
- The main treatment for most back disorders is rest, prolonged periods of up to 12 months being necessary. Some cases of soft-tissue injury to the back may be assisted by a course of oral phenylbutazone (Treatment No. 88) for several weeks, at a dose rate of 2.2 mg/kg once daily. In cases of sacroiliac pain, even prolonged rest may not result in the anticipated improvement. However, soft-tissue back injuries, particularly those which are muscular, may respond well.
- If there is evidence of overriding of the thoracic dorsal spinous processes, surgery is possible to resect one or more of the processes. The results of this surgery are not always predictable. Before such treatment is contemplated it is important to see an improvement after infusion of local anesthetic into the affected area.

- Standardbred pacers with sacroiliac pain have been assisted by a change in training. We have found that galloping these horses instead of hobbling them for their fast work may result in improvement in the clinical signs.

References

Jeffcott, L. B.: Guidelines for the diagnosis and treatment of back problems in horses: Thoracolumbar (TL) disorders. *Proc. 26th Conv. Am. Assoc. Equine Pract.*, 1980, p. 381.

Jeffcott, L. B.: The examination of a horse with a potential back problem. *Proc. 31st Conv. Am. Assoc. Equine Pract.*, 1985, p. 271.

Marks, D.: Notes on treatment and management of thoracolumbar pain in the horse. *Proc. 31st Conv. Am. Assoc. Equine Pract.*, 1985, p. 353.

General Musculoskeletal Abnormalities

Arthritis or Degenerative Joint Disease

Arthritis (degenerative joint disease, DJD) is a common condition, particularly in racehorses and other performance horses. It is usually thought of as a "wear and tear" disease most commonly affecting highly mobile joints such as the carpus and fetlock. While this has some validity, it is obviously much more complex, with factors such as conformation, bone maturity, exercising surface, and horse use playing important roles. A sequence of events thought to involve increasing degeneration of articular cartilage leads to cartilage erosion, altered permeability of the synovial membrane, and changes to the composition of synovial fluid. Once these changes occur, there is a "vicious cycle" of trauma and inflammation leading to further joint damage. In addition to the changes in the articular surface, there is also evidence of synovitis at all stages of the disease. This synovitis causes much of the painful response in the joint and is the target of many of the drugs used in therapy.

Aspects of Diagnosis

- The most common clinical sign is lameness in the affected limb, with or without some degree of swelling around the joint.
- Usually, there is some distension of the joint capsule and pain on extreme flexion of the joint. The joint capsule distension is best determined by direct palpation and comparison with the opposite joint.
- With DJD involving the fetlock, there is distension of the palmar or plantar pouches with some evidence of dorsal capsule distension. In the case of carpal joint disease, distension of the dorsal joint capsule over the middle carpal (intercarpal) and proximal carpal (radiocarpal) joints is characteristic. Thickening of the joint capsule can be detected on palpation of the affected carpal joint. Other joints, notably the small hock joints, coffin joint, and stifle may show few signs of capsule distension, and localization of a DJD problem is often difficult without intraarticular anesthesia.
- The lameness may be aggravated by flexion of the joint for 1 to 2 minutes, after which the horse is trotted off.

Diagnostic Tests

- Radiology is the most useful aid to diagnosis. The degree of narrowing of the joint space, the amount of periarticular new bone growth, and any calcification associated with origins or insertions of tendons and ligaments should be assessed. The dorsopalmar view is usually the best for assessing any reduction in the joint space, and it should be ensured that the primary beam is centered on the affected joint. Oblique views are necessary to discern periarticular new bone formation, which is usually found on the dorsomedial and/or dorsolateral aspect of the affected joint. The lateral view of an affected joint is helpful to assess the extent of soft-tissue swelling and changes in articular contours.

■ Intraarticular local anesthesia is important to confirm the particular joint as the site of lameness. Details of arthrocentesis are shown in Figures 3-24 to 3-49.

Therapeutic Options

The aim of therapy should be to attempt reestablishment of a normal joint environment and hence normal joint function. However, this is never achieved with the drugs that are currently available. The treatments of choice are those used intraarticularly (see below), with rest an important adjunct to therapy. Rest periods of 3 months appear to be the minimum to assist in the process of healing.

Sodium Hyaluronate (Treatment No. 60)—This is available in a variety of forms, but the most effective is the high-molecular-weight salt of hyaluronic acid, *Hylartin V*, which imparts viscosity to synovial fluid. This compound, a nonsulfated glycosaminoglycan that is derived from rooster combs, is a salt of hyaluronic acid, the component of synovial fluid that imparts viscosity and lubrication to the joint. In arthritis, the amount of hyaluronate in synovial fluid is decreased. Sodium hyaluronate administration aids in reestablishing local hyaluronate synthesis, as well as normalizing the internal joint environment. There also appear to be local anti-inflammatory effects that may be important in reducing the degree of synovitis. Therefore, decreasing lameness is due to improvement in joint function rather than purely suppression of inflammation and pain. This is a physiologic treatment, since it partially reestablishes the normality of the joint environment and enables normal hyaluronate synthesis to proceed in the affected joint. A 2-ml (20-mg) injection is given intraarticularly and may be combined with the simultaneous administration of intraarticular corticosteroids. We have found the combination of drugs useful in cases where there is evidence of capsulitis.

Synovial Fluid Transfer—This is a "poor man's" sodium hyaluronate. Between 4 and 10 ml of synovial fluid is collected from a healthy joint in the same horse and transferred to the diseased joint. The joint most commonly used for collection of the synovial fluid is the tarsocrural joint. The principle is similar to that for the use of sodium hyaluronate, although the concentrations of hyaluronate would be lower. The treatment seems to give the best results in horses in the early stages of arthritis, with no radiographic signs of joint disease. While there is a report in the literature of the efficacy of this therapy in Swedish trotters, in our experience, the results of treatment are disappointing.

Intraarticular Corticosteroids (Treatment Nos. 12, 13, 74, 106)—The corticosteroids have been the main intraarticular agents used to treat arthritis, being potent anti-inflammatory agents that inhibit lysosomal enzymes, collagenase, and prostaglandin release. While they have a favorable effect on soft-tissue injuries and result in relief of lameness associated with arthritis, corticosteroids may cause further cartilage degeneration. However, it may be that the latter disadvantage has been overemphasized in the past, with further deterioration because the horse is able to exercise on a compromised joint, rather than because of the presence of the corticosteroids and their effects on the cartilage. The benefits of reduced inflammation and decreased liberation of destructive enzymes should be considered. Intraarticular steroids are popular in racetrack practice because most trainers are under pressure to produce results, and the corticosteroids allow horses to return to training more quickly than most other forms of therapy. While corticosteroids have theoretical ill effects on articular cartilage, most equine practitioners find long-acting steroids to be greatly beneficial in both acute and chronic forms of arthritis. Steroid administration is ideally accompanied by 2 to 3 months of rest. It should be pointed out to owners and trainers that although intraarticular corticosteroids allow horses to remain in work, the damage to articular cartilage could be worsened as a result, and the long-term prognosis may be poor. However, we have had personal experience with a number of horses who have had six or more intraarticular injections over a period of 12 to 18 months and have not only remained in training but have had no demonstrable ill effects from repeated injections. Therefore, while the long-acting corticosteroids should be used with caution, it is clear that the detrimental effects may be less serious than were previously thought. An important consideration in states and countries with controlled medication laws, is that following intraarticular use of a long acting corticosteroid, detection of the drug is possible for as long as 6 to 8 weeks.

Polysulfated Glycosaminoglycans (PSGAGs) (Treatment No. 90)—The PSGAGs aim to improve joint function physiologically, in a similar manner to sodium hyaluronate. It is reported that they stimulate synthesis of hyaluronic acid and decrease loss of glycosaminoglycans from articular cartilage. Therefore, the PSGAGs may be useful in cases with damage to articular cartilage. However, PSGAG is thought to be chondroprotective rather than capable of healing large defects already present. The treatment regimen is usually as follows: weekly intraarticular injections of 250 mg PSGAG for 3 weeks. If PSGAGs are to be used after surgery, a period of several weeks should elapse prior to the first injection. Problems with septic arthritis have occurred following intraarticular PSGAGs in some cases where used close to the time of surgery. This may be due to alterations in the intraarticular environment that favor the growth of pathogenic bacteria such as staphylococci.

Intraarticular Orgotein (Treatment No. 79)—Orgotein is a water-soluble copper–zinc–metalloprotein complex. It affects superoxide dismutase activity as well as having anti-inflammatory effects. When used intraarticularly, it is thought to exert its effect on the joint capsule. Good results have been reported in cases of serous arthritis. In a limited number of cases we have had quite poor results with this drug and would hesitate to recommend its use.

Topical Application of Dimethylsulfoxide (Treatment No. 34)—Dimethylsulfoxide (DMSO) is a hydroxyl scavenger with some direct anti-inflammatory properties. It is applied topically to the affected joint and appears to be useful in all stages of arthritis. It can be used in conjunction with intraarticular treatments. It appears to be of most use in cases of serous arthritis where there is evidence of capsulitis rather than in cases where there are radiographic changes involving the joint. Because DMSO acts as a vehicle to take other products through the skin, some veterinarians choose to mix this product with other anti-inflammatory drugs such as phenylbutazone and flumethasone. In some countries there are commercial preparations of DMSO combinations that can be applied topically.

Other treatments that are used include systemic anti-inflammatory and analgesic drugs such as the nonsteroidal anti-inflammatories (see Chap. 17).

Azoturia

See Rhabdomyolysis

Cellulitis

Cellulitis is an infection of the soft tissues that occurs commonly in horses following local trauma, particularly due to wire cuts on the limbs. Such infections can spread to involve the bone and tendon sheaths, which can be extremely difficult to treat. In other cases, the infection can spread within soft tissues in the distal limb, resulting in a limb appearance similar to that in lymphangitis.

History and Presenting Signs

- Acute limb lameness
- Swelling of the affected limb
- History of trauma

Clinical Findings and Diagnosis

- Swelling and heat associated with soft-tissue inflammation in the affected area of the leg, usually the distal limb.
- Variable degrees of lameness are associated with the local cellulitis. However, unless closely related to a joint or tendon sheath, where infection of these structures can occur, the degree of lameness is usually minimal.
- Radiographs may be necessary to ensure that there are no changes in bony structures underlying the area of cellulitis. Reradiographing the affected area may be necessary about 14 days after the initial trauma because new periosteal bone growth may develop. If there has been a laceration that is deep enough to penetrate to the cortical bone, localized osteomyelitis may ensue (see p. 129). Radiographs will reveal signs of bone lysis and sequestrum formation.

Differential Diagnosis

- Osteomyelitis/Osteitis
- Tendon sheath infection
- Septic arthritis

Treatment

- Where the cellulitis is localized, local wound treatment using saline irrigation and povidone-iodine (see Disinfectants, Chap. 17) is effective in resolving the problem. This local treatment should be combined with bandaging the wound, using paraffin gauze applied to the site.
- Where there is more extensive tissue involvement, it is important to use appropriate antimicrobial therapy. Our experience is that most cases of cellulitis respond well to therapy with systemic penicillin. Sodium or potassium penicillin (20,000 IU/kg given IM) (Treatment Nos. 84 and 85) can be used to commence therapy, and this is followed by 15 mg/kg (15,000 IU/Kg) procaine penicillin (Treatment No. 83) administered IM twice daily for 3 to 5 days depending on the observed response.

Fistulous Withers

Fistulous withers is the term used to describe supraspinous bursitis, due mostly to localized infection with *Brucella abortus*. Occasionally, the organism will localize in the atlantal bursa, causing "poll evil." These conditions are seen quite infrequently in veterinary practice today. However, it is still a difficult condition to treat successfully, since many cases tend to recur because the infection localizes in various tissues surrounding the bursa.

Aspects of Diagnosis

- The first sign of fistulous withers is sensitivity over the wither region together with swelling.
- The swelling is usually localized and fluid-filled, although occasionally it is more diffuse.
- After a variable time course, a discharging sinus usually develops, with a purulent discharge.

Diagnostic Tests

- Diagnosis is possible from the clinical signs, although serum may be taken for *antibody titers* and purulent material aspirated for *microbiology*.

- In cases where there is a discharging sinus, swabs for microbiology are not worthwhile because a range of bacteria will be cultured. However, in the early stages of the condition, prior to development of a discharging sinus, it is possible to aspirate fluid from the supraspinous bursa for culture.

Differential Diagnosis

- Trauma
- Osteomyelitis
- Foreign body

Therapeutic Options

- If the condition is diagnosed before the discharging sinus develops, administration of oxytetracycline (Treatment No. 80) at a dose rate of 3 to 5 mg/kg twice daily for 7 days may achieve resolution. However, after a discharging sinus has developed, there is seldom a response to antibiotic therapy.
- Radical surgery, to establish effective drainage, is the only useful treatment, but the success rate is seldom better than 50%. Care must be taken regarding the discharge that contains *Brucella abortus* in low numbers. In particular, zoonotic infections should be avoided by rigorous hygiene.

Joint-III

See Septic Arthritis

Lymphangitis

Lymphangitis is a condition that results in swelling of the leg and is thought to be due to a restriction in lymphatic flow, possibly due to a bacterial infection. *Corynebacterium pseudotuberculosis* has been cultured from affected horses, but in many cases bacterial culture will be negative. It sometimes occurs in outbreak form, and we have seen up to 20% of horses affected in a mounted police stables. The mode of transmission and the etiologic agent could not be established.

Aspects of Diagnosis

KEY POINT ► By far the majority of cases affected involve the hindlimb(s), with swelling being apparent usually as far proximally as the hock and, occasionally, the stifle. In some cases, the distal limb may be enlarged up to two to three times normal size.

- Most horses will not show severe lameness of the affected limb, although they may show discomfort.
- There is usually no temperature rise or change in other cardinal signs.
- In most cases it is impossible to establish the causative agent.

Diagnostic Tests

- Ultrasonography, if performed, will reveal subcutaneous fluid accumulation only. There is also a loss of definition of some of the structures.
- Bacteriology may be useful if a fluid sample can be aspirated aseptically. In most cases, however, we have found it impossible to procure an adequate sample for bacteriology.

Differential Diagnosis

- Infection of the tendon sheaths
- Septic arthritis
- Cellulitis

Therapeutic Options

- Despite the use of a range of antibiotics, there has seldom been any response in most cases treated by us. In one outbreak at the mounted police stables, we found that the only antibiotic that resulted in improvement was oxytetracycline (Treatment No. 80). In other cases where this antibiotic has been used since, the results have been disappointing.
- Likewise, anti-inflammatory drugs such as phenylbutazone (Treatment No. 88) do not aid resolution.
- Cold hosing and pressure bandaging (Robert-Jones bandage) may be useful in the early stages.
- Some cases will improve temporarily following exercise, and some will resolve spontaneously with rest.
- Lymphangitis is a frustrating condition to treat.

Nutritional Secondary Hyperparathyroidism ("Big Head")

This disease is most common in horses grazing pastures that are predominant in tropical grasses such as buffel grass and setaria. These grasses contain oxalates that bind calcium, making it unavailable for absorption. Similar effects can be found from horses being fed high grain rations or diets with excessive phosphorus.

Aspects of Diagnosis

- A shifting lameness may be the first sign of a problem, followed by reluctance to move and, in severe cases, recumbency.
- Severely affected horses usually develop swellings of the maxilla and mandible.

Diagnostic Tests

Urinalysis will enable diagnosis of calcium deficiency or calcium–phosphorus imbalance by enabling assessment of dietary calcium level. The calcium concentration and specific gravity of urine should be determined, and then the following equation should be used:

$$\text{Ca excretion (mol/mosmol)} = \frac{\text{urine Ca concentration (mmol/L)} \times 0.04}{\text{specific gravity} - 0.997}$$

Calcium excretion values greater than 15 mol/mosmol indicate adequate dietary calcium.

Differential Diagnosis

- Epiphysitis
- Osteochondritis dissecans
- Hypertrophic pulmonary osteopathy

Therapeutic Options

- For horses grazing tropical grasses, a supplement of 1 kg of rock phosphate in 1.5 kg of molasses may be effective in prevention and treatment.
- In horses receiving excessive grain, the use of 20 to 40 g calcium carbonate, administered daily in the feed, is usually effective.

Osteochondrosis Dissecans

Osteochondrosis dissecans (OCD) is a term used to describe a defect in endochondral ossification whereby separation of cartilage and subchondral bone may occur within a joint. It is commonly found in growing horses and presents typically in yearlings and 2-year-olds. While the highest incidence is in thoroughbreds, it is also found in most other breeds, particularly fast-growing, athletic horses. A variety of joints have been reported to be affected, including the phalangeal, fetlock, carpal, shoulder, tarsal, and stifle joints. Joints within the vertebral column are also affected, most commonly the cervical spine. In addition to typical osteochondritis lesions, subchondral cystic lesions also have been described, although there is some debate as to whether they are part of the same syndrome or have a different pathogenesis.

KEY POINT ► Recent work has shown that diet plays a significant role in the etiology of OCD.

Diets that are high in energy and have calcium–phosphorus imbalance will result in a high incidence of OCD in a susceptible population. Furthermore, one study has shown that diets marginal in copper may contribute to a higher incidence of OCD lesions. Foals supplemented to give a dietary value of 55 ppm copper had fewer cartilage lesions than those fed a diet containing 15 ppm copper.

Aspects of Diagnosis

- Lameness and swelling and distension of the joint capsule are the main clinical signs. Effusion, which in some joints, notably the hock and stifle, is quite dramatic, is a consistent feature of OCD.

- Most commonly this will first become apparent in yearlings or 2-year-old horses.
- It is not uncommon for a horse to have several joints involved, and it is important to examine the joint contralateral to the affected one.
- In OCD involving the cervical spine, the resulting instability may lead to neurologic disease, with horses sometimes presenting as "wobblers."

Diagnostic Tests

- Radiographs are essential not only for diagnosis but also for prognosis.
- Arthroscopy is sometimes used as a diagnostic procedure, but in most cases radiographs are sufficient to establish the diagnosis.

Differential Diagnosis

- Degenerative joint disease
- Acute serous arthritis
- Traumatic osteochondral fragments

Therapeutic Options

- In mild cases, rest periods of 6 to 12 months will give resolution of the lameness in 50% to 70% of horses.

KEY POINT ► The treatment of choice in the majority of cases is arthroscopic surgery to remove the fragments of cartilage and bone.

- Most joints are now accessible using the arthroscope, and even quite large osteochondral fragments can be removed using arthroscopic visualization. Where there are extensive areas of damaged articular cartilage, the prognosis for athletic soundness is quite poor.
- In the young horse, it is important to reduce the dietary energy, and it may be of value to supplement the diet with copper to a total value of 55 ppm.

Osteomyelitis/Osteitis

Osteomyelitis is inflammation and infection of bone, which may result from either a localized infection following trauma or hematogenous spread. Hematogenous osteomyelitis is usually found in young foals, since they have well-vascularized bone, particularly in the region of the physis (growth plate). A wide range of bacteria may be identified by culture. Localized infection following trauma to the leg is particularly common in the metacarpus and metatarsus and usually involves only the cortical bone. It is referred to as osteitis.

Aspects of Diagnosis

- In localized osteitis following trauma (e.g., a wire cut to the distal limb), the most consistent finding is a purulent discharging sinus with a nonhealing wound.

- Horses with this type of bone infection do not usually show lameness, but there is localized swelling at the site of the discharge.
- If there has been hematogenous spread of infection, particularly to a growth plate, the foal will be very lame, and there is usually swelling of the affected area. In these cases, there will be no discharge. However, they may be concomitant septic arthritis involving the joint closest to the affected physis.

Diagnostic Tests

- Radiology is essential to confirm the diagnosis. Typical radiologic findings are a localized area of bone lysis with a surrounding area of sclerosis (increased bone density). There is usually a sequestrum of bone that is evident as an area of increased density within the area of bone lysis. Where the localized bone infection is the result of external trauma, there is usually substantial new periosteal bone growth associated with the area of bone lysis, which is usually located within the cortex.
- If there is infection of the growth plate, a 12-gauge needle may sometimes allow collection of a sample of material in an aseptic manner for bacterial culture and sensitivity.

KEY POINT ► If a discharging sinus is present, bacterial culture of the discharge should not be performed because the bacteria cultured will be secondary invaders. The results of such cultures lead to antibiotics being chosen that are likely to be worthless.

Differential Diagnosis

- Foreign body
- Localized cellulitis
- Local wound infection

Therapeutic Options

KEY POINT ► If a localized bone infection secondary to a limb wound is present, antibiotic therapy is of little or no value.

- There is usually a sequestrum of bone present, which has to be removed surgically. This is a simple technique that involves following the sinus tract and curetting the area of infected bone. Samples of bone from the infected area at surgery should be taken for microbiology rather than bacteriologic swabs. Penrose drains may be used, but most cases will resolve without drains being placed. Systemic antibiotic therapy is usually not necessary.
- In hematogenous osteomyelitis, it is very important to establish the specific causative bacteria and the antibiotic sensitivity patterns. Prolonged antibiotic therapy (see Chap. 17) for up to 3 to 4 weeks is necessary. If the horse is treated early

in the course of the infection, there may be resolution. Surgery is not advised if a growth plate is involved, because this may result in complete collapse of the leg.

Rhabdomyolysis ("Azoturia," Myoglobinuria, "Tying up," "Setfast")

Muscular problems are common in working horses and range from stiffness and mild cramps to recumbency with myoglobinuria. The terminology for these conditions has been variable and has included "Monday morning disease," "tying up," "setfast," and "azoturia." From the histopathologic findings on muscle biopsy samples, the term *rhabdomyolysis* is the most accurate. The basic mechanism for the condition remains unknown, although a common history in many cases is several days without exercise while fed on grain followed by vigorous exercise. It was thought that muscle glycogen accumulated during rest, and this was utilized during exercise with the production of excessive amounts of lactate. It now seems unlikely that this theory is correct, but the pathogenesis remains elusive. Clinical observations throughout the world have indicated that fillies and mares are affected much more commonly than stallions and geldings. Young horses may have only one or two attacks of the condition and no further problems, which is probably why clinicians have reported favorable responses to a variety of treatments. Single, acute episodes with significant muscle damage, myoglobinuria, and profound increases in muscle enzymes are found most commonly during endurance rides. The chronic, intermittent form of the disease is the most difficult to manage. Recently, it has been reported that there is a genetic component to the disease.

KEY POINT ► Studies from UK racing stables have indicated that chronic sodium and/or potassium deficiencies may be involved in the pathogenesis of chronic intermittent rhabdomyolysis.

These findings have been established from fractional excretion of urinary electrolytes, and there has been resolution following appropriate electrolyte supplementation. Although vitamin E deficiency has been incriminated in the etiology of rhabdomyolysis, it is now clear that vitamin E deficiency is not a cause of the classic disease.

Aspects of Diagnosis

- In mild cases (so-called tying up), hindleg stiffness and a shuffling hindleg gait are seen. There may be pain on palpation over the gluteal muscles, usually in both hindlegs. This form of the disease may occur when the horses have received very limited amounts of exercise.
- In some cases, horses may only need exposure to some form of stress (e.g., placing the horse in the starting barrier, transport, etc.). This type of

problem is more common in younger horses, where there may be a psychogenic factor involved.

- In some milder cases of rhabdomyolysis, poor performance may be the only feature of the disease.
- In more severe cases, there may be signs of severe pain with sweating, elevated heart rate, and reluctance to move. There also may be hard and painful locomotor muscles, the passage of dark-colored urine (myoglobinuria), and occasionally, recumbency. This is more common in horses during protracted exercise, where significant fluid and electrolyte alterations occur.

Diagnostic Tests

KEY POINT ▶ Diagnosis is possible usually on clinical signs alone, but in mild cases it is helpful to collect a blood sample for estimation of muscle enzyme activities in the serum.

- The most useful measurements are creatine kinase (CK or CPK) and aspartate aminotransferase (AST or GOT). These enzymes will be greatly elevated over normal values (see Hematology, Appendix 2), and in severe cases the values may be greater than 100,000 U/L. More commonly in horses with the mild acute or chronic, intermittent form of the disease, values are in the range 1500 to 10,000 U/L.
- Horses with chronic, intermittent rhabdomyolysis frequently demonstrate increases in serum or plasma CK and AST following an exercise test (10–15 minutes of lunging). Blood samples should be collected within 30 minutes of exercise and 4 to 6 hours after exercise. A positive result is indicated if CK values double after exercise.
- Because recent research has shown that a number of horses with mild, chronic, intermittent rhabdomyolysis have electrolyte deficiencies, urinary electrolyte excretions should be determined. Alterations in the excretion of sodium, potassium, calcium, and phosphorus have been reported. Simultaneous collection of urine and blood for electrolyte and creatinine determinations should be performed. Normal values must be established in the population studied because variations in feeding and management affect individual values.

Differential Diagnosis

- Aortoiliac thrombosis
- Colic
- Various causes of acute back pain
- Neurologic disease
- Laminitis
- Pleuropneumonia
- Muscle cramping

Therapeutic Options

A variety of different treatment regimens have been recommended, including thiamine, vitamin E and selenium, calcium borogluconate, anti-inflammatory drugs, tranquilizers, and muscle relaxants. In addition, many veterinarians have recommended the use of sodium bicarbonate in the feed to correct the purported acidosis. However, studies have demonstrated that metabolic acidosis is not a typical feature of horses with rhabdomyolysis, and bicarbonate use may not be justified.

Of all the treatments used to treat rhabdomyolysis, few have been examined critically for their efficacy. The treatments that appear to give consistent results are as follows:

Severe Cases—Intravenous fluids (see Fluid Therapy, Chap. 17) should be used if any signs of shock are present and also to ensure that myoglobin does not produce renal damage, particularly in the face of hypovolemia. In addition, 0.2 mg/kg dexamethasone (Treatment Nos. 29 and 30) intravenously is useful in aiding relief of clinical signs. The use of nonsteroidal anti-inflammatory drugs such as phenylbutazone (Treatment No. 88) at dose rates of 2.2 mg/kg twice daily for 3 to 5 days may be indicated. If horses are in severe pain, the use of drugs such as detomidine (Treatment No. 28) at dose rates of 10 to 20 μg/kg or xylazine (Treatment No. 108) at a dose rate of 0.2 mg/kg may be indicated. Because these drugs have a profound effect on blood pressure, they should not be used before correction of hypovolemia. After recovery, the horse should be rested for at least 6 to 8 weeks and then slowly brought back into training.

Mild Cases—Walking affected horses is sometimes useful, and most will recover without any further treatment. Intravenous thiamine and intramuscular vitamin E and selenium have been used widely in practice, and there is some empirical evidence that they may assist recovery. The use of nonsteroidal anti-inflammatory drugs such as phenylbutazone at dose rates of 2.2 mg/kg twice daily for 3 to 5 days may be indicated. Horses are usually rested for 3 to 4 days and then introduced to a gradually increasing exercise program. Lowering of the training intensity together with reduction of grain in the diet is often useful. Acepromazine (8–15 mg per 450-kg horse) can help alleviate the muscle spasm and promote peripheral vasodilatation in mild cases. In some cases, acepromazine at dose rates of 5 to 8 mg per 450-kg horse, administered prior to training, is useful in preventing further signs of the disease.

Chronic, Intermittent Cases—The administration of the intracellular calcium blocking agent dantrolene sodium (Dantrium) and the sodium and calcium channel-blocking agent phenytoin (Treatment No. 89) has been reported to aid in the prevention of recurrence of rhabdomyolysis. Dantrolene is expensive to use, difficult to achieve adequate circulating blood concentrations, and of questionable efficacy.

KEY POINT ► However, we have found phenytoin to be a useful adjunct to management changes in horses with the recurrent form of the disease.

Ideally, dosage schedules should be based on determinations of plasma concentrations, with therapeutic levels considered to be in the range 5 to 10 µg/ml. This is usually achieved by oral administration of 10 to 12 mg/kg phenytoin twice daily for 3 days, followed by 10 to 12 mg/kg once daily for 3 days. After this, the dose is reduced to 5 to 6 mg/kg once daily. The drug should be withdrawn at least 7 days prior to racing. The response to this drug is not consistent, and adverse effects include drowsiness, ataxia, and rarely, seizures. During the first 3 days on the high dose twice daily it is best to avoid serious training, since the horses usually become a little depressed. If urinary electrolyte clearances indicate marginal dietary sodium and/or potassium, electrolyte supplementation may be indicated. This usually involves adding 20 to 60 g sodium and/or potassium chloride to the feed.

Septic Arthritis

Septic arthritis may occur either in foals, where it is usually the result of septicemia and involves multiple joints ("joint-ill"), or in adult horses, where it results from penetrating injuries and is mostly monarticular. Owing to the destructive effects on articular cartilage of bacteria, high leukocyte concentrations, and resultant enzyme liberation, early diagnosis and treatment are essential if irreversible damage to the joint is to be avoided. The most common mistake made by equine practitioners in treating suspected septic arthritis is that of commencing antibiotic therapy prior to the collecting synovial fluid samples for culture and sensitivity testing. The use of antibiotics, even if ineffective, will make the subsequent culture of bacteria difficult.

Aspects of Diagnosis

■ The earliest clinical sign is a reluctance to bear weight associated with marked heat, swelling, and pain in the affected joint(s). Considerable joint effusion is found in all cases of septic arthritis.
■ There may be signs of a septicemia or bacteremia, including elevated heart rate and temperature, particularly in foals with "joint-ill." In the early stages of septic arthritis, horses appear depressed and may be inappetent. Temperature can fluctuate greatly during the course of the day but is usually in the range 39.0 to 40°C (102.5 to 104°F).

Differential Diagnosis

■ Fractures
■ Osteomyelitis (particularly of the epiphyses)
■ Infection of tendon sheaths
■ Foot abscess
■ Infection of the navicular bursa

Diagnostic Tests

Synovial Fluid Analysis

It is important that synovial fluid be collected in a completely sterile fashion, and this is best performed under general anesthesia. While synovial fluid can be collected in the conscious horse, there are often difficulties in obtaining uncontaminated samples. Because the affected joint(s) is inflamed and painful, horses are difficult to restrain for synovial fluid collection. A contaminated synovial fluid sample submitted for bacteriology is worse than no synovial fluid sample. Under general anesthesia, fluid samples can be collected in a completely sterile manner. This sample collection can be combined with lavage therapy.

Synovial fluid samples should be collected into EDTA for total and differential white cell counts and total protein measurement. White cell counts in excess of 5000/µL (5000 × 10⁶/L) with greater than 80% neutrophils and total protein values greater than 30 g/L (3 g/dL) indicate septic arthritis. In the acute stages of septic arthritis, prior to antibiotic therapy, white cell counts in synovial fluid are often greater than 30,000 × 10⁶/L, and the percentage of neutrophils is in excess of 95%.

Collection of a sterile sample for bacteriology is essential if an appropriate antibiotic is to be chosen for therapy. The synovial fluid should be handled in the following way:

(a) *The sample is centrifuged, and the supernatant is discarded.*
(b) *From the deposit, a Gram stain is made, and the remainder is placed in enrichment media (e.g., brain/heart broth).*
(c) *Subcultures are made at 12 and 24 hours after the deposit has been placed in the enrichment media.*
(d) *Antibiotic sensitivity tests are performed. For further details, see Clinical Bacteriology (Chap. 15).*

■ If antibiotics have been used prior to collection of the synovial fluid samples, antibiotic removal devices can be used to assist in recovery of bacteria.

Synovial Membrane Biopsy. In some cases, bacteria cannot be recovered from synovial fluid, particularly when antibiotics have been used prior to bacteriologic sampling. Synovial membrane biopsy can then be used to obtain tissue for bacteriologic culture and sensitivity testing. This is best performed using an arthroscope to visualize the area of synovial membrane to be biopsied. The sample should be submitted in a sterile container to the laboratory.

Therapeutic Options

- There is no possibility of predicting the type of bacteria involved without synovial fluid examination and culture. In both foals and adult horses, a range of gram-negative and gram-positive bacteria have been found. However, on the basis of the Gram stain, systemic therapy can be commenced (see Chap. 17). For example, for Gram-positive species, use penicillin (Treatment Nos. 83–85); for Gram-negative species, use gentamicin (Treatment No. 56) or amikacin (Treatment No. 4). The treatment can subsequently be modified when the complete bacteriologic results become known. If early treatment is undertaken, appropriate systemic antibiotic administration will result in good recovery of function.
- Irrigation of the joint with 3 to 4 L of a balanced electrolyte solution containing an appropriate antibiotic should be performed. This may need to be performed every other day in the first week. A minimum of 14 days of antibiotic therapy is usually necessary. Response to therapy can be monitored by synovial fluid white cell counts and Gram stains. A considerable reduction in synovial fluid white cell count may be found within 48 hours of instituting therapy.
- More recently, good results have been obtained by irrigating 4 to 5 L of a 20% solution of dimethylsulfoxide (Treatment No. 34) through an indwelling drain placed into the joint. This is usually followed by a povidone-iodine solution. This solution may be flushed through the joint overnight. Cases of septic arthritis improve much more rapidly than with the more traditional lavage using balanced electrolyte solutions.
- In more chronic cases, arthroscopic surgery may be required to remove debris from the joint and allow thorough lavage following initial systemic antibiotic therapy. We also have found in some cases that arthrotomy may be required to clear the debris from the joint. In some cases, 2 to 3 weeks of antibiotic treatment may be necessary.

- Some surgeons favor the use of through-and-through drains in the affected joint. Our experience with these is that it is difficult to obtain effective drainage, except possibly by drains inserted into the tarsocrural (tibiotarsal) joint. Furthermore, because of contamination of the drains, it is possible that the joint may become infected with additional bacteria, complicating the antibiotic therapy.
- Long-term follow-up in a range of horses presented to our clinic with septic arthritis has shown that even in horses that appear to respond well in the short term, low-grade lameness is often a subsequent finding. This is so because degenerative joint disease is a common sequel to infection as a result of the damage to articular cartilage.

References

Bertone, A. L., McIlwraith, C. W., Jones, R. L., et al.: Comparison of various treatments for experimentally induced equine infectious arthritis. *Am. J. Vet. Res.* 48:519, 1987.
Clyne, M. J.: Pathogenesis of degenerative joint disease. *Equine Vet. J.* 19:15, 1987.
Dyson, S.: Clinical questions concerning degenerative joint disease. *Equine Vet. J.* 19:6, 1987.
Firth, E. C.: Hematogenous osteomyelitis in the foal. *Proc. 33rd Conv. Am. Assoc. Equine Pract.*, 1987, p. 795.
Gibson, K. T., McIlwraith, C. W., Turner, A. S., et al.: Open joint injuries in horses: 58 cases (1980–1986). *J. Am. Vet. Med. Assoc.* 194:398, 1989.
Markel, M. D., Wheat, J. D., and Jang, S. S.: Cellulitis associated with coagulase-positive staphylococci in racehorses: Nine cases (1975–1984). *J. Am. Vet. Med. Assoc.* 189:1600, 1986.
Martens, R. J., Auer, J. A., and Carter, G. K.: Equine pediatrics: Septic arthritis and osteomyelitis. *J. Am. Vet. Med. Assoc.* 188:582, 1986.
McIlwraith, C. W.: Antibiotic use in musculoskeletal disease. *Proc. 32nd Conv. Am. Assoc. Equine Pract.*, 1986, p. 241.
Pool, R. R., and Meagher, D. M.: Pathologic findings and pathogenesis of racetrack injuries. *Vet. Clin. North Am.* 6:1, 1990.

CHAPTER 4

Respiratory System

Diseases of the respiratory system are common in horses, particularly in North America and Europe, where infectious respiratory conditions often result in significant wastage and poor performance in athletes. The combination of climate, the need for housing during the colder months resulting in close contact between animals, stressful activities such as racing and transport, and the presence of a variety of respiratory viruses results in the high incidence of respiratory disease. Infectious respiratory disease often produces the greatest morbidity in younger horses and frequently is a particular problem on stud farms and in racehorse populations.

Most infectious respiratory diseases are initiated by viral infections in which the affected horse becomes depressed, inappetent, and febrile. Commonly, the offending agent is cleared by the host. However, where the horse's defenses are compromised, secondary bacterial infections may result in more severe bronchitis, pneumonia, or possibly pleuropneumonia.

The challenge in respiratory disease is in making a specific diagnosis. Signs of respiratory tract involvement are usually self-evident and include respiratory noise during exercise, nasal discharge, cough, dyspnea, and fever. It is only after careful examination and utilization of relevant diagnostic aids that a correct diagnosis and therefore appropriate therapy can be instituted.

SIGNALMENT AND HISTORY

Signalment is important because younger horses often suffer from infectious diseases (e.g., *Rhodococcus equi* in foals and rhinopneumonitis in weanlings and yearlings), whereas older animals tend to be afflicted more commonly with chronic disorders (e.g., chronic allergic respiratory disease). A thorough history is essential when one is presented with a horse suspected of having a respiratory disorder. Determination of the exact complaint, duration of

the disorder, exposure to stress or other horses with similar signs, recent changes in management, vaccination schedules, and responses to treatment (if any) should all be determined. Some of the specific questions related to various respiratory disorders were outlined in Chapter 2.

EXAMINATION PROCEDURE

Respiratory disease frequently results in generalized systemic signs, making it important to assess carefully the animal's overall status in addition to a specific examination of the respiratory tract. Initial evaluation of a horse with respiratory disease should include assessments of alterations in general body condition, quality of the hair coat, rectal temperature, heart rate, pulse quality, and hydration status (see Chap. 1). Following these appraisals, a thorough examination of the respiratory tract should be performed. This is best performed initially at rest and in a location free from distracting outside noise.

Initial Inspection

The examiner should begin by gaining a general impression of the horse's respiratory rate, effort, pattern, and whether there is any evidence of inspiratory or expiratory noise. Abnormalities such as dyspnea, flaring of the nostrils, guarded inspirations, or a marked diphasic expiratory effort with an increased contribution by the abdominal musculature should be noted. The presence of a nasal discharge should also be investigated. Serous nasal discharge is common with viral respiratory infections, whereas mucopurulent exudate is more likely with a bacterial disease. It also should be noted whether the discharge is unilateral or bilateral, malodorous, or more profuse when the head is lowered or the horse is eating (as often occurs with guttural pouch empyema). It should be ascertained whether the horse has a cough, and if so, its frequency and character should be determined.

Detailed Examination

Examination begins with inspection of the head and neck for any obvious asymmetry. Care is taken to examine the nostrils for symmetry, equality of airflow, and presence of abnormal respiratory sounds, odor (which may indicate turbinate necrosis, guttural pouch disease, or pleuropneumonia), or palpable abnormalities in the nostrils. Examination of the mucous membranes should follow to check for cyanosis or hemorrhages. The area between the mandibles and the parotid region is then examined to determine if there is any enlargement of lymph nodes. Percussion of the maxillary and frontal sinuses should be performed to determine if there is any fluid present or associated pain. The maxillary sinuses lie dorsal to the facial crest, and the frontal sinuses lie on either side of the dorsal midline, with their centers approximately at the level of the eyes. Determination of alterations in the resonance of maxillary sinuses is greatly facilitated if the horse's mouth is opened by placing a finger in the interdental space, while percussing. The larynx is then palpated to determine if any asymmetry of the dorsal cricoarytenoid muscles can be felt. This is done by placing the index fingers under the tendon of the sternocephalicus muscle on either side of the neck and palpating the anterior dorsal part of the larynx. If there is atrophy of the dorsal cricoarytenoid muscle (as often occurs in idiopathic left laryngeal hemiplegia), the muscular process of the arytenoid cartilage will be very prominent on the affected side. Any scarring or thickening of skin that could suggest a previous laryngoplasty or laryngotomy should be noted. If there is any indication of excessive prominence of the left muscular process of the arytenoid cartilage, indicating laryngeal hemiplegia, a laryngeal adductor ("slap test") may be useful.

KEY POINT ▶ The "slap test" is done while palpating the muscular processes on left and right sides.

Slapping the left thorax gently with the open hand should result in the right muscular process adducting, and this can be felt as a "flicking" or movement of the process. Similarly, slapping of the right thorax should result in the muscular process of the left arytenoid cartilage "flicking." In horses with idiopathic left laryngeal hemiplegia, the "flicking" of the left muscular process does not occur or is reduced in response to the "slap test" on the right side of the chest. Squeezing firmly at the junction of the cricoid cartilage and trachea will induce a cough, and in horses with pharyngitis, laryngitis, or tracheitis, pressure in this region may evoke a paroxysm of coughing. Palpation of the cervical trachea should then be performed to assess for the presence of stenosis.

Auscultation

Careful auscultation of the chest on both left and right sides and over the cervical trachea is important if pulmonary disease is suspected. Auscultation should be performed in a quiet environment to optimize the chances of detecting abnormalities. The normal margins of the thoracic cavity are level with the tuber coxae at the eighteenth rib, midthorax at the thirteenth rib, shoulder at the eleventh rib, and then curving down to the level of the elbow.

KEY POINT ▶ Because of the quiet respiration of most horses (particularly fat animals), it may be helpful to accentuate the respiratory sounds by placing a large plastic bag over the horse's nose (Fig. 4-1).

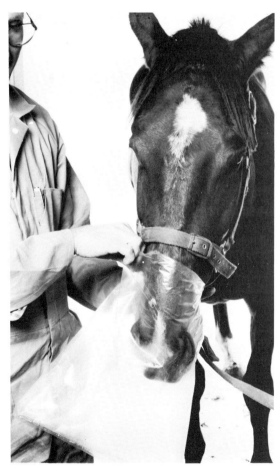

Figure 4–1. Auscultation of the chest using a rebreathing technique. A plastic bag is placed over the nose, and the resulting increase in arterial carbon dioxide tension and decrease in arterial oxygen tension results in an increase in tidal volume and respiratory rate.

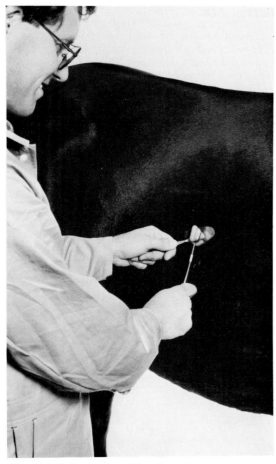

Figure 4–2. Percussion of the chest using a metal spoon as a plexor and a patellar hammer as a pleximeter.

This will stimulate increased rate and depth of respiration by lowering the inspired O_2 concentration and increasing the CO_2 concentration. The result is large respiratory excursions, and air movement through both large and small airways is more easily heard. Care should be taken when using this technique in horses with painful pleural conditions because the discomfort associated with deep respiratory efforts may be severe. Another complication associated with rebreathing bags is the induction of paroxysmal coughing, which occasionally occurs in horses with highly sensitive airways (e.g., chronic allergic respiratory disease). Such a reaction will preclude effective auscultation of the respiratory tract. Under normal conditions, inspiratory sounds are louder than expiratory sounds, with all sounds being slightly louder on the right side of the thorax. Sounds over the carina are more audible than those in other parts of the respiratory tract. Abnormalities include increases in the intensity of respiratory sounds (particularly if expiration is louder than inspiration), areas of dullness, radiation of

heart sounds over a greater area than normal, crackles (discontinuous sounds), wheezes (continuous sounds), and pleural friction rubs (loudest at the end of inspiration). A common normal finding when auscultating the chest is the presence of intestinal sounds within the thoracic cavity. Borborygmal sounds within the margins of the thoracic cavity are considered to be a normal finding.

Percussion

Percussion of the chest is a technique that is used less frequently, since the advent of ultrasonographic techniques, to assess horses with respiratory disease. However, percussion can be very effective, especially for detection of fluid or pleural pain. Percussion can be performed using a plexor and pleximeter or a rubber hammer as a plexor and a spoon as a pleximeter (Fig. 4-2) or by using the thumb and middle finger to flick the chest. By working along the chest in parallel lines from dorsal to ventral and anterior to posterior, the whole chest can be covered. Dull areas indicate consolidation near the lung surface or the presence of fluid.

DIAGNOSTIC AIDS
Endoscopy

Direct visual examination of the respiratory tract with flexible endoscopes is widely practiced in equine medicine. Most endoscopes in use today have an external diameter of 8 to 10 mm and range in length from 60 cm to 3 m. Examination is best performed with the horse restrained in stocks (if possible). Sedation is usually not necessary and may influence the findings of some examinations, because function of the arytenoid cartilages may be modified following administration of sedatives. Following application of a twitch, the endoscope is passed up the ventral nasal meatus. Depending on the indication, examination of the nasal passages, nasomaxillary ostium of the paranasal sinuses, ethmoid region, pharynx, larynx, guttural pouch openings (and the internal linings of the pouches), trachea, and some other parts of the lower airways can be carried out. A line drawing showing the normal larynx and pharynx as viewed from the nasopharynx is presented in Figure 4-3. Longer endoscopes can be passed distally as far as some of the mainstream bronchi. Endoscopy is a particularly valuable tool for examination of the upper respiratory tract and enables diagnosis of laryngeal hemiplegia, aryepiglottic entrapment, pharyngeal cysts, and lymphoid hyperplasia. The technique is also often integral to the detection of nasal tumors, polyps, and mycoses; ethmoidal hematomas; guttural pouch empyema and mycosis; pus or blood draining from the nasomaxillary opening; exercise-induced pulmonary hemorrhage; and the accumu-

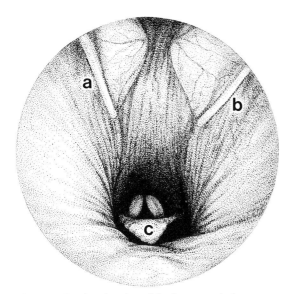

Figure 4–3. Line drawing of the larynx and pharynx as seen via an endoscope positioned in the nasopharynx. The soft palate lies ventrally under the epiglottis (c), and dorsally the right (a) and left (b) guttural pouch openings are visible.

lation of large volumes of abnormal fluid or pus within the trachea.

Laryngeal function tests that are useful during endoscopy include partial nostril occlusion to stimulate laryngeal abductor movement and flushing water through the endoscope to stimulate swallowing. The normal endoscopic appearance of the larynx at rest and after nostril occlusion is shown in Fig. 4-4.

Catheterization of the Guttural Pouches

This procedure is useful for collecting samples for bacterial and fungal culture and for irrigating the pouches. There are two methods for catheterization of the pouches, *blind* and *endoscope-guided*. When using the blind technique, a Chamber's or plastic mare uterine infusion catheter is used with approximately 3.75 cm at the end bent at about 20 degrees. The distance the catheter is to be passed to gain access to the guttural pouch can be determined by measuring the distance between the lateral canthus of the eye and the nostril. A mark is placed on the catheter as a reference point when it is inserted. The catheter is passed down the ventral meatus, with the tip pointed down. When inserted to a depth of about 2 to 5 cm from the mark, the catheter is rotated laterally through about 150 degrees, and the end of the catheter in the nostril is moved into a dorsal and lateral position over the alar fold. The catheter is advanced, and contact with the pharyngeal wall can be sensed. When the horse swallows, the guttural pouch openings will dilate, and the catheter can be passed into the pouch. Once the catheter passes through the opening, it can continue to be advanced with less resistance than if it were pushing into the pharyngeal wall. Passage of the catheter is achieved more easily if an endoscope is passed up the contralateral nostril and the catheter is observed as it is passed into the pouch opening. Samples for microbiologic analysis can then be collected by infusion of a sterile lavage solution (e.g., normal saline) with subsequent aspiration. Obviously, this technique also provides a mechanism by which solutions for therapy can be infused into the pouch.

A number of methods have been described for

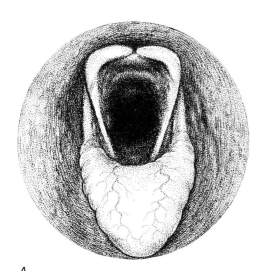
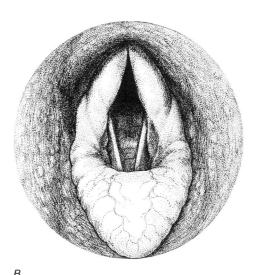

A   *B*

Figure 4–4. Line drawing of the endoscopic appearance of the larynx in the horse during quiet breathing (*B*) and after respiratory stimulation showing arytenoid abduction (*A*).

the placement and maintenance of indwelling catheters in the guttural pouch. These include Foley catheters (27F) with the balloon inflated with saline when in the pouch. Alternatives include an intra-uterine catheter with a "rams horn" tip or a catheter with a curled grapple at the tip constructed from polyethylene (PE 240) tubing. The grapple is made by heating the tubing in hot water and then wrapping it around the barrel of a 30-ml syringe. Although these catheters provide an excellent means for repeated pouch infusions, they may induce considerable local irritation to the mucosa of the guttural pouch.

Transtracheal Aspiration

A number of techniques have been described for lavage and aspiration of the tracheobronchial tree. Transtracheal aspiration allows aseptic collection of samples from the lower respiratory tract, for cytology and microbiology.

KEY POINT ▶ For collection of samples under the most aseptic conditions for microbiology, a transtracheal wash and aspirate is the optimal method.

Contamination of sampling catheters and aspirates with bacteria from the nasal passages and pharynx is avoided, and the findings are more likely to reflect the real situation. To perform the technique, an area over the middle to lower trachea is clipped and shaved. Although this is not an intrinsically painful procedure, horses may require application of a twitch or administration of a small dose of sedative prior to the procedure. A small volume of local anesthetic is injected under the skin over the trachea (Fig. 4-5), and a small stab incision is made (Fig. 4-6). The operator applies surgical gloves, and the trachea is palpated and stabilized with one hand. A 12- or 14-gauge needle or catheter is inserted in a downward direction through the skin incision into the lumen of the trachea (Fig. 4-7), taking care to penetrate between the tracheal rings and not to damage the tracheal rings on the opposite side of the trachea. If resistance to passage of the needle or catheter into the trachea is detected, this may indicate that the needle or catheter is against a tracheal ring. A 5F or 6F sterile dog urinary catheter is then passed down the trachea to the level of the carina (Fig. 4-8). Because the ends of these catheters are sealed, it may be useful to cut off the end to allow passage of tenacious secretions. An alternate method utilizes a 60-cm drum catheter/needle combination (Deseret Co., Sandy, Utah). The catheter should be inserted 50 to 60 cm—at least to the level of the thoracic inlet (where the trachea lies in the horizontal plane and secretions may accumulate). Sterile saline (50 ml) is injected into the trachea (Fig. 4-9), and aspiration is performed (Fig. 4-10). If there is little or no yield of fluid on aspiration, the catheter can be repositioned

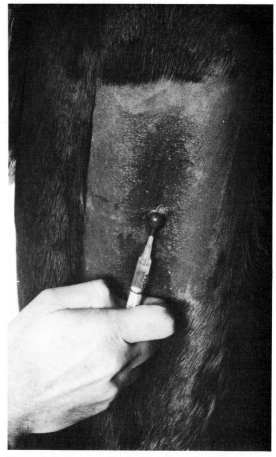

Figure 4–5. Transtracheal aspiration. The skin over the ventral midline of the midcervical region is clipped, and after disinfection, a bleb (1–2 mL) of local anesthetic is injected.

slightly, and aspiration can be repeated. If this is still unsuccessful, the flushing/aspiration procedure can be repeated. In addition, the horse's head can be lowered to further improve the chance of a successful aspiration. Some horses will cough during infusion of saline, which may increase the yield of mucopurulent material. If there is severe coughing, the catheter may be dislodged proximally to lie around the laryngeal opening.

Following collection of the sample, the urinary catheter is removed first, followed by the introducer. This sequence may not be possible if a needle is used as an introducer, because retrograde movement of the catheter may result in severance of the catheter tip in the trachea.

Complications of the procedure include:

■ Damage to the tracheal rings, which can be reduced if care is taken when the needle is inserted.
■ Breakage of the catheter within the trachea. This is rare, and most horses cough up the catheter within 30 minutes with no untoward side effects.

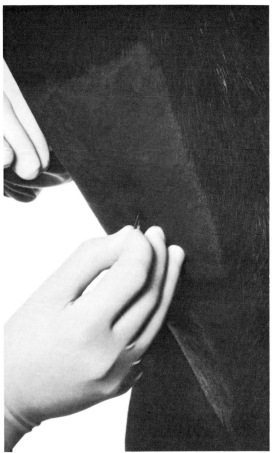

Figure 4–6. Transtracheal aspirate. After clipping and appropriate skin disinfection, a stab incision is made through the skin and subcutaneous tissues with a no. 11 scalpel blade.

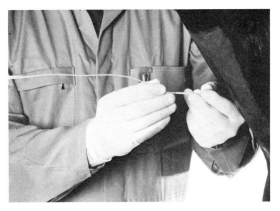

Figure 4–8. Transtracheal aspirate. A sterile dog urinary catheter (8Fr) is inserted through the needle into the trachea so that is comes to lie around the area of the carina.

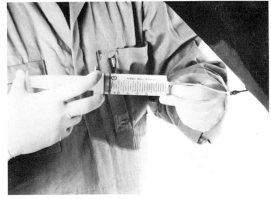

Figure 4–9. Sterile phosphate-buffered saline (50–200 mL) is injected through the urinary catheter.

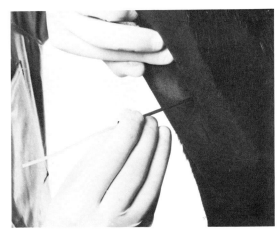

Figure 4–7. Transtracheal aspirate. A large-bore (12-gauge) needle is inserted between the tracheal rings into the lumen of the trachea.

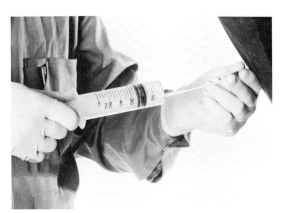

Figure 4–10. Aspiration of mucopurulent material from the lower airway.

■ Cellulitis at the site of tracheal puncture. This is probably the most common adverse effect and may be reduced in severity if the catheter is removed prior to extirpation of the introducing needle and a bandage is applied for 24 hours after the procedure. Systemic antibiotics should be administered if malodorous or purulent material is harvested or if the initial Gram stains indicate bacterial infection. If swelling does occur, local therapy with hot packs and topical DMSO may be useful.

KEY POINT ▶ Samples may be collected for cytology via a catheter inserted into the lower airway through the biopsy channel of a flexible endoscope.

However, because there is contamination by bacteria resident in the upper respiratory tract, such samples are unreliable for microbiology. The operator can visualize the areas of accumulated mucoid or purulent material, direct the catheter appropriately, and harvest samples using a similar technique to that described for the transtracheal method. Overall contamination of samples is reduced if the endoscope is disinfected prior to the procedure.

Recently, "guarded" catheters for insertion through the nasopharynx for collection of tracheobronchial aspirates have been described (Darien microbiol-ogy aspiration catheter, Mill-Rose Labs., Inc, Mentor, Ohio). These catheters decrease the chance of contamination of samples but do not eliminate the possibility entirely.

Following collection, the aspirate is placed in a sterile container (or kept in the sterile syringe) and subjected to cytologic, bacteriologic, and possibly mycologic examination (see Chap. 15).

Bronchoalveolar Lavage (BAL)

This procedure has been used much more widely in recent years and is designed to collect fluid and cells from the distal airways and alveoli. It is a simple technique that often provides useful information with respect to the integrity and constituents of the lower respiratory tract. BAL can be performed "blind" or with a flexible fiberoptic endoscope. When the endoscopic technique is used, the horse is sedated (xylazine at a dose rate of 0.2–0.4 mg/kg is suitable), and the tip of the endoscope is passed into the lower respiratory tract and wedged in the smallest possible airway. With the "blind" technique, an equine BAL tube (Bivona, Inc., Gary, Ind.) is passed into the lower airway and wedged into position (Fig. 4-11). Passage of the tube into the trachea is facilitated if an assistant extends the horse's head. Obviously, the operator has little

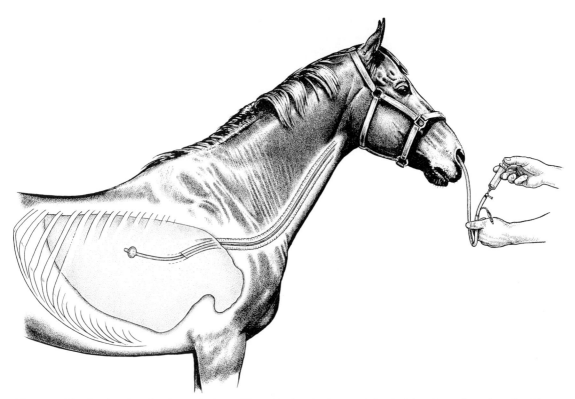

Figure 4–11. Line drawing showing technique of bronchoalveolar lavage. After lodging the catheter in a distal bronchus, the balloon on the catheter is inflated with 5 ml air. Sterile saline (50 mL) is then flushed into lung and aspirated for cytologic analysis.

knowledge of which respiratory unit the lavage tube is wedged in. Between 50 and 300 ml of saline is infused in 50-ml aliquots, and it is aspirated immediately following infusion.

Subsequent to collection, samples are observed for color and subjected to cytologic (total and differential nucleated cell counts) examination.

KEY POINT ▶ BAL will only provide information about the portion of the lung sampled. This *may not* be indicative of the overall condition of the lung.

Ultrasound Examination

Over the past decade, the advent of portable ultrasound equipment has made this form of examination of a horse's thorax feasible. As a result, ultrasound is now widely used by equine practitioners, particularly in cases where lower respiratory tract pathology is suspected. Ultrasound is most suitable for detection of accumulations of fluid within the pleural space, consolidation of the lung parenchyma, and the presence of abscessation. In addition, if fluid has accumulated within the thorax, some indications regarding the quality of that fluid can be obtained. Both linear and sector scanners can be used to examine the equine thorax. Sector scanners provide the best-quality images but are more expensive than linear scanners (commonly used for pregnancy diagnosis). Both types of scanners can provide quite acceptable images of the equine lung and pleural space. It is important to clip the hair over the region to be imaged because intact hair traps air, which dramatically interferes with the quality of the image (Fig. 4-12). A suitable acoustic coupling gel should then be applied. The boundaries of the lung were described earlier in this chapter. Such anatomic landmarks are important when imaging the thorax. Fluid containing small amounts of particulate matter may create little

acoustic reflection (anechoic), whereas accumulations of inflammatory debris (cells and fibrin) are echogenic. Anaerobic infections may be reflected by the appearance of gas bubbles within pleural fluid accumulations.

Thoracocentesis

If a dull area or fluid line is suspected by auscultation or percussion or fluid is imaged with ultrasound examination or radiography, thoracocentesis is indicated to reveal (1) if fluid is present and (2) the cytologic and microbiologic characteristics of that fluid. In general, thoracocentesis should be performed in the ventral third of the thorax, with care being exercised to avoid the heart. Although not imperative, ultrasound-guided thoracocentesis is the optimal method. For initial sampling, if only a small amount of fluid is suspected, a 6- to 7.5-cm teat cannula can be used.

KEY POINT ▶ Aseptic technique is very important, and therefore, an area of skin over the sixth, seventh, and eighth intercostal spaces about 7.5 to 10 cm above the level of the olecranon is clipped, shaved, and aseptically prepared.

Local anesthetic is infused subcutaneously and into the intercostal muscles and sufficiently deep to include the parietal pleura. A stab incision is made in the skin with a small blade, and the cannula is inserted cranial to the rib border to ensure that the intercostal vessels and nerves, which course down the caudal aspects of the ribs, are not damaged. The cannula is advanced into the pleural space, and fluid is aspirated (Fig. 4-13). If large amounts of fluid are present, or if the fluid has a high concentration of fibrin material, larger-bore catheters can be utilized. Blunt-tipped thoracic drainage tubes designed for human use are ideal and are available

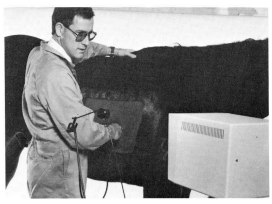

Figure 4–12. Ultrasound examination of the chest to determine the presence of fluid. Note that the hair over the chest wall must be clipped to permit good-quality images.

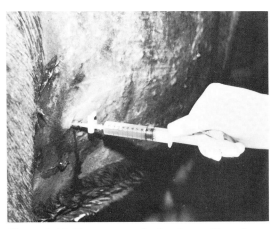

Figure 4–13. Thoracocentesis showing position of cannula in the eighth intercostal space.

in a variety of sizes. These may be sutured in place and plugged if repeated drainage is required. Thoracocentesis should be performed on both sides of the thorax, because different bacteriologic results can be found.

The quantity and quality of fluid obtained during this procedure may provide valuable information for the clinician. In the normal horse, little or no fluid is obtained from the thorax. In conditions where pathology exists, more than 25 L fluid may be drained from each hemithorax. In addition to fluid volume reflecting pathology, the color of the fluid, degree of opacity, presence of fibrinous material, and odor are all useful indicators of the severity of disease. With infectious causes of pleural effusion, the fluid will often become more opaque, malodorous, and contain fibrin clots. The presence of a fetid odor often reflects the presence of anaerobic bacteria.

Cytologic examination of normal pleural fluid reveals a sterile fluid with a total protein concentration below 30 to 35 g/L (3 to 3.5 g/dL) and a nucleated cell count of less than the peripheral white cell count and usually less than 8000 to 10,000 nucleated cells $\times$ 10^6/L (8000 to 10,000/μL). Of these cells, less than 60% to 70% should be neutrophils, with the balance being macrophages and lymphocytes. With pleuropneumonia, the volume of fluid increases, as does the cell count (predominantly neutrophils) and total protein concentration. The pH and glucose content of pleural fluid also may be a good indicator of disease. Under normal conditions, pleural fluid pH is similar to that of peripheral blood (7.4), with the glucose concentration being greater than 2 mmol/L (40 mg/dL). In cases of pleuropneumonia, pH and glucose concentrations often fall below these values.

Thoracic fluid should be placed into appropriate preservatives for cytologic and microbiologic examinations. For cytologic examination and protein determination, samples should be placed in EDTA tubes used for preservation of peripheral blood samples. Samples to be submitted for determination of glucose concentration should be submitted in fluoride oxalate preservative. Methods for management of samples for bacteriology are described in Chap. 15. Particular care must be taken when anaerobic infections are suspected.

Radiography

Radiographic examination of the respiratory tract can be helpful in the diagnosis of sinusitis, nasal masses (e.g., neoplasia and ethmoid hematomas), tooth-root problems, guttural pouch disorders (e.g., empyema and chondroids), and tracheal stenosis. If the clinician has access to equipment of suitable size and power, thoracic disorders (e.g., pneumonia, abscessation, pleural effusion, neoplasia, etc.) can be diagnosed. Radiography of the thorax of foals can be particularly helpful if pneumonia (e.g., *Rhodococcus equi*) is suspected.

Arterial Blood Gas Analysis

Assessments of pulmonary function—in particular, ventilation—can be made by the measurement of the partial pressures of oxygen and carbon dioxide within the arterial blood. Measurement of the partial pressure of carbon dioxide in the arterial blood ($PaCO_2$) reflects alveolar ventilation and is therefore a valid and easily determined indicator of airway obstruction, especially in diseases creating an impediment to lower respiratory tract airflow (e.g., chronic obstructive pulmonary disease). In contrast, the PaO_2 is related to the inspired oxygen tension, alveolar ventilation, and the effectiveness of gas exchange across the alveolar–capillary membrane. Thus, in an animal breathing ambient air, with a normal $PaCO_2$ (reflective of normal alveolar ventilation), hypoxemia indicates impaired efficiency of gas exchange within the lung. An example is provided by diseases causing severe lung consolidation (e.g., pneumonia), where there is mismatching between ventilation and perfusion to large areas of the lung.

Although many veterinary practices do not own blood gas machines, most hospitals have this apparatus and are willing to process samples for veterinarians for an arranged fee. Samples can be stored on ice for several hours following collection, making this procedure one worthy of consideration, even for the busiest of practitioners.

The two most frequently used sites for collection of arterial blood samples from the conscious horse are the common carotid artery and the transverse facial artery. Collection of a sample from the *carotid artery* is undertaken following aseptic preparation of the skin dorsal to the jugular groove on the right side of the neck. The carotid artery can be palpated as a cord-like structure deep to the jugular vein on the dorsal side of the groove (no pulse will be detected), and a 3.75-cm, 18- to 19-gauge needle is directed into the vessel. It may be necessary to perform several manipulations with the needle following penetration of the skin to obtain access to the lumen of the artery. Once the needle is in place, blood will be expelled from the vessel under pulsatile pressure (Fig. 4-14). The needle is stabilized with the fingers of one hand, and a 2- or 5-ml syringe is connected to the hub. This syringe should have been heparinized, with a small volume of 1000 IU/ml sodium heparin filling the dead space.

KEY POINT ► Following collection of the sample, the syringe should have all air bubbles expelled from the lumen, and a needle should be attached.

This is necessary because air bubbles lead to spurious results during analysis. After expulsion of the air, the needle should be capped with a rubber

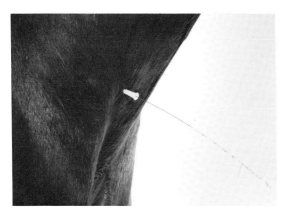

Figure 4–14. Position of 18-gauge, 3.75-cm needle in the right carotid artery to permit arterial blood gas sampling.

stopper (a Vacutainer lid is ideal), and the sample should be assayed immediately or stored in an ice bath until analysis. Samples remain stable in an ice bath for 4 to 6 hours after collection. The horse's body temperature should be taken at the time of collection of the sample to allow for correction during the assay procedure. Following removal of the needle, pressure should be maintained over the arteriopuncture site for several minutes to reduce the possibility of hematoma formation.

An alternate site for collection of samples in the conscious, standing horse is the *transverse facial artery*. This vessel is located just lateral to the lateral canthus of the eye and is easily palpated. The site is aseptically prepared, the artery is stabilized with the fingers of one hand, and a 21- to 23-gauge, 1- to 2.5-cm needle is inserted into the vessel lumen. Deposition of 0.2 to 0.3 ml lidocaine under the skin over the vessel using a 25-gauge needle may prevent sensitive horses from moving their heads during arteriopuncture. Collection and assay of the sample are performed as described for samples obtained from the carotid artery.

In foals, an arterial sample can be collected from the great metatarsal artery in a laterally recumbent foal.

At sea level, normal horses have PaO_2 values in the range of 85 to 100 mmHg and $PaCO_2$ values in the range of 35 to 45 mmHg. Hypoxemia ($PaO_2 < 80$ mmHg) usually occurs with derangements in ventilation–perfusion matching (e.g., severe consolidating pneumonia or general anesthesia) or in response to high altitude. Hypoxemia in association with hypercapnia ($PaCO_2 > 45$ mmHg) reflects hypoventilation. In horses, the most common disease-induced cause of hypoventilation is chronic allergic respiratory disease.

Sinuscentesis

In the adult horse, the dorsal margin of the maxillary sinus is a line from the infraorbital foramen caudally running parallel with the facial crest. Rostrally, the limit is a line from the facial crest to the infraorbital foramen, and the caudal margin lies in a transverse plane on the rostral side of the root of the orbital process of the zygomatic bone. In the foal, the ventral limit is much higher owing to incomplete eruption of the teeth. The maxillary sinus is divided into two compartments (rostral and caudal) by a complete oblique septum.

The frontal sinus is also paired. The rostral limit is defined by the point where the facial bones diverge. The caudal limit is near the level of the temporomandibular joint.

Sinuscentesis of the maxillary and frontal sinuses is performed under local anesthesia with the horse sedated. An area of skin is shaved and aseptically prepared, and local anesthetic is infiltrated under the skin. A stab incision is made in the skin and a sterile Steinmann pin is used to puncture the bony roof of the sinus (Figs. 4-15 and 4-16). A small sterile urinary catheter is introduced through the hole,

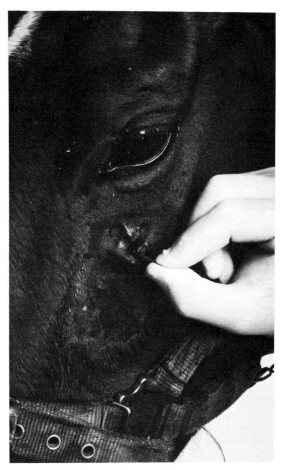

Figure 4–15. Sinuscentesis. Stab incision through a bleb of local anesthetic that has been previously placed in the skin and subcutaneous tissues over the caudal compartment of the maxillary sinus.

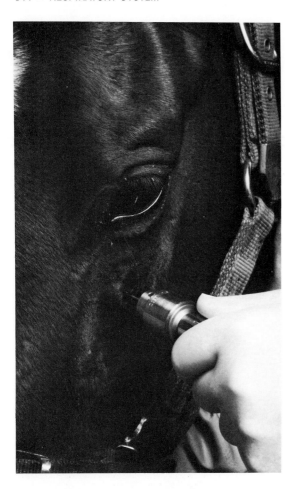

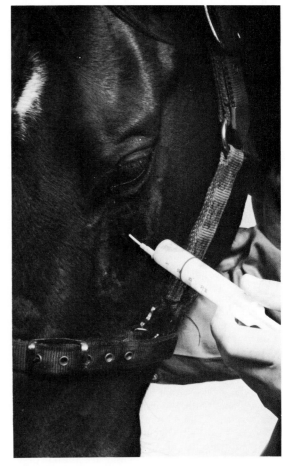

Figure 4–16. Sinuscentesis. A hole is drilled into the maxillary sinus with a Steinmann bone pin.

Figure 4–17. Sinuscentesis. A catheter is placed in the maxillary sinus to permit aspiration of any fluid.

and aspiration is performed (Fig. 4-17). The sample can be submitted for microbiologic and cytologic examination. Radiographic identification of fluid accumulations prior to sinuscentesis may assist in obtaining a diagnostically useful sample. Following collection of the sample, the catheter is removed, and a single skin suture is inserted. A technique for visual inspection of the sinus using a bronchoscope or arthroscope also may provide an indication of the characteristics of the sinus lumen.

Upper Respiratory Tract Diseases

GENERAL NOSE AND THROAT PROBLEMS

Atheroma

Atheroma is a sebaceous cyst that creates a firm round swelling in the nasoincisive notch (false nostril).

History and Presenting Signs

- Swelling near nostril
- Young horse

Clinical Findings and Diagnosis

- Atheromas usually occur unilaterally in young horses.
- Lesions are painless, may enlarge with time, but rarely cause obstruction to airflow.
- They are easily diagnosed, because external swelling is evident over the dorsal aspect of the nasal diverticulum or false nostril.
- The contents of the cyst are usually fluid.

Differential Diagnosis

- Congenital defects of the nostril
- Local infections (e.g., abscesses)
- Tumors (e.g., sarcoids)

Treatment

KEY POINT ▶ Because of their location, atheromas seldom have any effect on airflow, but treatment is usually requested from a cosmetic point of view.

- The atheroma can be removed surgically in the standing, sedated horse following regional infusion of local anesthetic or induction of an infraorbital nerve block. Alternatively, general anesthesia can be induced and the cyst removed.
- An incision is made over the dorsal aspect of the cyst, and the lining is carefully dissected away from the subcutaneous tissues. The skin incision is then sutured.
- An alternative method involves incising into the cyst from the undersurface. The cyst lining is

then removed, and routine closure is performed. This procedure, although a little more complicated, results in less chance of postoperative scarring. It is important to ensure ventral drainage.

Chondritis of the Arytenoid Cartilages

Chondritis is a condition most commonly affecting young racehorses in which one or both of the arytenoid cartilages undergo dystrophic changes, including enlargement, inflammation, mineralization, and the deposition of granulation tissue. The net result of these changes is a reduction in the laryngeal luminal diameter. The cause of the condition is not known, although trauma to the cartilages, particularly by stomach tubes and infection, has been implicated.

History and Presenting Signs

- Decreased exercise capacity and an inspiratory stridor are the most common signs. Signs are shown during higher-speed exercise and are the result of restricted airflow at the larynx.
- Onset of signs is often progressive.
- In severe cases, dyspnea may be present at rest.

Clinical Findings and Diagnosis

- Palpation of the larynx may reveal abnormalities in the shape of the affected cartilage.
- Diagnosis is usually confirmed during endoscopic examination of the larynx. Changes may be mild, but they often include a change in shape of the arytenoid cartilage, reduction in the size of the laryngeal opening, ulcers on the mucous membranes, and possibly granulation tissue.
- Unilateral involvement is most frequently observed, but bilateral lesions also occur. In severe cases, the affected cartilage will be noticeably thickened, with the dystrophic tissue intruding into the laryngeal lumen.
- Lateral radiographs of the larynx may reveal mineralization of the affected tissues.

Differential Diagnosis

- Idiopathic left laryngeal hemiplegia
- Subepiglottic/pharyngeal cysts
- Neoplasia of the larynx/pharynx, including hypertrophic dystrophy of the arytenoid cartilages

Treatment

KEY POINT ► In acute forms, where laryngeal obstruction is almost complete, a temporary tracheostomy and systemic antibiotic and anti-inflammatory therapy may give transient relief of the problem.

- Removal of the affected cartilage is the treatment of choice for long-term relief of the problem. A number of techniques have been described, including arytenoidectomy, subtotal arytenoidectomy, and partial arytenoidectomy.
- Unilateral arytenoidectomy is the most frequently utilized technique in racehorses, with the success rate for return to athletic endeavors reported to be about 45% to 60%. Mild dysphagia is a common complication of this procedure.
- If the problem is bilateral and removal of both arytenoid cartilages is required, the prognosis for return to racing is poor.

Epiglottic Entrapment

Epiglottic entrapment is a relatively common disorder in which the aryepiglottic folds (thick bands of mucous membrane that attach to the ventral surface of the epiglottis and extend caudodorsally to merge with mucous membranes that join the corniculate processes) envelop the epiglottis. This derangement can occur because the subepiglottic epithelium is relatively loose, thereby allowing for elevation of the epiglottis during swallowing. Entrapment occurs when this loose tissue folds over the apex and lateral aspects of the epiglottis.

KEY POINT ► Entrapment may result in a functional obstruction to airflow and a variety of clinical signs, but in mild cases it may result in no functional problems.

It has been suggested that this condition has a congenital basis, particularly in horses with epiglottic hypoplasia.

History and Presenting Signs

- Respiratory noise
- Thoroughbred and standardbred horses
- Coughing

Clinical Findings and Diagnosis

- Signs are variable, with some horses showing no clinical manifestations of the disorder and entrapment only being demonstrated during a routine rhinolaryngoscopic examination.
- When entrapment does result in clinical manifestations, one of the major signs is turbulent airflow resulting in respiratory stridor (inspiratory and expiratory noise) and poor athletic performance.

- The severity of clinical signs is dependent on the degree of occlusion of the airway due to the entrapment. This is a function of the amount of tissue that is entrapped, the inflammatory response occurring in the surrounding tissues, and whether there is coexisting dorsal displacement of the soft palate.
- In some cases, the entrapment causes no problems, since the condition has been found during routine examinations of horses.
- Diagnosis can only be made by rhinolaryngoscopy, where the entrapped epiglottis can be seen to have a distinctive V-shaped aryepiglottic fold lying over its dorsal aspect. The normal crenated appearance of the edges of the epiglottis disappears, and the vessels normally apparent on the dorsal epiglottis cannot be seen.

Differential Diagnosis

- Soft palate displacement
- Idiopathic left laryngeal hemiplegia
- Subepiglottic cysts
- Laryngeal chondritis
- Ethmoid hematomas
- Diseases causing nasal deformity/obstruction
- Rostral displacement of the palatopharyngeal arch

Treatment

- If the performance of the horse is not affected, no treatment is necessary. In one survey of approximately 500 normal thoroughbred horses that were examined endoscopically, 10 had entrapment. None of these animals had evidence of decreased performance.
- If performance is impeded, surgery to divide the aryepiglottic membrane is indicated. Methods of correction include the use of bistouries, electrocautery, and, more recently, the Nd:YAG laser. Some surgeons perform the procedure in the standing horse; others, via the oral or nasal route in the anesthetized animal.
- Occasionally, the epiglottis is hypoplastic, and in these cases, dislocation of the soft palate may be a subsequent result, causing continued respiratory noise and impaired performance.
- Radiographs (lateral projections) of the larynx and epiglottis prior to performing surgery for correction of the entrapment may provide the clinician with an indication of whether hypoplasia of the epiglottis exists. This allows the practitioner the ability to provide the owner or trainer with a clearer idea of prognosis prior to surgery being undertaken.

Epistaxis

Epistaxis, or bleeding from the nose, is a relatively common disorder, particularly in racehorses, as one of the sequels to exercise-induced pulmonary hemorrhage. In some cases, there is no doubt about the cause, where, for instance, epistaxis follows the passage of a stomach tube. However, in many cases, the source of the blood may be difficult to determine, requiring a thorough investigation of the horse's respiratory tract. The possible sites of origin include the following:

1. *Nasal Cavity*
   a. *Trauma** (e.g., blunt trauma, nasogastric entubation/endoscopy)
   b. *Infection* (e.g., sinusitis, conchal necrosis, fungal granuloma)
   c. *Polyps*
   d. *Amyloidosis*
   e. *Iatrogenic*—passage of a stomach tube or endoscope
2. *Ethmoid Labyrinth*
   a. *Progressive hematoma** (also may occur in sinuses)
3. *Guttural Pouches*
   a. *Guttural pouch mycosis**
   b. *Empyema*
4. *Lungs*
   a. *Exercise-induced pulmonary hemorrhage**
   b. *Abscess*
   c. *Neoplasia*
   d. *Fungal pneumonia*

History and Presenting Signs

- Blood discharging from one or both nostrils. Can vary from being a trickle and intermittent to being profuse and life-threatening.
- Signs can be associated with exercise.
- There may be a history of trauma to the head or nose.

Clinical Findings and Diagnosis

- Blood at the nostrils is self-evident. The important factors to be determined are the characteristics of the discharge, its volume, and the relationship of the discharge to any recent event (e.g., exercise, nasal intubation, etc.).
- Epistaxis may occur as frank blood, and this is often seen following trauma to the nasal conchae or hemorrhage from the guttural pouches.
- Serosanguinous fluid often accompanies conditions where chronic inflammatory changes occur in association with the hemorrhage. Examples are ethmoidal hematomas, sinusitis, hemorrhage from neoplasms, and abscesses.
- It is important to determine whether the epistaxis occurs in association with other systemic signs, such as fever, depression, inappetence, cough, etc.
- Diagnosis is based on careful accumulation of information from the history and physical examination. Important details of the history include whether the hemorrhage occurs in association with exercise or subsequent to an infectious or traumatic process involving the respiratory tract. A thorough inspection of the nares and other parts of the upper respiratory tract, including percussion of the sinuses and palpation over the guttural pouches and larynx and trachea, should be undertaken.
- Endoscopy is often vital in determining the site of hemorrhage. A careful and thorough examination of the airway is necessary, paying particular attention to ensuring that sites are examined from which hemorrhage is common. These include the nasal meati, nasomaxillary openings, ethmoid labyrinth, guttural pouch openings (and possibly the pouches themselves if hemorrhage is detected), and the trachea.
- Additional diagnostic aids include radiography of suspected sites of hemorrhage, possibly ultrasound examinations, transtracheal lavage and aspiration if previous hemorrhage from the lungs is suspected, and judicious use of clinical laboratory data to assess the degree of systemic response if the problem appears to be more generalized.
- The conditions described in this section that are known to cause epistaxis are dealt with as individual conditions elsewhere in this chapter.

Differential Diagnosis

- Trauma (e.g., blunt trauma, nasogastric entubation/endoscopy)
- Infection (e.g., sinusitis, conchal necrosis, fungal granuloma)
- Nasal polyps
- Amyloidosis
- Progressive hematoma of the ethmoid or sinuses
- Guttural pouch mycosis or empyema
- Exercise-induced pulmonary hemorrhage
- Pulmonary abscess
- Respiratory tract neoplasia
- Fungal infections of the respiratory tract

Treatment

Treatments for the individual conditions are described in the relevant sections.

Ethmoid Hematoma

Hematomas of the ethmoid and paranasal sinuses are slowly progressive tumors that resemble hemangiomas in many ways but apparently are not neoplastic. The most common location for such lesions is in the ethmoid (labyrinthal) region, with the paranasal sinuses being less commonly affected. Given the progressive nature of the disease, older horses are most commonly affected.

---

*Most common causes.

History and Presenting Signs

- Nasal discharge that may be unilateral or bilateral
- Epistaxis

Clinical Findings and Diagnosis

- Intermittent epistaxis apparent at rest and after exercise in an older horse is the most consistent clinical sign. This is usually mild and unilateral and occurs because the progressive enlargement of the tumor results in its outstripping its blood supply. As a result, the surface necroses and hemorrhage is common.
- Severe cases may invade the surrounding tissues, resulting in dyspnea, particularly during exercise.
- Endoscopy is useful to determine the location of the tumor, which is usually located dorsally in the nose. The surface of the hematoma usually glistens and is green/red in color. Hemorrhage may be seen originating from the tumor. Bleeding is common if the hematoma is traumatized by the endoscope. If a horse has a history of unilateral epistaxis, the ethmoid region should always be examined for the presence of a progressive hematoma.
- Radiography is an integral part of the diagnosis to assist in outlining the soft-tissue mass. If lesions are present in the paranasal sinuses, radiography provides the most effective means for delineation of the tumor.
- Histopathologic examination of a biopsy specimen or samples collected following removal of the lesion reveals tissue types consistent with those described for ethmoidal hematomas. The tissue is vascular with evidence of repeated hemorrhage and reorganization. Surface tissue is composed predominantly of epithelium and fibrous tissue.

Differential Diagnosis

- Guttural pouch mycosis/empyema
- Trauma
- Primary or secondary sinusitis
- Foreign body
- Fungal infection
- Neoplasia (e.g., fibroma/fibrosarcoma, squamous cell carcinoma, adenocarcinoma, etc.)
- Conchal necrosis
- Amyloidosis
- Exercise-induced pulmonary hemorrhage

Treatment

KEY POINT ► Surgical removal of the tumor masses may provide palliation of the disease for variable periods. Unfortunately, recurrence is common, particularly when the tumor is only excised or removed with a wire snare.

- Surgical approach to the tumor is often difficult, requiring a frontonasal flap or sinus flap, and is complicated by the potential for significant blood loss. This may be reduced by using temporary bilateral carotid artery occlusion.
- Cryofreezing of the tumor and removal of the mass while still frozen have been advocated to decrease the chance of hemorrhage and improve the potential for removal of most of the diseased tissue. Cryosurgery also has the advantage of producing cell death in residual tumor tissue. At least three freeze-thaw cycles are advocated to optimize cellular destruction. Freezing to $-20°C$ provides the most satisfactory results. Disadvantages of cryosurgery are possible damage to local healthy tissues, including mucosa, the infraorbital nerve, and possibly the cribriform plate. In addition, nasal discharge may persist for weeks postoperatively.

GUTTURAL POUCH PROBLEMS

The guttural pouches communicate with the pharynx through the slit-like epipharyngeal orifices on the lateral walls of the pharynx. The function of these pouches is unclear, but because of their location and the fact that the epipharyngeal orifices open during swallowing, extension of bacterial upper respiratory infections into the guttural pouches may take place. Several disorders involving the guttural pouches may occur and can limit performance.

History and Presenting Signs

- Nasal discharge
- Epistaxis
- Distension in the region of Viborg's triangle

Guttural Pouch Empyema

Bacterial infection and pus accumulation in the guttural pouch can occur as a secondary event to upper respiratory tract infections, particularly infections due to *Streptococcus equi* ("strangles").

Clinical Findings and Diagnosis

KEY POINT ► Apart from poor performance, the major clinical manifestation of guttural pouch empyema is a persistent unilateral or bilateral nasal discharge.

- This discharge is usually increased when the horse swallows, lowers its head, or the region of the guttural pouches is palpated.
- There may be little or no swelling in the region of Viborg's triangle and few other systemic signs.
- The condition can be diagnosed on endoscopic examination of the pharynx. Purulent material can be seen discharging from the guttural pouch

opening, particularly when the horse's head is lowered or after swallowing.

- At times, passage of the endoscope into the pouch may be necessary to confirm the diagnosis.
- Radiography of the pharynx also may confirm the presence of fluid or accumulated material within the guttural pouches.
- Aspiration of a sample of purulent material via a catheter may be very useful for confirmation of the diagnosis (cytology, Gram stain) and culture of the offending bacteria.

Differential Diagnosis

- Primary or secondary sinusitis
- Ethmoidal hematoma
- Guttural pouch mycosis
- Trauma
- Foreign body
- Fungal infection
- Neoplasia (e.g., fibroma/fibrosarcoma, squamous cell carcinoma, adenocarcinoma, etc.)
- Conchal necrosis
- Amyloidosis

Treatment

KEY POINT ▶ The most common infections are *Streptococcus* spp., particularly *Strep. equi*, var. *zooepidemicus*. These organisms are sensitive to penicillin, so local lavage and systemic therapy are often successful.

- Parenteral procaine penicillin G (Treatment No. 83) at a dose rate of 15 mg/kg (15,000 IU/kg) q12h, combined with local irrigation with warm isotonic polyionic solutions containing crystalline penicillin (Treatment Nos. 84 and 85) once or twice daily for 5 days will usually resolve the infection.
- Catheterization of the guttural pouch is performed using a plastic mare uterine infusion catheter with the tip bent (see Guttural Pouch Catheterization, p. 137). Catheters can be inserted blind or with the aid of an endoscopic view of the pharynx.
- In severe cases, particularly those where the purulent material has become caseous, surgical drainage of the guttural pouch may be required. A number of techniques providing surgical access to the guttural pouch have been described. The most common technique is performed through Viborg's triangle. However, we have found that the dorsal approach just cranial to the atlas gives better exposure.

Guttural Pouch Mycosis

Guttural pouch mycosis occurs more commonly in the northern than southern hemispheres. When fungi invade the guttural pouch, the mycosis com-

monly involves the medial compartment of the pouch and can therefore damage a number of structures and result in a variety of clinical signs. For example, in some cases there is erosion through the carotid artery, resulting in severe and sometimes fatal epistaxis.

Clinical Findings and Diagnosis

KEY POINT ▶ The most common signs associated with guttural pouch mycosis are epistaxis and dysphagia due to involvement of cranial nerves VII, IX, X, and XI, which traverse the region of the guttural pouches.

- Other signs include parotid pain, nasal discharge, abnormal head posture, and Horner's syndrome.
- Positive diagnosis is made on the basis of history, clinical signs, and endoscopy, in particular by introducing the endoscope into the guttural pouch, where a typical diphtheritic membrane, hemorrhage, and discharge are seen.
- The specific fungal pathogen producing the infection is often not identifiable, although *Aspergillus* spp. (ubiquitous fungi) are commonly cultured from affected pouches.

Differential Diagnosis

- Primary or secondary sinusitis
- Ethmoidal hematoma
- Guttural pouch empyema
- Trauma
- Foreign body
- Fungi infection of the nasal passages or paranasal sinuses
- Neoplasia (e.g., fibroma/fibrosarcoma, squamous cell carcinoma, adenocarcinoma, etc.)
- Conchal necrosis
- Amyloidosis

Treatment

- Topical treatment using the same methods described for empyema may be attempted.

KEY POINT ▶ Because lesions are often confined to the dorsal aspect of the pouch, delivery of medications (e.g., 1% miconazole [Treatment No. 76] 1% to 5% ketoconazole [Treatment No. 65], enilconazole [Treatment No. 37], amphotericin B [Treatment No. 7]) to the site of infection can be difficult, and response is often slow. Daily infusions for 4 to 6 weeks are often necessary.

- If the internal carotid artery is involved, ligation of this vessel is critical, because profuse, life-threatening hemorrhage can occur. This provides the most useful and effective means for controlling epistaxis in affected animals. Several techniques are described; however, the use of a balloon catheter inserted into the artery to a point beyond the area of fungal infection and ligation of the vessel proximal to the lesion appear to provide the most satisfactory results. In severe cases of epistaxis, blood transfusions may be required.

■ Systemic treatment of guttural pouch mycosis with intravenous ketoconazole (Treatment No. 65) has been reported, although this agent has no specific in vitro activity against *Aspergillus* spp. Amphotericin B (Treatment No. 7) also may be a possible drug for systemic administration, although a number of untoward side effects have been reported with prolonged use. These include nephrotoxicity, phlebitis near the site of injection, anorexia, and depression.

Guttural Pouch Tympany

This condition is a developmental disorder and so is most common in foals. The precise etiology of the disease has not been defined, and it has been suggested that this disease has a functional rather than a mechanical basis, such that air is trapped within the guttural pouch or pouches, producing tympany. Suggestions have been made that the disease occurs because of a malformation of one or both epipharyngeal orifices, resulting in air becoming trapped in the guttural pouch. This has not been proven.

Clinical Findings and Diagnosis

KEY POINT ▶ Marked, nonpainful distension of one or both sides of the neck in the region of Viborg's triangle in foals or weanlings is a common finding.

■ Percussion over the swollen area will reveal tympany.
■ If the enlargement is sufficiently great, obstruction to airflow may occur, producing dyspnea. In severe unilateral cases, swelling may extend to the opposite side of the neck despite an absence of the disorder in that pouch. Complications include dysphagia, nasal discharge, secondary infections of the pouch (empyema), and aspiration pneumonia.
■ Affected foals may make a "snoring" sound when sucking.
■ Diagnosis is usually made based on the physical examination and pathognomonic appearance of the swollen pouch.
■ Apart from swelling extending into the pharynx, endoscopic findings are usually unremarkable.
■ Radiographs, in the dorsoventral plane, are helpful if there is a question as to whether the condition is unilateral or bilateral.
■ Additionally, aspiration of air from a distended pouch may assist in diagnosis.

Differential Diagnosis

■ Guttural pouch empyema
■ Congenital malformations

Treatment

■ Temporary relief may be afforded by insertion of a catheter into the pouch via the nasopharynx, needle aspiration, or digital pressure on the pouch.
■ A commonly practiced, potentially permanent method of treatment involves surgical correction of the problem.
■ In unilateral cases, fenestration of the septum between the two pouches often affords relief.
■ In bilateral cases, the treatment of choice is enlargement of the pharyngeal openings of one or both guttural pouches. This is done using a procedure in which the pouch is entered via Viborg's triangle. If only one opening is enlarged, fenestration of the septum is imperative. An alternate and less traumatic method involves insertion of a balloon-tipped catheter into the pouch via the nasopharyngeal opening. This catheter is left in place for several weeks or longer, with the intention of producing a permanent ostium into the pouch.
■ The prognosis for this disorder is often good if the foal does not have significant complications (e.g., aspiration pneumonia) and if the condition is unilateral.

NASAL PASSAGE PROBLEMS

There are a number of disorders that can involve the nasal passages. These include foreign bodies, amyloidosis, fungal diseases, disorders of the nasal septum, neoplasia, polyps, and necrosis of the conchae.

History and Presenting Signs

■ Nasal discharge
■ Respiratory noise
■ Dyspnea

Clinical Findings and Diagnosis

KEY POINT ▶ Manifestations of diseases of the nasal passages may include epistaxis, nasal discharge, malodor, alterations in airflow, and respiratory noise.

■ Careful collation of the information obtained from the history and physical examination is invaluable if a correct diagnosis is to be made.
■ Judicious use of diagnostic aids (e.g., endoscopy, radiography, biopsy, and collection of samples for cytologic and microbiologic examination) is important.

Characteristics of the specific disorders include the following:

Foreign Bodies

- Often induce head shyness, epistaxis, and obvious discomfort for the horse.
- Malodorous nasal discharge is common.
- Endoscopy and radiography are often useful for diagnosis.

Amyloidosis

- Horses of all ages have been reported to deposit glycoprotein in various body organs in response to continued immunologic stimulation, often a chronic infection.
- A common site for deposition of amyloid is the upper airway, including the nasal passages, particularly the nasal septum and conchae.
- Clinical manifestations include nasal discharge, epistaxis, reduced exercise tolerance, and possibly dyspnea and weight loss.
- Lesions are firm and nodular or plaque-like with fragile, smooth walls.
- Diagnosis can be made by clinical examination, endoscopy, evidence or a history of chronic antigenic stimulation, biopsy, and histopathology.

Fungal Infections

- Although quite rare, fungal diseases of the upper airways are more common in tropical and subtropical regions.
- Fungi implicated include *Conidiobolus, Cryptococcus, Coccidioides, Aspergillus,* and *Rhinosporidium.*
- Clinical signs of fungal infections of the upper airway may include mucopurulent and possibly malodorous nasal discharge, epistaxis, dyspnea, respiratory noises, and submandibular and parotid lymphadenopathy.
- Diagnosis is based on clinical signs, endoscopic appearance, smears and culture of the nasal discharge and of material from the lesions, and histopathology.

Disorders of the Nasal Septum

- Usually congenital disorders that become obvious when the horse undertakes exercise and there is respiratory stridor
- Attention may be directed toward septal disorders earlier in the horse's life if they involve malformations of the other nasal bones.
- Other causes of nasal septum dysfunction include trauma, septal and conchal necrosis secondary to severe respiratory tract infections, amyloidosis, and fungal infections.
- The most common clinical manifestation is respiratory stridor (louder on inspiration) and dyspnea during exercise.
- Facial deformity may be present.
- Diagnosis is based on a history of trauma, infection, or evidence of facial deformity.
- Deformities in the rostral portion of the septum can be detected by palpation and direct and inspection. Lesions located more caudad may require inspection with an endoscope.
- Dorsoventral radiographs also may provide useful information with respect to the degree of tissue derangement present.
- Biopsy samples collected from local lesions may help identify specific etiologic agents in certain cases.

Differential Diagnosis

- Ethmoid hematoma
- Tooth-root abnormalities
- Trauma or fractures of the nasal region
- Atheroma
- Epistaxis
- Tracheal stenosis
- Idiopathic laryngeal hemiplegia
- Arytenoid chondritis

Treatment

Foreign Bodies

- Removal with forceps with or without the aid of an endoscope may be possible.
- In severe cases, more invasive procedures may be indicated.

Amyloidosis

- Removal of the chronic antigenic stimulus may reduce the continued deposition of amyloid. However, it is likely that this has no effect on the glycoprotein already deposited.
- If the amyloid deposits are restricted to well-defined, circumscribed lesions, surgical removal of the lesions can be beneficial.
- Corticosteroid administration appears to provide no benefit to affected horses.

Fungal Infections

- In many cases, surgical removal of the masses is successful.
- The antifungal agents amphotericin B (intravenously and locally; Treatment No. 7) and ketoconazole (intravenously; Treatment No. 65) may be effective in lesions that are not extensive. Ketaconazole is often the drug of choice and is administered at a dose rate of 300 mg/kg IV q12h for 7 to 10 days.

Disorders of the Nasal Septum

- Surgical removal of the septum is indicated if respiratory stertor causes reduced performance or if there are areas of necrotic tissue present.
- Resection of the septum is a relatively complex procedure, and blood loss can be profuse.

Nasal Polyps

Nasal polyps are slow-growing, pedunculated tumors originating from the nasal mucosa, septum, and on occasion the tooth roots. Lesions are frequently unilateral and result from proliferation of connective tissue in response to chronic inflammation or from hypertrophy of the mucosa.

History and Presenting Signs

- Occurs in horses of all ages.
- Progressive dyspnea, particularly with exercise, is common.
- Nasal discharge, frequently malodorous, is common. Epistaxis is rare.
- In some cases, owners, trainers, or handlers may see a polyp in the naris of the affected side.

Clinical Findings and Diagnosis

- Diagnosis can be made on direct inspection of the nasal cavity if the polyp extends to near the external naris. As polyps grow, they may invade the entire lumen of the nasal cavity on the affected side and even protrude out the nostril. Lesions up to 30 cm in length have been reported.
- Polyps are usually creamy white in color, pedunculated, and have a smooth surface.
- Diagnosis can be confirmed with endoscopy. In extensive cases, polyps may be seen extending caudally beyond the nasal meati when viewed through the opposite nostril.
- Radiographs also may assist in delineation of the margins of the mass.
- Confirmation of the diagnosis may be made with biopsy, which will reveal mature and immature fibrous tissue covered with epithelium.

Differential Diagnosis

- Neoplasia (e.g., fibroma/fibrosarcoma, squamous cell carcinoma, adenocarcinoma, etc.)
- Foreign body
- Fungal infection
- Amyloidosis
- Nasal malformations
- Conchal necrosis

Treatment

- Surgical removal is the treatment of choice and is often quite feasible. Methods employed vary according to the size and location of the polyp.
- Because of the potential for regrowth if all abnormal tissue is not removed, most procedures involve direct access to the lesion and complete excision.
- Access to a polyp near the external naris can be gained by opening the nostril between the false nostril and nasoincisive notch. Polyps located further caudad usually require trephination or use of a bone flap though the nasal bones to the site of the polyp.
- It must be remembered that polyps have an excellent vascular supply, and hemorrhage is often extensive, requiring packing of the nostrils.
- Removal of lesions via the external nares using a wire snare often provides only temporary relief because the polyps regrow as a result of inadequate resection using this technique.

LARYNGEAL, PHARYNGEAL, AND TRACHEAL PROBLEMS

Idiopathic Left Laryngeal Hemiplegia (ILH)

Idiopathic laryngeal hemiplegia (ILH) is a disorder occurring mainly in young, large thoroughbred horses and affecting the left side of the larynx. The incidence of ILH is probably in the range of 3% to 8% in this group of horses. ILH results from demyelination of the left recurrent laryngeal nerve (and some other long peripheral nerves), denervating the muscles of the larynx, particularly the cricoarytenoideus dorsalis (CAD), which is responsible for abduction, and the cricoarytenoideus lateralis (CAL), the adductor. Although it is known that the lesion results from repeated bouts of segmental demyelination resulting in a distal axonopathy, the pathogenesis of the disorder remains obscure. In left laryngeal hemiplegia, atrophy of the left CAD muscle often can be determined by palpation. The result of the failure of abduction of the left arytenoid cartilage is a partial upper respiratory tract obstruction, which produces an inspiratory dyspnea. It usually becomes evident at 2 or 3 years of age. A heritable basis for the disease has been proposed but not definitively established.

History and Presenting Signs

- Respiratory noise during fast exercise
- Poor performance
- Thoroughbred horse, 2 years old

Clinical Findings and Diagnosis

- The first sign of laryngeal hemiplegia is a respiratory noise, usually evident during fast exercise, and/or reduced performance capacity.
- The noise may vary from a whistle to a roar.
- The condition is progressive, and therefore, the noise becomes evident at slower gaits.

KEY POINT ► On clinical examination, the larynx also should be palpated to determine if atrophy of the dorsal cricoarytenoid muscle can be felt.

- If present, the muscular process of the left arytenoid cartilage will be more prominent than on the right side, and this is felt as a bump (see Fig.

1-14). Note should be taken of any scarring or thickening of skin that could suggest a previous laryngoplasty or laryngotomy.

- If there is any indication of more prominence of the left muscular process of the arytenoid cartilage, a laryngeal adductor test ("slap test") should be performed while palpating the muscular process on left and right sides. Slapping the left thorax gently with the open hand should result in the right muscular process adducting, and this can be felt as a "flicking" or movement of the process. Similarly, slapping of the right thorax should result in the muscular process of the left arytenoid cartilage "flicking." In horses with ILH, the "flicking" of the left muscular process does not occur or is reduced in response to the "slap test." The response also may be lost in horses with cervical spinal cord disease.
- The laryngeal depression test is useful in horses immediately following exercise. With this procedure, the muscular process of each arytenoid cartilage is depressed while the horse's respiratory effort remains elevated after exercise. Horses with ILH will often make a more profound stertorous sound when the left side is depressed as compared with the right side.
- Positive diagnosis is only possible using a rhinolaryngoscope, where an atypical appearance of the larynx will be found. Features include an asymmetric appearance, a kink in the aryepiglottic fold, and a failure to abduct the left arytenoid cartilage, which may be most obvious immediately after the horse swallows. Use of the "slap test" during endoscopic examination (with the horse not sedated) improves the chances of diagnosis of ILH by allowing direct observation of adductor function.
- Asynchronous movement of the arytenoid cartilages is a normal finding in some horses and does not progress to clinical laryngeal hemiplegia.
- The availability of high-speed treadmills has provided a vehicle whereby endoscopy can be performed during exercise. This procedure may assist in the diagnosis of ILH, particularly in those cases where diagnosis is equivocal at rest.

Differential Diagnosis

- Soft palate displacement
- Epiglottic entrapment
- Subepiglottic cysts
- Laryngeal chondritis
- Rostral displacement of the palatopharyngeal arch
- Diseases causing nasal deformity/obstruction (e.g., sinusitis, neoplasia)

Treatment

- Surgical treatment is possible, and the combination of laryngoplasty ("tie back") and ventriculectomy gives the best results currently. The current technique of laryngoplasty involves insertion of material such as Mersilene, Dacron, Polydek, or Ethibond to mimic the action of the atrophied left cricoarytenoideus dorsalis muscle so that the left arytenoid cartilage is permanently abducted. A ventriculectomy is performed to create adhesions between the thyroid and arytenoid cartilages, since the suture material usually pulls through the cartilage in 2 to 3 months.
- While the initial appearance of the larynx after surgery is often good, the left arytenoid cartilage often sags inward after several months, causing a partial obstruction.
- The major complication of surgery is chronic coughing, which results from food particles entering the trachea and causing a chronic tracheitis.
- The result of this procedure is that 50% to 60% of horses will have no or markedly reduced inspiratory noise following surgery, and most horses will have improvement in airflow. Most horses require 3 months rest following surgery, before recommencing training.
- Recently, the technique of nerve pedicle grafting has been described. This has a major disadvantage in that up to 12 months is required postoperatively for improvement in laryngeal function.

Pharyngeal Lymphoid Hyperplasia (PLH)

Pharyngeal lymphoid hyperplasia (PLH) is a condition commonly afflicting young horses in training. The disorder promotes controversy, because disagreement exists as to the significance of the lesions, although many now seem to agree that PLH is a normal physiologic finding in younger horses. It is thought PLH is a manifestation of an immunologic response of the mucosa within the pharynx. Since young horses have the greatest density of lymphoid follicles within the pharynx, it is not surprising that PLH is more common in this age group. Possibly viruses that damage the upper respiratory tract, inhaled irritants, and pollutants contribute to the induction of hyperplasia. Classically, horses with PLH have a chronic cough and poor performance, which may be a sequel to a viral upper respiratory tract infection.

History and Presenting Signs

- Horses may have a chronic cough.
- Reduced performance may be reported in some horses.
- PLH may be an incidental finding on endoscopic examination of the upper airway.

Clinical Findings and Diagnosis

- Diagnosis of PLH is made by rhinolaryngoscopic examination, which reveals hyperplasia of the lymphoid tissue ("follicles") on the roof of the pharynx.

■ The degree of hyperplasia can be graded (see below). There also may be some discharge associated with a general inflammatory response.

KEY POINT ▶ Care must be taken in interpretation of endoscopic findings with regard to PLH, because there are a number of studies that demonstrate that PLH has little or no effect on respiratory gas exchange.

■ Racing performance is unlikely to be impaired by PLH under most circumstances, although in severe cases (grades III to IV), decrements in performance and a chronic cough may occur.

Grades of Pharyngeal Lymphoid Hyperplasia

Grade I—Very few, small, inactive follicles in the pharynx.

Grade II—More follicles with a wider distribution than seen in grade I. Follicles can be seen on the dorsal and lateral pharynx. Some follicles are edematous.

Grade III—Many more, larger, pink/red follicles than in grade II. The pharyngeal tonsillar tissue is often hyperplastic. Follicles may be seen on the soft palate.

Grade IV—More severe manifestation of the changes seen in grade III. Many large, edematous follicles with a wide distribution, including the dorsal and lateral pharyngeal walls, soft palate, and possibly the epiglottis. Small polyp-like lesions may be observed.

Differential Diagnosis

■ Idiopathic laryngeal hemiplegia
■ Soft palate dislocation
■ Epiglottic entrapment
■ Subepiglottic cysts
■ Viral respiratory disease
■ Retropharyngeal abscessation

Treatment

■ A number of treatments have been described for more severely affected horses. Often a rest period of 8 to 12 weeks is sufficient to resolve the problem.
■ In North America, surgical management of PLH using cryosurgery, chemical cautery, and electrocautery is often utilized.
■ However, because PLH is often self-limiting, such treatments may only be indicated in the most severe cases.
■ Most treatments require a period of convalescence/reduced training of 4 to 6 weeks.

Retropharyngeal Abscessation

The most common cause of retropharyngeal abscessation in the horse is severe lymphadenopathy that accompanies *Streptococcus equi* ("strangles") infections. A much less common cause of cellulitis and abscessation in this site is pharyngeal trauma. Owing to the pyogenic nature of the organisms that often induce this pharyngeal abscessation or cellulitis, systemic manifestations of these disorders are common.

History and Presenting Signs

■ Retropharyngeal abscessation often follows a history of "strangles" in the affected animal or the herd.
■ Signs frequently result from the presence of a space-occupying lesion and include local swelling and possibly dyspnea.
■ In severe cases, dysphagia, and nasal discharge may be present in addition to respiratory embarrassment.

Clinical Findings and Diagnosis

■ Diagnosis is based on history, clinical manifestations, and clinical pathology findings.
■ Palpation of the retropharyngeal region often reveals pain and swelling. Most commonly this is unilateral and manifests as a reduction in the lumen size of the nasopharynx.
■ Systemic manifestations including fever, depression, inappetence, and lower respiratory tract disorders (possibly due to aspiration). Coughing may be present.
■ Endoscopy may reveal distortion of the pharynx and possibly the larynx. If the endoscope can be passed into the guttural pouch, distortion of the medial compartment on the affected side is the most frequent observation.
■ On radiographic examination of the pharyngeal area, a large soft-tissue density impinging on the pharynx and larynx is often visible.
■ Clinical pathology may reveal a leukocytosis, hyperfibrinogenemia, hyperproteinemia, (hyperglobulinemia) and other changes depending on the degree of systemic involvement.

Differential Diagnosis

■ *Streptococcus equi* infection ("strangles")
■ Pharyngeal trauma
■ Diseases causing upper airway obstruction (e.g., subepiglottic cysts, guttural pouch empyema, laryngeal paralysis, laryngeal chondritis)
■ Guttural pouch tympany

Treatment

■ In most cases, medical management of retropharyngeal abscessation provides an acceptable outcome, although the treatment often needs to be maintained for several weeks.

■ Administration of appropriate doses of antimicrobial agents is the mainstay of this form of therapy (see Chap. 17). Most cases are the result of infections with *Streptococcus* spp. Penicillin is the drug of choice against these organisms because it is bactericidal, adequate concentrations can be achieved in the circulation and in the diseased tissue, and the drug is inexpensive. Procaine penicillin administered intramuscularly at a dose rate of 15,000 to 20,000 IU/kg (15–20 mg/kg) q12h is appropriate (Treatment No. 83).

■ Signs of depression, inappetence, and retropharyngeal pain may respond favorably following the administration of nonsteroidal anti-inflammatory drugs (see Chap. 17). These should only be used after the initial fever abates, because a decrease in temperature is a useful indicator of response to antimicrobial treatment.

■ In cases where severe airway obstruction is present, a tracheostomy may be indicated.

■ Surgical drainage of the abscess cavity may be required in some severe cases.

Soft Palate Dislocation (Dorsal Displacement of the Soft Palate)

The soft palate is long in horses, and dorsal displacement of the soft palate causes a narrowing of the nasopharyngeal airway, creating turbulence on inspiration and expiration. Soft palate displacement may be intermittent or persistent. The intermittent form is most common in racehorses, causing temporary obstruction of the airway at high speeds. The soft palate normally forms an airtight seal around the larynx, together with the pharyngeal arch, to allow efficient movement of air down the respiratory tract during exercise.

KEY POINT ▶ If dislocation of the soft palate occurs, it becomes displaced from its normal position under the epiglottis and lies over the opening of the larynx. This results in turbulent and inefficient airflow with a great reduction in performance.

Severely affected horses may become weak and attempt to mouth breathe. Swallowing (repeated attempts may be required) usually results in replacement of the soft palate to its normal position. Although soft palate displacement may be a sequel to a variety of inflammatory diseases of the upper airway and hypoplasia of the epiglottis, in most cases the cause for the displacement is not defined. It may be due to caudal displacement of the larynx associated with activity of the sternothyrohyoideus and omohyoideus muscles during exercise.

History and Presenting Signs

■ Gurgling noise during fast exercise
■ Usually in racehorses

Clinical Findings and Diagnosis

KEY POINT ▶ Soft palate displacement usually occurs during fast exercise, particularly when the horse is pulling hard.

■ Trainers, jockeys, and drivers often describe horses as making a gurgling noise or "choking up," and there is a dramatic reduction in their performance.

■ Endoscopic examination at rest usually shows no abnormalities.

■ Endoscopic examination following high-intensity exercise may reveal soft palate dislocation. However, on many occasions no abnormalities are detected, since the dislocation usually occurs during high-speed exercise.

■ Manual occlusion of the nostrils may assist in inducing displacement of the soft palate. Diagnosis is therefore often made by exclusion of other upper respiratory problems, together with the typical history.

■ Treadmill endoscopy, with a bit in the horse's mouth and the use of long reins, may result in palate displacement.

Differential Diagnosis

■ Idiopathic laryngeal hemiplegia
■ Epiglottic entrapment
■ Subepiglottic cyst
■ Pharyngeal lymphoid hyperplasia
■ Sinus cyst
■ Guttural pouch empyema/abscess
■ Nasal polyp
■ Atheroma

Treatment

KEY POINT ▶ In some cases, application of a tongue tie or use of a straight bit will result in elimination of the problem.

■ Where these techniques are not successful, surgery can be performed to remove the sternothyrohyoideus and omohyoideus muscles. Myectomy of the sternothyrohyoideus muscle can be performed with the horse standing, and training can be resumed within 12 to 14 days in most cases. Myectomy of both muscles requires greater dissection, and general anesthesia is indicated. Approximately 50% of horses can be expected to show improvement after the myectomy procedure (assuming the epiglottis is not hypoplastic). However, the efficacy of the surgery is still not completely clear.

- In cases where the myectomy provides little or no relief, a staphylectomy can be performed. This involves resection of a portion of the caudal border of the soft palate. This procedure results in improvement in some horses, although the exact reason for this benefit is unknown. There is a strong contraindication for this procedure if the epiglottis is hypoplastic, because the operation will only worsen the problem.

Subepiglottic Cysts (Pharyngeal Cysts)

The most common location for cysts within the pharynx is in the subepiglottic area, although cysts have been reported near the larynx, soft palate, and other sites within the pharynx. It has been proposed that subepiglottic cysts are the result of a defect in embryologic development. In all cases, cysts usually contain a viscous yellow–tan mucus-like material. Cysts are most frequently reported in standardbred and thoroughbred racehorses. A congenital form of the disorder occurs in foals.

History and Presenting Signs

- Respiratory stridor during exercise and reduced performance are common.
- Dysphagia may be reported but is rare.
- A chronic cough, dyspnea, and dysphagia may be reported in foals with the disorder.

Clinical Findings and Diagnosis

KEY POINT ▶ The most common clinical signs in older horses (2–5 years old) that are associated with subepiglottic cysts are reduced performance capacity and an inspiratory and expiratory respiratory noise that is often only prominent during exercise.

- The dyspnea becomes more pronounced with increasing exercise intensity.
- Dysphagia and nasal discharge are uncommon manifestations of this disease in adult horses.
- Subepiglottic cysts have been reported infrequently in foals. In this age group, the cysts are often extremely large when diagnosed and produce dyspnea at rest and, possibly, nasal discharge, dysphagia and an increased potential for aspiration pneumonia.
- Subepiglottic and pharyngeal cysts are diagnosed on endoscopic examination. In adults, the cysts are usually 1 to 5 cm (0.5 to 2 in) in diameter and are smooth-walled, lying under or lateral to the epiglottis. When examining the pharyngeal area, it is important to make the horse swallow, since some cysts may not be visible until this maneuver is accomplished.
- Lateral radiographs of the laryngeal/pharyngeal region also may be of value in defining cystic lesions.
- In foals, the cysts are often much larger at the time of diagnosis and are usually obvious during endoscopic examination. If there is dysphagia, careful examination of the chest should be undertaken for signs indicative of aspiration pneumonia. If there is a suspicion of pneumonia, radiographs of the thorax may be useful.

Differential Diagnosis

Adults

- Idiopathic laryngeal hemiplegia
- Epiglottic entrapment
- Pharyngeal lymphoid hyperplasia
- Sinus cyst
- Guttural pouch empyema/abscess
- Nasal polyp
- Atheroma

Foals

- Congenital deformities of the upper airway
- Disorders resulting in dysphagia and dyspnea (e.g., guttural pouch tympany, retropharyngeal abscessation)
- Viral or bacterial pneumonia

Treatment

- Therapy involves removal of the offending cyst. Currently, several techniques are available.
- One surgical treatment involves a ventral laryngotomy so that direct access to the cyst is achieved, and it is dissected free from the surrounding tissue. Healing is by second intention, and convalescence is about 4 to 8 weeks. This is the technique of choice in foals and horses with particularly large lesions.
- The alternate technique involves removal of the cyst via an oral approach using short-term general anesthesia, an oral speculum, and a wire snare. Although the surgeon gains less favorable visual access to the cyst, because of the nature of the lesions, recurrence is rare, and this procedure has been made more popular by some clinicians because the postoperative convalescence period is greatly reduced, being only 1 to 3 weeks before the horses can return to training. This technique is not suitable for all cases because access to the cyst is dependent on its size and location and the lumen diameter of the horse's mouth.
- The use of Nd:YAG lasers for extirpation of the cysts via an oral approach also has been reported.

Tracheal Stenosis

Also referred to as "scabbard" trachea or dorsoventral flattening of the trachea, tracheal stenosis is a condition that most commonly has a congenital origin. Ponies and miniature horses constitute the breeds most frequently afflicted. In the congenital form of the disease, much of the length of the trachea is involved. Acquired forms of tracheal stenosis may result from direct trauma to the cervical trachea, resulting in a partial narrowing and hence a restriction to airflow.

History and Presenting Signs

Demonstration of a collapsed trachea is often an incidental finding; however, presenting complaints by owners may include poor performance, dyspnea (during exercise), and chronic, paroxysmal coughing, particularly in association with exercise.

Clinical Findings and Diagnosis

KEY POINT ▶ Clinical manifestations of a collapsed trachea are relatively rare, with the diagnosis often being made as an incidental finding at necropsy. In animals in which clinical signs are apparent, stertorous respiration with some degree of respiratory stridor is usually present.

- Chronic, paroxysmal bouts of coughing may be stimulated by tracheal palpation or exercise.
- Some animals show clinical manifestations similar to those seen in horses suffering from chronic obstructive pulmonary disease (COPD).
- Diagnosis can be made by palpation of the cervical trachea, which may reveal a flattening at the site of the abnormality.
- Endoscopic examination of the lumen of the trachea is a valuable diagnostic tool, as are lateral radiographs of the cervical trachea.

Differential Diagnosis

- Chronic obstructive pulmonary disease (COPD)
- Retropharyngeal abscessation
- Pneumonia
- Upper airway obstruction (e.g., foreign bodies, neoplasms, sinus cysts, etc.)

Treatment

- Several reports exist that describe attempts to correct the stenosis. These are difficult, often fraught with complications, and are usually only undertaken by specialist surgeons.
- If the animal is not required to perform athletic endeavors and is not coughing too severely, the best advice is not to attempt correction of the problem. Retirement of animals to a more sedentary lifestyle may result in palliation of the signs.

SINUS PROBLEMS

Sinus Cysts

Sinus cysts are fluid-filled cavities developing principally in the maxillary sinuses. The cause of the cysts is unknown, although most cysts have an epithelial lining. The proposal has been proffered that sinus cysts have a similar pathogenesis to ethmoidal hematomas, but this appears unlikely. A congenital form has been described in foals.

History and Presenting Signs

- Long-term, clear, unilateral nasal discharge is commonly reported.
- History of progressive facial swelling is common.
- Dyspnea and exercise intolerance may occur.

Clinical Findings and Diagnosis

- The most common findings on examination are a clear to mucoid nasal discharge, facial swelling, and dyspnea.
- There appear to be two groups of animals affected by sinus cysts: animals less than 1 year old (probably a congenital form) and mature horses (>9–10 years old).
- Despite the propensity of nasal cysts to distort the paranasal sinuses and tooth roots, they rarely invade the nasal cavity.
- Involvement of the frontal sinuses is rare.
- Diagnosis is based on the signalment, history of progressive swelling in the paranasal sinus region, physical examination findings, and the results of diagnostic tests.
- The two most important diagnostic tests are endoscopy and radiography.
- Endoscopic examination of the paranasal sinuses can have the appearance of impinging into the airway. This is reflected by the ventral concha being enlarged.
- Radiography of the affected area usually reveals fluid-filled cavities within the sinuses. The multiloculate form of the cysts is most common, although single fluid-filled cavities may be identified in some horses.
- Sclerosis of surrounding bone is common, as is displacement of tooth roots.
- Sinuscentesis may reveal moderately viscous fluid of a flaxen–amber color. There are few cells on cytologic examination and no bacteria.

Differential Diagnosis

- Primary or secondary sinusitis
- Congenital malformations of the nasal cavity or facial bones other than sinus cysts
- Neoplasia of the paranasal sinuses (e.g., squamous cell carcinoma, fibroma/fibrosarcoma, adenocarcinoma, etc.)

- Mucocele (young horses)
- Ethmoidal hematoma
- Trauma

Treatment

- Extirpation of the sinus cyst is the treatment of choice. An incision and bone flap are used to gain access to the affected sinus.
- The cyst and its lining are then dissected free of the surrounding sinus tissues. Considerable hemorrhage may accompany the procedure.
- In many cases, the postoperative course is relatively uncomplicated, with the incidence of recurrence being relatively low.
- Aesthetically favorable facial remodeling after extirpation of the cyst frequently occurs, making the longer-term prognosis more promising than might have been expected on initial diagnosis.

Sinusitis

The maxillary and frontal sinuses have communications with the nasal cavity, and the caudal compartment of the maxillary sinus communicates with the frontal sinus via the frontomaxillary opening. As a result, upper respiratory tract infections can extend into these regions, resulting in primary sinusitis.

KEY POINT ► Primary sinusitis occurs most frequently in younger horses, since the incidence of infectious respiratory tract disorders is greater in this age group.

In addition, the last four upper cheek teeth extend into the maxillary sinus, so infection of the tooth roots can be manifested as a secondary sinusitis (see Tooth-Root Abnormalities).

History and Presenting Signs

- Chronic, persistent, unilateral, mucopurulent nasal discharge that increases during exercise is commonly reported.
- Some horses demonstrate dyspnea, particularly in response to exercise.

Clinical Findings and Diagnosis

- Distortion of the facial contours is rare but can be seen in chronic cases.
- Stertorous breathing during exercise may occur.
- Systemic signs (e.g., fever, inappetence, weight loss) occur occasionally, as does epiphora.
- Extension of infection in severe cases of frontal sinusitis has been associated with meningitis and neurologic dysfunction.
- Diagnosis of primary sinusitis can be supported by a history of upper respiratory tract infection and the clinical signs.

- An oral examination should be performed if secondary sinusitis due to tooth-root problems is suspected.
- Accumulation of fluid in the sinuses may be indicated by a change in resonance when percussing the sinuses.
- Endoscopy may reveal pus draining from the nasomaxillary opening.
- Radiography is frequently of great assistance in revealing fluid within the sinus. Chronic cases may show osteolysis and mineralization on radiography.
- Sinuscentesis is a valuable tool for confirmation of infection and elucidation of the causative organisms. *Streptococcus equi* var. *zooepidemicus* and *Streptococcus equi* var. *equi* are implicated most frequently.

Treatment

KEY POINT ► Systemic antibiotics are rarely successful in resolving the problem. However, in some mild cases, they may give remission.

- Penicillin (procaine or aqueous) is the drug of choice for infections due to *Streptococcus equi* var. *zooepidemicus* and *Streptococcus equi* var. *equi* (Treatment Nos. 83 to 85).
- More aggressive therapy involves lavage and drainage of the sinus with polyionic solutions (0.5–2 L warmed to near body temperature) infused once or several times per day through a catheter or polyethylene tubing inserted through a trephine hole. Catheters can be sutured in place for repeated lavage. Lavage provides mechanical flushing of the sinus and is often an effective method for removal of the purulent material and debris.
- In more extensive infections of the maxillary sinus, a maxillary bone-flap technique may be used to gain access to the entire sinus for removal of mineralized and necrotic tissue. Postoperative care requires lavage and appropriate systemic antibiotics.

Tooth-Root Abnormalities and Secondary Sinusitis

Because the roots of the upper premolar and molar teeth project into the maxillary sinus and are close to the ventral nasal meatus, any disorders involving the tooth roots may lead to narrowing of the nasal cavity, obstruction to airflow, local infections (including pulpitis), and secondary sinusitis. Conditions such as fractures, patent infundibula, chronic ossifying alveolar periostitis, tooth displacement, dental malposition, tumors of the tooth roots, or dental malposition can cause such problems. Dental disease is most common in mature horses.

History and Presenting Signs

- Nasal discharge that is often unilateral and malodorous is common.
- Dyspnea may be reported. This occurs secondary to narrowing of the nasal passages

Clinical Findings and Diagnosis

KEY POINT ▶ Nasal discharge, dyspnea (respiratory stertor), malodorous breath, and, rarely, sinus tracts to the skin may indicate tooth-root problems, particularly those involving local infections.

- Distortion and swelling over the maxillary region may be seen.
- Dysphagia is rare.
- Diagnosis is aided by thorough oral examination (often requiring sedation and use of a mouth gag), endoscopic examination, and radiography.
- When performing an oral examination in a horse with suspected tooth-root problems, specific things to be checked for are evidence of cracked teeth, dental malposition, fetid breath, drainage of purulent material from around tooth roots, patent infundibula, or pulpitis.
- Evidence of nasal obstruction may be revealed by passage of a stomach tube.
- Absence of signs on physical examination does not preclude the existence of tooth-root disease.
- Endoscopy may reveal purulent material draining from the ventral compartment of the maxillary sinus into the nasal cavity via the nasomaxillary opening, if secondary sinusitis exists, and distortions of the nasal passages.
- Radiographs often reveal the presence of a tooth-root or apical granuloma. A zone of local osteolysis is common with a sclerotic margin.
- Diagnosis of the obstruction is possible by passage of a stomach tube, which will meet an obstruction at the site of narrowing of the ventral nasal meatus.
- *Micronema delatrix,* a saprophytic nematode found in decaying humus, may invade the nasal passages and paranasal sinuses on occasion and result in clinical manifestations similar to those described in this section. There appears to be a high risk of spread of the organisms to other organs, including the lower mandible, brain, and kidneys. Diagnosis is based on the results of biopsy examinations.

Differential Diagnosis

- Primary sinusitis
- Sinus cysts
- Congenital malformations of the nasal cavity or facial bones
- Trauma
- Foreign body
- Ethmoidal hematoma
- Nematode infection (e.g., *Micronema delatrix*)
- Neoplasia (e.g., fibroma/fibrosarcoma, squamous cell carcinoma, adenocarcinoma, etc.)
- Conchal necrosis
- Amyloidosis

Treatment

- Most tooth-root problems usually develop slowly, and by the time the horse presents for examination, removal of the diseased tooth and other infected local tissues is the most appropriate course of action. This is a difficult procedure and is most easily performed via a sinus flap. Postoperative care includes antibiotic coverage (see Chap. 17) and local wound therapy. The latter may consist of packing the alveolar socket with gauze. The packing is changed every other day, and the socket is flushed with warm saline or dilute antiseptic. New gauze is wedged back in the socket. Umbilical tape is tied around the pack before insertion, and the loose end of the tape is directed to exit at the skin surface, where it is secured to another gauze roll. This procedure requires a mouth gag, and most horses require sedation. A less risky procedure involves packing the alveolar socket with acrylic at the time of surgery. Securing the acrylic in the socket can provide a challenge. The aim of both procedures is to allow the socket to fill with granulation tissue while preventing the egress of food from the mouth into the socket or sinus. In summary, tooth removal is often time-consuming, and complications occur relatively frequently.
- *Micronema delatrix* is sensitive to Ivermectin (200 μg/kg PO; Treatment No. 62); however, the propensity for this organism to invade other tissues may make therapy unrewarding.

References

Archer, R. M., Lindsay, W. A., and Duncan, I. D.: A comparison of techniques to enhance the evaluation of equine laryngeal function. *Equine Vet. J.* 23(2):104, 1991.

Beech, J.: *Equine Respiratory Disorders.* Philadelphia: Lea & Febiger, 1991.

Belknap, J. K., Derksen, F. J., Nickels, F. A., et al.: Failure of subtotal arytenoidectomy to improve upper airway flow mechanics in exercising standardbreds with induced laryngeal hemiplegia. *Am. J. Vet. Res.* 9:1481, 1990.

Cook, W. R.: Some observations on form and function of the equine upper airway in health and disease: I. Pharynx. *Proc. 27th Conv. Am. Assoc. Equine Pract.,* 1981, p. 355.

Cook, W. R.: Some observations on form and function of the equine upper airway in health and disease: II. Larynx. *Proc. 27th Conv. Am. Assoc. Equine Pract.,* 1981, p. 393.

Dean, P. W.: Diagnosis, treatment, and prognosis of arytenoid chondropathy. *Proc. 36th Conv. Am. Assoc. Equine Pract.,* 1990, p. 415.

Ducharme, N. G., and Hackett, R. P.: The value of surgical treatment of laryngeal hemiplegia in horses. *Compend. Contin. Educ. Pract. Vet.* 13:472, 1991.

Finn, S. T., and Park, R. D.: Radiology of the nasal cavity and paranasal sinuses in the horse. *Proc. 33d Annu. Conv. Am. Assoc. Equine Pract.*, 1987, p. 383.

Greet, T. R. C.: Outcome of treatment of 35 cases of guttural pouch mycosis. *Equine Vet. J.* 19:483, 1987.

Haynes, P. F.: Obstructive disease of the upper respiratory tract: Current thoughts on diagnosis and surgical management. *Proc. 32d Annu. Conv. Am. Assoc. Equine Pract.*, 1986, p. 283.

Haynes, P. F., Snider, T. G., and McClure, J. R.: Chronic chondritis of the equine arytenoid cartilage. *J. Am. Vet. Med. Assoc.* 177:1135, 1980.

Honnas, C. M., Schumacher, J., and Dean, P. W.: Epiglottic entrapment: The techniques for diagnosis and surgical treatment. *Vet. Med.* 85:613, 1990.

Honnas, C. M., Schumacher, J., and Dean, P. W.: Identifying and correcting displacements of the soft palate and pharyngeal tissues. *Vet. Med.* 85:622, 1990.

Lane, J. G., Longstaffe, J. A., and Gibbs, C.: Equine paranasal sinus cysts: A report of 15 cases. *Equine Vet. J.* 19:537, 1987.

Morris, E., and Seeherman, H.: The dynamic evaluation of upper respiratory function in the exercising horse. *Proc. 34th Annu. Conv. Am. Assoc. Equine Pract.*, 1988, p. 159.

Morris, E. A., and Seeherman, H. J.: Evaluation of upper respiratory tract function during strenuous exercise in racehorses. *J. Am. Vet. Med. Assoc.* 196:431–438, 1990.

Raker, C. W., and Boles, C. L.: Pharyngeal lymphoid hyperplasia in the horse. *J. Equine Med. Surg.* 2:202, 1978.

White, S. L., and Williamson, L.: How to make a retention catheter to treat guttural pouch empyema. *Vet. Med.* 82:76, 1987.

Lower Respiratory Tract Diseases

Bacterial Pneumonia

Bacterial pneumonia is one of the most common diseases affecting the lower respiratory tract in adult horses. Bacterial pneumonia is frequently the result of some stressful event that produces some degree of immunocompromise and is often secondary to viral respiratory disease.

History and Presenting Signs

KEY POINT ► History of exposure to stressful situations is common (e.g., transport, anesthesia, training, weaning, congregations of large numbers of horses).

■ The horse will usually have a history of signs consistent with a previous viral respiratory tract infection

Clinical Findings and Diagnosis

KEY POINT ► Increases in respiratory rate, heart rate, dyspnea, fever, mucopurulent nasal discharge, depression, and inappetence are all common features of this disease.

■ In racehorses, poor performance (acute onset) may be noted, as are signs of distress after racing or training.

■ Auscultation of the thorax may reveal harshness, wheezes, and "gurgling" respiratory sounds, and these may be accentuated by the use of a rebreathing bag.

■ Definitive diagnosis is obtained with the use of transtracheal lavage and aspiration (see p. 138). This procedure allows for cytologic and bacteriologic analysis of samples collected. Appropriate antibiotic selection can then be made on the basis of culture and sensitivity results.

■ Bronchoalveolar lavage also may provide a very useful indication of the cytologic and to a lesser extent bacteriologic (due to the potential for contamination by bacteria resident in the upper airway when the tube is passed) characteristics of the airway in the caudal lung region. The most common aerobic bacterial species involved in the induction of pneumonia in horses are members of the families Lactobacillaceae (gram-positive) and Enterobacteriaciae (gram-negative).

■ Anaerobic bacteria are being implicated with greater frequency as causative agents in bacterial pneumonias in adult horses. As a result, submission of samples for anaerobic culture, particularly in cases with severe clinical manifestations, is indicated (see Chap. 15).

■ Hematology will give some guide to the severity of the infection in acute cases. Anticipated abnormalities include a leukocytosis, with neutrophilia, and increased serum fibrinogen and globulin concentrations if the disease process has been active for more than a few days.

KEY POINT ▶ Pleuropneumonia and pleural effusion often occur secondarily to pneumonia, and therefore, additional physical examinations (including careful auscultation) should be undertaken in horses not showing a favorable clinical response to therapy. Particular consideration should be given to repeating the transtracheal aspiration, ultrasound examinations, and/or thoracocentesis if there is a lack of response to therapy.

Differential Diagnosis

■ Viral respiratory tract infections
■ Pleuropneumonia
■ Acute respiratory distress

Treatment

■ Systemic antibiotic therapy at maximum therapeutic dose rates should be undertaken.

■ Selection of antibiotic therapy "in the dark" or use of "shotgun" antibiotic treatment is unlikely to prove effective because it is difficult in many cases to predict the organism involved.

■ Therapy can be started with gentamicin (2 mg/kg IV q12h; Treatment No. 56), and crystalline penicillin (20,000 IU/kg IV or IM q6h; Treatment Nos. 84 and 85) in horses showing signs consistent with acute bacterial pneumonia is usually indicated.

■ Procaine penicillin [15,000–20,000 IU/kg (15–20 mg/kg) IM q12h; Treatment No. 83] is also a good choice to follow initial therapy with crystalline penicillin.

KEY POINT ▶ The procaine in procaine penicillin G may take up to 6 weeks to be eliminated in racehorses following administration.

■ Other potentially suitable antibiotics include trimethoprim–sulphonamide (15 mg/kg of combined agent PO q12h; Treatment No. 107) and ceftiofur (Treatment No. 18).

■ Following the return of bacterial culture and sensitivity results, the appropriate antibiotic selections can be made.

■ Other therapies for pneumonia may include bronchodilators, mucolytics, nonsteroidal anti-inflammatory drugs, reduction of stress, and good nursing care.

■ The most commonly employed and effective bronchodilators are aminophylline (5–10 mg/kg PO q12h; Treatment No. 5) and clenbuterol HCl (0.8 μg/kg IV or PO q12h; Treatment No. 27). These agents appear to reduce the respiratory effort required by many horses with acute bacterial pneumonia and improve the clearance of mucopurulent secretions from the lower airways.

■ Nonsteroidal anti-inflammatory drugs (see Chap. 17) may be required in horses showing significant debility as a result of the pneumonia to afford them a little more comfort and to increase their interest in eating and drinking.

KEY POINT ▶ Anti-inflammatory drugs may mask fever, and it is therefore important not to discontinue antimicrobial therapy too soon or return the horse to work too rapidly if the horse is receiving nonsteroidal anti-inflammatory drugs.

■ Withdrawal of the affected animal from a training program during periods when there is clinical evidence for the existence of pneumonia is also vital.

■ The ongoing stress of training in the face of bacterial pneumonia is one of the most frequent causes of severe complications such as pleuropneumonia.

■ Provision of a high-quality, palatable, digestible diet is important in animals that are debilitated by the systemic effects of bacterial pneumonia.

■ Appropriate attention to the fluid and electrolyte needs of the animal is also critical in the successful management of horses with pneumonia.

Chronic Obstructive Pulmonary Disease (COPD, "Heaves")

Chronic obstructive pulmonary disease (COPD) is a condition found mainly in older horses that are kept in box stalls. It is the result of an allergic bronchitis and bronchiolitis from exposure to various molds or dust in straw and hay.

KEY POINT ▶ The condition is common in the northern hemisphere because horses are stalled in barns for prolonged periods.

Owing to different housing and management conditions, COPD is rare in the southern hemisphere.

History and Presenting Signs

KEY POINT ▶ Chronic cough, dyspnea, and exercise intolerance in older horses are the most common complaints by owners.

Clinical Findings and Diagnosis

- The most common signs are increased respiratory effort and dyspnea after strenuous exercise and a soft cough, particularly in association with feeding and exercise.
- Clinical examination may reveal a biphasic expiratory effort, and in long-standing cases, there will be a "heave line" along the ventral rib cage.
- In addition to decreased exercise tolerance, horses with COPD may exhibit dyspnea and coughing during exercise.
- Auscultation of the chest reveals wheezing sounds that are most easily heard if a rebreathing bag is used.
- Arterial blood gas analysis will reveal low oxygen partial pressures in arterial blood, with values usually less than 80 mmHg at rest.
- Hematology and serum or plasma biochemistry are usually unremarkable.

Differential Diagnosis

- Viral respiratory disease
- Bacterial pneumonia
- Pleuropneumonia
- Other causes of dyspnea/respiratory noise during exercise (e.g., idiopathic laryngeal hemiplegia, epiglottic dislocation, pharyngeal cysts)

Treatment

- This is a management-related disease, so the main aspect of treatment is to remove the predisposing cause, i.e., remove the horse from the stable (if possible) and turn it out to pasture. Most horses respond quite quickly to rest while housed outdoors. Recurrence is common when they are returned to the stable environment. Reduction of dust in bedding and feed (wetting down food prior to it being offered to the horse) also will assist in reducing the severity of signs.
- Bronchodilator therapy using clenbuterol (Treatment No. 5) is quite effective, although long-term treatment may be required.
- The use of oral corticosteroids (prednisolone; Treatment No. 92) also can provide good symptomatic relief. Both drugs need to be withdrawn prior to racing.
- A form of the disease exists in the southern states of the United States in which allergens in pastures during summer months produce signs similar to those in stabled horses. In these cases, the treatment is to remove the horses from pasture into stables.

Exercise-Induced Pulmonary Hemorrhage (EIPH)

EIPH is a common disorder, particularly in thoroughbred and quarter horse racehorses, where the incidence is likely to be between 50% and 75%. Standardbreds probably have an incidence in the range of 40% to 60%, whereas in polo ponies the incidence is probably about 10%. EIPH is rare in endurance horses.

KEY POINT ▶ From these findings it seems apparent that the incidence of EIPH is directly related to the absolute intensity of exercise that horses are required to undertake.

Hemorrhage originates in the lungs, probably in the thoracophrenic region. This origin for the hemorrhage is supported by necropsy examinations of horses with a known history of EIPH. Although many hypotheses (at least five are currently under discussion) as to the pathogenesis of EIPH have been proposed, no clear mechanism has been defined.

History and Presenting Signs

- Horses with EIPH are frequently reported to perform poorly. The effects of EIPH on performance are not clear.
- Respiratory distress and an increased rate of swallowing after exercise can occur. The swallowing is presumably to clear blood ascending from the lower airway.
- On rare occasions, blood discharges from the nostrils

Clinical Findings and Diagnosis

- The predominant clinical manifestation of EIPH is blood in the ventral part of the tracheobronchial tree, visible via endoscopy. Only about 1% to 10% of horses with EIPH ever demonstrate epistaxis.
- Coughing also may occur, but this is a nonspecific sign associated with many conditions of the upper and lower respiratory tracts. In severe cases there may be noticeable alterations in the breathing pattern during the postexercise period.
- Diagnosis is usually based on the history and endoscopic findings. Blood in the trachea will be most obvious 30 to 60 minutes after strenuous exercise.
- Other procedures that may assist in the diagnosis of EIPH are transtracheal lavage and aspiration or bronchoalveolar lavage for the demonstration of hemosiderophages.
- Hemosiderophages clear slowly from the lungs, and their recovery in respiratory secretions can be anticipated for prolonged periods after the hemorrhagic episode.

■ Special stains (e.g., Sano's trichome) may increase the likelihood of visualizing hemosiderophages on appropriate smears. Increases in the proportion of neutrophils and eosinophils also occur in horses with a history of EIPH. Increases in the bronchointerstitial pattern in chest radiographs, particularly in the caudodorsal lung fields, may be visualized in horses with EIPH. This finding is not consistent in all horses with EIPH, however.

Differential Diagnosis

■ Other causes of dyspnea/respiratory embarrassment during exercise (e.g., idiopathic laryngeal hemiplegia, epiglottic dislocation, pharyngeal cysts)
■ Viral respiratory disease
■ Pharyngeal lymphoid hyperplasia
■ Other causes of epistaxis (e.g., guttural pouch disease, nasal tumors, ethmoid hematoma)
■ Chronic obstructive pulmonary disease (COPD)

Treatment

■ Veterinarians and horse people are particularly inventive individuals. As a result, a plethora of remedies for EIPH have been described. Unfortunately, few, if any, of these provide good palliation of the condition.

KEY POINT ► Furosemide (0.3–0.6 mg/kg IV 3–4 hours prior to racing; Treatment Nos. 54 and 55) is widely prescribed in the United States in horses prior to racing.

■ Based on the observations of skilled observers, there seems little doubt (at least on the basis of a large volume of empirical evidence) that this medication reduces the severity of EIPH in approximately 50% of the horses it is administered to prior to racing.
■ Furosemide does not eliminate the hemorrhage; it just reduces the severity. The mechanism by which the agent exerts these effects is not clear.

Lungworm

Dictyocaulus arnfeldi is the lungworm in the horse that may be a cause of chronic coughing. The donkey or donkey crosses (mule and ass) are the natural hosts for lungworm. Natural hosts show few, if any, clinical signs of infestation. The condition in horses is usually found in those which have been in the company of donkeys, mules, or asses. Clinical signs usually become manifest in horses in the fall or winter following exposure to primary hosts in the summer months. Infective larvae are sensitive to low ambient temperatures, and the cold temperatures common to the frost belt of North America and northern England and Europe kill many of the infective larvae on pasture. As a result,

new infections and clinical signs in horses are often noticed following the warmer months of the year.

KEY POINT ► Patent infections are quite rare in horses.

History and Presenting Signs

■ Chronic cough, particularly in the late summer, fall, or early winter
■ A history of the horse living with donkeys

Clinical Findings and Diagnosis

■ Coughing, often of several weeks' duration, and possibly signs referable to a condition producing lower respiratory tract obstruction in the late summer or fall are the most common indicators of clinically significant disease.
■ Since patent infections are rare, examination of feces for eggs by the Baermann flotation procedure may be unrewarding. However, use of this technique in donkey or donkey-cross animals that have been in contact with the horse suspected of having the disease may provide evidence of patent infection. This may be sufficient evidence to strongly suspect *D. arnfeldi* infestation in the horse in question.
■ Transtracheal aspiration can be helpful in diagnosis in some cases where a large number of eosinophils are observed in smears of the aspirate.

Differential Diagnosis

■ Chronic obstructive pulmonary disease (COPD)
■ Viral respiratory infection
■ Bacterial pneumonia

Treatment

Ivermectin at a dose rate of 200 μg/kg PO (Treatment No. 62) appears to be the drug of choice for treatment of lungworm infection in horses.

Pleuropneumonia (Infectious Pleural Effusion, Pleuritis)

KEY POINT ► Pleuritis or pleural effusion is a condition that results in the production of large volumes of fluid in the thoracic cavity, usually secondary to a bacterial pneumonia.

Stress (e.g., transport, racing, surgery) is often an integral part of the history of horses afflicted with this disorder. Less common causes of infectious pleural effusion include blunt trauma to (with or without foreign-body penetration of) the thoracic cavity. In many cases where fluid is present in the chest, careful clinical evaluation is required to determine its presence. Aggressive therapy is required in order to limit the progression of this serious disease.

History and Presenting Signs

- Depression, inappetence, and a prior history of stress (e.g., transport is common)
- A history of what appeared to be a viral respiratory tract infection is common.
- Reluctance to move, sweating, and apparent anxiety may be reported.
- In chronic cases, weight loss and ventral edema may be noted.

Clinical Findings and Diagnosis

- Horses may have similar presenting signs to those described for pneumonia.
- At rest, a variable degree of dyspnea may be present, and the respiration is often shallow and rapid.
- Respirations often appear to be painful, and affected horses may "grunt" when required to move.
- The gait is often stiff due to this pain (pleurodynia), because the parietal pleura are well endowed with pain sensing fibers. This is often mistaken
as being indicative of laminitis, a myopathy, or colic.
- There is usually an elevated heart rate and increased rectal temperature.
- A soft cough, mucopurulent nasal discharge, and fetid breath are common.
- On auscultation of the chest, there may be abnormal lung sounds in the dorsal regions, such as wheezes, crackles, rales, and harshness, with muffled or absent sounds in the ventral regions.
- Auscultation with a rebreathing bag is often useful in helping define abnormal lung sounds. Pleural friction rubs may be detectable. In addition to auscultation, percussion of the chest can be a useful and inexpensive means for establishing the presence of pleural effusion. Other more sophisticated techniques include thoracic ultrasonography (the technique of choice) and radiography.

KEY POINT ► In any horse suspected of having a pleural effusion, thoracocentesis should always be performed (on *both* sides of the chest). Ultrasound examination will greatly assist in appropriate placement of the needle or cannula. Cytologic and bacteriologic examination of this fluid is *imperative*.

- If the horse has had the pleuritis and pleural effusion for more than 1 to 2 weeks, there may be evidence of weight loss, ventral edema (particularly in the pectoral region), and a history of intermittent pyrexia.

KEY POINT ► Inappetence is not a common feature in horses with pleuropneumonia.

- Clinical pathology on peripheral blood usually shows leukocytosis, neutrophilia, profound hyperfibrinogenemia, and so on.

Differential Diagnosis

- Viral or bacterial pneumonia
- Chronic obstructive pulmonary disease (COPD)
- Thoracic neoplasia with effusion
- Conditions causing signs of generalized pain (e.g., laminitis, colic, myopathy)
- Thoracic foreign body
- Severe exercise-induced pulmonary hemorrhage

Treatment

- Thoracic drainage to aspirate fluid and necrotic material from the chest is usually necessary, particularly if more than a few liters of fluid are in the thoracic cavity. This may be done with a teat cannula if the volume of fluid is small and the fluid contains little fibrinous material.
- When there is a large volume of flocculent fluid, it should be drained with a relatively large bore chest tube (20–28F blunt-tipped chest tube).

KEY POINT ► Fluid is allowed to drain via gravity (suction is contraindicated because as it aspirates flocculent material into the tube, thereby blocking the lumen). Tubes may be fixed in place with a purse-string suture, and a one-way valve can be made from a latex condom with the tip cut off that is taped to the end of the tube.

- If the volume of fluid is not thought to be too great, intermittent drainage every day or every other day can be considered.
- Parenteral antibiotics are integral to the treatment of these horses. It is important that a bactericidal rather than a bacteriostatic antibiotic be used (see Pneumonia).

KEY POINT ► From a bacteriologic point of view, pleuropneumonia does not usually constitute a medical emergency.

- As a result, treating the horse with anti-inflammatory drugs until appropriate samples for bacterial culture and sensitivity are obtained is a far superior practice than commencing "shotgun" therapy in the absence of pertinent bacteriologic data.
- Once samples have been collected (fluid from both thoracic cavities and from a transtracheal wash and aspirate), empirical antimicrobial therapy can be commenced until culture and sensitivity results come to hand. Penicillin and aminoglycoside antibiotics (see Chap. 17) are usually the drugs of choice in pleuropneumonia because they (1) are active against the vast majority of organisms encountered in this disease, (2) are bacteri-

cidal, (3) provide good plasma and tissue concentrations, (4) have a reasonably broad therapeutic index, and (5) are relatively cost-effective.

- Since many cases will have anaerobic bacteria involved, the use of metronidazole (10 mg/kg PO q6h; Treatment No. 75) should be strongly considered if the culture results indicate penicillin-resistant *B. fragilis* (see Chap. 17).
- Anti-inflammatory therapy is also important in an attempt to limit the degree of debility inflicted by the disease. A number of agents are readily available. Examples include flunixin meglumine (Treatment No. 52), phenylbutazone (Treatment No. 88), and ketoprofen (Treatment No. 66). Care should be exercised in horses with associated dehydration because the nephrotoxic potential of these agents is increased.
- In cases where significant systemic manifestations of the disease exist (e.g., toxemia, dehydration, etc.), fluid therapy is also indicated (see Chap. 17). The degree of volume contraction is reflected by physical findings (e.g., skin turgor, mucous membrane color, and capillary refill time) and appropriate clinicopathologic measurements (e.g., PCV, TPP, urea, creatinine).
- Following initial replacement of deficits, oral fluid supplementation can usually cover ongoing losses.
- Good nursing care is also vital in the management of pleuropneumonia. This includes limitation of stress, provision of a highly palatable and digestible diet, and constant surveillance for such complications as lung abscessation, anterior thoracic masses/abscesses, pulmonary infarction, bronchopleural fistulas, pericardial effusion, and laminitis.
- In acute cases with limited effusion, the prognosis for full recovery is likely to be reasonable if appropriate therapy is undertaken. However, in long-standing or complicated cases that have significant sequelae, the degree of damage to the contents of the thoracic cavity is often quite severe. Although salvage in many cases is possible if aggressive therapy is maintained for appropriate periods, prognosis for return to a successful athletic career must remain much more guarded.

Rhodococcus equi Infection ("Rattles")

This is a debilitating disease of foals with predominantly respiratory signs. There are two forms of pneumonia: *subacute,* with diffuse miliary pyogranulomatous pneumonia that usually has a fatal outcome, and *chronic,* where foals have pneumonaia and are unthrifty for relatively protracted periods. The disorder is much more prevalent in foals kept in large populations. Morbidity worldwide is about 10%, with mortality rates greater than 50%. Since this disease is restricted almost entirely to foals 1 to 6 months of age, the disease process is discussed in greater detail in Chapter 8.

Streptococcus equi var. *equi* Infection ("Strangles")

"Strangles" is a highly infectious bacterial respiratory disease in horses caused by *Streptococcus equi* var. *equi.* Infection is by inhalation or ingestion of the organism with subsequent localization in the mandibular and pharyngeal lymph nodes. The disease is most common in young horses (1–5 years of age). The organism is spread in nasal discharges or by contaminated grooming utensils, rugs, feed bins/utensils, or humans (e.g., on hands, clothes, stomach tubes). Animals incubating or recovering from the disease are the usual source of introduction of the organism to a naive population. Horses chronically shedding the organism are rare. Periodic outbreaks of strangles, characterized by a high incidence in young horses, occur on stud farms and race training complexes.

The incubation period is 3 to 10 days, with morbidity being variable depending on the age, immune status, and management of the herd. At times, morbidity may approach 100% in some susceptible populations. Mortality in well-managed outbreaks is usually less than 5%.

History and Presenting Signs

- Acute onset of depression, inappetence, and nasal discharge, often in a number of younger horses in a population
- Outbreaks may occur.
- In more advanced cases, swelling in the submandibular region may be noted.

KEY POINT ► Submandibular swelling is often the first sign of the disease noticed by the owner.

Clinical Findings and Diagnosis

KEY POINT ► Initial clinical signs in addition to inappetence, depression, and serous nasal discharge are fever (>40°C), pain, and swelling in the pharyngeal region.

- Dysphagia or dyspnea may occur as a result of swelling in the "throatlatch"—hence the name "strangles." Coughing is a feature of some cases.
- Clinical signs may persist for days to months. In most cases, once affected nodes have abscessed and drained, recovery is uneventful.
- Major clinicopathologic changes may include evidence of dehydration in the early phases of the disease, leukocytosis, and an increase in fibrinogen.
- Abscessation in a variety of other body sites is possible, including the periorbital area, retropharyngeal lymph nodes, guttural pouches, lungs/thorax, abdominal cavity (e.g., mesentery, liver,

spleen, and kidney), brain, and joints. These metastases are referred to as "bastard strangles."
■ Horses with metastatic abscesses often demonstrate chronic weight loss.
■ Affected lactating mares may have significant reductions in milk production.
■ Purpura hemorrhagica is a relatively rare but potentially fatal complication. Signs include fever, peripheral edema, depression, and possibly petechial hemorrhages evident on the mucosae.

KEY POINT ► Diagnosis is best made on the basis of clinical signs (e.g., depression, fever, lymphadenopathy) and isolation of *Streptococcus equi* var. *equi*. Nasal swabs, purulent discharges, and direct aspiration of material from abscesses that have not yet discharged (the optimal site for collection of samples) are suitable for isolation of the organism.

■ Diagnostic success is increased if samples from a variety of sites are cultured (e.g., swabs from draining lymph nodes and the nasal or pharyngeal mucosa). Use of an appropriate transport medium (Streptswab, Medical Wire and Equipment Co., Cleveland, Ohio) improves the recovery rate of organisms from samples, particularly those which are likely to be delayed in transit to the laboratory.
■ "Bastard strangles" may be suspected on the basis of physical examination findings (e.g., rectal examination, endoscopy) and the use of other diagnostic aids (e.g., radiography, ultrasonography, abdominal or thoracic paracentesis, joint-fluid analysis, etc.). Anemia of chronic disease, persistent leukocytosis, and hyperfibrinogenemia are common features of this disease.

Differential Diagnosis

■ Viral respiratory tract disease
■ Bacterial pneumonia
■ Guttural pouch empyema
■ Abscessation due to bacteria other than *Streptococcus equi*

Treatment

KEY POINT ► Affected horses should be quarantined to prevent exposure to naive horses.

■ The presence of clinical signs may have no relationship to the potential a horse has for spreading the disease. Previously affected horses may still spread the disease for 1 to 2 months after disappearance of clinical manifestations. In some cases, horses may be able to transmit the disease for up to 8 months. Horses should remain isolated for 4 to 5 weeks after disappearance of signs.

■ Negative results from three culture swabs taken over 7 to 10 days are recommended before a horse is assumed to have cleared the infection.
■ Personal hygiene is important for those handling horses. For example, handlers of infected horses should not, if at all possible, be in contact with uninfected horses. Scrupulous hand and boot washing and the use of disposable overclothing are recommended. Disinfection of food and grooming materials and reusable veterinary equipment is imperative.

KEY POINT ► Penicillin G is the drug of choice.

■ Appropriate doses must be used (15,000–20,000 IU/kg [15–20 mg/kg] procaine penicillin IM q12h or crystalline penicillin 20,000 IU/kg IV q6h; Treatment Nos. 83–85). Administration of the agent must be continued for 5 to 7 days after clinical signs have resolved. Failure to do so may result in recrudescence of the disease. Other drugs that have been used are the semisynthetic penicillins (ampicillin, amoxycillin), trimethoprim–sulfonamide combinations, and oxytetracycline. All have activity against *Streptococcus equi* but are less effective than penicillin G.
■ Routine monitoring of animals at risk by measurement of rectal temperature (once or twice a day) and aggressive administration of penicillin to those showing evidence of fever appear to reduce the severity of disease in many situations.
■ Most mild cases of strangles probably do not require antibiotic therapy and resolve without incident.
■ In some cases, drainage of purulent material from localized lymph node infections may be required. Exudate should be disposed of appropriately.
■ "Bastard strangles" often requires protracted antimicrobial therapy (4–6 weeks) and specific local therapy (e.g., abscess drainage, etc.).
■ Purpura hemorrhagica requires aggressive long-term antibiotic and anti-inflammatory therapy. Initial treatment with penicillin (Treatment Nos. 83–85) and dexamethasone (0.06–0.1 mg/kg q24h; Treatment Nos. 29 and 30) is indicated. Reduction of the steroid dose as soon as possible after clinical improvement occurs is advised. Dexamethasone appears to be more effective than prednisolone. Phenylbutazone (Treatment No. 88) or flunixin meglumine (Treatment No. 52) also can be useful.

Prophylaxis

■ The chance of prevention of strangles is improved if stringent quarantine measures are employed.
■ There is a report in which the morbidity due to strangles in foals in the face of an outbreak was decreased when benzathine penicillin was administered (5000 IU/kg IM q48h) for 3 weeks (Treatment No. 82).
■ Several vaccines are available. One vaccine con-

tains the M-protein to *Streptococcus equi* (Treatment No. 114), whereas the other contains an purified enzyme extract of *Streptococcus equi* (Treatment No. 114).

- Vaccination has been shown to reduce morbidity and severity of clinical signs but *does not* prevent the disease. Best immunity appears to be afforded by a course of vaccinations. Annual booster vaccinations are recommended.
- Swelling at the site of injection and some mild systemic signs (e.g., depression, inappetence) are relatively common following vaccination.

Thoracic Neoplasia

Neoplasia in the thoracic cavity is rare in the horse. Most commonly, thoracic neoplasia involves metastasis from another site.

History and Presenting Signs

- Weight loss is commonly reported.
- Older horses are often affected.
- Respiratory distress, particularly in response to exercise, may be a feature.

Clinical Findings and Diagnosis

KEY POINT ▶ Affected horses may have evidence of weight loss, dyspnea, tachypnea, cough, nasal discharge, and epistaxis.

- Diagnosis is based on clinical signs and the results of specific diagnostic tests, including endoscopy, radiography, thoracocentesis, and possibly biopsy. Examination of other body systems may provide evidence of generalized systemic involvement of the neoplasm. Results of blood analyses frequently show nonspecific evidence of disease (e.g., anemia of chronic disease).
- Often diagnosis is not confirmed until a postmortem examination is performed. Discovery of a thoracic neoplastic process may be an incidental finding during a routine necropsy.

Treatment

In general, thoracic neoplasia is untreatable.

Viral Respiratory Disease

Viral respiratory disease is common in the horse and provides a frequent cause of horse owners seeking veterinary attention for affected animals. A number of viral agents have been implicated, with influenza (A/equine 2) and herpesvirus (rhinopneumonitis, equine herpesvirus 4) being the most prominent causes of infirmity. Other viral agents that have been implicated in equine respiratory disease include other strains of influenza virus, equine herpesvirus 2, equine viral arteritis, adenoviruses, rhinoviruses, and parainfluenza viruses. The signif-

icance of the latter two virus groups in the pathogenesis of respiratory disease in horses is limited. Respiratory viral infections generally occur in young animals that are stabled together, with spread between animals the result of direct contact, aerosol, fomites, and, in some cases (e.g., equine viral arteritis), venereal.

KEY POINT ▶ Outbreaks of viral respiratory disease may cause a high degree of wastage and poor performance in the racing industry. Valuable training time is lost while horses recover from infection.

Vaccines are now available for equine herpesvirus 1 and 4 (EHV-1 and EHV-4), the A/equine 1 and 2 strains of influenza virus, and equine viral arteritis virus, although the efficacy of vaccination programs remains open to question.

Adenovirus is a normal inhabitant of the upper respiratory tract and generally only causes infection in immunocompromised foals, such as Arabians with combined immunodeficiency (CID) or other horses that have been under significant stress.

History and Presenting Signs

- Inappetence and depression are two of the most commonly reported presenting signs.
- Outbreaks of the disease may occur, particularly in young horses or those housed under intensive conditions (e.g., racing and training facilities).
- Viral respiratory disease frequently causes poor performance.

Clinical Findings and Diagnosis

- Viral respiratory infections cause a variety of clinical manifestations that vary depending on the type of virus involved and the age and susceptibility of the host.

KEY POINT ▶ The most common signs include inappetence, fever, depression, and a slight nasal discharge in the early stages of infection.

- Within 24 to 48 hours the nasal discharge is often more copious, and a cough, due to pharyngitis and/or laryngitis, may be detected.

Equine Influenza

- The most debilitating effects of viral respiratory infections are commonly associated with equine influenza virus.

KEY POINT ▶ Spread is rapid, and morbidity is often high, with horses in training and those amassed in large populations (e.g., racetracks, training stables, etc.) being most at risk. Younger animals (2–3 years of age) appear to be most susceptible.

- Signs include fever (up to 41°C), inappetence, nasal discharge, depression, and a reduced willingness to move around. Harsh lung sounds may be detected.
- Uncomplicated infections tend to show improvement in clinical signs in 4 to 7 days. Complications, including secondary bacterial invasion, cardiomyopathy, and persistently poor performance, also may occur.
- Horses exposed to continued stress or immune compromise may experience secondary complications (e.g., bacterial pneumonia or pleuropneumonia).

Equine Herpesvirus 1 and 4

- Respiratory disease is a sequel to infection with either of these viral strains; however, most cases of herpesvirus respiratory disease are the result of infection with EHV-4.

KEY POINT ► The clinical manifestations tend to be less severe and morbidity lower than that resulting from infection with influenza virus.

- In young foals, clinical signs are often relatively restricted and transient. However, in older foals, in whom maternal antibody titers have waned and who are exposed to high levels of stress (e.g., weaning), clinical manifestations may be more severe, including fever, serous nasal discharge, pharyngeal lymphoid hyperplasia, lymphadenopathy, and an increase in the intensity of respiratory sounds.
- Secondary bacterial complications are common in foals exposed to continued stress throughout the course of the viral infection.

KEY POINT ► Infection of pregnant mares with EHV-1 in the last trimester may cause abortion or the birth of weak foals that die soon after birth with degenerative lesions in the respiratory tract, liver, and lymphoid tissue.

- Neurologic dysfunction, specifically ataxia, has been reported in horses subsequent to infection with EHV-1.

Equine Herpesvirus 2

- Fever, nasal discharge, lymphadenopathy, inappetence, pharyngeal lymphoid hyperplasia, and failure to thrive have been reported in foals in response to infection with EHV-2.
- Keratoconjunctivitis also has been associated with infections with this strain of equine herpesvirus.

Equine Viral Arteritis

- The clinical manifestations of infection with this virus are variable, with respiratory signs occurring on occasion.

- The most common indications of infection include fever, inappetence, peripheral edema, conjunctivitis, nasal discharge, possibly abortion, and diarrhea, and frailty.

Diagnosis

Diagnostic procedures for identification of the etiologic agent in horses with respiratory disease of suspected viral origin are often not performed because of the self-limiting nature of the disease in most cases. However, when an outbreak of severe respiratory disease occurs, the attending clinician may wish to pursue a specific diagnosis, and the index of suspicion may be increased by the utilization of virus isolation (from nasal mucus, nasal/nasopharyngeal and conjunctival swabs and scrapings), immunofluorescence, electron microscopic serologic, and histopathologic techniques. Serologic tests are used most commonly for confirmation of respiratory viral infections and require the collection of acute and convalescent serum samples. If specific procedures are to be undertaken, the clinician should consult with a suitable diagnostic laboratory to determine the methods most applicable for diagnosis of the suspected viral agent and appropriate methods for handling samples.

Treatment

KEY POINT ► Most uncomplicated viral infections in racehorses run a natural course of 7 to 14 days, with spontaneous resolution.

- In some cases, secondary bacterial infection may give rise to more severe clinical signs of lower respiratory disease.
- There is no specific effective treatment for viral respiratory disease.

KEY POINT ► Good nursing care, reduction of stress, decrease or cessation of the training stimulus, and minimization of potential complications should be the strategy employed in horses with suspected viral respiratory disease.

- Infected horses can shed large amounts of virus in nasal secretions and can provide a significant reservoir of infection for other horses. Isolation of affected horses is indicated and should be encouraged.
- Some practitioners suggest that antibiotics should be administered to horses with suspected viral respiratory tract infections to prevent secondary complications. This practice is controversial, since viruses are not sensitive to antibiotics and the vast majority of viral respiratory tract infections are self-limiting. In addition, indiscriminate use of antibiotics encourages the selection of resistant strains of bacteria and can result in untow-

ard side affects in horses being treated (e.g., diarrhea). As a result, we rarely use antibiotics in horses with suspected viral respiratory tract infections. Good nursing care and reduction of stress are likely to provide a better clinical response than antibiotics.

- Additional therapeutic considerations may involve the use of bronchodilator drugs (e.g., clenbuterol, aminophylline, or terbutaline; Treatment Nos. 27, 5, and 102).

Prophylaxis

- Isolation of infected animals (if possible), reduction of stress, and a clean, well-ventilated environment probably provide the best mechanism for reducing the incidence and severity of viral respiratory tract infections.
- Killed and modified live virus vaccines for EHV-1 and EHV-4 are currently available in the United States (Treatment No. 110). The efficacy of these vaccines in preventing rhinopneumonitis has been questioned, but it does appear that they decrease the severity of clinical signs and the duration of viral shedding. One of the benefits of vaccination may be a reduction in the spread of the disease by limiting the amount of virus being liberated into the environment by infected horses.
- Vaccination of pregnant mares with EHV-1 antigens (Treatment No. 110) at 5, 7, and 9 months of gestation reduces the incidence of abortions due to infection with this virus.
- Inactivated virus vaccines for equine influenza A/equine 1 and A/equine 2 strains are available (Treatment No. 111). Two primary doses are usually given several weeks apart when the horse is 4 to 8 months old. Booster injections are prescribed subsequently. The recommendation by manufacturers is for annual or semiannual boosters; however, many veterinarians prescribe 3 to 4 monthly boosters. The efficacy of vaccination schedules for reducing the incidence or severity of equine influenza has been clearly established.
- A modified live virus vaccine for protection against equine viral arteritis is available (Treatment No. 117). The vaccine is effective in reducing the severity of signs, degree of viral shedding, and extent of spread of the disease.

KEY POINT ▶ Mild febrile reactions, inappetence, and local pain and swelling may occur following vaccination with any of the respiratory virus vaccines. This may reduce owner and trainer enthusiasm when veterinarians prescribe this form of prophylaxis.

References

Beech, J.: Therapeutic strategies for diseases of the lower respiratory tract. *Proc. Annu. Conv. Am. Assoc. Equine Pract.*, 1984, vol. 30 p. 275.
Beech, J.: Diagnosing chronic obstructive pulmonary disease. *Vet. Med.* 6:614, 1989.
Beech, J.: *Equine Respiratory Disorders.* Philadelphia: Lea & Febiger, 1991.
Brumbaugh, G. W.: Respiratory therapy: Clinical applications of bronchodilatory and expectorant medications in horses. *Proc. 36th Annu. Conv. Am. Assoc. Equine Pract.*, 1990, p. 133.
Burch, G. E., and Jensen, B.: The use of cytology in the diagnosis of equine respiratory infections. *Equine Pract.* 2:7, 1987.
Derksen, F. J., Brown, C. M., Sonea, I., et al.: Comparison of transtracheal aspirate and bronchoalveolar lavage cytology in 50 horses with chronic lung disease. *Equine Vet. J.* 21:23, 1989.
Lamb, C. R., and O'Callaghan, M. W.: Diagnostic imaging of equine pulmonary disease. *Compend. Contin. Educ. Pract. Vet.* 9:1110, 1989.
Liu, I. K. M.: Update on respiratory vaccines in the horse. *Proc. 32d Annu. Conv. Am. Assoc. Equine Pract.*, 1986, p. 277.
MacNamara, B., Bauer, S., and Iafe, J.: Endoscopic evaluation of exercise-induced pulmonary hemorrhage and chronic obstructive pulmonary disease in association with poor performance in racing Standardbreds. *J. Am. Vet. Med. Assoc.* 3:443, 1990.
Mair, T. S.: Value of tracheal aspirates in the diagnosis of chronic pulmonary diseases in the horse. *Equine Vet. J.* 5:463, 1987.
Murray, M. J.: Respiratory problems in horses: Dealing with lower airway disease. *Vet. Med.* 1:105, 1989.
Ostlund, E. N., Powell, D., and Bryans, J. T.: Equine herpesvirus 1: A review. *Proc. 36th Annu. Conv. Am. Assoc. Equine Pract.*, 1990, p. 387.
Raphel, C. R., and Beech, J.: Pleuritis secondary to pneumonia or lung abscessation in 90 horses. *J. Am. Vet. Med. Assoc.* 181:808, 1982.
Robinson, N. E.: Pathophysiology of coughing. *Proc. 32d Annu. Conv. Am. Assoc. Equine Pract.*, 1986, p. 263.
Schott, H. C., and Mansmann, R.: Respiratory disease: Thoracic drainage in horses. *Compend. Contin. Educ. Pract. Vet.* 2:251, 1990.
Semrad, S. D., and Byars, T. D.: Pleuropneumonia and pleural effusion: Diagnosis and treatment. *Vet. Med.* 6:627, 1989.
Spurlock, S. L.: Antimicrobial use in equine respiratory disease. *Proc. 32d Annu. Conv. Am. Assoc. Equine Pract.*, 1986, p. 229.
Sweeney, C. R., Benson, C. E., Whitlock, R. H., et al.: *Streptococcus equi* infection in horses, parts I and II. *Compend. Contin. Educ. Pract. Vet.* 9:689 and 9:845, 1987.
Sweeney, C. R., Sweeney, R. W., and Benson, C. E.: Bacteriology of guarded endoscope tracheal swabs compared to percutaneous tracheal aspirates in the horse. *J. Am. Vet. Med. Assoc.* 195:1225, 1989.
Thomson, J. R., and McPherson, E. A.: Chronic obstructive pulmonary disease in the horse. *Equine Pract.* 7:31, 1988.
Timoney, P. J., and McCollum, W. H.: Equine viral arteritis. *Can. Vet. J.* 28:693, 1987.

CHAPTER 5

Cardiovascular System

Diseases of the cardiovascular system are relatively uncommon in horses as compared with other species. However, in athletic horses required to perform at their peak, minor disturbances of cardiovascular function can result in significant decreases in exercise capacity. It is natural for clinicians to focus on the heart, and therefore, auscultation forms one of the key parts of the clinical examination, but evaluation of vessel function also should be a key part of cardiovascular assessment. Over the last 10 years, we have been involved in assessments of a variety of competitive horses—thoroughbred and standardbred racehorses and endurance and eventing horses—for reduced performance. We became aware that while cardiovascular assessment at rest was valuable, it was often difficult to determine the clinical significance of minor degrees of cardiovascular dysfunction. The availability of treadmills has resulted in the capacity to monitor various aspects of cardiovascular function at different exercise loads up to intensities similar to those of racing. Under these circumstances, it is sometimes possible to evaluate the significance of a low-grade heart murmur as well as to diagnose abnormalities that may not be apparent at rest. Some aspects of cardiovascular function during exercise will be discussed later in this chapter.

The cardiac reserve in the horse is notable. While the heart rate at rest is usually in the range 30 to 40 beats per minute, during exercise, the maximum heart rate (HR_{max}) increases to up to 240 beats per minute. There is little increase in stroke volume during exercise, and in an average 450-kg thoroughbred racehorse, the stroke volume will average 1 to 1.5 L per beat. Thus the cardiac output will increase from around 40 L/min at rest to 240 to 350 L/min during maximal exercise. Because of this reserve, clinical signs of heart disease that are commonly found in other species may not be obvious in the horse until the end stage of disease, when cardiac dysfunction produces compromise even at rest. Considerable care must be exercised when evaluating the cardiovascular system and in providing assessments of abnormal findings, which may be subtle but have significant effects on exercise capacity. Apart from primary cardiovascular disease, of greater significance in daily clinical practice is secondary cardiovascular dysfunction. Problems such as fluid and electrolyte disturbances, colic, endotoxemia, and grain overload can result in major disturbances to cardiovascular function, chiefly due to fluid movement out of the vascular compartment.

CARDIOVASCULAR EXAMINATION

A detailed cardiovascular examination takes time, although a brief examination may be acceptable in horses presenting with a problem that is not likely to involve the cardiovascular system. After appropriate history taking, the physical examination is conducted (see Chap. 1). One advantage of starting at the front and working to the rear of the horse is that different aspects of the cardiovascular system are examined: mucous membranes, peripheral perfusion, pulse quality and regularity (head), jugular venous distension (neck), and heart sounds (chest).

History

Specific aspects of history related to the cardiovascular system will depend on the presenting sign and the use of the horse. If the horse is a performance horse, it is useful to have specific documentation of its race or competition times to assist in determination of the time of onset of the problem. It also may help to determine whether the problem relates to a decrease in performance or the horse simply evidences a lack of ability. History related to training schedules and duration of training is helpful in establishing whether the owner or trainer considers the horse to be at peak fitness. In our experience, such details are difficult to obtain from many horse trainers. Because some cardiovascular problems are secondary to such problems as respiratory disease, fluid and electrolyte imbalances, and muscular problems, details of the previous medical history are important to the assessment.

KEY POINT ► Of particular importance in the history is whether the problem for which the horse is presented is a progressive disorder, a constant problem, or an isolated event in the midst of apparent normality.

Isolated problems, with sudden collapse, unsteadiness on the legs, and abrupt decrease in performance, are more difficult to diagnose than problems that have a consistent and progressive history. The most important aspect of signalment is the age of the horse, because a young horse (<3 years old) presenting with signs of cardiovascular disease is more likely to have a congenital cardiac problem, whereas an older horse (>3 years old) is likely to have valvular or electrical disturbances.

General Inspection

During the general inspection that is a routine part of the clinical examination, some details are of particular importance in assessing cardiovascular function. The attitude of the horse will help to indicate whether there is systemic disease that could result in secondary cardiovascular dysfunction. Note also should be taken of some of the major veins, particularly the jugular and saphenous veins. A prominent jugular pulse with distension of the vein should alert the clinician to the possibility of congestive heart failure.

Detailed Examination
Mucous Membrane Examination

Mucous membrane color gives a basic guide to tissue oxygenation and peripheral perfusion. The mucous membranes of the mouth are usually the most easily accessible, and the color is normally pale pink. Usually there have to be severe disturbances to peripheral perfusion and/or gas exchange for the mucous membranes to change color.

KEY POINT ► In horses with severe shock or congenital heart disease and foals with severe pneumonia, the mucous membranes can have a bluish (cyanotic) color.

In horses in which there are fluid and/or electrolyte disturbances with dehydration or with endotoxemia, the mucous membranes will have a darker reddish color that is usually described as "injected." The mucous membranes of the nasal cavity also can be examined at the most rostral site and are usually slightly darker in color than the mucous membranes of the mouth. Anemia may result in pale mucous membranes, but this may be difficult to assess.

Capillary refill time is a helpful clinical tool for assessing the peripheral circulation. This is usually evaluated by pressing firmly with the index finger on the mucous membrane of the gum above a corner incisor tooth. This will result in blanching of the mucous membrane, after which blood will refill the area over 1 to 2 seconds. If the test is repeated in the same area several times, there will be a decrease in the capillary refill time. Prolongation of capillary refill time may indicate a decrease in peripheral perfusion. However, care must be taken in interpretation of capillary refill time. In septic or toxemic states, there may be dilatation of the arterioles, and despite a reduction in peripheral perfusion, the capillary refill time will be normal. It is also worrying to note that on examination of the capillary refill time in several horses after death, we found that the refill time was excellent!

Assessment of Peripheral Pulse

The *character of the pulse* provides an important subjective guide to the state of the cardiovascular system. Pulse character is dependent on vessel size, distance away from the heart, and difference between systolic and diastolic pressures. Because there can be heightening of the pulse wave as it moves peripherally, the pulse may be more easily detectable in the digital artery than in the carotid artery. Assessment of the pulse character in the digital artery is part of the normal evaluation of the limbs, and digital pulses usually are more prominent when there is an inflammatory disease in the distal limb. Increased digital pulse is often used as an indication of early laminitis. An exaggerated pulse in the central circulation is common in association with aortic insufficiency. A decrease in pulse pressure (hypokinetic pulse) is often the result of shock and hypovolemia.

The pulse is most easily detected in the facial artery as it rounds the mandible, although the transverse facial artery, near the lateral canthus of the eye, is also a good site for palpation. The different sites for detecting the peripheral pulse were shown in Chapter 1. The normal pulse character is a prolonged, full wave that is easily palpated with mild digital pressure.

KEY POINT ► Of greatest clinical significance is a decreased pulse pressure, which is detected as a weak peripheral pulse and usually indicates decreased systemic arterial pressure and shock.

Pulse rhythm is important to assess when the character of the pulse is being evaluated. Abnormalities of rhythm, while not always easy to detect, will alert the clinician to the possibility of a primary cardiac disturbance.

Assessment of the Venous Circulation

Evaluation of the venous circulation is difficult because of its low pressure. Of most significance is the jugular pulse, which reflects right atrial and thoracic pressure changes. Because the average right atrial pressure is around 4 mmHg, the pressure wave does not progress far up the jugular vein. Normally, the jugular pulse is only visible around the thoracic inlet and for up to 10 cm rostrally. The jugular pulse is most evident in the normal horse toward the end of diastole, when the stage of rapid ventricular filling is complete. However, if the head is lowered below the level of the right atrium, or if there is an increase in right atrial pressure, which may be the situation in right-sided congestive heart failure, the pulse in the jugular vein becomes more prominent, together with jugular venous distension.

In racehorses, because many medications are given via the jugular veins, it is important to check for the presence of thrombophlebitis by palpating along the length of the vein. In some cases, thrombophlebitis can progress to occlude the affected jugular vein. Facial vein distension may be found in horses with thrombophlebitis of the jugular vein, particularly following exercise. Saphenous vein distension is normally found in horses at rest and after exercise. In cases of iliac thrombosis, a lack of saphenous vein distension has been noted on the affected side immediately after exercise.

Palpation

Palpation of the apex beat is useful to note a change in location that could indicate heart enlargement. The apex beat is most easily palpable over fourth and fifth intercostal spaces of the lower third of the left chest wall. In most horses it is not possible to palpate an apex beat on the right side of the chest.

KEY POINT ▶ In the case of significant heart murmurs, it may be possible to palpate a thrill.

However, many clinically significant heart murmurs will not be accompanied by a thrill, particularly in a horse that is heavily muscled. We have noted that a thrill is usually seen more often in young horses with congenital cardiac disease.

The *extremities and ventral abdomen* also should be palpated as part of the cardiovascular examination. In a horse that has been at rest for some time, the finding of cool to cold extremities, particularly the lower limbs and ends of the ears, may indicate decreased peripheral perfusion. Edema referable to congestive heart failure is most common in the ventral abdomen, and without careful palpation, this can sometimes be missed on simple observation, particularly in horses with thick hair coats.

Auscultation of the Heart

Once the more peripheral parts of the circulation have been examined, careful auscultation of the heart should be performed on both sides of the chest. This should be carried out in a quiet area away from traffic noise and, hopefully, without the owner or trainer talking to you. We have noted a remarkable tendency for owners to want to carry out a conversation as soon as you place the earpieces of the stethoscope in your ears.

Initial Auscultation. Auscultation should be undertaken using a good-quality stethoscope and tubing not longer than 40 cm because the heart sounds will be attenuated. The examination usually begins over the area of the apex beat, just caudal to the triceps muscles and ventral to the level of the point of the shoulder. Over 60 to 90 seconds, a general impression of the heart sounds and rhythm should be gained. In many horses the heart rate (HR) will be elevated initially but will settle to a true resting rate of 25 to 40 beats per minute over 30 to 60 seconds. Abnormal heart sounds or murmurs will be detectable, as will gross disturbances to rhythm. However, a longer period of auscultation is necessary for more subtle findings.

Detailed Auscultation. After the initial assessment, the entire cardiac region should be auscultated. The stethoscope should be pushed well forward under the triceps muscle as far cranially as possible, after which the stethoscope bell is gradually withdrawn caudally. In the dorsoventral plane, auscultation should take place from a point level with the point of the elbow dorsally to a region below a horizontal line through the point of the shoulder. Ejection murmurs, which are common in many fit performance horses, are usually heard in a localized region well forward on the left chest wall. The same procedure should be performed on the right side, although it may be more difficult to hear the heart sounds as distinctly as on the left because of the lower pressures on the right side of the circulation.

Normal Heart Sounds

Heart sounds that can be heard easily are restricted to the first and second sounds, although in many horses three sounds can be heard, and in some, all four. The significance of the heart sounds is as follows:

Fourth or Atrial Heart Sound (S_A)—The first sound heard, and it occurs toward the end of diastole, when the stage of rapid ventricular filling is complete. It is most audible well forward and with the stethoscope at the dorsal limit of the cardiac field. In some horses, S_A is followed so closely by S_1 that these may be indistinguishable. In others, although the period of separation is brief, it is quite distinct, and S_A and S_1 can be heard as separate sounds.

KEY POINT ► These separate sounds have led to some clinicians mistakenly diagnosing a "split" first heart sound.

First Heart Sound (S₁)—Louder and of longer duration than S_2. The point of maximum intensity of the sound is located ventrally, usually over the region of the apex beat. S_1 is associated with closure of the atrioventricular (A-V) valves and turbulence in the larger vessels during early systole. S_1 occurs just after the QRS complex on an electrocardiogram (ECG).

Second Heart Sound (S₂)—A higher pitch and of shorter duration than S_1. It is most easily heard toward the base of the heart. The sound arises from events associated with closure of the aortic and pulmonic valves.

Third Heart Sound (S₃)—Infrequently heard, occurring immediately after the second heart sound. The sound is associated with events during early diastole, with opening of the A-V valves and rapid ventricular filling.

Abnormal Rhythms (Dysrhythmias or Arrhythmias)

The terms *dysrhythmia* and *arrhythmia* are often used interchangeably. However, in a strict sense, *dysrhythmia* means a disturbance of rhythm, whereas *arrhythmia* indicates an absence of rhythm. Some dysrhythmias (e.g., atrial fibrillation) are immediately recognizable within seconds of placing the stethoscope on the chest wall. Others are more subtle and, if intermittent, may be missed on auscultation. For this reason, it is important to auscultate for several minutes to assess rhythm abnormalities. The following details should be noted:

- Ventricular rate—normal, bradycardia, or tachycardia
- Rhythm of first and second heart sounds—regular or irregular
- Presence of "dropped" or premature beats

The most common dysrhythmias are second-degree atrioventricular block and sinus dysrhythmia. Both these dysrhythmias are considered to be within the normal range of findings, but an ECG may be required to make the diagnosis.

Heart Murmurs

A *heart murmur* is an abnormal sound that results from disturbance to normal laminar flow. This can arise from a variety of situations, and while valvular abnormalities are the most common cause of heart murmurs, a number of other problems can cause the abnormal sounds. For example, an increase in blood velocity or a decrease in blood viscosity can cause a heart murmur.

KEY POINT ► A variety of problems can result in heart murmurs.

Some problems resulting in heart murmurs are:

- Decreased viscosity—most commonly anemia and/or hypoproteinemia
- Conditions that produce increases in cardiac output (e.g., excitement, exercise, high temperature)
- Abnormal blood flow as typically occurs with valvular incompetence
- Interruption of blood flow across cardiac chambers (e.g., aortic stenosis)

We also have noted a temporary heart murmur in some horses with colic. The reason for this transient murmur is not clear.

Physiologically Normal Murmurs

"Normal" murmurs are found with problems that produce a decrease in viscosity as well as with conditions that result in an increase in cardiac output.

KEY POINT ► It is relatively common to find fit racehorses with localized low-grade heart murmurs heard well forward on the left chest wall. This occurs presumably because of high resting stroke volumes. Such murmurs are usually termed *ejection murmurs*.

Pathologic Murmurs

These murmurs are usually the result of either valvular stenosis or incompetence. Murmurs are also common in horses with intra- or extracardiac communications, such as found in septal defects or patent ductus arteriosus.

Grading of Murmurs

Murmurs should be described in the following ways to allow evaluation of their significance:

- *Timing*—in relation to S_1 and S_2 (i.e., systolic or diastolic)
- *Intensity* and *location* of murmur—graded as soft, medium or loud; localized or widespread over the cardiac field, left or right side
- Murmur *type*—ejection, blowing, machinery, regurgitant

A grading system has been advocated to indicate the intensity of the heart murmur:

Grade 1—Softest murmurs, usually well localized and only heard after detailed examination

Grade 2—Soft murmur that is audible after brief examination

Grade 3—Murmur that is heard immediately upon auscultation and is present over quite a large area of the chest wall

Grade 4—A louder murmur that radiates quite widely but does not produce a palpable thrill

Grade 5—Similar to grade 4, except that a palpable thrill is evident

Grade 6—Audible when the stethoscope is removed from the chest wall; always accompanied by a definite thrill

This grading system for murmurs is useful in describing the intensity of sounds heard because the pathologic significance of the murmurs increases with an increase in grade.

DIAGNOSTIC AIDS

From the physical examination it should be clear whether the problem involves the central or peripheral circulation. A range of diagnostic aids then can be employed depending on the facilities and equipment available. In some cases, it may be clear that the problem is an electrical one, and therefore, an ECG is needed. In others, the history may be suggestive of primary cardiac disease, but auscultatory findings are normal and there are no abnormal findings on physical examination. In these cases, it may be necessary to undertake a range of diagnostic procedures, including ultrasound examination and telemetry electrocardiography during exercise, to establish a diagnosis.

Electrocardiography

The most easily accessible of the diagnostic aids for cardiovascular problems is the electrocardiogram (ECG). However, it must be remembered that the ECG has somewhat limited value because it provides information about the electrical activity of the heart rather than its mechanical function.

The ECG machine can be thought of as a type of galvanometer that is used in such a way that the potential difference is measured between two electrodes situated on the surface of the body.

Recording Technique

To record an ECG, one needs a quiet place with minimal interference. A rubber mat for the horse to stand on has been suggested, but in most cases this can be dispensed with, provided that there are no major sources of electrical interference.

KEY POINT ▶ The best place for recording an ECG is the horse's own box stall, if available.

In such surroundings the horse is usually quiet and relaxed, and a good-quality tracing can be recorded. Care must be taken to ensure that the site where the horse stands during recording is completely dry. The ECG machine used should have fil-

ters to avoid interference, particularly from skin movement and electrical activity.

The ECG machine used should be portable and enable recording without an immediate mains power supply by using rechargable batteries. Recordings are usually made at a paper speed of 25 mm/s and a sensitivity of 1 cm = 1 mV.

The configurations of both QRS and T-wave complexes are affected by limb position and heart rate. Therefore, to allow standardized interpretation, the ECG should always be recorded with the left forelimb slightly in front of the right forelimb and the heart rate less than 42 beats per minute.

The recording system used is usually one of two main types:

1. *Metal electrodes that are connected to the legs by rubber straps.* To permit good conductivity, an electrode paste is applied under the electrodes. Usual electrode placement on the forelimb is on the caudal aspect of the distal radius, just proximal to the accessory carpal bone, whereas electrodes are applied to the cranial aspect of the distal tibia, just above the point of the hock, in the hindlimbs. The chest electrode is secured using a rubber girth strap so that the lead lies 5 cm behind the point of the elbow on the left ventral thorax. If the electrodes are applied directly to the skin by alligator clips, this can be performed by attachment to the skin just below the olecranon in the forelimbs and just below the stifle in the hindlimbs. The machine should be able to record leads I, II, III, aVR, aVL, aVF, and V (the exploring electrode). This system is criticized on the basis that for a quadruped, the frontal lead system is inaccurate because it is based on the three recording leads (left foreleg, right foreleg, and left hindleg) being part of an equilateral triangle (Einthoven's triangle), which is obviously not the case. For determination of conduction disturbances, it does not matter if this system or the Y lead described below is used. More complex vectorcardiography has been described, but it appears to provide little extra information to the clinician than the more simple recording systems.

2. *A bipolar lead system using the Y lead.* This is the most commonly used system for general ECG examination, and this or a base–apex system, as is shown in Figure 5-1, may be used. To record the Y lead, the positive lead is attached over the xiphisternum and the negative lead over the manubrium. The ground, or earth, lead (brown) can be attached over the point of the shoulder. Mostly this is performed using alligator clips attached directly to the skin, with ECG paste being applied to the sites to increase conductivity. An alternative to commercial paste is alcohol, but a cheap ECG paste also can be made up by mixing salt with an obstetrical lubricant. Some horses object to the alligator clips, and in these horses the metal electrodes and rubber straps will permit a better recording to be made than with the clips applied directly to the skin.

complexes, and T waves are present for each heartbeat throughout the trace.
■ Assess individual wave formations, and measure the intervals.

Analysis of the ECG should be performed using an $8\times$ to $10\times$ magnifier to assist in accuracy of interval measurement. In the frontal lead system described above, the following intervals are normal for measurements in lead 2.

P-wave duration	<0.17 s
P-wave peak interval	<0.08 s
PR interval	<0.44 s
QRS complex duration	<0.17 s
ST interval	<0.60 s

Measurement of the various intervals is shown in Figure 5-2.

It should be noted that the PR and QT intervals are heart rate–dependent, with the intervals shortening considerably when there is an increase in heart rate. A normal ECG tracing using a frontal lead system and recording the various leads is shown in Figure 5-3. A typical tracing using the Y lead is shown in Figure 5-4.

Evaluation of ECG Waveforms and Intervals

P Wave. The P wave represents atrial depolarization and will vary in appearance. Most commonly it has an M-shaped appearance, but it can appear diphasic, as shown in Figure 5-5. It is quite common to have a number of different waveforms within the same ECG lead, the appearance varying from beat to beat. This is normal and is referred to as *wandering pacemaker.*

PR Interval. The PR interval is from the beginning of the P wave to the beginning of the QRS complex. The interval is dependent on heart rate and shortens as the heart rate increases. As horses get older, the PR interval progressively lengthens. Therefore, a longer than normal PR interval (first-degree A-V block) is of little clinical significance.

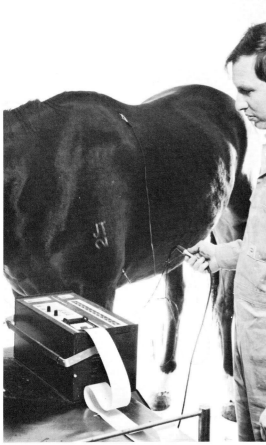

Figure 5–1. ECG recording being taken from a horse using a typical base–apex lead system. The most widely used recording technique for assessing waveforms is the Y lead, in which electrodes are placed over the manubrium and xiphisternum.

Interpretation of the ECG

It is important to obtain several minutes of ECG recording to allow assessment of changes in rhythm and to determine the presence of conduction abnormalities. The most obvious findings will relate to rhythm disturbances. Obvious abnormalities in individual waveforms can be recognized, as can missing components of the ECG, for example, a P wave not followed by a QRS complex or T wave, indicating second-degree atrioventricular (A-V) block. Some findings, such as ventricular premature contractions, only may be found as an isolated event on a recording and may be missed unless the tracing is evaluated carefully. The following sequence for ECG investigation is useful:

■ Examine the complete tracing to note any abnormal rhythm.
■ Determine whether complete P waves, QRS

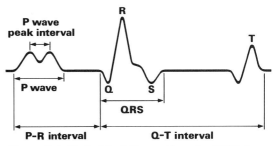

Figure 5–2. Typical lead II recording of an ECG showing the different waveforms and their measurement.

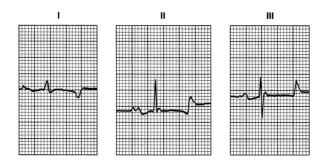

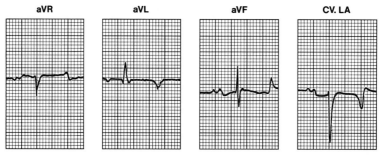

Figure 5–3. Normal frontal-lead ECG recording, from leads I, II, III, aVR, aVL, aVF, and CV.LA (chest lead), showing typical waveforms. Recording was made at 25 mm/s and an amplitude of 1 mV/cm. The chest lead (CV.LA) is recorded with the electrode located approximately 5 cm caudal to the point of the elbow.

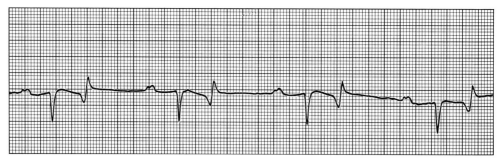

Figure 5–4. Typical recording using the Y lead, with electrodes placed over the manubrium (positive) and xiphisternum (negative).

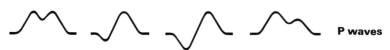

Figure 5–5. Range of normal appearances of the P wave in an ECG recording.

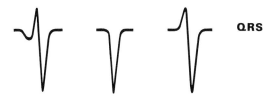

Figure 5–6. Range of normal appearances of the QRS complex in an ECG recording.

QRS Complex. The QRS complex represents ventricular depolarization, and depending on the particular lead, some of the components may not be present. The Q wave is often missing, and the S wave is variable in appearance. Some of the variations in QRS waveforms are shown in Figure 5-6.

T Wave. The T wave represents ventricular repolarization. It is extremely sensitive to changes in heart rate, there being changes in both amplitude and polarity. As the heart rate increases, usually there is an increase in both the amplitude of the T wave and a change in direction so that it becomes positive, particularly in the unipolar V lead. While some clinicians regard changes in the T wave as abnormal, the extreme lability of the T wave makes interpretation rather difficult. There is evidence that T waves will change polarity with training state, with waves in the chest leads becoming pos-

itive and peaked (>1 mV). The following T-wave directions have been found to be normal using the frontal lead system:

Lead	T wave direction
Lead I	Negative or diphasic
Lead II	Positive or diphasic
Lead III	Positive or diphasic
Lead aVR	Positive or diphasic
Lead aVL	Negative
Lead aVF	Positive or diphasic
Chest leads	Diphasic

A typical ECG tracing in a horse with "abnormal" T waves in a number of leads, recorded using the frontal system, is shown in Figure 5-7.

QT Interval. This interval, from the beginning of the QRS complex to the end of the T wave, is of little clinical significance. The interval will shorten with an increase in heart rate.

The Heart-Score Concept

The concept of heart score was developed by Dr. Jim Steel in Australia in the late 1950s. The *heart score* is an indirect method for assessing heart size and is determined by measuring the QRS complex duration in milliseconds in leads I, II, and III and averaging the result. A horse with QRS complex durations of 100, 120, and 110 ms, respectively, in

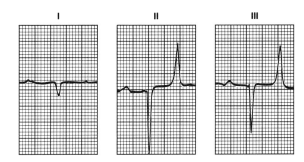

Figure 5–7. ECG tracing from a horse with "abnormal" T waves recorded using the frontal system. Recording was made at 25 mm/s and an amplitude of 1 mV/cm.

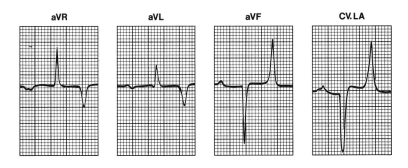

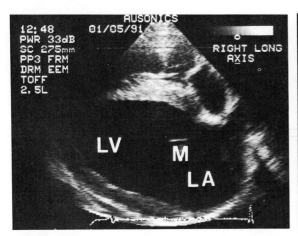

Figure 5–8. Echocardiogram recorded from a 5-year-old thoroughbred horse on the right side of the chest using a long-axis view. The left ventricle is shown (*LV*) along with the left atrioventricular (mitral) valve (*M*) and the left atrium (*LA*). (Recording courtesy of Dr. Karon Hoffman.)

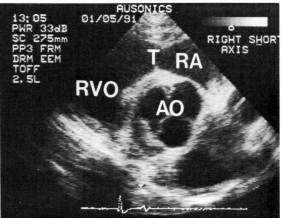

Figure 5–10. Echocardiogram recorded from a 5-year-old thoroughbred horse on the right side of the chest using a short-axis view. The right ventricular outflow tract (*RVO*) can be seen together with the aortic valve (*AO*), right atrioventricular (tricuspid) view (*T*), and right atrium (*RA*). (Recording courtesy of Dr. Karon Hoffman.)

leads I, II, and III has a heart score of 110. Average heart score values in mature thoroughbred horses are 113 to 116, whereas values over 120 are considered to be indicative of above-average heart size. This is based on the good correlation ($r = 0.89$) noted by Steel between heart score and heart weight. There was also an association between heart score and prize money won by thoroughbred horses, although the correlation coefficient was only 0.44. From the measurement of heart score, veterinarians have made predictions about performance potential. Other studies have shown correlations with performance in standardbred pacers and endurance horses.

While heart-score measurement is used extensively in some countries (Australia, New Zealand, South Africa, and France), various authorities have described the measurement as being unphysiologic and of no value. Apart from the difficulty in measurement of QRS complex duration, Steel's data show that only 80% of the variation in heart score is due to changes in heart weight. Furthermore, no allowance is made for variations in individual horse's body weights.

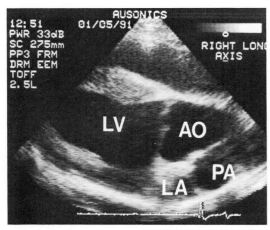

Figure 5–9. Echocardiogram recorded from a 5-year-old thoroughbred horse on the right side of the chest using a long-axis view. The left ventricular outflow tract is shown. Structures that can be visualized include the left ventricle (*LV*), left atrium (*LA*), pulmonary artery (*PA*), and aorta (*AO*). (Recording courtesy of Dr. Karon Hoffman.)

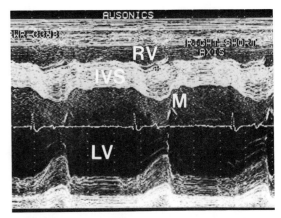

Figure 5–11. Echocardiogram recorded from a 5-year-old thoroughbred horse on the right side of the chest using M-mode. The right (*RV*) and left ventricles (*LV*) can be seen, together with the interventricular septum (*IVS*) and part of the left atrioventricular valve (*M*). (Recording courtesy of Dr. Karon Hoffman.)

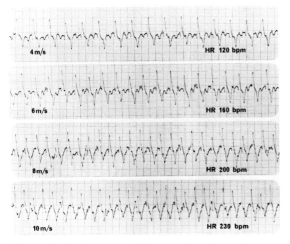

Figure 5–12. Telemetric ECG recording from a 3-year-old thoroughbred horse during exercise on a treadmill at a slope of 6 degrees (10%) and at speeds varying from 4 to 10 m/s. Recording was made at 25 mm/s and an amplitude of 1 mV/cm.

KEY POINT ▶ Therefore, while it can be said that horses with low heart scores (<100) are likely to have lower cardiac capacity and horses with high heart scores (>120) are likely to have higher capacity, it is difficult to be more precise.

The heart-score concept has been overemphasized by some veterinarians because of the assumption that heart size is the only factor of importance in determining athletic performance. Heart size is, of course, only one element, and other factors, including respiratory function, muscle function, biomechanics, and oxygen-carrying capacity, all play important roles in performance. The heart score is therefore of some value in providing a broad indication of heart size, but limited significance should be given and care should be taken in providing predictions of performance.

Echocardiography

Echocardiography has been used widely in academic institutions for the last 10 to 12 years but has been utilized infrequently in equine practice. This situation has changed with the decrease in price of ultrasound machines and their widespread use in stud-farm practice as well as for evaluation of tendon and ligament injuries. For cardiac examination in adult horses, a 1.6- or 2.5-MHz transducer is necessary. The most common mode used for echocardiography has been M-mode, which provides a one-dimensional image of the heart. This is the technique used for measuring various chamber dimensions as well as for assessing valve movement. Two-dimensional real-time ultrasound provides a cross-sectional view of the heart in motion. More recently, pulsed-wave Doppler echocardiography has become available and is combined with two-dimensional echocardiography to enable evaluation of flow disturbances in cases of valve dysfunction or congenital heart problems. For most of the cardiac views, the transducer is placed over the fourth intercostal space on the right chest wall. Typical images are presented in Figures 5-8 to 5-11.

Exercise Testing and Telemetry Electrocardiography

In some cases, the significance of resting ECG or auscultatory findings may be difficult to assess. In these cases, exercise or "stress" testing can be of value in determining the prognosis and treatment.

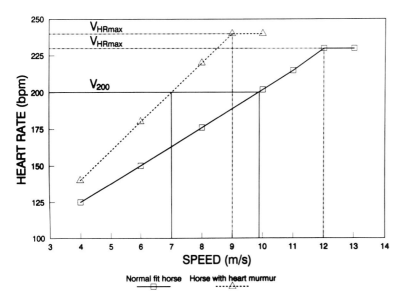

Figure 5–13. Heart-rate response to exercise in two horses on a high-speed treadmill during an incremental exercise test at a slope of 6 degrees (+10%). Note the elevated heart response at all stages in the horse with the heart murmur compared with the normal, fit thoroughbred. The steeper slope of the heart-rate versus speed line is also quite obvious. Two useful reference points are the speed (velocity) at a heart rate of 200 beats per minute (V_{200}) and the speed at maximum heart rate (V_{HRmax}) that are shown on the graph. In the normal, fit horse, the V_{200} is 9.8 m/s and the V_{HRmax} is 12.0 m/s. In contrast, the horse with the heart murmur has a V_{200} of 7.0 m/s and a V_{HRmax} of 9.0 m/s.

Treadmill exercise testing is of most value because conditions can be standardized and an array of information can be gained under conditions where the workload is precisely known. We have conducted clinical exercise testing on several hundred thoroughbred and standardbred racehorses, as well as on endurance and pleasure horses. The tests are all performed with the treadmill inclined at a slope of 6 degrees (10%), and the horses progress through trotting, cantering, and galloping (or pacing) at speeds up to 12 m/s. Recording of the ECG by telemetry (Fig. 5-12) is useful to determine whether abnormalities occur and can be most easily visualized in the first 30 to 60 seconds after the horse stops fast exercise. Alternatively, much information can be gained from the horse's heart-rate response to exercise, and the heart rate can be measured using a cardiotachometer, of which several types are commercially available (EQB, Philadelphia, Pa.; Hippocard, Zurich, Switzerland). The heart-rate responses to exercise of a normal, fit thoroughbred racehorse and a horse with a systolic cardiac murmur are shown in Figure 5-13.

Cardiovascular Diseases

CARDIAC DYSRHYTHMIAS OR ARRHYTHMIAS

Dysrhythmias of various types are quite common in the horse, although the majority of these may not be of pathologic significance. Investigation of dysrhythmias must include an ECG. Services such as Cardiopet are available that allow the ECG to be transmitted by telephone for analysis. Most of the "normal" dysrhythmias are regularly occurring, with the normal heart rhythm being regularly interrupted by an absence of a beat.

History and Presenting Signs

- Poor racing performance
- Dyspnea
- Slow recovery after exercise
- Prepurchase or routine examination finding

Clinical Findings and Diagnosis

- Dysrhythmias affecting cardiac function during exercise will usually be pronounced and cause irregular heart sounds.
- With some dysrhythmias (e.g., second-degree A-V block), there may be no history of a presenting problem, but an abnormality of rhythm may be noted on clinical examination.

KEY POINT ▶ An ECG recording should be performed, and it may be useful to vary the degree of vagal tone during recording by application of a twitch to decrease the heart rate and by stimulating the horse so that the heart rate increases.

Differential Diagnosis

- Second-degree A-V block
- Third-degree A-V block
- Sinoatrial block
- Atrial fibrillation
- Paroxysmal atrial fibrillation
- Atrial premature contractions
- Ventricular premature contractions
- Sinus dysrhythmia
- Ventricular tachycardia
- A-V dissociation

Treatment

For the majority of the dysrhythmias, there is little that can be done in the way of therapy. Some cases, where there is a viral myocarditis, will resolve with rest. Others may require various forms of therapy. Specific treatments are indicated in the following section, which provides details of each of the common dysrhythmias.

Atrioventricular Block

Atrioventricular (A-V) block, of which there are three types, is the most common of the atrial dysrhythmias. *First-degree A-V block* is diagnosed on the basis of progressive lengthening of the PR interval to values greater than 0.44 s. This upper limit of normal is arbitrarily defined, and the PR interval will lengthen with increasing age. No abnormalities are detected on auscultation. First-degree A-V block has no pathologic significance.

Second-degree A-V block is the most common dysrhythmia and is characterized by a P wave that is not followed by a QRS complex or T wave (Fig. 5-14). There are two types of second-degree A-V block, the most common being associated with a progressive lengthening of the PR interval until the blocked beat occurs (Wenkebach type). In the other type of A-V block, the PR interval is regular in length. Second-degree A-V block usually occurs regularly, every 4 to 8 beats, but it may be intermittent. On careful auscultation, the atrial (S_A or S_4) sound can be heard without the following S_1 and S_2 sounds.

KEY POINT ▶ While some clinicians regard second-degree A-V block as being abnormal, most would regard this block as normal and a consequence of the high vagal tone in the resting horse.

The block always disappears when the heart rate increases. However, there have been some studies demonstrating histopathologic changes in the myocardium of horses with second-degree A-V block. From the ECG findings in several thousand horses that we have undertaken, we think that if this block occurs frequently during a trace and is found in a young horse, there should be an index of suspicion about the pathologic significance.

Third-degree A-V block is quite rare in the horse and represents a complete block in conduction between the atria and the ventricles. The atria beat at a normal sinus rate, whereas the ventricles have a slower rate. On auscultation, this block is characterized by a very low heart rate (15–20 beats/min) and a prominent jugular pulse. In some cases, third-degree A-V block can be the cause of syncopal attacks.

There is no treatment for the various types of A-V block, and the prognosis will vary with the type found. Third-degree A-V block obviously has a poor prognosis for athletic performance and tends not to resolve with time. First- and second-degree A-V blocks are usually of no pathologic significance.

Atrial Fibrillation

Atrial fibrillation is a dysrhythmia most commonly found in standardbred horses, although it also has been found in a variety of other breeds, including Clydesdales. In many cases it can occur during a race and causes a severe decrease in the horse's performance.

KEY POINT ▶ On auscultation, the condition is characterized by an irregular heart rhythm with a series of rapid heart beats followed by no heart sounds, and a presumptive diagnosis can be made by auscultation alone.

If the pulse rate is taken at the same time as the heart rate, there may be a pulse deficit. The resting heart rate is usually higher than normal and may range from 30 to 100 beats per minute. In some cases there may be signs of an increased jugular pulse, indicating congestive heart failure.

If a dysrhythmia indicates the probability of atrial fibrillation, an ECG recording is the method of choice for diagnosis. The ECG is characterized by the presence of *f*, or flutter, waves between irregularly spaced QRS complexes (Fig. 5-15).

KEY POINT ▶ If there are no signs of congestive heart failure, often it is possible to correct the abnormality using quinidine sulfate (Treatment No. 98) administered by stomach tube.

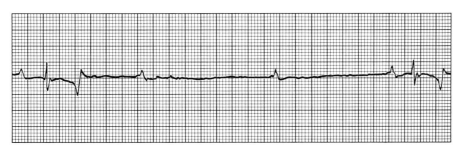

Figure 5–14. ECG tracing (lead II) from a horse with second-degree A-V block showing isolated P waves. Note the progressive lengthening of the PR interval in the beats prior to the block. Recording was made at 25 mm/s and an amplitude of 1 mV/cm.

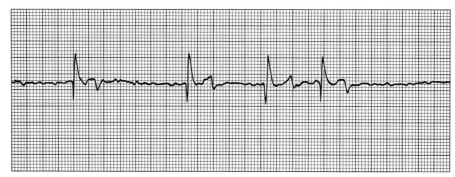

Figure 5–15. ECG tracing (lead Y) from a 3-year-old standardbred horse presented with poor racing performance. Note the irregular spacing of the QRS complexes and the presence of flutter waves. This is typical of atrial fibrillation. Recording was made at 25 mm/s and an amplitude of 1 mV/cm.

Most clinicians use a test dose of quinidine sulfate at a dose rate of 15 to 20 mg/kg prior to the treatment schedule. Quinidine is usually available in 200-mg tablets, which should be crushed and suspended in water. While there are a number of possible protocols for quinidine sulfate administration, we have found that a simple and effective technique is a dose of 10 g for an adult horse (22 mg/kg) given every 2 hours until there is cardioversion to normal sinus rhythm. The total amount of quinidine sulfate usually required is 30 to 60 g. However, in some horses, a dose of up to 90 g may be required. Once the total dose has exceeded 60 g, the risk of toxicity is increased, and considerable care is required. If the horse fails to convert, treatment can be restarted the next day, and some horses may require several days of therapy prior to conversion. In a few cases where blood levels have been measured, it appears that at least some of the variability in response is due to poor absorption of the administered drug. Plasma concentrations in the range 2 to 4 μg/ml are usually necessary for cardioversion, and toxicity is found at concentrations greater than 5 μg/ml.

Quinidine treatment of atrial fibrillation is very successful, with most horses returning to previous athletic capacity once sinus rhythm has been reestablished. Toxicity from quinidine therapy is unusual, but we have had one horse die in ventricular fibrillation after a total dose of 80 g. Most commonly, horses will show signs of dullness or depression and sweating, and there may be gastrointestinal signs, including colic and diarrhea. Nasal congestion also has been reported as a common sign of toxicity. Quinidine causes a substantial increase in heart rate, and after doses of 40 to 50 g, heart rates around 100 beats per minute are quite common.

Quinidine gluconate, given IV, has been recommended in cases where the history suggests a recent (less than 1 week) onset of the problem. Quinidine gluconate is given at a dose rate of 1.5 mg/kg every 10 minutes until cardioversion occurs, for a maximum of six treatments.

Paroxysmal Atrial Fibrillation

KEY POINT ▶ Paroxysmal atrial fibrillation is a form of atrial fibrillation that disappears spontaneously, usually within several hours of its occurrence.

It is most common in racehorses and is responsible for a dramatic decrease in performance during a race. Monitoring of the ECG in the immediate postrace period in horses that have suffered poor racing performance has shown that paroxysmal atrial fibrillation is more common than was previously thought. The greatest difficulty in cases of paroxysmal atrial fibrillation is in making the diagnosis. Horses that are examined the day after racing because of poor performance may have normal ECG findings despite suffering atrial fibrillation at the time of the race. Therefore, horses with racing form reversals or poor performance that have dysrhythmias on auscultation after competing should have an ECG performed soon after the race or event. Paroxysmal atrial fibrillation also has been reported in newborn foals. There is no treatment for the condition, which usually resolves spontaneously. Some cases may go on to permanent atrial fibrillation, whereas others may reoccur intermittently.

Atrial Premature Contractions

KEY POINT ▶ Atrial premature contractions cause a dysrhythmia due to generation of impulses in an ectopic pacemaker located in the atria.

This type of dysrhythmia is quite rare in the horse. Horses with atrial premature contractions usually are presented for poor racing performance. Auscultation will reveal a largely regular rhythm with an occasional premature beat. An ECG is necessary for diagnosis, and a typical example of the problem is shown in Figure 5-16. There is little that can be done apart from rest for 3 to 6 months followed by a further ECG to assess progress. The

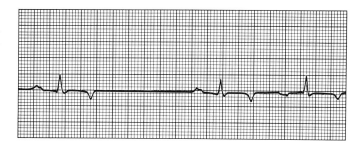

Figure 5–16. ECG tracing from a 4-year-old thoroughbred horse with an isolated atrial premature contraction (lead II). There were no other ECG abnormalities, and the condition did not appear to be associated with cardiac pathology. Recording was made at 25 mm/s and an amplitude of 1 mV/cm.

condition may be of little clinical significance if it occurs as an isolated event, but if it is more frequent during an ECG recording, it may reflect atrial pathology.

Atrioventricular Dissociation

Atrioventricular (A-V) dissociation can occur in cases of parasystole, third-degree A-V block, and ventricular tachycardia. If the dissociation is intermittent, an irregular dysrhythmia is usually heard on auscultation. A tracing from an 8-year-old endurance horse presented because of poor heart-rate recoveries is presented in Figure 5-17, and it demonstrates that some of the P waves and QRS complexes are unrelated.

KEY POINT ▶ Problems that lead to A-V dissociation are quite severe, and the prognosis should be guarded.

Rest for 8 to 12 weeks followed by rerecording of the ECG should be undertaken to assess changes in the condition.

Bundle-Branch Block (Intraventricular Block)

This disorder is difficult to diagnose, and there is disagreement about whether the condition truly occurs in the horse. It does not result in any dysrhythmia but is characterized by a prolongation of the QRS complex duration to greater than 0.16 s.

KEY POINT ▶ Poor racing performance is the main clinical sign of intraventricular block, and therefore, it needs to be distinguished from other causes of poor performance.

We have seen several cases where sequential ECG recordings over 1 to 2 months indicating a prolongation of the QRS complex have enabled a diagnosis to be made. This disorder appears not to resolve and has a very poor prognosis for successful athletic performance.

Intraatrial Block

KEY POINT ▶ As with intraventricular block, intraatrial block does not cause any dysrhythmia, and there are no abnormalities on auscultation.

It can be diagnosed only by an ECG. The main clinical sign is a reduction in racing performance. Clinical examination and auscultation do not reveal any abnormalities. The ECG will reveal a P-wave duration in lead II of more than 0.17 s and a P-wave peak interval of more than 0.08 s (Fig. 5-18). Intraatrial block cannot be treated, and there have been no cases of spontaneous resolution. The condition appears to have an adverse effect on athletic performance.

Sinoatrial Block

KEY POINT ▶ Sinoatrial block is characterized by a regularly "dropped" beat and on auscultation may appear similar to second-degree A-V block.

In contrast to second-degree A-V block, no atrial (S_4) sound can be heard when the block occurs. Diagnosis is made by ECG in which there is a doubling of the normal PP interval when the block occurs so that there is a gap on the ECG trace with

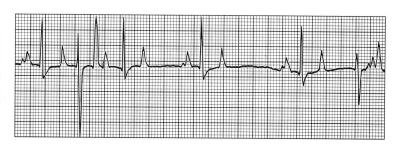

Figure 5–17. ECG tracing (lead II) from an 8-year-old endurance horse presented because of poor heart-rate recoveries. Note the A-V dissociation. Recording was made at 25 mm/s and an amplitude of 1 mV/cm.

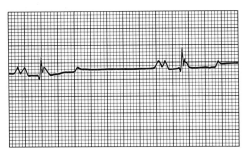

Figure 5–18. ECG tracing (lead II) from a 4-year-old thoroughbred racehorse presented with poor racing performance. Note the prolonged P-wave duration (0.19 s) and P-wave peak interval (0.09 s), which are typical of intraatrial block.

no P wave, QRS complex, or T wave (Fig. 5-19). This may be difficult to distinguish from sinus dysrhythmia (a normal phenomenon), but in such situations, the PP interval is not exactly doubled. Sinoatrial block is abolished when the heart rate is elevated (as during exercise). While some veterinarians regard sinoatrial block as a normal finding, reflecting increased vagal tone, we think that this dysrhythmia may have adverse effects on performance. We find that sinoatrial block is found infrequently, in contrast to second-degree A-V block. We also have noted that horses with sinoatrial block often have a history of poor racing performance despite few other abnormal findings on clinical examination.

KEY POINT ► This dysrhythmia should therefore be viewed with some suspicion, and a guarded prognosis should be given for high-intensity athletic performance.

It is of value to assess the heart-rate response to a graded incremental exercise test, as described previously. There is no treatment that is worthwhile, however.

Sinus Dysrhythmia

The horse's heart rate is normally quite regular, with little variation in the interval between successive heart beats. In some cases, there may be variation in the interval between beats, and on the ECG tracing the time between the RR intervals is somewhat irregular.

KEY POINT ► In some horses we have noted pronounced sinus dysrhythmia during the first 1 to 2 minutes of recovery after treadmill exercise tests (Fig. 5-20).

Our impression is that in horses where this response is pronounced, the heart-rate response to exercise is higher than normal. Further work is necessary to determine if there is an association between the finding of postexercise sinus dysrhythmia and reduced performance capacity.

Ventricular Premature Contractions

The problem of occasional ventricular premature contractions (VPCs) is a relatively common cause of cardiac dysrhythmias in the horse. On auscultation, the abnormal beat usually results in a louder S_1.

KEY POINT ► A VPC is easily diagnosed on ECG by the characteristic premature nature of the beat in relation to normal sinus rhythm and the unusual QRS waveform, as shown in Figure 5-21.

Our experience is that VPCs are of clinical significance and indicate myocardial irritation. It may be useful in cases where there are only one or two isolated VPCs on a resting ECG to perform a telemetric ECG during exercise to determine whether more abnormal beats occur and whether the heart-rate response to exercise is abnormal. There may be an association with some upper respiratory tract infections, particularly equine influenza. Horses with VPCs should be rested for 8 to 12 weeks, and in many cases the dysrhythmia will resolve.

Ventricular Tachycardia

Ventricular tachycardia occurs most commonly in the horse in a paroxysmal form.

KEY POINT ► The problem is characterized by a very much higher heart rate than

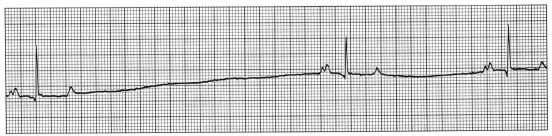

Figure 5–19. ECG tracing (lead II) from a horse with a sinoatrial block showing the doubling of the RR interval, with no P wave, QRS complex, or T wave. Recording was made at 25 mm/s and an amplitude of 1 mV/cm.

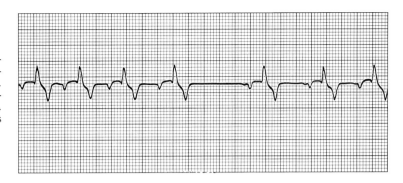

Figure 5–20. Telemetry ECG recording from a horse at the completion of a treadmill exercise test. Note the marked sinus dysrhythmia in the period after exercise. Recording was made at 25 mm/s and an amplitude of 1 mV/cm.

normal and a characteristic abnormal ECG tracing.

The QRS complexes are abnormal in appearance, and P waves may not be apparent. The T waves are large and follow immediately on from the QRS complex. These features are shown in an ECG tracing from a 3-year-old standardbred pacer in Figure 5-22, where the waveform changes suddenly to normal sinus rhythm. Ventricular tachycardia is a particularly severe arrhythmia but in many cases is secondary to other metabolic disturbances, such as electrolyte and acid–base abnormalities. We have seen this problem most commonly under general anesthesia and in the immediate postexercise period after high-intensity exercise.

Wolff-Parkinson-White Syndrome

The condition, also known as *preexcitation syndrome,* is unusual in the horse and usually occurs together with other abnormal ECG findings.

KEY POINT ▶ The condition is characterized by a very short PR interval together with a prolonged QRS complex duration.

It can often appear in an intermittent form, interspersed by normal sinus rhythm. The pathologic significance is debatable, but if the problem is persistent, it is likely to have significant deleterious effects on athletic performance.

CONGENITAL HEART DISEASES

Congenital heart disease is relatively common in horses, but many cases do not become evident until the horse is first trained or at the time of an insurance or prepurchase examination. The most common congenital heart disorder is a ventricular septal defect (VSD), which, if small, may not result in adverse clinical signs until the horse is required to perform competitively. Signs of congenital cardiac disease will vary with the extent of the problem and whether there are abnormal passages that result in shunting of blood away from its normal course through the cardiovascular system.

One finding that can be confusing for the clinician inexperienced in examining foals is that a systolic murmur often is present from shortly after birth until the foal is 3 to 4 months old. This murmur is not associated with a patent ductus arteriosus but appears to be an ejection-type murmur, similar to that found in some fit racehorses. The murmur is usually localized well forward on the left chest wall and is not of clinical significance.

History and Presenting Signs

- Dyspnea
- Poor growth rate
- Exercise intolerance

Figure 5–21. ECG tracing (lead II) from the 5-year-old standardbred gelding presented because of poor racing performance. Note the bizarre QRS complex in an otherwise normal ECG recording. This is typical of ventricular premature contractions. Recording was made at 25 mm/s and an amplitude of 1 mV/cm.

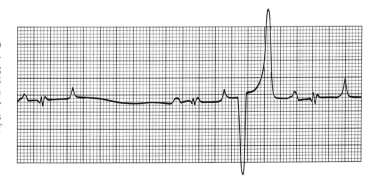

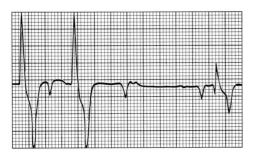

Figure 5–22. ECG tracing (Y lead) from a 3-year-old standardbred pacer presented for routine evaluation of fitness by treadmill exercise testing. The ventricular tachycardia occurred in a paroxysmal form, interspersed by periods of normal sinus rhythm, immediately after exercise. Recording was made at 25 mm/s and an amplitude of 1 mV/cm.

- Cyanosis
- Jugular vein distension
- No presenting signs

Clinical Findings and Diagnosis

- With the majority of congenital cardiac abnormalities, a murmur is heard. In some cases, this murmur may be loud and continuous (e.g., persistent patent ductus arteriosus) or may be more localized, as in the case of VSDs.
- Careful auscultation to determine the relation of the murmur to the phase of the cardiac cycle is important if an accurate diagnosis is to be made. The resting heart rate will provide a broad guide to the degree of the problem. Horses with congenital cardiac problems that cause little cardiac dysfunction or arterial hypoxemia will have a normal resting heart rate, whereas those in which there is severe cardiac dysfunction will have rapid heart rates.
- Careful note should be made of signs of jugular venous distension, which can indicate cardiac decompensation.
- Echocardiography is often useful to define problems such as septal defects. However, considerable experience is necessary to obtain good-quality images and for interpretation of changes in chamber dimensions.
- Arterial blood gas sampling is often useful to determine the extent of arterial desaturation. In foals, this can be accomplished via the great metatarsal artery with the foal in lateral recumbency (see Chap. 8). In adults, arterial blood samples can be obtained from the carotid artery. Normal arterial blood gas values together with details of sampling are discussed in Chapters 4 and 8.
- Recording of the ECG is not helpful in many cases, but where there is cardiac enlargement, gross changes in electrical axis will be demonstrable even using a frontal lead system.

- Cardiac catheterization may be performed at specialist clinics and institutions. Catheterization of the right side of the heart, with measurement of central venous pressure and pressures in the right atrium, right ventricle, and pulmonary artery, can be of considerable use in reaching a diagnosis.

Differential Diagnosis

- Ventricular septal defect
- Persistent patent ductus arteriosus
- Atrial septal defect
- Tetralogy of Fallot
- Tricuspid valve atresia

Treatment

In the absence of an increased jugular pulse and other signs of congestive heart failure, the prognosis for survival may be quite good. If the arterial blood gases are normal and there is no evidence of cardiac enlargement on echocardiography, horses can go on to lead normal lives. However, with most congenital cardiac abnormalities, the horse will not be a useful athlete.

Patent Ductus Arteriosus

The ductus arteriosus, a fetal connection between the pulmonary artery and the aorta, is usually patent for a short period after birth. However, in almost all foals, the ductus closes within the first 24 hours after birth. A persistent ductus will result in a loud "machinery" type of murmur that radiates extensively on auscultation. A systolic murmur is commonly present for several months after birth in foals, and some clinicians mistake this murmur for a ductal murmur. Patent ductus arteriosus is unusual in the horse and is associated most commonly with a variety of other congenital cardiac abnormalities. Because of this, it carries a poor prognosis.

Ventricular Septal Defects

Ventricular septal defect (VSD) is probably the most common significant congenital cardiac abnormality in the horse. It also can occur together with a range of other less common cardiac abnormalities, such as tetralogy of Fallot, patent ductus arteriosus, atrial septal defects, and tricuspid atresia. Simple VSD may result in few abnormal findings, but there is usually a significant systolic heart murmur.

KEY POINT ► Most VSDs occur relatively high in the heart, immediately below the aortic valve and therefore can sometimes be difficult to visualize on echocardiography, particularly if the lesion is small. With large defects, clinical signs are quite pronounced and the foals are hypoxemic.

Tetralogy of Fallot

This is an uncommon complex congenital cardiovascular disorder that consists of ventricular septal defect, dextrorotated aorta, pulmonic stenosis, and right ventricular hypertrophy. There is often right-to-left shunting of blood through the septal defect, and arterial hypoxemia is severe.

Atrial Septal Defects

Many atrial septal defects are asymptomatic, and there may not be a heart murmur present because of the low pressure and blood flow in this region. In large septal defects, pulmonary hypertension can occur, and right-sided heart failure may be the end result. Some cases may show splitting of S_2 on auscultation. This also may be heard in cases of pulmonic stenosis.

Tricuspid Atresia

In combination with tricuspid atresia, there is an atrial septal defect and right ventricular hypoplasia. The cases reported also have included a ventricular septal defect and in some cases a patent ductus arteriosus. Foals are usually poorly grown, and there is severe hypoxemia. Because of the range of anomalies, there is a loud murmur, usually systolic, that radiates widely.

Other Cardiovascular Disease

Most other heart disease that does not primarily involve conduction disturbances is associated with valve disorders and sometimes disorders of the great vessels. Most cases of heart disease are not responsive to treatment, making the treatment options limited. Of greatest interest to horse owners and trainers is the prognosis. While there are a large number of possible disorders affecting the heart and vessels, most of these are unusual in a normal practice setting. The cardiovascular disorders described below are those which are most likely to be found in equine practice.

Aortic Rupture

Aortic rupture is uncommon but often spectacular, particularly if it occurs in association with exercise. Aortic rupture may be the result of a weak point such as an aneurysm in the vessel wall or may occur spontaneously around the level of the aortic valve. In some cases in which histopathology has been done, necrosis has been found involving the media of the aortic wall.

History and Presenting Signs

Sudden death

Clinical Findings and Diagnosis

■ If the problem occurs at rest, the horse will be found dead

KEY POINT ▶ If the problem occurs during exercise, most horses will show a sudden decrease in speed, become ataxic, and collapse. In most cases there is sufficient warning that there is something wrong for the rider to dismount prior to the horse collapsing.

■ Necropsy reveals large amounts of blood in the thorax. In one case this was localized within the pericardium so that cardiac tamponade resulted.

Differential Diagnosis

■ Snake bite
■ Lightning strike

Treatment

Stand out of the way!

Endocarditis

KEY POINT ▶ Endocarditis is an uncommon disease that is usually the result of bacterial localization in the endocardium and may involve the valves.

History and Presenting Signs

- Coughing
- Depression
- Ventral edema

Clinical Findings and Diagnosis

- Horses are usually depressed and may have intermittent fever.
- If localization of the problem is in the wall of the endocardium and there is no valvular involvement, there may be no heart murmur.
- There may be signs of heart failure late in the course of the problem.
- If there is valvular involvement, case studies have shown that the aortic and left A-V valves are the most common valves affected.
- If there is a heart murmur, it is most commonly a diastolic murmur because aortic valve lesions are most common.
- Vegetative lesions of the valves can often be detected on echocardiography if the valves are thickened.
- Hematology and plasma biochemistry may show anemia, neutrophilia, and hyperfibrinogenemia.
- Blood culture can be helpful to determine the bacteria involved. This is most useful in the acute stages when there is usually fever and bacteremia. *Streptococcus* spp. are most commonly involved.

Differential Diagnosis

- Valvular insufficiency
- Congenital heart problems
- Thrombophlebitis
- Pleuritis

Treatment

- Treatment is often unrewarding.
- Assessment of the degree of cardiac compromise is important for prognosis.
- Antimicrobial therapy may be useful in the acute stages of endocarditis, and the results of blood culture may be helpful in deciding which drug to use. If no bacteriologic results are known, therapy with penicillin (20,000 IU/kg of Na or K penicillin given IV or IM qid [Treatment Nos. 84 and 85]) and gentamicin (3 mg/kg tid) (Treatment No. 56) may be used.

Jugular Thrombosis

KEY POINT ▶ Thrombosis and thrombophlebitis are common problems in horses, particularly racehorses, because of the range of medications administered via the jugular vein.

In horses that require prolonged jugular catheterization, thrombophlebitis is not infrequent. Predisposing factors include endotoxemia, bacteremia, and mechanical factors such as irritation by the catheter or drugs. The perivascular injection of irritant drugs such as thiopentone, phenylbutazone, and aminoglycosides can lead to intense local phlebitis.

History and Presenting Signs

- Prolonged catheterization
- Systemic infection
- Repeated injections of irritant drugs
- Perivascular injections

Clinical Findings and Diagnosis

- The most consistent sign is swelling around the jugular vein, with vein thrombosis being palpable as a hard, cord-like structure.
- There may be swelling around the proximal part of the neck and the head because of the venous compromise. However, in most cases the collateral venous circulation is sufficient to resolve the congestion.
- Horses may have an elevated body temperature and show signs of depression and anorexia in the acute phase of the disease.
- Septic thrombophlebitis may be characterized by a draining tract over the vein, but this is uncommon.
- Ultrasound examination is useful to determine whether the vein is patent or occluded.
- A hemogram and fibrinogen estimation are useful to determine whether there is evidence of infection. In early cases where there is intermittent fever, blood culture is useful to isolate significant bacteria.

Differential Diagnosis

Localized cellulitis

Treatment

- Because many cases of thrombosis and thrombophlebitis are secondary to intravenous catheterization, it is important to use good technique (see Chap. 17). In this way, problems of thrombophlebitis may be avoided.
- Local anti-inflammatory therapy can include cold or warm compresses to the site, depending on the stage at which the problem is found. Nonsteroidal anti-inflammatory drugs such as phenyl-

butazone (Treatment No. 88) at a dose rate of 4.4 mg/kg bid orally for 4 to 7 days and topical dimethylsulfoxide (Treatment No. 34) can be useful.

KEY POINT ► Despite an occluded jugular vein, many athletic horses perform satisfactorily and have no adverse effects once the initial active inflammatory process has resolved.

■ Antimicrobial therapy is important and may have to be maintained for several weeks. Where possible, this should be based on results of culture and sensitivity tests, although culture of a discharging sinus will not result in useful information. Procaine penicillin (Treatment No. 83) given intramuscularly at a dose rate of 15,000 IU/kg (15 mg/kg) and gentamicin (Treatment No. 56) given intravenously at a dose rate of 2 to 3 mg/kg are the antibiotics of choice.
■ Surgical "stripping" of the affected vein is indicated in severe cases that are refractory to medical therapy. This is a major procedure and is best undertaken at an institution or a major referral practice.

Pericarditis

KEY POINT ► Pericarditis is not common in horses, and when it does occur, it may be the result of extension of pneumonia and pleuritis.

Pericarditis produces a range of severe clinical abnormalities, and the problem can be suspected where there are signs of a severe and progressive cardiac disorder. The cause for the pericarditis is mostly unknown, but cases have been reported associated with trauma, chest infections, and systemic viral or bacterial infections.

History and Presenting Signs

■ Ventral edema
■ Prominent jugular venous distension
■ Dyspnea
■ Usually found in mature horses

Clinical Findings and Diagnosis

■ The majority of horses will have an increased heart rate, and the pulse is weak and thready.
■ The classical sign of pericarditis is muffled heart sounds.
■ Because of the direct pressure on the heart, venous obstruction is a common finding. The end result is jugular vein distension and ventral edema. These findings are typical of many cases of congestive heart failure, and therefore, pericarditis must be distinguished from other causes.
■ Most horses show signs of dyspnea, and there may be alterations in the appearance of the mucous membranes, with some horses showing cyanosis. Prolongation of capillary refill time is common, indicating poor peripheral perfusion.
■ Diagnosis is made by the typical signs together with ultrasound examination of the heart (see Echocardiography, p. 179). Fluid can be seen on the echocardiogram.

KEY POINT ► To establish a definitive diagnosis, pericardiocentesis should be performed.

■ This can be done using ultrasound guidance but is also possible "blind." Pericardiocentesis is best performed a little caudal to the heart, over the sixth intercostal space. At this location there is less risk of trauma to the heart compared with a more anterior site.

Differential Diagnosis

■ Pleuritis
■ Endocarditis
■ Congestive heart failure
■ Thrombophlebitis

Treatment

■ Drainage of the pericardial sac should be performed using a 12- to 14-gauge catheter that is at least 12.5 cm long. In most cases there is a substantial amount of fibrin deposition, and therefore, the catheter may become blocked.
■ Great care should be taken when advancing the catheter because if the stylet damages the surface of the myocardium, the horse may die. The most direct access is over the fourth or fifth intercostal space, but great care must be taken in this location.
■ If there is profound fluid accumulation in the pericardium, it may be difficult to distinguish the fluid from that found in pleuritis.
■ Some horses will recover following drainage of fluid from the pericardium, but the prognosis is poor for the majority of horses.

Valvular Disorders

While stenoses of the various heart valves have been reported in individual case studies, such lesions are unusual in clinical practice.

KEY POINT ► By far the majority of valvular disorders involve insufficiency rather than stenosis. The most common abnormalities affect the left A-V (mitral) and aortic valves.

History and Presenting Signs

■ Decreased exercise tolerance
■ Poor recovery rates after exercise

Clinical Findings and Diagnosis

- Heart murmurs are heard in all cases and are usually grade II or III if there are no overt signs of heart failure.
- Because of the large cardiac reserve of the horse, heart failure is uncommon and is usually found toward the end stage of disease.

KEY POINT ► Right-sided heart failure is more common than left-sided failure and is manifested by prominent jugular vein distension and possibly edema of the ventral abdomen.

- Left-sided heart valve lesions are found more commonly than those on the right side of the heart.
- Echocardiography is useful, in gross valvular abnormalities, to determine the extent of the changes. Unfortunately, in the majority of horses in which valvular disorders are suspected, nothing abnormal may be found on echocardiography. However, it is always useful to determine chamber sizes so that it is clear whether compensatory enlargement has occurred. Doppler echocardiography can be of use in demonstrating the flow disturbances across the valves.
- ECG examination is not usually of value unless there is gross cardiac enlargement, in which there will be a shift in the cardiac axis.

Left Atrioventricular Valve Insufficiency

KEY POINT ► Left A-V valve insufficiency is the most common valvular problem and is associated with a systolic heart murmur that has its maximal intensity on the left thorax around the fifth intercostal space, a little below the level of the point of the shoulder.

Cases of chordae tendinae rupture associated with left A-V valve insufficiency result in a more severe systolic heart murmur.

Aortic Valve Insufficiency. Aortic valve insufficiency is the other common valvular disorder in the horse. It causes a diastolic heart murmur that begins just after S_2. The murmur is usually of greatest intensity over the left chest wall, just below the level of the point of the shoulder around the fourth to fifth intercostal space. In some cases there will be a characteristic prominent pulse because of the increase in end-diastolic volume associated with reflux of blood into the left ventricle.

Right A-V Valve Insufficiency. Right A-V valve insufficiency is encountered more rarely than that of the left A-V and aortic valves. We see one to two cases a year that are presented with a decrease in performance, and the only clinical finding is a localized right-sided systolic heart murmur. Few of

these horses develop congestive heart failure in the short term.

Differential Diagnosis
(in order of likelihood of occurrence)

- Left A-V (mitral) valve insufficiency
- Aortic valve insufficiency
- Right A-V (tricuspid) valve insufficiency
- Pulmonic valve insufficiency
- Valvular stenosis (very uncommon)

Treatment

- No long-term treatment is possible in valvular insufficiency. However, if there are signs of congestive heart failure, some treatment that may relieve the clinical signs is possible.
- By the time edema of the ventral abdomen develops, it is difficult to give any worthwhile therapy. However, the use of a diuretic such as furosemide (Treatment No. 55) is helpful, and digoxin (Treatment No. 33) may be considered.
- Digoxin may be given intravenously at a loading dose of 14 µg/kg, followed by a maintenance dose of 3.5 µg/kg twice daily. Alternatively, the drug may be given orally at a loading dose of 70 µg/kg once daily, followed by 12 hourly dosing at dose rates of 35 to 40 µg/kg. Because of great variability in the absorption of digoxin when given orally, it is helpful if plasma concentrations can be measured. Effective plasma concentrations of digoxin are in the range 0.5 to 2.0 ng/ml.

Viral or Bacterial Myocarditis

Myocarditis, a localized inflammatory response in the myocardium, is diagnosed infrequently and is not common. In the past it has been diagnosed on the basis of abnormalities of the T wave. However, it is now apparent that such a diagnosis is incorrect.

KEY POINT ► While there have been few confirmed cases, the equine veterinary literature often mentions myocarditis as a sequel to equine influenza, African horse sickness, and strangles.

This may be because a percentage of horses that recover from these conditions show a decrease in exercise capacity following infection. It is likely that the reason for the reduced performance in such cases is respiratory rather than cardiovascular in origin.

History and Presenting Signs

- Previous respiratory infection
- Usually in young horses
- Exercise intolerance

Clinical Findings and Diagnosis

- Exercise intolerance is the most common history, there usually being evidence of distress following hard exercise.
- On auscultation, there may be an dysrhythmia if the myocarditis involves one of the conducting pathways. An ECG will be necessary to determine the precise nature of the electrical disturbance.
- Auscultation of the heart may not indicate rhythm disturbances, but there may be alterations in electrical activity, with abnormalities of conduction, such as bundle-branch block or intraatrial block, or abnormalities during repolarization.
- If the resting ECG is normal, it may be valuable to record the ECG during exercise, since dysrhythmias may be more obvious during or immediately after strenuous exercise.
- In the acute stages of myocarditis, we have found increases in serum concentrations of lactate dehydrogenase (LDH) and creatine phosphokinase (CPK). However, because few laboratories measure LDH isoenzymes, it is difficult to be sure that elevations in serum or plasma CPK or LDH indicate myocardial damage.
- Echocardiography is not useful for diagnosis.

Differential Diagnosis

- Lower respiratory tract disease
- Endocarditis
- Minor ECG conduction abnormalities

Treatment

- No treatment is likely to be useful if there is myocarditis, apart from rest and time. In some cases, we have seen the ECG return to normal after 3 to 6 months of rest.
- If there is evidence of systemic bacterial infection, it may be useful to give a course of an antibiotic such as procaine penicillin (Treatment No. 83) at a dose rate of 15,000 IU/kg (15 mg/kg).
- If there are indications of severe cardiac disease, including heart failure, the prognosis is very poor.

References

Adams, H. R.: New perspectives in cardiology: Pharmacodynamic classification of antiarrhythmic drugs. J. Am. Vet. Med. Assoc. 189(5):525, 1986.

Bonagura, J. D., and Miller, M. S.: Normal ECG complexes. J. Equine Vet. Sci. 5(4):200, 1985.

Bonagura, J. D., and Miller, M. S.: Junctional and ventricular arrhythmias. J. Equine Vet. Sci. 5(6):347, 1985.

Bonagura, J. D., and Miller, M. S.: Common conduction disturbances. J. Equine Vet. Sci. 6(1):23, 1986.

Bertone, J. J., and Wingfield, W. E.: Atrial fibrillation in horses. Compend. Contin. Educ. Pract. Vet. 9(7):763, 1987.

Carlsten, J. C.: Two-dimensional, real-time echocardiography in the horse. Vet. Radiol. 28(3):76, 1987.

Evans, D. L., and Rose, R. J.: Method of investigation of the accuracy of four digitally displaying heart rate meters suitable for use in the exercising horse. Equine Vet. J. 18(2):129, 1986.

Foreman, J. H., Bayly, W. M., Grant, B. D., and Gollnick, P. D.: Standardized exercise test and daily heart rate responses of thoroughbreds undergoing conventional race training and detraining. Am. J. Vet. Res. 51(6):914, 1990.

Glazier, D. B.: Congestive heart failure and congenital cardiac defects in horses. Equine Pract. 8(9):20, 1986.

Holmes, J. R., Henigan, M., Williams, R. B., and Witherington, D. H.: Paroxysmal atrial fibrillation in racehorses. Equine Vet. J. 18(1):37, 1986.

Miller, M.: The equine electrocardiogram: Usage in equine practice. Proc. 34th Conv. Am. Assoc. Equine Pract., 1988, p. 577.

Miller, M. S., and Bonagura, J. D.: Atrial arrhythmias. J. Equine Vet. Sci. 5(5):300, 1985.

Physick-Sheard, P. W.: Diseases of the cardiovascular system. In P. T. Colahan, I. G. Mayhew, A. M. Merritt, and J. N. Moore, (Eds.), Equine Medicine and Surgery, 4th Ed. Goleta, Calif.: American Veterinary Publications, 1991, p. 165.

Rantanen, N. W., Byars, T. D., Hauser, M. L., and Gaines, R. D.: Spontaneous contrast and mass lesions in the hearts of race horses: Ultrasound diagnosis—Preliminary data. J. Equine Vet. Sci. 4(5):220, 1984.

Reef, V. B., and Spencer, P.: Echocardiographic evaluation of equine aortic insufficiency. Am. J. Vet. Res. 48(6):904, 1987.

Reef, V. B., Levitan, C. W., and Spencer, P. A.: Factors affecting prognosis and conversion in atrial fibrillation. J. Vet. Intern. Med. 2(1):1, 1988.

Alimentary System

EXAMINATION OF THE ALIMENTARY TRACT

A thorough and careful examination of the digestive system is particularly important when evaluating horses with suspected gastrointestinal tract disorders. In general, as with the examination of any other body system, a logical sequence of events is followed during the examination procedure. Following collection of appropriate information relating to signalment, history, and duration of signs (see Chap. 2), examination usually begins at the head and proceeds caudally (see Chap. 1). We base our approach on the comprehensive examination procedure described by Adams.

History

Important questions relating to gastrointestinal dysfunction include the following:

- Is the horse eating normally?
- Does the horse lose food from its mouth when eating?
- Does the horse salivate excessively when eating?
- Is there evidence of weight loss?
- Is there evidence of abdominal pain?
- What is the duration of the problem?
- Is this the only animal on the premises showing these abnormalities?
- What is the vaccination and deworming history of this and other animals on the farm?
- Is the horse stabled or does it live outdoors?
- Is the horse hand fed or does it eat pasture?
- Does the horse live in an environment where there is a lot of sand?

Following collection of the history, the clinician then undertakes the physical examination.

Initial Inspection

Examination of a horse with suspected alimentary tract disease has a number of components, including general physical examination, auscultation,

rectal examination, passage of a nasogastric tube, clinical pathology, and other diagnostic aids. Initial inspection involves determination of the cardinal signs (i.e., heart rate, respiratory rate, capillary refill time, pulse quality, mucous membrane color, and body temperature), followed by specific examination of the alimentary tract. Examination begins at the mouth, with evidence of malocclusion of the jaws being investigated. In addition, the presence of sharp edges on teeth and damage to the lips and gums should be explored. Nasal discharge, excessive salivation, and other abnormalities (e.g., swellings) are then searched for. Next, the neck and external abdominal contours are determined, with note being made if distension of the flanks is present. This is usually the result of gas accumulation within the large bowel. The presence of edema or other abnormalities (e.g., hernias) also should be noted.

DIAGNOSTIC AIDS

Auscultation

Following initial inspection, auscultation of the abdomen is performed. The left and right sides of the abdomen should be auscultated; approximately 4 to 5 minutes is required to perform this procedure thoroughly. Normal sounds are often referred to as "rumbling," "bubbling," and "splashing" sounds. The clinician should note the tone, intensity, and duration of sounds. Large intestinal sounds are often of lower intensity and deeper than those originating from the small intestine. Examination begins in the region of the paralumbar fossa, subsequently moving to the middle to ventral abdominal regions (see Figs. 1-20 and 1-21). In the right paralumbar fossa, ileocecal sounds can be heard, which are a high-pitched rumble that is said to sound like water rushing down a drainpipe. Ileocecal sounds occur approximately one to three times per minute in the normal horse. When the lower side of the abdomen is auscultated, small intestinal sounds often can be detected. These are referred to as *borborygmi* and are low-pitched fluid sounds.

Repeated auscultation is vital when monitoring horses with acute abdominal pain. Although auscultation alone will not be diagnostic, a progressive decline in the frequency or intensity of intestinal sounds may be associated with an unfavorable prognosis. Although sounds may be temporarily reduced in some cases of colic, a persisting absence of gut sounds is often ominous. In contrast, increased intensity of gastrointestinal sounds and evidence of the presence of large amounts of gas may be indicative of spasmodic colic.

In horses that have gaseous distension of the abdomen, simultaneous auscultation and percussion may reveal a resonant ping.

KEY POINT ▶ Repeated auscultation in horses with colic is essential.

Rectal Examination

Rectal examination is useful in horses with suspected gastrointestinal tract disease, particularly those suffering from abdominal pain. Any horse with a history of persistent or recurrent colic, chronic weight loss, fever of unknown origin, or chronic diarrhea should be considered a candidate for rectal examination. The clinician should be thorough and systematic when performing this examination, since it can provide valuable diagnostic information. In addition, care is required because of the risk of irritation or rupture of the rectum. Appropriate restraint of the horse is necessary, and this may be done using stocks, a stall door, hay bales, or hobbles. The operator should wear a thin plastic sleeve that should be well lubricated prior to insertion in the rectum. We find methylcellulose to be the best lubricant. The examiner should be patient, introducing the arm into the rectum slowly. It is important not to fight the horse's peristaltic movements when performing this procedure. Following evacuation of the rectum of feces, if the horse still continues to strain, 30 to 60 ml of lidocaine (Treatment No. 67) alone or mixed with an equal volume of obstetrical lubricant can be infused into the rectum. This will provide local analgesia and help reduce straining. We examine the pelvic structures first, and then survey the left side of the abdomen, sweep across the midline, and finish the examination on the right side. In the normal horse, the following structures may be identified: bladder; female reproductive tract; inguinal rings; small and large colon, including pelvic flexure; spleen, left kidney, nephrosplenic ligament, mesenteric root, aorta, ventral band, and dorsal attachment of the cecum; and the peritoneal surface.

KEY POINT ▶ The following points should be considered when examining organs per rectum: position; size; mobility; thickness; evidence of edema, tight mesenteric bands, or distension due to gas; and presence of fluid or ingesta.

Adams and White note the following points:

Feces—May be dry, hard, or contain blood, mucous, or sand.

Rectal Mucosa—Should be smooth and folded. Significant abnormal changes include roughening or thickening of the rectal wall.

Inguinal Rings—Normally located about 10 cm (4 in) lateral to the midline on the brim of the pelvis. One of the most common abnormalities of the inguinal rings in colts and stallions is herniation and incarceration of small intestine through the inguinal canals. This can be detected by palpating the loops of bowel passing through the internal inguinal ring.

Small Colon—Detected by palpation of fecal balls within its lumen. The small colon has marked sacculations, is relatively mobile, and has a prominent antimesenteric band. Abnormalities in the small colon include distension and impaction.

Small Intestine—Usually cannot be examined in the normal animal. However, if examination of the middle portion of the abdomen indicates some form of space-occupying structure that is not easily identifiable, it is usually the small intestine. Distended loops of small intestine are commonly found in association with strangulation of the small bowel and anterior enteritis. At times, intussusception of the small intestine can be palpated, with the bowel becoming thick, turgid, and feeling somewhat like a sausage. Taut mesenteric bands in the small intestine also can be suggestive of pathology.

Pelvic Flexure—May be identified in the caudoventral portion of the abdomen near the midline, usually on the left-hand side. One of the most common abnormalities associated with the pelvic flexure is impaction, and firm masses may be indented on digital palpation. Impactions due to sand often give evidence of a gritty sensation. In these cases, sand can frequently be found in the feces.

Large Colon—Distension associated with taut bands and pain may be suggestive of large colon torsion or malposition.

Spleen—Can be identified on the left side of the abdomen next to the abdominal wall near the level of the last rib. It is usually firm and has a distinct shape with a sharp caudal edge. Splenomegaly may be reflective of neoplasia, abscessation or disorders in the reticuloendothelial system.

KEY POINT ▶ One should always palpate from the spleen dorsally toward the midline, across the nephrosplenic ligament, to the caudal pole of the left kidney, since at times the colon may displace dorsally and lodge in the nephrosplenic ligament area.

Mesenteric Root—Difficult to palpate. Enlargement is usually the result of increased size of lymph nodes or lymph node abscessation. This is one of the most common sites for internal abscessation in horses.

Right Dorsal Colon—May be palpable in some horses but is not normally detected unless the colon is distended due to gas or fluid accumulation. One of most common causes of distension of the right dorsal colon is enteroliths causing luminal blockage of the small colon.

Ventral Band of the Cecum—Descends from dorsal to ventral on a right to left diagonal path. In addition, the dorsal attachment of the cecum can be identified in the region of the right dorsal abdominal wall. The base and body of the cecum are usually only detected when the cecum is distended with gas or ingesta. Cecal impactions may be noted as firm, doughy masses. The ileum is usually not palpated as it passes into the cecum unless there is an impaction or intussusception.

Peritoneum—Should be the final structure examined during the rectal examination. Evidence of nodules, roughening, and response to pain or adhesions can be valuable indicators of dysfunction when evaluating a horse with evidence of gastrointestinal tract disease.

Passage of a Nasogastric Tube

Nasogastric intubation is vital in the approach to a horse with suspected alimentary tract disease. Passage of a tube is used for several major functions. These include decompression of the proximal gastrointestinal tract to prevent rupture of the stomach, assistance in the location of obstructions (e.g., "choke"), and administration of fluids and medications. The tube is introduced, via the ventral nasal meatus, into the pharynx and then into the esophagus (Figs. 6-12 and 6-11).

KEY POINT ▶ Passage of a nasogastric tube is indicated in all horses exhibiting signs of moderate to severe abdominal pain that persists for more than 15 mintues.

It is important to ensure that the tube is passed into the stomach if decompression is to occur. However, spontaneous decompression will not always occur, and it is necessary to prime the tube

Text continues on p. 199

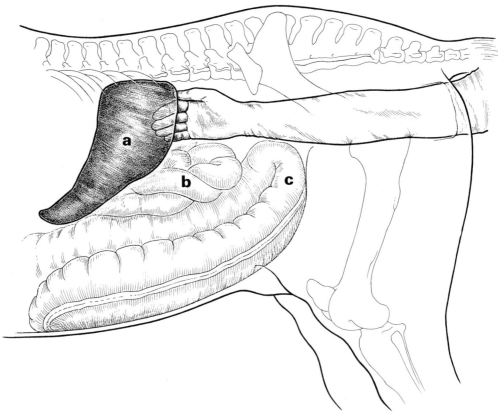

Figure 6–1. Rectal examination. Position of examiner's arm in the rectum when palpating the spleen (*a*). The spleen normally lies in the dorsal part of the abdomen on the left hand side adjacent to the body wall. The tapering posterior edge of the spleen is most easily palpable. The small intestine (*b*) and pelvic flexure (*c*) are shown.

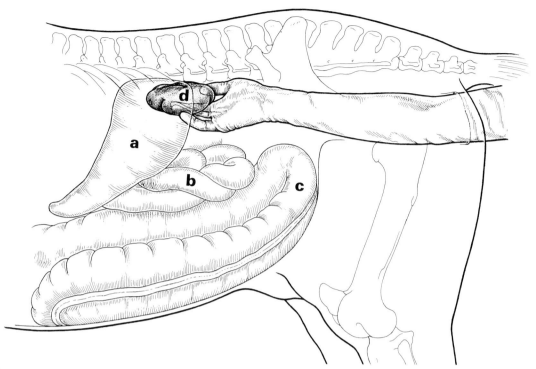

Figure 6–2. Rectal examination. Position of examiner's arm in the rectum when palpating the left kidney (*d*). The kidney is dorsal and medial to the spleen and is attached to the body wall. The aorta lies medial to the kidney. The spleen (*a*), small intestines (*b*), and pelvic flexure (*c*) are shown.

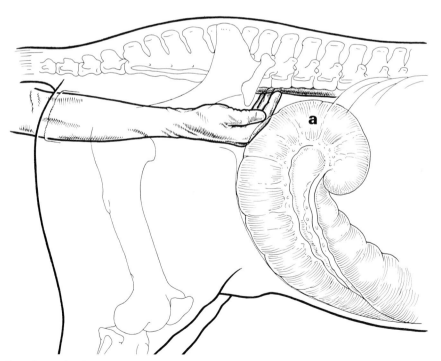

Figure 6–3. Rectal examination. Position of examiner's arm in the rectum when palpating the aorta. It lies in the midline attached to the dorsal body wall. A pulse should be felt. Moving caudad, the bifurcation of the aorta is palpable. The base of the cecum (*a*) is shown.

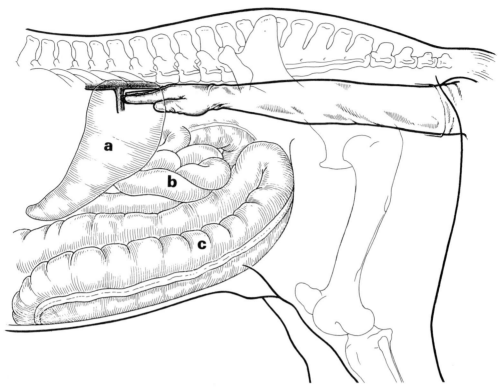

Figure 6–4. Rectal examination. Position of examiner's arm in the rectum when palpating the mesenteric root. The arm should be inserted as far into the rectum as possible. The mesenteric root is a taut structure running dorsoventrally in the middle of the abdomen. The spleen (*a*), small intestine (*b*), and left ventral colon (*c*) are shown.

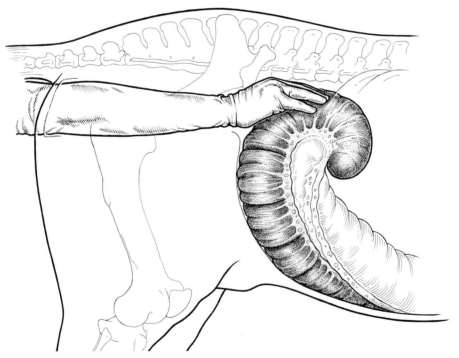

Figure 6–5. Rectal examination. Position of examiner's arm in the rectum when palpating the cecum. The taenia on the body of the cecum can be felt on the dorsum of the cecum coursing ventromedially.

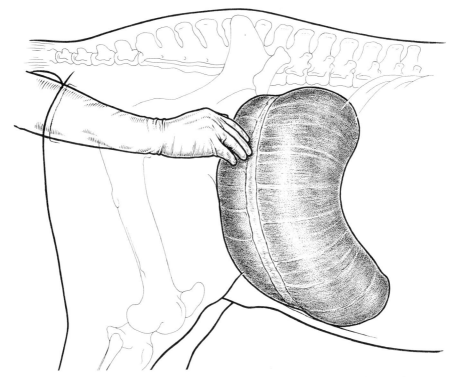

Figure 6–6. Rectal examination. Position of examiner's arm in the rectum when palpating cecal tympany. The cecum is distended and moves caudally to the pelvic inlet. The ventral band is taut and curves dorsoventrally from left to right.

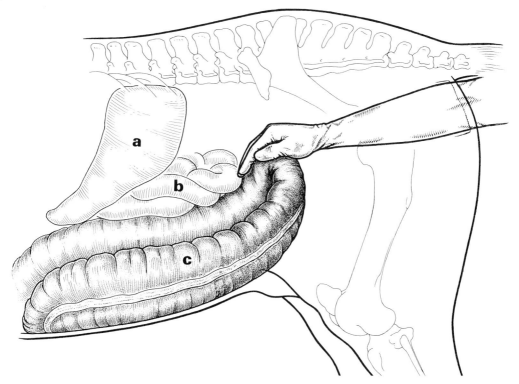

Figure 6–7. Rectal examination. Position of examiner's arm in the rectum when palpating the pelvic flexure of the large colon. It lies just over the pelvic brim on the left-hand side of the midline on the ventral abdominal wall. The spleen (*a*), small intestine (*b*), and left ventral colon (*c*) are shown.

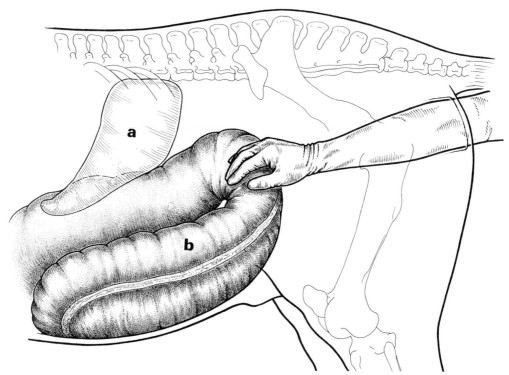

Figure 6–8. Rectal examination. Position of examiner's arm in the rectum when palpating an impaction of the large colon. The usual location is in the left or right ventral quadrants, although position is variable. The spleen (*a*) and left ventral colon (*b*) are shown.

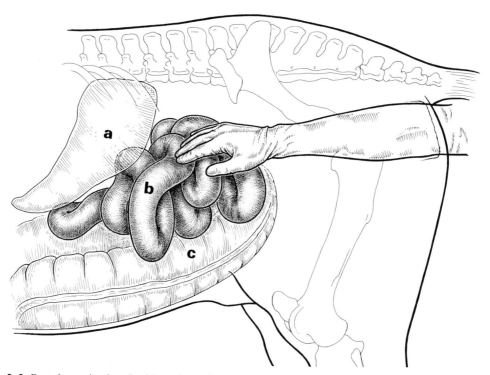

Figure 6–9. Rectal examination. Position of examiner's arm in the rectum when palpating a small intestinal strangulation. Taut loops of gas- and fluid-filled small intestine are often palpable (*b*). In some cases only one loop is palpable, whereas in others many loops are involved. The spleen (*a*) and left ventral colon (*c*) are shown.

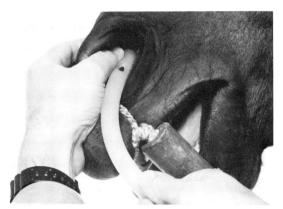

Figure 6–10. Passage of a nasogastric tube showing introduction of the tube into the ventral nasal meatus.

with water. This can be done by flushing about 500 ml of water into the tube using gravity feed with a funnel, fluid pump (Fig. 6-12), or garden hose. After the water is infused, the gastric fluid is then allowed to siphon off (Fig. 6-13). We have found that up to a dozen flushes may be required to ensure that the stomach is fully decompressed. The presence of particulate matter in the stomach will block the tube, making it essential to pass a large tube that has a number of fenestrations in the distal end. Examination of the fluid obtained following gastric reflux may provide some indication of the cause of the problem. The quantity, smell, content, and pH of the reflux should be assessed.

Abdominocentesis

The composition of abdominal fluid is determined by the condition of the organs that are bathed by this fluid. As a result, evaluation of abdominal fluid can provide vital information in the assessment of horses with alimentary tract disease.

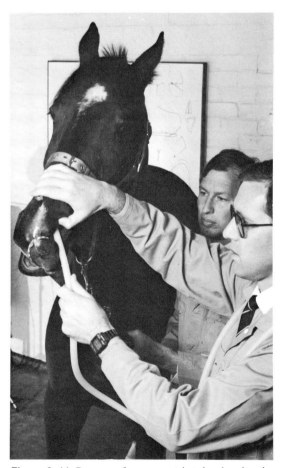

Figure 6–11. Passage of a nasogastric tube showing the position of the handler and veterinarian.

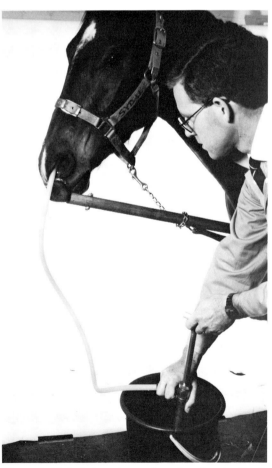

Figure 6–12. Infusion of water into the tube, the distal tip of which has been placed in the stomach. This is to assist in reflux of any excess fluid present in the upper gastrointestinal tract.

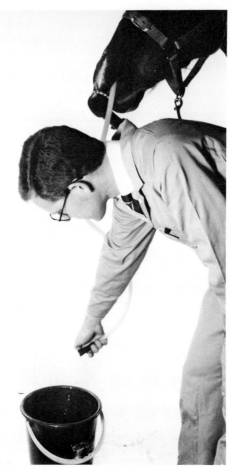

Figure 6–13. Reflux of water from the stomach tube following infusion of several hundred ml water.

KEY POINT ► Abdominocentesis is indicated in horses with a history of acute or recurrent colic, chronic weight loss, or chronic diarrhea.

Abdominocentesis is a safe procedure with a very low complication rate. Puncture of the bowel is relatively common but results in exceedingly few problems to the horse. Fluid is usually collected from the most dependent site of the ventral abdomen. Hair along the midline is clipped and shaved, and the skin is prepared. A small bleb of local anesthetic can be infused under the skin using a 25-gauge, 15-mm (5/8-in) needle (Fig. 6-14). However, these procedures, with the exception of skin disinfection, are not necessary if an 18-gauge, 3.75-cm (1.5-in) needle is to be used for abdominocentesis. In most horses, an 18-gauge, 3.75-cm needle is adequate for collection of abdominal fluid (Fig. 6-15). With the clinician standing in a position where he or she is least likely to be kicked by a hind leg, the needle is inserted rapidly through the skin and into the abdomen. If no fluid is obtained, the needle

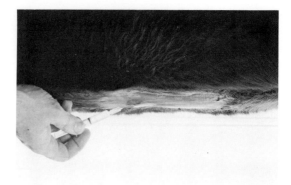

Figure 6–14. Abdominocentesis. Injection of local anesthetic into the most dependent point of the ventral abdomen.

should be repositioned. On occasion, rotation of the needle, injection of air with a sterile syringe, or insertion of several other needles assists in drainage of fluid. In larger breeds and fat horses, a teat cannula, stainless steel bitch urinary catheter, or spinal needle may be required to penetrate the layer of fat that lies on the internal side of the linea alba. When using this technique, local anesthetic is infiltrated subcutaneously, and a stab incision using a no. 11 or 15 scalpel blade is required (Fig. 6-16) to allow insertion of the cannula. Following the stab incision, contamination of the sample with blood is a potential problem. This can be overcome by inserting the cannula through a gauze sponge prior to insertion of the needle through the abdominal wall (Fig. 6-17). When peripheral blood contamination does occur, the fluid draining from the cannula is clear but is streaked with swirls of blood. In contrast, splenic puncture yields fluid with a high PCV (greater than that of peripheral blood), whereas diapedesis from nonviable bowel wall results in fluid with a low PCV (<0.05 L/L).

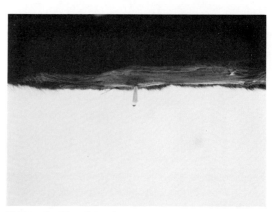

Figure 6–15. Abdominocentesis. Position of an 18-gauge, 3.75-cm needle inserted through the ventral abdominal midline. Abdominal fluid can be seen dripping from the needle.

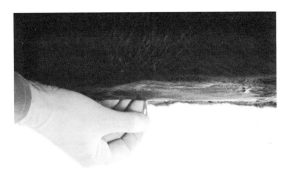

Figure 6–16. Abdominocentesis. Stab incision through the skin and subcutaneous tissues over the midline of the ventral abdomen prior to insertion of a teat cannula.

Laboratory Analysis of Abdominal Fluid

Abdominal fluid is collected into (1) a tube containing EDTA as an anticoagulant and (2) a sterile tube if bacteriology is required. Usual determinations include total red cells, total and differential nucleated cells, and total protein. Changes in abdominal fluid for a variety of diseases are represented in the Table 6-1.

Endoscopic Examination of the Upper Alimentary Tract

Endoscopic examination of the alimentary tract has become more popular in recent years with the advent of flexible fiber endoscopes. However, most endoscopes are made for human use and are not long enough for examination of the lower esophagus and stomach in the horse. The readily available endoscopes are up to 180 cm (70 in) in length and

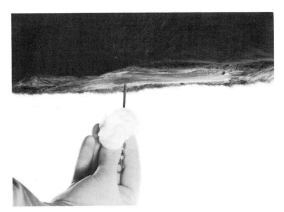

Figure 6–17. Abdominocentesis. Insertion of a teat cannula into the abdomen via the ventral midline. Note that a sterile gauze swab has been used to prevent blood contamination of the sample from blood associated with the skin incision.

13.5 mm (0.6 in) in diameter. With these, examination of the nasal passages, larynx, pharynx, and proximal esophagus in adult horses is possible. The use of longer endoscopes [360 cm (140 in)], allowing examination of the distal esophagus and stomach, is described, but this equipment is usually custom-made and is therefore restricted to use in large referral hospitals. Indications for endoscopy of the upper alimentary tract include discharge of food or other material from the nares, dysphagia, excessive salivation, abnormal discharge from the mouth, dyspnea, and suspected "choke." The endoscope is normally passed down the ventral meatus in a manner similar to that described for a stomach tube. Following examination of the nasal passages, pharynx (including the guttural pouch openings), and larynx, the endoscope is passed into the cervical esophagus. The esophagus is dilated with air, and the lumen and mucosa of the esophagus are examined.

KEY POINT ▶ Evidence of esophageal obstruction ("choke"), ulceration, diverticula, and at times perforation or strictures can be gained from endoscopic examination.

However, when considering esophageal strictures, it has been our experience that they may not be visible because the folded contours of the esophageal mucosa may disguise their presence. On occasion, material that is lodged in the esophagus can be removed by the use of small, flexible forceps which are passed down through the biopsy port of the endoscope. With the use of longer, custom-made endoscopes, there are many reports of gastric ulceration in adult horses. Similarly, use of smaller-diameter endoscopes has allowed more routine access to the gastric mucosa in foals.

Radiography

With care and patience, high-quality radiographs of the head and cervical esophagus can be obtained using readily available portable veterinary radiographic equipment. A number of disorders that affect the upper alimentary tract can be diagnosed using this technique. These include tooth root abscessation, alveolitis, impacted or fractured teeth, dentigerous cysts, fractures of the mandible/maxilla or hyoid apparatus, fibromas, bony neoplasms, and in some cases disorders of the pharynx (e.g., retropharyngeal abscessation).

KEY POINT ▶ Signs of retropharyngeal abscessation are dyspnea, dysphagia, and radiographic evidence of compression of surrounding tissues.

Radiography of the cranial esophageal region is indicated in cases where there is regurgitation of food from the nares, dysphagia, or suspected "choke." In cases where obstruction of the esophagus has occurred, it may be possible to visualize

TABLE 6–1. Changes in Abdominal Fluid with Different Abdominal Disorders

Condition	Gross Appearance	Total Nucleated Cell Count ($\times$ 10^6/L or per μl)	Total Protein Concentration (g/L)	Cytologic Appearance
Normal	Clear to yellow	<7,500 (<peripheral WBCC)	<20 (<2.0 g/dl)	Neutrophils 40–80% Mononuclear cells 20–50%
Abdominal abscess	Yellow to light brown, ± turbid, blood tinged	15,000–250,000	40–65 (4.0–6.5 g/dl)	Predominantly neutrophils with mild degenerative changes, ± intracellular Gram + cocci
Simple large bowel impaction or small intestinal obstruction (no devitalized tissue)	Yellow, clear	3000–15,000	<30 (<3.0 g/dl)	Predominantly neutrophils, good morphologic condition
Small intestinal strangulation (prerupture)	Red to brown, turbid to opaque, ± blood tinged	>5000–50,000	25–60 (2.5–6.0 g/dl)	Neutrophils predominant, degenerative changes moderate/severe
Anterior enteritis	Yellow, turbid, possibly serosanguinous	<10,000	30–45 (3.0–4.5 g/dl)	Predominantly neutrophils, fair morphologic condition
Bowel necrosis (rupture)	Orange to brown to green tinged, turbid, ± particulate matter	>150,000	50–65 (5.0–6.5 g/dl)	Highly cellular > 95% neutrophils, degenerative, many bacteria: Gram − and +, intra- and extracellular
Intestinal contents (sample from bowel lumen)	Green, turbid, much particulate matter	<1000	Variable	Relatively few cells, many *free* bacteria: Gram − and +

the site of the obstruction radiographically. Certainly, if there is rupture of the esophagus and localized cellulitis, this will be notable by the accumulation of gas in the periesophageal region. Contrast radiography using barium sulfate also may assist in providing diagnostically useful radiographs of the upper alimentary tract. When attempting to highlight the esophagus, we favor administration of the barium using a small-bore stomach tube that is inserted approximately 10 cm (4 in) into the esophagus. The dose of barium (about 500 ml for an adult horse) is then injected into the esophagus with a 1-L stomach pump. We find contrast radiography to be useful when attempting to define esophageal strictures and diverticula in adult horses and megaesophagus in foals. Although contrast techniques have been described for the diagnosis of gastric ulcers in foals, we have found this procedure unrewarding. Techniques for radiographic demonstration of enteroliths and sand impactions in adult horses have been reported but require equipment that is usually limited to large referral practices.

Ultrasound Examination

With the increased availability and reduced cost of ultrasound machines, this form of examination has become more popular in recent years. How-

ever, the technique is still restricted, particularly in large horses, because the beam will only penetrate to a maximum of about 30 cm. In general, sector scanners provide the best images, with 3.0- and 5.0-MHz heads being the most frequently used. The 3.0-Mhz scan head provides greater tissue penetration than the 5.0-MHz head, but this occurs at the expense of image quality. We have found that transabdominal ultrasound examination of the abdomen readily helps in identification of the liver, diaphragm, kidneys, spleen, peritoneal surfaces, and gut wall. For best images, the hair should be clipped and liberal amounts of coupling gel applied. We routinely use ultrasound guidance when performing biopsies of the liver, kidneys, and spleen. At times, organs in the caudal abdomen also may be imaged after passing the probe into the rectum.

KEY POINT ► Ultrasound examination provides evidence of increased fluid accumulation within the abdominal cavity, fibrinous accumulations on the peritoneal wall, and, at times, the presence of masses in the liver, spleen, or kidneys.

The liver can be imaged on the right side along the ventral border of the diaphragm between the seventh and fifteenth intercostal spaces. If there is a reduction in the hepatic mass, detection of the presence of the liver on this side may be more difficult. On the left side, the liver is located between the seventh and ninth intercostal spaces. Some indication of hepatic dimensions and architecture can be obtained with ultrasound examination. Other abnormalities that may detected include evidence of dilated bile ducts and dilated veins, the presence of choleliths, and in some cases the presence of hepatic tumors or abscesses. The spleen is located on the left side between the eighth and seventeenth intercostal spaces caudal to the liver. It is located in the cranioventral portion of the abdomen near the diaphragm and rises to a caudodorsal position lateral to the left kidney. We often find it difficult to obtain useful ultrasound information relating to the gastrointestinal tract because the gas within the lumen interferes with ultrasound waves.

Clinical Pathology

Clinical pathology examinations often provide an invaluable adjunct to diagnosis when attempting to define the cause or severity of alimentary tract disease. Logic dictates that these examinations be used to support the clinician's impressions based on the results of history and physical examination findings rather than being a sole means of diagnosis. However, judicious use of well-chosen clinical laboratory tests may have a significant influence on the clinician's diagnostic suspicions.

Hematology

Measurement of the hematocrit (PCV) is one of the most frequently performed laboratory tests in equine practice. An increase in the PCV (and red blood cell numbers) often occurs in association with abdominal disease in the horse. Circulating red blood cell numbers increase following splenic contraction, a response to catecholamine release, or as a result of a decrease in the plasma volume due to fluid loss.

KEY POINT ▶ Hemoconcentration is common in association with abdominal diseases, including gastrointestinal obstructions, peritonitis, diarrhea, and endotoxic shock.

Anemia, which is reduction in the red blood cell mass, may occur as a result of blood loss or as a consequence of bone marrow suppression. Blood loss from the alimentary system can occur as a result of parasitism, gastroduodenal ulcers, or gastric carcinoma. In contrast, bone marrow suppression is common in horses as a response to chronic inflammatory conditions (e.g., neoplasia and persistent infections) and is referred to as *anemia of chronic inflammatory disease*.

Alterations in the white blood cell count may be reflective of stress, inflammation, and infection. Stress (e.g., transport, exercise, or abdominal pain)

is the most common cause of a mature neutrophilia that is associated with reductions in the numbers of eosinophils and lymphocytes. This manifestation is referred to as a *stress leukogram*. In contrast, inflammation and infection will produce an increase in the neutrophil count with more limited changes in the numbers of other white cells. However, when extreme demand is placed on the horse's capacity to produce neutrophils, as may occur with severe enteric diseases, a neutropenia with *toxic neutrophils* may result.

Serum or Plasma Protein Concentration

Plasma protein is composed of three main fractions that are easily measured in the laboratory. The predominate fractions are albumin and globulins, with a lesser, but still important contribution by fibrinogen. Total plasma protein concentration will increase in response to dehydration and contraction of the plasma volume. Reduced water intake and disorders producing abdominal pain and shock may result in dehydration. In these conditions there is normally an increase in both albumin and globulin fractions. Hyperproteinemia also may occur as a result of increases in the globulin concentration in response to chronic antigenic stimulation. Hypoproteinemia occurs in response to protein-losing enteropathy and possibly liver disease. Loss of protein from the bowel may accompany enteritis, parasitism, neoplasia, and nonsteroidal anti-inflammatory drug toxicity.

KEY POINT ▶ Fibrinogen, the third major fraction of total plasma protein that is routinely measured, reflects the severity and duration of an inflammatory disease.

The normal serum fibrinogen concentration is 2 to 4 g/dl (200–400 mg/dl), which may increase to more than 8 g/L (800 mg/dl) in response to severe inflammation.

Serum Biochemistry

Determination of the plasma or serum concentration of electrolytes; activities of a number of cellular enzymes, minerals, bilirubin, bile acids; and acid–base balance is done in horses with suspected alimentary tract disease. With the exception of acid–base measurements, samples can be collected into serum or lithium heparin tubes. If there is to be a delay of more than a few hours before analysis, the samples should be centrifuged and the serum or plasma decanted and refrigerated until analysis is performed. Horses with acute diarrhea will often experience hyponatremia, hypochloremia, hypokalemia, and metabolic acidosis. The extent of these changes will depend on the severity of the diarrhea and whether the horse continues to drink water, thereby further diluting the concentrations of these electrolytes within the plasma. Hypocalcemia and hypomagnesemia also may occur with enteritis, particularly anterior enteritis, where there is loss of these ions with the fluid that is sequestered into the bowel lumen. Elevations in the serum activities of hepatic enzymes are often reflective of hepatic dysfunction. γ-Glutamyl transferase (GGT) is the best screening enzyme for liver disease, but there will also be elevations in the activities of alkaline phosphatase (AP), aspartate aminotransferase (AST), lactate dehydrogenase (LDH), and sorbitol dehydrogenase (SDH). It should be noted that the extent of the increases in activity does not always correlate with the degree of hepatic dysfunction. Increases in the serum concentration of bile acids will often accompany increases in the activities of hepatocellular enzymes. The concentration of bilirubin is relatively labile in the horse, undergoing mild elevations in response to inappetence, with more marked elevations accompanying liver or hemolytic diseases. Acid–base abnormalities are relatively common in association with acute gastrointestinal tract disorders.

KEY POINT ► The most common change is acidosis due to intestinal bicarbonate loss in association with severe enteritis and diarrhea.

In contrast, metabolic alkalosis may occur in diseases where there is substantial loss of hydrogen ions from the gut (e.g., anterior enteritis).

Fecal Examination

Detection of parasite ova using flotation in salt solutions is commonly employed for determination of parasitic infestation. In addition, feces may be examined for parasitic organisms, blood, and bacteria. Specific bacterial species can, at times, be isolated from feces (see Chap. 15). These include *Salmonella* spp., *Campylobacter* spp., *Clostridium* spp., and *Escherichia coli*. In addition, electron microscopy and use of ELISAs for determination of viral infection, particularly rotavirus in foals, also may be undertaken.

Liver Function Tests

The excretion of sulfobromophthalein (BSP) has been used as an indication of liver dysfunction. However, with the advent of techniques to measure serum bilirubin concentrations and, more recently, serum bile acid concentrations, the value in determining the excretion of BSP has been lessened. Alterations in specific liver function tests are discussed in the section on liver diseases.

Liver Biopsy

Liver biopsy is particularly useful for defining the cause, severity, and prognosis in horses with suspected hepatopathies. The site for insertion of the biopsy needle is the twelfth to fourteenth intercostal spaces of the right thorax on a line drawn be-

tween the tuber coxa and the point of the shoulder. An area of skin is clipped, shaved, and aseptically prepared. Local anesthetic (5 ml) is injected subcutaneously and into the intercostal muscles with a 23-gauge, 2.5-cm needle. A stab incision is made with a no. 11 or 15 scalpel blade. A biopsy needle (Tru-Cut, Baxter Travenol, St. Louis, Mo.; Franklin-modified Vim Silverman, Mueller and Company, Chicago, Ill.) is inserted and directed craniad and ventrad. The needle is passed through the diaphragm and 10 to 13 cm into the liver parenchyma (Figs. 6-18 and 6-19). The chances of a successful biopsy are improved if ultrasound is used to locate the liver and guide the biopsy needle. If ultrasound is available, biopsies also may be attempted in other sites, including the left side of the horse. Following collection, samples should be placed in formalin for subsequent histopathologic examinations or submitted for bacterial culture and sensitivity (if indicated). The skin wound can be left to heal by second intention or is sutured. Contraindications for liver biopsy include evidence of coagulopathies and suspicion of liver abscessation.

Small Intestinal Absorption Tests

KEY POINT ► Absorptive capacity of the small intestine is commonly evaluated using either the D-glucose or D-xylose absorption tests.

The D-glucose absorption test is easy and inexpensive to perform but is less specific than the D-xylose test because blood glucose concentration is affected by the horse's metabolic rate and a number of endocrine factors. To perform the test, the horse is fasted of food and water for approximately 12 hours prior to and during the test. This ensures

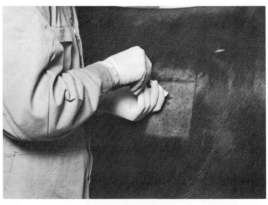

Figure 6–18. Liver biopsy. Position of biopsy needle. The needle has been inserted through the right fourteenth intercostal space, with the tip of the biopsy needle pointing toward the opposite elbow. The needle has been placed along a line drawn between the tuber coxae and the point of the shoulder.

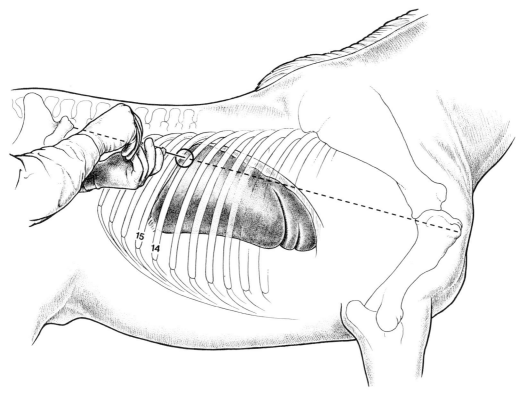

Figure 6–19. Liver biopsy. Line drawing showing position of needle in the liver.

that food does not delay the passage of glucose into the small intestine or otherwise influence the blood glucose concentration. Glucose is administered at a rate of 1 g/kg as a 20% solution via a nasogastric tube. A normal response is reflected by an increase in blood glucose concentrations of more than 100% over baseline values within 1 to 2 hours (Fig. 6-20).

Xylose is a sugar that is not normally found in equine plasma. Since plasma D-xylose concentration is not influenced by metabolic status, this test is proposed to be a more specific indicator of small intestinal absorptive capacity when compared with the D-glucose test. Disadvantages of the procedure include increased cost and restricted availability of the assay in many laboratories. The horse is fasted of food and water for 12 hours and 0.5 g/kg of D-xylose is given via a nasogastric tube. A D-xylose concentration of at least 1.0 mmol/L (15 mg/dl) should have occurred within 1 to 2 hours in normal horses (Fig. 6-21).

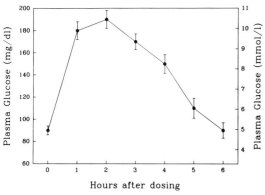

Figure 6–20. Oral D-glucose absorption test. Typical curve of plasma glucose values in adult horses after administration of 1.0 g/kg of D-glucose by stomach tube.

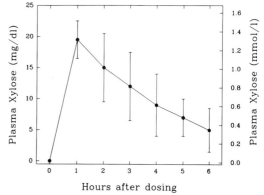

Figure 6–21. Oral D-xylose absorption test. Typical curve of plasma D-xylose values in adult horses after administration of 0.5 g/kg of D-xylose by stomach tube.

Examination and Approach to Treatment of the Horse with Abdominal Pain ("Colic")

Over 70 causes of colic in the horse have been identified. This discussion does not address all the known causes but rather will focus on abdominal pain in a problem-oriented fashion. With careful consideration of the history, signs, and appropriate laboratory data, it is hoped that this approach will help the clinician logically define what is the most likely cause of the colic. We base our examination technique on procedures described by White, and Bramlage.

Causes of Colic

- Impaction—usually large intestine
- Spasmodic (hypermotility)—usually small intestine
- Intussusception, telescoping of bowel—most commonly in ileocecal region
- Volvulus, rotation and twisting—usually of small intestine
- Torsion, twisting of bowel—most commonly large colon
- Strangulation, interruption to blood supply—may occur with volvulus and torsion
- Tympany, excessive gas production—particularly involving the cecum and large colon
- Colitis/enteritis—inflammatory disorder of intestine
- Thromboembolic (verminous)—chronic damage to cranial mesenteric artery due to *S. vulgaris.* There are several types, including segmental infarction, thrombosis without occlusion, and diffuse (stasis).

Anatomic Factors Predisposing the Horse to Colic

- Horse cannot vomit.
- Unfixed position of left colon.
- Long mesentery of small intestine.
- Upward movement of ingesta and narrowing of lumen at the pelvic flexure.
- Cecum is a blind sac.
- Termination of right dorsal colon into much narrower small colon.

History

The following general points are important to consider when gastrointestinal disease (colic) occurs:

- Husbandry—diet and diet changes
- Habitat—box stall, pasture, sandy soil, and weather changes
- Routine—changes in training, exercise, transport
- Vices—cribbing, windsucking, indiscriminant appetite
- Medical history—this and other horses'
- Parasite control

Specific Historical Aspects Pertaining to Colic

- Attitude—depressed, alert
- Signs—onset, duration
- Intensity and nature of pain
- Possible causes—if known
- Therapy—type and response
- Defecation—frequency, composition
- Pregnancy, breeding history

PHYSICAL EXAMINATION

Initial Inspection

- Determination of cardinal signs—temperature, pulse, respiration
- Presence of abdominal distension—usually reflective of cecal or large colon distension
- Signs seen—pawing, rolling, recumbency, abrasions (eyes, head, tuber coxae, and limbs)

KEY POINT ► It is important to be thorough and systematic when undertaking the examination and to assess the whole horse, not just one or two measurements.

A checklist to assist the clinician undertaking an examination of a horse with abdominal pain is provided as Table 6-2.

TABLE 6–2. Examination of the Horse with Abdominal Pain

Date: _____

Time: _____

CHECKLIST

1. Previous medication _____

2. Attitude _____

3. Severity of pain ☐ Severe ☐ Moderate ☐ Mild

4. Heart rate _____ beats/min

   Rectal temperature _____ degrees

   Respiratory rate _____ breaths/min

   Capillary refill time _____ seconds

   Mucous membrane color _____

5. Peristalsis Left side _____ Right side _____

6. Rectal palpation ☐ Yes ☐ No Result _____

7. Passage of nasogastric tube ☐ Yes ☐ No Result _____

8. Abdominal paracentesis ☐ Yes ☐ No Result _____

9. Packed cell volume _____ % Total plasma protein _____ gm/dl

Assessment of Pain

- Horses readily display signs of abdominal discomfort.
- Pain is the response to stimulation of receptors in the gut wall. Regardless of the lesion, the manifestations of pain consist of pawing, rolling, lying down, kicking at the abdomen, looking at the flanks, sweating, and attempts to urinate.
- Type of pain. Intense continuous pain is often associated with the most severe lesions, particularly proximal obstructions or strangulations.
- Obstruction of the bowel leads to accumulation of gas and fluids, resulting in pain and possibly shock. Pain is often more severe if the small intestine is involved, since this organ has a limited capacity for distension when compared with the large intestine.

KEY POINT ▶ Rule of thumb:

- Severe pain = proximal lesion with strangulation and fluid accumulation.
- Mild/moderate pain = nonobstructive lesions without strangulation.
- Extraluminal obstructions lead to ischemic bowel and reductions in lumen size, resulting in severe, often continuous pain with toxemia and subsequently shock. Intraluminal obstructions lead to an obstructed lumen with an intact blood supply, resulting in pain of moderate intensity. Pain is

often intermittent, since it is exacerbated by peristaltic movements.
- Acute, moderately intense pain may be associated with spasmodic contractions of the intestinal wall in stressed or excitable horses.
- Spontaneous remission of severe pain may accompany resolution of the problem; however, it should always be remembered that gastrointestinal decompression (and a dramatic reduction in the manifestations of pain) may accompany rupture of a viscus. Rupture of the stomach is a good example of this process.

Pulse and Heart Rate

- Pulse rate and strength are related to pain, vascular volume, and response to endotoxemia.
- The pulse can be felt in the facial, digital, brachial, and great metatarsal arteries (Fig. 1-13).
- Pulse rate is important to assist in the evaluation of cardiovascular status. Pulse rate and strength usually indicate the severity of the cardiovascular dysfunction occurring in response to the disease.
- A weak, thready, or absent pulse is related to a poor prognosis.
- Severe pain usually increases heart rate more than 80 beats per minute.
- Simple obstruction usually increases the heart rate to 40 to 65 beats per minute, strangulating obstructions from 50 to 100 beats per minute, and enteritis up to 90 beats per minute. This response will be influenced by the site of the lesion, vol-

ume of fluid loss, degree of toxemia, and duration of the problem.
- Spasmodic colic results in an intermittent increase in heart rate, often associated with increased gut motility.
- Pulse rate may indicate the severity of the disorder but may not help in making a diagnosis.
- Dehydration and shock result in increased heart rate and constriction of the peripheral vasculature in an attempt to maintain the central circulatory volume and cardiac output.

KEY POINT ► When examining a horse with colic, it is a good idea to:

- Take the heart rate with a stethoscope while concurrently measuring the pulse rate.
- Assess the pulse at several sites.
- Assess (if possible) the blood pressure.

Blood pressure is simply measured in the coccygeal artery using a Doppler device and pressure cuff applied to the tail. Normal systolic blood pressure in the adult horse is 100 to 125 mmHg. Results of a study equating systolic blood pressure with survival in horses with colic revealed that horses with a systolic pressure of less than 80 mmHg generally have a poor prognosis. Often, however, the outcome in these cases is related to the therapy employed. *Note:* Prolonged hypotension (systolic pressure <70 mmHg) for several hours will lead to irreversible tissue damage.

Peripheral Perfusion

- Best assessed by color and refill time of mucosae of the gingiva and orifices using digital pressure (see Fig. 1-2).
- Normal color is pale pink.
- Normal refill time is approximately 1.5 seconds.
- Dehydration and endotoxemia will be associated with altered perfusion and cardiovascular dysfunction.

Gut Sounds

- Normal sounds are gurgling and fluid mixing with gas.
- Auscultate at least four sites, including the dorsal and ventral abdomen, on both sides of the horse (see Figs. 1-20 and 1-21).
- Altered sounds may indicate the severity of involvement.
- In the right paralumbar fossa, ileocecal sounds, or "water down a drain pipe," are heard, one to three per minute.
- Obstructions cause decreased peristalsis.
- Spasmodic contractions result in hyperperistalsis.
- Absence of gut sounds is usually associated with a poor prognosis.

KEY POINT ► Gastrointestinal sounds should be reassessed frequently in a horse with continuing abdominal pain.

Rectal Examination

- Rectal examination is an integral part of the approach to a horse with colic, particularly in cases showing signs of severe or protracted pain.
- The clinician should have a routine for the examination which should always be undertaken in a thorough and systematic manner in horses with colic.
- Adequate restraint and lubrication are imperative.
- In horses who strain, infusion of local anesthetic into the rectum may be useful.

KEY POINT ► Be careful and patient when performing the rectal palpation.

- Determine size, shape, texture, position, and relation of organs with each other. Also note sensitivity to pressure and palpation (see Rectal Examination, p. 193).

Important Points Relating to Signs of Colic

Things to feel per rectum:

- Distended bowel, altered texture, tight bands
- Peritoneal surfaces—rough texture and fibrin tags indicate pathology.
- Location of the base of the cecum, feeling for the presence of tympany or impactions
- Medial displacement of the caudal edge of the spleen, which occurs when the large colon is displaced laterally and dorsally over the nephrosplenic ligament
- Alterations associated with the pelvic flexure

KEY POINT ► Always attempt to locate and examine the pelvic flexure, since it is a frequent site of impaction. This structure is mobile and may reside in a number of positions but is not necessarily displaced.

- Inguinal rings, especially in stallions, checking for herniation

DIAGNOSTIC AIDS
Passage of a Stomach Tube

- Since the horse cannot vomit, entubation allows decompression of the stomach and anterior gastrointestinal tract.
- Introduction of a tube into the stomach will provide a passage for reflux of gas and fluid. This reduces pain associated with distension and aids in prevention of gastric rupture. Regular manipulation of the tube and priming with water are necessary to ensure gastric decompression (see Passage of a Stomach tube, p. 194, and Figs. 6-10 to 6-13).
- In horses with severe pain, nasogastric entubation should be performed at the initiation of the examination to prevent gastric rupture.

- In cases where reflux persists, the tube can be left indwelling by taping it to the halter or suturing it to the nostril.
- In general, proximal lesions result in the most rapid accumulation of fluid.

KEY POINT ▶ It is important not to force medications into the stomach via the nasogastric tube.

Abdominocentesis

- Abdominocentesis is an easy and reliable way of assessing the condition of the abdominal contents (see p. 199).

KEY POINT ▶ Abdominocentesis is indicated in all cases of severe, persistent, or recurrent colic.

- The procedure is normally performed using an 18-gauge, 3.5-cm (1.5-in) needle inserted at the most dependent point of the abdomen. Complications are rare.
- Useful information is gained from gross and laboratory analysis of the fluid. Altered cell numbers and protein concentration will reflect the health of the bowel (see Table 6-1).

ASSESSMENT FOLLOWING INITIAL EXAMINATION

KEY POINT ▶ Most horses with colic recover spontaneously or respond to simple medical management and do not require surgery.

The most common manifestations include mild, intermittent pain with moderate elevations in heart rate and normal gut sounds. Blood pressure remains normal or is mildly elevated, the capillary refill time and mucous membrane color are normal. There are no abnormalities detected on rectal examination or reflux when gastric entubation is performed. Several studies have shown that less than 2% of horses afflicted with colic subsequently require surgical intervention. Therefore, although advances in fluid therapy, anesthesia, and surgery have increased survival rates in horses with severe

colic in recent years, animals requiring surgery still represent a minority of colic cases.

Following the initial examination, it is more the exception than the rule to have arrived at a definitive diagnosis. Usually the clinician will have sorted out a list of problems and their possible causes and have arrived at a plan for subsequent therapeutic and/or diagnostic measures.

ADDITIONAL DIAGNOSTIC TESTS

Depending on the severity of the case, other diagnostic tests may be indicated.

Hematocrit and Total Protein

- These procedures provide a relatively easy and accurate method for assessing the hydration status.
- Rules of thumb when assessing PCV and TPP are presented in Table 6-3.

Blood Gas Analysis

- Many gastrointestinal abnormalities will produce a metabolic acidosis with respiratory compensation. Typical values are pH 7.3 units, pCO_2 35 mmHg, and HCO_3^- 15 mmol/L (mEq/L).
- Arterial samples are preferable and are relatively easily collected from the carotid artery (see Fig. 4-11).
- Rapid deterioration in acid–base status is often associated with a poor prognosis.

Serum Electrolyte and Chemistry Profiles

- Since colic usually has a relatively rapid course and fluid losses are generally isotonic, substantial alterations in plasma electrolyte values are relatively unusual. Some exceptions exist: *Gastric dilatation* produces sequestration of fluids and HCl, leading to dehydration, hypochloremia, and alkalosis. *Anterior enteritis* leads to substantial gastric reflux with large fluid, electrolyte, and protein losses. Hypocalcemia may accompany these changes. *Large colon obstructions* produce progressive dehydration and a decrease in plasma Cl due to sequestration in the gut lumen.

TABLE 6–3. Interpretation of Hematocrit and Total Protein Changes Associated with Colic in Horses

PCV (%)	Total Plasma Protein (g/L)	Indications for Fluid Therapy
<40	<75 (<7.5 g/dl)	None required; observe for deterioration
40–45	75–85 (7.5–8.5 g/dl)	Intravenous isotonic fluids indicated (20–40 ml/kg); note any continued deterioration
45–55	85–95 (8.5–9.5 g/dl)	Intravenous fluids definitely required (40–60 ml/kg)
>55	>95 (>9.5 g/dl)	Rapid and large-volume intravenous fluid therapy required (60–100 ml/kg)

Note: Few horses with PCVs > 60% and TPPs > 100 g/L (10 g/dl) survive, regardless of therapy.

- Prerenal azotemia, due to increases in serum urea and creatinine concentrations, is common in horses with complicated abdominal disease. This is usually due to the combined effects of hypovolemia and endotoxemia.
- Serum enzyme changes may be reflective of certain disorders in horses with colic. Increased serum alkaline phosphatase (AP) activity results from its liberation from damaged intestinal walls and white blood cells. This is a common feature of complicated abdominal disease in the horse.
- Increases in serum γ-glutamyl transferase (GGT) activity provides a good screening test for hepatic dysfunction.
- Increased bilirubin concentration may reflect inappetence, hemolysis, or a hepatopathy. Mild increases are a feature of reductions in feed intake, whereas larger elevations often accompany hepatopathies and hemolysis.
- Elevations in the serum bile acid concentration accompany cholestasis.
- Muscle damage associated with pain and self-inflicted trauma may result in increased serum creatine phosphokinase (CPK), aminoaspartate transferase (AST), and lactate dehydrogenase (LDH) activities.

Is Surgery Necessary?

Some guidelines relating to the decision to refer for surgery are given in Table 6-4.

MEDICAL MANAGEMENT OF COLIC

In addition to abdominal pain, gastrointestinal diseases result in alterations in gut motility, obstructions, vascular compromise of affected abdominal organs, endotoxemia, and shock. If un-

treated, these processes may lead to debility or death of the patient. Considering these factors, a clinician must approach the medical management of colic in a logical manner and utilize appropriate medications.

Control of Pain

Analgesia is one of the most important aspects in the management of colic. Although analgesics relieve many of the physical signs of pain, administration of these agents must be tempered, given that they may mask signs of progression of the disorder.

Nonsteroidal Anti-Inflammatory Drugs

Nonsteroidal anti-inflammatory drugs (NSAIDs) inhibit cyclooxygenase, an enzyme involved in the arachadonic acid cascade, which is integrally involved in the production of prostaglandins, many of which are potent mediators of abdominal pain in horses. NSAIDs constitute one of the most frequently utilized groups of drugs in the treatment of abdominal pain. They exert their effect by reducing the concentration of inflammatory mediators at the site of the lesion, decreasing the perception of pain by the central nervous system, and reducing fever. Phenylbutazone (Treatment No. 88), flunixin meglumine (Treatment No. 52), dipyrone (Treatment No. 36), and ketoprofen (Treatment No. 66) are the most commonly used NSAIDs. Dosage schedules are provided in Tables 6-5 and 17-4. Phenylbutazone and dipyrone have mild effects when used to relieve abdominal pain, whereas flunixin meglumine and ketoprofen exert more profound analgesic effects. Flunixin meglumine is the most potent NSAID for control of visceral pain, with effects lasting 1 to several hours. A disadvantage of flunixin meglumine is its ability to mask the signs of endotoxemia. As a result, the drug may disguise the

TABLE 6–4. Guidelines for Referral for Possible Surgical Intervention

Referral for Surgery Indicated	Sign/Clinical Manifestation	Continued Medical Management Indicated
Depressed	Attitude	Alert, responsive
Moderate-severe, progressive	Severity of pain	Mild-moderate, transient
HR > 75/min, pulse—weak, CRT > 2.5 s, injected mucous membranes, cold extremities, "shock"; normal/slightly increased temperature	Cardinal signs	HR < 55/min, pulse—strong, CRT < 1.5 s, pink mucous membranes, warm extremities; pyrexia—persistent
Ileus, no feces passed	Peristalsis	Peristalsis present, passage of feces
> 5 L ± rapid reaccumulation of fluid	Nasogastric reflux	< 2 L
Bowel distension/displacement	Rectal palpation	No abnormalities detected
See Table 6–1	Abdominal paracentesis	See Table 6–1
Moderate-severe elevation (see Table 6–3)	PCV and TPP	Mild elevation (see Table 6–3)
Poor: continuing pain, metabolic deterioration, progressive CNS depression	Response to therapy	Good: decreased pain, improved cardinal signs and hydration status

clinical manifestations of potentially devastating gastrointestinal lesions, in particular strangulations. Drugs that mask signs and therefore delay the decision for referral for surgery are contraindicated. In an attempt to overcome this problem, reductions in dose rate and increases in dosage frequency of flunixin meglumine provide a valuable means of reducing the adverse effects of endotoxemia (fluid shifts, cardiovascular compromise, shock, etc.) while providing some limited analgesic effects. This treatment strategy allows frequent reassessment of the horse's condition and appropriate decisions to be made. Ketoprofen blocks cyclooxygenase and lipooxygenase, an enzyme responsible for induction of other inflammatory mediators. In particular, lipooxygenase stimulates mediators capable of promoting neutrophil chemotaxis, which is a potent mechanism for local cellular damage. Ketoprofen is not as effective as flunixin meglumine for alleviating abdominal pain in the horse.

Sedative/Analgesics

Xylazine (Treatment No. 108) and detomidine (Treatment No. 28) are α_2-adrenoceptor agonists that induce analgesia (by suppression of CNS neurotransmission) and muscle relaxation. At high doses (1.1 mg/kg IV or IM), xylazine is a potent drug for the control of abdominal pain, with effects lasting up to 45 minutes. In many cases where pain is less intense, lower doses (0.3–0.7 mg/kg IV or IM) provide effective analgesia. Many clinicians routinely use lower doses, since the short duration of action allows for repeated assessment of the animal's condition without long-term masking of signs. The most potentially serious side effects of α_2-adrenoceptor agonist drugs are hypotension, decreased cardiac output, ileus, and decreased intestinal blood flow, all of which are dose-dependent. Detomidine is more potent than xylazine, with analgesia and sedation lasting up to 90 minutes. Although this drug produces similar side effects to xylazine, doses producing equipotent analgesic effects induce fewer detrimental effects on cardiovascular function and gastrointestinal motility. Dosage information for xylazine and detimodine are provided in Tables 6-5 and 17-4.

Narcotics

Although nonnarcotic analgesics (e.g., flunixin meglumine and xylazine) are now used more commonly for the treatment of abdominal pain in horses, narcotics retain a place in the treatment of abdominal pain because of their potent analgesic and sedative effects. Morphine, oxymorphone, and meperidine have all been used. Two other agents, butorphanol (Treatment No. 15) and pentazocine (Treatment No. 86) have the most predictable analgesia and freedom from adverse side effects, although pentazocine is now rarely used because of its limited and short-lived analgesic effects.

KEY POINT ► Butorphanol provides good analgesia that lasts for 10 to 90 minutes depending on dose and cause of the pain.

Many clinicians combine xylazine (up to 0.2–0.4 mg/kg IV) with butorphanol (0.02–0.1 mg/kg IV) to provide improved analgesia in horses with severe abdominal pain (Table 6-5). Morphine, oxymorphone, and meperidine are potent analgesics but have the unfortunate side effects of paradoxical excitation, increased activity/agitation, and a reduction in gastrointestinal transit time.

Laxatives/Lubricants

KEY POINT ► Softening (hydration) and lubrication of impactions in the large colon are the usual indications for administration of lubricants.

Hydration and passage of intraluminal obstructions/impactions are usually achieved by a combination of fluid therapy (intravenous or oral) and administration of inert lubricating agents.

KEY POINT ► Care should be taken not to administer oral fluids to horses with gastric reflux.

Large volumes (100–120 ml/kg) of intravenous fluids are effective in softening many impacted masses. Methods for administration and objectives of fluid therapy are discussed elsewhere in this chapter and in Chapter 17.

Mineral oil (Treatment No. 77) is the lubricant of choice of many equine clinicians. It is a surface lubricant that facilitates the passage of ingesta through the gastrointestinal tract by direct lubricant effects and reduction of intestinal water absorption. The latter effect increases the hydration of intraluminal contents. The therapeutic efficacy of mineral oil is limited to the treatment of mild obstructions. Dose rates of 5 to 10 ml/kg PO q12–24h are usually prescribed (see Table 6-5).

Psyllium hydrophilic mucilloid (Treatment No. 97) is administered orally and absorbs water, acting as a laxative by increasing the water content and bulk of the fecal mass. Psyllium can be administered safely up to four times per day. The most common indication for this agent is in the management of sand ingestion. Following diagnosis of sand impaction (see p. 232), psyllium (1 g/kg PO q24h) should be prescribed for several weeks to encourage the expulsion of sand from the large colon. Longer-term therapy is thought to result in decreased effectiveness owing to a more rapid microbial degradation of the mucilloid in the colon.

Dioctyl sodium sulfosuccinate (DSS) (Treatment No. 35) is a detergent designed to decrease the surface tension of intraluminal masses and allow increased penetration of water and ions. The dose rate is 10 to 20 mg/kg PO q48h as a 5% solution (see Table 6-5).

TABLE 6–5. Drugs Utilized for the Medical Management of Colic

Drug	Action/Drug Group	Dosage	Side Effects
Phenylbutazone	NSAID	2.2–4.4 mg/kg IV q12–24h	Gut mucosa and renal toxicity
Flunixin meglumine	NSAID	0.25 mg/kg IV, IM q6–8h 0.5–1.1 mg/kg IV, IM q12–24h	At higher doses may mask signs of endotoxemia; gut mucosa and renal toxicity
Dipyrone	NSAID	5–22 mg/kg IV, IM q12–24h	Limited pain relief
Xylazine	Sedative/analgesic	0.3–1.1 mg/kg IV, IM as required	Hypotension, decreased cardiac output, ileus, ↓ GIT blood flow
Detomidine	Sedative/analgesic	10–30 μg/kg IV as required	Hypotension, ↓ cardiac output, ileus, ↓ GIT blood flow
Butorphanol	Opioid analgesic	0.05–0.1 mg/kg IV, IM as required 0.02–0.1 mg/kg IV, IM in combination with xylazine (0.2–0.4 mg/kg IV, IM)	Excitement at higher doses, possibly ↓ GIT motility
Mineral oil	Laxative	5–10 ml/kg PO q12–24h	Contraindicated when reflux or complete obstruction present
Psyllium hydrophilic mucilloid	Laxative	1 g/kg PO q6–24h	Prolonged use may result in ↓ efficacy
Dioctyl sodium sulfosuccinate	Detergent/laxative	10–20 mg/kg PO q48h as a 5% solution	Concentrated solutions and increased dosing frequency may result in diarrhea
Neostigmine	GIT motility stimulant	0.02 mg/kg SC q30min for up to 5 doses	↑ Pain, sweating, inappropriate changes in motility
Bethanechol	GIT motility stimulant	0.025 mg/kg SC q6–8h for 3–4 doses Then 0.3–0.4 mg/kg PO q6–8h	Sweating, ↑ pain, inappropriate GIT motility
Dimethyl sulfoxide	Anti-inflammatory agent, free radical scavenger	0.5–0.9 g/kg IV q12–24h as a 10–20% solution for 2–3 days	Hemolysis

KEY POINT ▶ Higher dose rates, more frequent administration, or the use of more concentrated solutions can result in diarrhea.

Magnesium sulfate has been a popular laxative in years past. It is now infrequently used because of its potential toxic effects on the gastrointestinal mucosa.

Agents Affecting Gastrointestinal Motility

Reduction in gastrointestinal motility (ileus) is a frequent side effect of diseases of the abdominal cavity. Peritonitis, local derangements in blood flow, and endotoxemia are all potentially potent inducers of ileus. As a result, attempts have been made to find agents that assist in returning gastrointestinal motility to normal (see Table 6-5).

Neostigmine (Prostigmin, Hoffmann-LaRoche, Nutley, N.J.) in doses of 0.02 mg/kg SC q30min increases the concentration of acetylcholine and thereby directly stimulates gastrointestinal motility. The major side effect of neostigmine is the induction of disorganized, segmental contractions that are likely to be of little benefit in increasing gastrointestinal progression of ingesta. Other side effects include increases in abdominal pain and sweating. As a result, the overall efficacy of neostigmine for the treatment of ileus is questionable.

Bethanechol (Urecholine, Merck Sharp & Dohme, Rahway, N.J.) in doses of 0.25 mg/kg SC q6–8h for two or three doses, followed by maintenance doses of 0.3 to 0.4 mg/kg PO q6–8h, has been prescribed to increase gastric emptying. Quite variable results have been reported. Increased salivation is a common side effect.

Metoclopramide (Reglan, AH Robbins, Richmond, Va.) has been utilized as a potential gastrointestinal stimulant because of its action as a nonspecific dopaminergic antagonist at a dose rate of 0.25 mg/kg IV q6–8h. Dopaminergic hyperactivity is regarded as an integral factor in the genesis of ileus.

KEY POINT ▶ Unfortunately, when administered at dose rates necessary to alleviate ileus, metoclopramide frequently results in central nervous system stimulation.

Nonsteroidal anti-inflammatory drugs inhibit some of the toxic side effects of endotoxemia invoking ileus. Flunixin meglumine (Treatment No. 52) is regarded as the most potent NSAID exerting antagonism to the effects of endotoxemia. As mentioned earlier, administration of lower doses (0.25 mg/kg q6–8h IV) of this drug results in a reduction of many of the untoward effects of endotoxemia without posing the risk of prolonged masking of signs or toxicity.

Dimethyl sulfoxide (DMSO; Treatment No. 34) is a solvent that is thought to exert good tissue penetration and anti-inflammatory effects. This latter effect is purported to be the result of the scavenging of free radicals produced by inflammatory cells. Empirical studies indicate that DMSO given to horses with endotoxemia and subsequent to bowel ischemia (0.1–0.5 g/kg q24h IV as a 10% to 20% solution) may improve the chances of survival when compared with untreated horses.

Fluid Therapy

Large-volume fluid therapy must be strongly considered in horses with severe abdominal pain or gastrointestinal disease showing evidence of compromise of cardiovascular function. Fluid therapy is discussed elsewhere in this chapter and in Chapter 17.

KEY POINT ▶ Fluid therapy is also valuable when treating intraluminal obstructions, particularly impactions of the large colon.

In these cases, therapy is designed to augment cardiovascular function and to assist in increasing the volume of fluid in the gastrointestinal tract. This increase in fluid serves to assist in hydration and maceration of the impacted mass. In cases where there is only partial obstruction of the lumen, as evidenced by the passage of small amounts of feces, and no gastric reflux, oral fluids may provide a convenient and inexpensive means of providing fluid support. An adult horse can tolerate volumes of 6 to 8 L of isotonic fluid administered via nasogastric tube every hour.

KEY POINT ▶ If complete obstruction or gastric reflux is present, fluids should not be administered by nasogastric tube.

Diseases of the Oral Cavity

Cleft Palate

Cleft palate is a disorder that is most commonly recognized in young foals resulting in ill thrift and discharge of food from the nostrils. The etiology of this disorder is unknown; however, it is a congenital condition.

History and Presenting Signs

■ Foals usually presented because of milk or water discharging from nares.

■ Failure to gain weight at an appropriate rate.

Clinical Findings and Diagnosis

■ On physical examination, foals are frequently in poor body condition, may have secondary pneumonia due to inhalation of material into the lungs, and as a result, lung sounds can be harsh and there also can be nasal discharge.

■ When foals attempt to drink, milk often discharges from the nares.

- The disorder is usually diagnosed on the basis of clinical signs and by visual inspection.
- A cleft palate can vary in degree from fissures in the soft and hard palates to only a small cleft in the posterior soft palate.
- Lesions can be defined either by oral examination or via endoscopic examination of the mouth and palate.

Differential Diagnosis

- Pneumonia from other causes
- Dysphagia
- Megaesophagus
- Choke

Treatment

- The fundamental principle of treatment is surgical repair of the deficit in the palate. Usually this is successful only in cases where there is a small cleft in the soft palate.
- Since access to the palate requires a mandibular symphysiotomy, it is important to assess the foal's general state of health prior to general anesthesia.
- This assessment will involve determination of the degree of aspiration pneumonia that may have occurred, a process usually requiring careful auscultation, hematology, and thoracic radiographs.

KEY POINT ► The surgical procedure is relatively complex and has a reasonably high degree of complications. As a result, most foals with a cleft palate that are likely candidates for surgical repair are sent to referral centers for treatment.

Cystic Sinuses

This is a condition in which there appears to be multiple cyst formation, usually within the nasal turbinate region.

History and Presenting Signs

Usually occurs in young animals.

Clinical Findings and Diagnosis

- Maxillary, mandibular, or facial distortion
- In severe cases, the nares become partially occluded, resulting in dyspnea. In such cases, "kissing" lesions in the nasal mucosa may produce secondary ulceration.
- Diagnosis is based on radiographic changes, and in early cases, differentiation between dentigerous cysts and cystic sinus disease can be difficult.

Differential Diagnosis

- Dentigerous cysts
- Secondary hyperparathyroidism
- Dental tumors

- Trauma
- Retained tooth caps
- Paranasal sinus cysts

Treatment

- In severe cases, attempted treatment is usually unrewarding.
- Some animals survive for protracted periods if the cysts are small and relatively noninvasive.

KEY POINT ► Surgery via maxillary and/or frontal sinus flaps to enable curettage of the cysts and associated structures may give excellent results in many milder cases. Note that hemorrhage in such cases can be severe.

Dentigerous Cysts

Dentigerous cysts are tumor-like structures of epithelial origin that frequently contain structures with tooth-like appearance. When cysts occur on the head, they are considered important because of their potential to disfigure the affected animal.

History and Presenting Signs

- Usually in younger animals
- Presence of a lump or facial/mandibular distortion is commonly reported.

Clinical Findings and Diagnosis

- The most common site for dentigerous cysts is in the area near the ear, where they are referred to as *temporal cysts*.
- Discharge from these cysts draining either into or near the ear may be seen.
- Other sites for dentigerous cysts include the maxillary sinus and elsewhere on the face.

KEY POINT ► Diagnosis is based on the presence of characteristic lesions in younger horses. The lesions are usually located in temporal, aural, or maxillary sinus regions.

- In some cases, a draining tract may be present.
- Radiographs usually reveal a cystic cavity with a high likelihood of dental-like structures within the cavity.

Differential Diagnosis

- Retained tooth caps with secondary alveolar periostitis
- Dental or paranasal sinus tumors
- Other causes of maxillary or facial deformity (e.g., nutritional secondary hyperparathyroidism)
- Local abscesses
- Trauma
- Paranasal sinus cysts

Treatment

- Resection of the dentigerous cyst is the usual course of action, with particular care being taken to remove all the lining of the cystic cavity.
- Following removal, the cavity is packed and the dead space is allowed to heal by second intention.

Gingivitis/Stomatitis

A number of conditions, including bacterial, viral, and mycotic diseases, can cause primary stomatitis, whereas other diseases (e.g., periodontal disease) may result in secondary manifestations of stomatitis.

History and Presenting Signs

- Inappetence or reluctance to eat
- Depression
- Salivation
- History of phenylbutazone administration

Clinical Findings and Diagnosis

- Generalized swelling and redness with ulceration noticed around the stomal and gingival tissues
- In severe cases, there can be large ulcerative lesions that result in increased salivation and substantial discomfort to the horse, producing a reluctance to eat and drink.
- Severely affected animals may become progressively dehydrated owing to their reluctance or inability to consume fluids.
- The most common causes of stomatitis in horses are vesicular stomatitis, horse pox, candidiasis, and possibly infections by *Pseudomonas* and *Rhodococcus* spp.
- Secondary stomatitis may accompany phenylbutazone toxicity, photosensitization, uremia, and possibly mercury toxicity. Other causes of stomal lesions may include lampas, where there is a swelling of the palate just caudal to the incisors. This process occurs in young horses during eruption of the permanent incisors. Lampas has clinical manifestations similar to those occurring in horses with stomatitis. Affected animals may be reluctant to eat and may salivate excessively when eating.

Differential Diagnosis

- Primary or secondary stomatitis
- Lampas
- Neoplasia
- Dental problems (e.g., retained tooth caps, malocclusion, enamel points, periodontal disease)

Treatment

- If treatment of primary stomatitis is undertaken, it involves attempts to reduce the local inflammatory response, including lavage of the mouth with mild antiseptic solutions (e.g., povidone-iodine).
- In cases where phenylbutazone toxicosis is the cause of the stomatitis, the drug should be discontinued.
- In animals that are severely affected, systemic nonsteroidal anti-inflammatory therapy and antibiotic coverage may be required. We commonly use phenylbutazone at a dose rate of 2.2 mg/kg q12h and procaine penicillin at 15,000 to 20,000 IU/kg (15–20 mg/kg) q12h.
- Those animals reluctant to eat or drink may require fluid administration, either via a nasogastric tube or intravenously (see Chap. 17).
- Horses with secondary stomatitis require diagnosis and treatment of the primary disease process to allow management of the secondary manifestation.
- Lampas is temporarily debilitating and resolves spontaneously.

Oral Ulceration

A number of conditions result in oral ulceration in the horse. Ulcers can be asymptomatic or cause dysphagia and painful mastication, thereby producing inappetence. Lesions are described by a variety of terms, including *vesicals, ulcers, crusts,* and *growths.* Sites where lesions occur include the lips, tongue, gingiva, palate, and pharynx.

History and Presenting Signs

- The main infectious cause of oral ulceration is the vesicular stomatitis virus.
- Other causes include phenylbutazone toxicity, yellow bristle grass ingestion, ulcers due to plant thorns, and oral foreign bodies.
- Other causes include the ingestion of toxic chemicals (e.g., when horses lick mercury blisters off their legs following ingestion of blister beetles), as a consequence of periodontal disease, and also possibly as a result of uremia.

Clinical Findings and Diagnosis

- Horses with vesicular stomatitis first develop small vesicles in the mouth, and then these vesicles turn into large ulcers. The tongue is often severely involved.
- There may be excessive salivation and fever associated with the early stages of the condition.
- Diagnosis is usually based on the presence of lesions within the mouth, on the lips or gums, or in the pharynx. In the case of toxicity, there is a history of ingestion of toxic materials such as high doses of phenylbutazone.
- The oral cavity should always be checked for plant thorns and foreign bodies, as well as for the presence of periodontal disease.

216 ■ ALIMENTARY SYSTEM

- Horses that have ingested blister beetles will often have other systemic signs, such as enteritis, polyuria, and hypocalcemia.
- Clinical pathology will readily determine the presence of uremia.

Differential Diagnosis

- Vesicular stomatitis
- Phenylbutazone toxicity
- Foxtail or plant thorn stomatitis
- Oral foreign body
- Ulcers secondary to yellow bristle grass
- Chemical stomatitis
- Periodontal disease
- Blister beetle toxicosis
- Uremia

Treatment

KEY POINT ▶ Vesicular stomatitis has an appearance similar to foot and mouth disease, and it is important that this highly contagious disease be appropriately diagnosed.

- If foot and mouth disease is suspected, veterinarians are obliged to make contact with state and federal authorities to confirm the diagnosis and undertake appropriate quarantine measures.
- If vesicular stomatitis is not suspected and another cause of oral ulceration is most likely, treatment strategies will involve local therapy to relieve the oral irritation, such as mouthwashes, removal of plant thorns or foreign bodies if present, and removal of any chemical irritants that may be causing oral ulceration (e.g., phenylbutazone).
- If the oral ulceration is secondary to periodontal disease, appropriate dental prophylactic measures (e.g., removal of affected teeth) should be undertaken.

Salivary Gland Diseases

Diseases of the salivary glands or their ducts are relatively rare, with the most common disorder being trauma to the parotid duct.

History and Presenting Signs

- History of trauma (e.g., kicks, wire cuts, etc.) or surgery to the parotid or guttural pouch region.
- Owners may report salivary discharge, particularly in association with feeding.

Clinical Findings and Diagnosis

- Affected horses will usually have evidence of trauma to the area of the mandible. Discharge of saliva from the wound is common.
- Trauma to the parotid salivary gland also may occur if the animal receives an injury caudal to the angle of the mandible near the location of the guttural pouch.
- The discharge of saliva from the wound is most profuse when the animal eats, since saliva production is at its greatest during this activity.
- If the duct ruptures subcutaneously following trauma, saliva may accumulate in that area, and the horse may be presented with a swelling in the mandibular region.
- Diagnosis is usually based on a history or evidence of previous trauma and the discharge of saliva from the wound. If the fluid is accumulating subcutaneously, a salivary mucocele can be differentiated from a seroma by aspiration of the fluid.
- By laboratory analysis, saliva has much higher concentrations of calcium and potassium than is found in most other fluid accumulations.

Differential Diagnosis

- Trauma (e.g., seroma, hematoma, or fracture)
- Bone sequestrum and local osteitis
- Mandibular or guttural pouch abscessation
- Neoplasia

Treatment

- Wounds to the parotid gland usually require appropriate cleansing, debridement of devitalized tissue, and suturing.
- In order to promote healing and decrease gland secretion, the horse is usually fed via a nasogastric tube and given an electrolyte mix and gruels for several days to decrease parotid gland secretion.

KEY POINT ▶ Salivary gland fistulas occurring as a result of trauma to the parotid duct will often heal spontaneously.

- However, those which do not heal after several weeks probably require surgical management with the aim to either (1) attempt to reestablish the duct or (2) destroy the salivary gland.
- An incision is made down to the duct, an appropriate-diameter medical-grade silicone tube is passed into the caudad portion of the duct and then into the rostrad portion of the duct and out into the salivary papilla in the cheek. The duct ends are then sutured together with fine suture material such as 5-0 Dexon, and the piece of the tube emerging from the salivary papilla is sutured to the cheek. The tube is allowed to remain in place for approximately 2 weeks and is then removed. If this procedure appears too complex, an alternative method involves ligation of the proximal end of the duct near the gland. An incision is made down to the duct, and the duct is ligated with umbilical tape, with care not to tie the ligature too tightly. This ensures that the lig-

ature does cut the duct before the gland atrophies. This method will promote gland atrophy and provide resolution of the problem.

Trauma to the Lips and Tongue

The most common injuries to the lips and tongue involve direct chemical irritation from exposure to caustic substances or injury to these structures by foreign-body penetration or direct trauma. The tongue and lips are often injured by wire, nails, pieces of wood, plant thorns, and so on. Injury can be iatrogenic secondary to dental procedures or overzealous manipulation of the tongue. Most injuries are minor, but at times damage can be severe.

History and Presenting Signs

- Reluctance to eat
- Blood or saliva discharging from the mouth
- History of trauma or overzealous grasping of the tongue during oral/dental procedures

Clinical Findings and Diagnosis

- Increased salivation. Sometimes the mouth will remain open, and evidence of trauma will be obvious. The tongue may hang out.
- Lacerations and foreign bodies within the tongue usually produce substantial pain in the horse. There may be reluctance to eat, evidence of salivation, or evidence of blood coming from the mouth.
- In some cases, the damage to the tongue will be readily obvious.
- Given the extensive blood supply to the tongue, the potential for hemorrhage following lacerations is relatively great.
- Diagnosis of lingual lacerations or foreign bodies is usually made on the basis of careful visual and physical examination.
- Lacerations are usually self-evident.
- Foreign bodies (e.g., wire or wood) in the tongue or lips may be difficult to locate. The only clinical sign may be local swelling and a draining sinus. Careful palpation of the tongue is often required to define the presence of a foreign body.
- Palpation of the region and possibly radiographs using contrast techniques following infusion of contrast media into the draining tract may be required to confirm the diagnosis.
- Tears, swelling, and pain in the region of the frenulum of the tongue may be visualized. Sublingual cellulitis also may be present. Sublingual cellulitis commonly occurs following damage to the frenulum resulting from overzealous, forceful ex-

teriorization of the tongue during dental or oral procedures. Diagnosis is based on visualization of damage to the frenulum and local swelling.
- Ingestion of yellow bristle grass. Thorns from the grass lodge in the oral cavity and produce granulating wounds.
- Diagnosis of injuries to the tongue is usually based on direct physical examination.

Differential Diagnosis

- Trauma to the tongue
- Lingual foreign bodies
- Sublingual cellulitis
- Primary or secondary stomatitis
- Oral ulceration
- Lampas
- Periodontal disease
- Dysphagia
- Botulism
- Nigropallidal encephalomalacia

Treatment

- Most lacerations of the lips and tongue, if small, will heal spontaneously with little direct treatment. However, severe contusions of these structures require wound debridement and suturing.
- Suturing the tongue is important to ensure good apposition of the various layers of tissue.
- In some very severe cases of tongue laceration, where the tip of the tongue is almost severed, partial glossectomy may be indicated.
- When performing the partial glossectomy, care should be taken to ensure that large vessels are appropriately ligated to prevent the potential for significant hemorrhage. If the lesion is small, only a wedge-shaped segment of the tongue may need to be removed.
- Healing of the tongue appears to occur rapidly and is often uncomplicated.
- Foreign bodies require surgical extirpation and suturing of the wounds.
- Additional treatment involves nonsteroidal antiinflammatory therapy such as phenylbutazone (Treatment No. 88) at a dose rate of 2.2 mg/kg q12h for 4 to 7 days. In severe cases, antibiotic coverage is indicated. Procaine penicillin (15,000–20,000 IU/kg [15–20 mg/kg] q12h; Treatment No. 83) or trimethoprim–sulfonamide combinations (15 mg/kg of combined agent IV q12h; Treatment No. 107) are good choices.
- Nursing care is important, with provision of adequate fluids and palatable, nutritious foods indicated.

Diseases of the Teeth

Dental disorders are relatively common in horses and frequently require veterinary attention. As a result, the attending veterinarian must have a good working knowledge of the dental formulas, structure of the teeth, and normal times for tooth eruption. Horses have an initial set of deciduous teeth that are subsequently replaced by permanent teeth. The times at which the deciduous teeth erupt in the foal are presented in Table 6-6, whereas the times for eruption of permanent teeth can be found in Table 6-7. Integral to the successful diagnosis of dental problems is the clinician's ability to perform a safe, thorough, and expedient examination of the dental arcades and oral cavity.

Because of their potential to interfere with the animal's ability to eat, dental problems often manifest as either a reluctance to eat or a spillage of food from the mouth during mastication. Sometimes the sharp edges on teeth may cause pain when the horse is being ridden with a bit in its mouth. Affected horses may show behavioral changes such as head shaking, failure to respond to commands, and other refractory behavior.

DENTAL EXAMINATION

An appropriate history should be obtained outlining the dietary habits, any evidence of quidding (spillage of food from the mouth during mastication), vices, or foul breath and taking note of the animal's age. A thorough dental examination is then performed. It is important that the horse is relatively relaxed, and in anxious individuals, mild tranquilization may be necessary. The first part of

TABLE 6–7. Times for Eruption of Permanent Teeth in the Horse

Tooth	Time of Eruption
Incisors	
1st Permanent (I1)	2.5 years (in wear 3 years)
2nd Permanent (I2)	3.5 years (in wear 4 years)
3rd Permanent (I3)	4.5 years (in wear 5 years)
Canine	
Permanent (C)	4–5 years
Premolars	
1st Permanent (wolf tooth)	~6 months
2nd Permanent (P2)	2.5 years
3rd Permanent (P3)	3 years
4th Permanent (P4)	4 years
Molars	
1st Permanent (M1)	~12 months
2nd Permanent (M2)	2 years
3rd Permanent (M3)	~4 years

the examination involves visual inspection of the incisors, with note being made of abnormalities in bite, such as "parrot mouth" or "sow mouth," and whether there are deciduous teeth still present. If so, it should be determined whether those teeth are about to be shed. The veterinarian also should check for the presence of supernumerary teeth and sharp edges on the incisors. Some indication of the presence of sharp edges on the buccal edges of the cheek teeth, particularly those in the upper arcade, can be obtained by external palpation through the cheeks. Following this initial examination, a more thorough visual and manual examination of the buccal cavity is performed. Several methods can be employed. One method involves the use of a mouth gag or speculum (see Figs. 1-5 to 1-7), whereas the other involves a manual technique without a mouth gag. Techniques not utilizing mouth gags are divided into a two-handed and a one-handed procedure.

Two-Handed Teeth Examination. With the two-handed procedure, the tongue is grasped on one side of the mouth through the interdental space and held in position on that side. The operator's other hand is then inserted into the mouth to feel the teeth and dental arcades on the opposite side to that to which the tongue is being held. When the tongue

TABLE 6–6. Times for Eruption of Deciduous Teeth in the Foal

Tooth	Time of Eruption
Incisors	
1st Deciduous	By 1 week
2nd Deciduous	1–2 months
3rd Deciduous	6–9 months
Premolars	
1st Deciduous	All within 2 weeks
2nd Deciduous	
3rd Deciduous	

is held to the side, the horse will usually have its mouth open, and a flashlight can be used to enhance visual examination of teeth on the opposite side.

KEY POINT ▶ Care must be exercised when pulling out the tongue not to be too aggressive, since damage to the frenulum on the ventral side of the tongue may occur resulting in sublingual cellulitis.

The operator then inserts a hand between the dental arcade and the cheeks with the knuckles toward the cheek and the palm toward the teeth. The cheek teeth are then palpated using the fingers. The idea of this procedure is to have the tongue held in a position between the teeth on the opposite side so that if the horse attempts to bite the operator's hands, it will bite onto its own tongue first. Under *most* circumstances, this procedure will prevent the horse from biting the operator's fingers.

One-Handed Teeth Examination. An alternative method involves the one-handed technique, whereby the operator inserts his or her hand through the interdental space with the back of the hand forcing the tongue between the opposite dental arcade. The palm is then facing toward the teeth that the operator wishes to examine (see Figs. 1-3 and 1-4). Therefore, the hand will be lying between the lingual surface of the cheek teeth to be examined and the tongue. After insertion of the hand, the operator is able to use a thumb and forefinger to palpate the buccal, lingual, and table surfaces of the teeth. The operator also can examine areas of mucosa, gingiva, and parts of the tongue using this procedure. Following examination of one side, the other hand is inserted through the opposite interdental space to facilitate examination of the opposite dental arcade. By inserting a hand, particularly the first finger and thumb, into the interdental space, the wolf teeth (first premolar teeth) and first upper and lower cheek teeth can be palpated. Particular note should be made of the presence of wolf teeth and whether there is any local irritation or the presence of sharp edges on the first cheek tooth.

Examination with the Aid of a Mouth Gag. If use of a mouth gag is favored, we have found the Swale's gag to be the most useful for examination of the teeth (see Figs. 1-6 and 1-7). This gag is safe for the veterinarian and horse and functions by forcibly holding the arcades open, allowing the operator to examine the dental arcade on the opposite side.

Examination of Teeth and Mouth under General Anesthesia. On occasion, the only means by which a satisfactory examination of the mouth and dental arcades can be achieved is following the induction of short-term general anesthesia (see Chap. 17). This allows more thorough evaluation because patient compliance is ensured.

Radiography. Radiographs of the head and teeth also may form an integral part of the dental examination. With care, adequate radiographs of the head and teeth can be obtained using portable equipment in the standing tranquilized horse. The quality of radiographs of the head and teeth has improved in recent years because of the advent of appropriate grids, films, and rare-earth screens. If greater detail is required and oblique or dorsoventral views seem indicated, these procedures should be performed with the horse under general anesthesia (see Chap. 17).

TREATMENT PROCEDURES

Tooth Floating. Veterinarians are frequently required to undertake routine dental procedures such as tooth floating. Adequate attention to dental prophylactic procedures will provide a horse with much more satisfactory function when it is masticating and also will potentially prevent the onset of untoward sequelae such as gingivitis. Floating is usually performed without a mouth gag, and the mouth is opened by holding a thumb on the hard palate on the side opposite to that in which the clinician wishes to insert the float. Once the float is inserted, the hand can often be withdrawn from the head/hard palate because the float will tend to maintain the mouth in an open position. An alternative method involves insertion of a gag (see Fig. 6-22).

KEY POINT ▶ It must be remembered that when performing teeth floating in horses, the operator may have to stand directly in front of the horse and is thus vulnerable to being kicked or struck.

If the veterinarian feels particularly vulnerable, a horse rug can be tied around the neck of the horse, providing a shield if the horse attempts to strike (see Fig. 1-28).

In general, it is not necessary to grasp the horse's tongue when attempting to perform tooth floating.

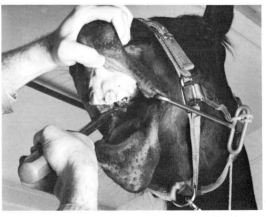

Figure 6–22. Rasping of upper premolar teeth using an angled rasp. Note that the rasp is positioned on the labial surface of the upper premolar teeth.

The objective of tooth floating is to remove enamel points or sharp projections on teeth that are causing problems with mastication or irritation to the horse's gums or lips. When floating the upper arcade, the buccal (labial) aspect of the arcade should be rasped at approximately a 60-degree angle, whereas on the lower arcade, the lingual aspect of cthe arcade should be floated. An angled float is used for the first few upper premolars, and a straight float is used on the caudal premolars, molars, and lower arcade. Particular care should be taken when rasping the teeth not to injure the mucosa. It is important to remove any sharp points or hooks that may be present on the rostral aspect of the first upper cheek tooth. This is usually done with a 45-degree float or a small hand-held file. In general, better control of the procedure is achieved if the float or file is held very close to the horse's head.

Removal of Deciduous Teeth/Caps and Wolf (First Premolar) Teeth. Wolf teeth can be present on both the upper and lower arcades but are most commonly found on the upper arcade.

KEY POINT ▶ There is often a strong and most likely unfounded belief within the equine industry that wolf teeth will create problems for young horses when working with a bit in their mouth.

As a result, wolf-teeth extraction is a commonly practiced procedure, but one for which there is little sound basis. Logic would seem to dictate that wolf teeth probably only need to be removed if they are impacted, causing gingival irritation or damage to the lips, or if they are displaced in some way. If wolf teeth require removal, several techniques have been described. In most circumstances, a dental elevator is used to loosen the tooth, and the tooth is then removed using a pair of forceps.

Retention of deciduous caps frequently occurs in young horses. One indication for removal of caps is the presence of sharp edges on them (which can be detected by palpation) causing irritation to the gingival and buccal mucosa. Another indication for removal of caps is the significant periosteal reaction and pain that occurs in association with the emergence of the permanent premolars in the maxillary and mandibular arcades. This reaction is often associated with local deformation, pain, and difficulty for the young horse when eating. Caps are usually prised off using a bone elevator, a pair of forceps, or a pair of bone-cutting forceps. An alternative lies in the use of a high-quality screwdriver. In horses that resent manipulation of the oral region, injection of local anesthesia around the gum line of the affected tooth or application of topical anesthetic sprays can be used.

Large hooks and sharp points may require cutting with tooth cutters or a chisel or grinding with a dental grinder.

KEY POINT ▶ When attempting to remove sharp points and hooks with tooth cutters or

chisels, it must be emphasized not to try and cut too much of the tooth at one time because there is a high risk of cracking the remaining healthy tooth.

Tooth Removal. In cases where there is severe periodontal disease, affected cheek teeth may be loose enough to allow removal using a pair of large animal tooth forceps. The procedure usually requires general anesthesia, and if the attempt to remove the tooth with the forceps is unsuccessful, repulsion of the teeth using trephine techniques and retrograde removal of the tooth are usually the next course of action. This procedure is rather more complex than attempting to remove the tooth with tooth forceps, and procedures for tooth removal are described in a variety of equine surgical texts.

Dental Caries (Apical Infections, Pulpitis)

Dental caries is a disease in which there is destruction of the cementum in teeth by food and microorganisms resulting in destruction of the integrity of the tooth. This is similar to the situation occurring in humans. Dental caries is a common disorder in older horses.

History and Presenting Signs

- Commonly in horses over 5 years of age
- Often only noticed when there is maxillary or mandibular swelling
- Affected horses may have a history of quidding, pain on mastication, and/or foul breath.

Clinical Findings and Diagnosis

- Caries/pulpitis may be obvious on oral examination.
- Most common in second and third cheek teeth
- May see broken teeth
- Pain associated with the affected tooth may be a feature.
- Nasal discharge, halitosis, and pain and swelling of paranasal sinuses occur in some cases.
- Diagnosis of secondary complications is frequently confirmed with radiographs.

Differential Diagnosis

- Dental/bone tumors
- Dentigerous cysts
- Periodontal disease
- Sinus cysts
- Paranasal sinusitis
- Trauma/osteomyelitis

Treatment

- Pulpitis is best prevented by regular dental attention to ensure appropriate mastication.
- Once disease has clinical manifestations (e.g.,

pulpitis, periostitis, or osteomyelitis), removal of the affected tooth and diseased tissue is the treatment of choice.

Enamel Points, Hooks, and Sharp Edges

The normal masticatory action of the horse produces wear on the teeth, often resulting in sharp enamel points on the premolars and molars.

KEY POINT ▶ Teeth in the upper arcade are slightly wider apart than those in the lower arcade, thereby producing a greater number of sharp points on the outside of teeth (labial surface) in the upper arcade and on the inside (lingual surface) of lower arcade.

These points result in injury to the insides of the cheeks and/or lateral aspects of the tongue during mastication. Pain during mastication also may be obvious. Enamel points are a common cause of unusual (e.g., head shaking) or refractory behavior when a horse is being ridden because of pain induced by the bit.

History and Presenting Signs

- "Quidding" or spillage of food from the mouth during eating
- Refractory behavior when a bit is in the horse's mouth

Clinical Findings and Diagnosis

- Evidence of pain when eating
- Abrasions on the insides of the cheeks and lateral aspects of the tongue
- Sharp points detected by visual and manual examination of the teeth

Differential Diagnosis

- Malocclusion
- Supernumerary teeth
- Impacted cheek teeth
- Gingivitis
- Periodontal disease
- Stomatitis

Treatment

- Rasping the outside of the upper arcade and inside of the lower arcade as required
- Removal of the hook (if present) on the rostral edge of the first upper cheek tooth and last lower cheek tooth
- Topical treatment of oral ulcers/abrasions if required
- Treatment includes mouthwashes and provision of soft, palatable foods.

Excessive/Disproportionate Dental Wear

Abnormal mastication due to malformations of the mandible or maxilla or the absence of teeth can result in a variety of dental disorders. Common problems include "wave mouth," "step mouth," "shear mouth," and "smooth mouth."

History and Presenting Signs

- Usually horses more than 6 years of age
- Often most severe in older horses
- "Quidding" and evidence of pain when eating
- May show weight loss

Clinical Findings and Diagnosis

- "Wave mouth," from uneven wear of the surfaces of dental arcades, resulting in more pronounced ridges and valleys of the dental surfaces
- Abnormal wear of incisor teeth is often secondary to stable vices (e.g., "cribbing") or chronic ingestion of sand or soil.
- "Step mouth" is due to long premolars/molars and may involve individual or multiple teeth. Usually this is the result of absence or damage to teeth on the opposing arcade.
- Sharp edges are normally found on the lateral aspect of upper arcade and medial aspect of lower arcade (see above).
- "Shear mouth" is due to the upper arcade being markedly wider than the lower arcade.
- Abrasions on the inside of the cheeks and lateral aspects of the tongue are found with sharp edges.
- Horses may have a worsening of normal wear patterns or unusual wear patterns if the degree of malocclusion is complicated by "parrot mouth."
- In old age, the teeth may be worn down to near the gum level. This is referred to as "smooth mouth." This problem can be exacerbated in horses eating off sandy soils.

Differential Diagnosis

- Fractured/damaged teeth
- Periodontal disease
- Dental caries/calculus
- Supernumerary teeth
- Impacted teeth
- Stomatitis

Treatment

- Vigorous rasping of the teeth should be done to remove sharp points and edges in an attempt to correct malocclusion.
- Correction of the underlying problem may be required, such as prevention of "cribbing" and strategies to reduce ingestion of sand by feeding out of a manger or on large rubber mats.
- Excessively long permanent teeth may require surgical cutting/grinding.

- Frequent dental attention (every few months) is usually required in horses with serious manifestations of abnormal wear patterns.

Periodontal Disease

Periodontal disease results from abnormal occlusion of teeth leading to gingivitis, which allows the accumulation of feed in the gingival sulcus. This, in turn, leads to erosion of the sulcus, alveolar sepsis, and finally, tooth loss.

History and Presenting Signs

- Occurs in horses of all ages; however, those over 5 years of age are most commonly affected.
- Halitosis
- "Quidding"
- Weight loss
- Nasal discharge, sinusitis, and colic are less common features.

Clinical Findings and Diagnosis

- Oral examination is the key to diagnosis. This is best done using a mouth gag.
- Gingivitis, alveolar sepsis, and erosion can be evident. In severe cases, tooth loss is possible.
- Radiographs may help confirm secondary changes.

Differential Diagnosis

- Diseases causing abnormal occlusion or shearing forces
- Fractured teeth
- Dental caries/pulpitis
- Stomatitis
- Gingivitis
- Primary or secondary paranasal sinusitis

Treatment

- Routine dental care should be undertaken to ensure appropriate occlusion and to decrease the potential for periodontal disease.
- Mouth washing can be used to assist in flushing necrotic material from pockets of infection.
- If the teeth are severely affected, those involved should be removed.
- For horses with inappetence and weight loss, high-energy palatable feeds should be provided (see Chap. 16).
- Anti-inflammatory drug therapy may be useful to reduce oral sensitivity. Phenylbutazone (Treatment No. 88) given at dose rates of 2.2 mg/kg PO q12h is useful.

- Horses with severe problems and oral inflammation may show a favorable response to antibiotic therapy. Procaine penicillin G (15,000 IU/kg or 15 mg/kg IM q12h) (Treatment No. 83) or trimethoprim–sulfonamide combinations (15–20 mg/kg of combined agent IV q12h) (Treatment No. 107) are usually active against many of the bacteria involved in periodontal disease.

Supernumerary Teeth

The reason for the occurrence of this disorder is not known. However, it is thought to be the result of division of the permanent tooth germ.

History and Presenting Signs

- Usually occurs in horses more than 3 years old because of the requirement for permanent teeth to be present
- There is often no relevant history, although evidence of pain when eating, "quidding," and changes in behavior are reported.

Clinical Findings and Diagnosis

- Supernumerary teeth are often found on routine dental examination.
- Incisors are most commonly affected. The first premolar (wolf) and other cheek teeth are affected in some animals.
- There may be evidence of local injury in association with the offending tooth.

Differential Diagnosis

- Malocclusion
- Impacted cheek teeth
- Gingivitis
- Periodontal disease
- Dental caries
- Stomatitis

Treatment

- No treatment is necessary if only an incisor is involved and there is no interference with mastication.
- In cases where supernumerary teeth are elongated or wear abnormally, cutting, grinding, or removal of the offending teeth may be required.
- Supernumerary cheek teeth should be removed owing to their potential to induce impaction, malocclusion, and further dental problems.

Diseases of the Esophagus

Esophageal Obstruction ("Choke")

There are a variety of esophageal diseases resulting from obstructive, traumatic, inflammatory, neoplastic, and congenital disorders, all of which may result in partial or complete obstruction. Obstruction can be due to intraluminal causes ("choke"), strictures of the esophageal wall, esophageal compression due to extraluminal causes, and diverticulae of the esophageal wall. Dysphagia is the most frequently observed clinical manifestation of esophageal diseases.

History and Presenting Signs

- Inappetence/anorexia
- Pain and retching when attempting to swallow
- Extension of the neck, particularly when attempting to swallow
- Increased salivation (ptyalism)
- Halitosis
- Nasal discharge
- Cervical swelling

Clinical Findings and Diagnosis

KEY POINT ▶ Dysphagia is the most common physical finding in horses with esophageal obstructions.

- When horses attempt to eat, food may be discharged from the nares.
- Swelling in the neck may be apparent. Warm, painful swelling is often indicative of a cervical abscess or cellulitis. Such lesions may cause a primary extraluminal esophageal obstruction. Perforation of the esophagus may result in a local cellulitis, crepitus, and possibly draining tracts.
- Acute onset of dysphagia and excessive salivation is often the result of acute feed or foreign-body impactions, whereas an insidious onset of dysphagia may be the result of progressive esophageal stricture, neoplasia, or an extraluminal mass.
- Secondary aspiration pneumonia may occur with associated signs present (e.g., dyspnea, increased lung sounds, foul breath).

KEY POINT ▶ Diagnosis of "choke" is confirmed by passage of a nasogastric tube. However, care must be exercised to avoid rupture of the esophagus, because tissue devitalization may have occurred.

- Plain radiographs of the throat and cervical region can assist in identifying the problem. Lateral radiographs are most useful for diagnosis. Accumulated air and feed material may be imaged. Esophageal rupture results in accumulation of periesophageal emphysema.

KEY POINT ▶ Contrast radiography may be necessary to confirm the diagnosis.

- Barium sulfate (50–200 ml) administered orally or via a nasogastric tube can be used to outline intra- and extraluminal obstructions, dilatations, strictures, inflammatory disorders, or diverticulae of the esophagus.
- Esophagoscopy using an endoscope suitable for rhinolaryngoscopy is useful to visualize lesions/obstructions and provides a mechanism by which biopsy samples of suspicious lesions can be obtained. In some cases, foreign bodies can be retrieved with the aid of an esophagoscope.
- Auscultation of the thorax, transtracheal aspiration or brohoalveolar lavage, thoracic radiographs, and hematology may assist in the diagnosis of secondary aspiration pneumonia. Mixed bacterial infections are common in cases where aspiration has occurred, with anaerobic organisms frequently implicated.

Differential Diagnosis

KEY POINT ▶ Acquired intraluminal esophageal obstruction due to impaction of feed material is the most common cause of "choke."

- External esophageal compression due to retropharyngeal or cervical lymphadenopathy (e.g., "strangles") is the second most common cause of "choke."
- Esophageal stricture, inflammatory disease, or ulceration
- Congenital esophageal disorders (e.g., megaesophagus)
- Dysphagia due to other causes (e.g., cranial nerve deficits, nigropallidal encephalomalacia, rabies)
- Oral foreign bodies

- Stomatitis
- Dental problems
- Gastroduodenal ulceration

Treatment

- Acquired intraluminal esophageal obstructions often resolve spontaneously. Those requiring treatment may respond to administration of sedatives and muscle relaxants, such as xylazine (0.5 mg/kg IV; Treatment No. 108), detomidine (20 μg/kg IV; Treatment No. 28), or acepromazine (0.04 mg/kg IV; Treatment No. 1).
- Deposition of a small amount of local anesthetic (20–50 ml lidocaine; Treatment No. 67) onto the impacted mass can promote esophageal relaxation and decrease discomfort for the horse.
- Lavage of the impaction using warm water administered with a dosing syringe via nasogastric tube can be helpful.

KEY POINT ▶ During lavage, ensure that the horse's head is lowered to allow passive drainage of fluid from the nose and prevent aspiration.

- Prior sedation assists in maintaining the horse's head in this lowered position. This lavage process may need to be repeated with intermittent periods of rest to achieve success. External massage of the esophageal mass may be of value. The affected horse should be prevented from having access to feed and bedding during this time. Cuffed nasogastric or small-gauge endotracheal tubes also may be used for delivery of the lavage solution. Inflation of the cuff helps ensure that effluent fluid exits via the tubal lumen.
- In refractory cases, conservative therapy should be continued with the horse under general anesthesia. An endotracheal tube should be inserted, the cuff inflated, and the head placed in a lowered position to reduce the potential for aspiration. In some cases, foreign material can be removed with forceps guided into position with an esophagoscope.
- Esophagostomy should be considered a last resort for treatment of esophageal impaction. A number of techniques are described in surgery texts. Healing is usually by second intention, slow, and often complicated. If an esophagostomy is required, referral to a specialized surgical facility should be considered.
- Some cases of esophageal obstruction require fluid therapy support. Isotonic polyionic fluids (see Chap. 17) with added potassium at the rate of 20 to 30 mmol/L (mEq/L) given intravenously are the fluids of choice.

- Judicious use of nonsteroidal anti-inflammatory drugs such as phenylbutazone (Treatment No. 88) or flunixin meglumine (Treatment No. 52) may be of value to decrease esophageal inflammation and local pain.
- Following mild obstructions, few food restrictions need apply. Horses with moderate to severe obstructions with subsequent mucosal damage benefit from feed being withheld for up to 3 days to allow mucosal healing to begin. Feed with high moisture content (e.g., fresh cut green grass) or slurries (e.g., alfalfa gruels or bran mashes) are then slowly introduced to the diet. The progress of mucosal healing can often be assessed using repeat esophagoscopy.
- Management of aspiration pneumonia should be based on the bacterial organisms involved. A transtracheal wash is indicated to define the cause and antimicrobial therapy based on these results. Procaine penicillin [15,000 IU/kg (15 mg/kg) IM q12h; Treatment No. 83], gentamicin sulfate (2–3 mg/kg IV or IM q8–12h; Treatment No. 56), and metronidazole (15 mg/kg PO q6h; Treatment No. 75) are good choices for broad-spectrum coverage prior to sensitivity results being available. Metronidazole is added to the regimen because anaerobic bacteria are frequently involved in aspiration pneumonia.
- Horses with esophageal perforation or requiring an esophagostomy are treated by allowing the wound to heal by second intention. Broad-spectrum antimicrobial coverage as detailed above and drainage of the local area (in cases of perforation) are indicated. Fluid and nutritional support is provided initially by an esophagostomy tube and then as healing occurs via a nasogastric tube.
- Medium- to long-term complications of esophageal obstruction include mucosal ulceration, diverticulae, and strictures.
- Extraluminal esophageal obstructions due to lymph node abscessation (i.e., secondary to infection with *Streptococcus equi var. equi*, "strangles") require long-term antimicrobial therapy. Procaine penicillin G [15,000 IU/kg (15 mg/kg) IM q12h; (Treatment No. 83) for 14 to 28 days], followed by trimethoprim–sulfonamide combination (15–20 mg/kg of the combination PO q12h; Treatment No. 107) for another 14 to 28 days, is indicated. Administration of nonsteroidal anti-inflammatory drugs is also indicated to help reduce pain and local swelling. Horses with respiratory embarrassment due to reduction in tracheal diameter may require a tracheostomy to reduce dyspnea. Drainage or aspiration of the offending mass is possible under some circumstances but is often difficult.

Diseases of the Stomach

Gastric Impaction, Dilatation, and Rupture

Impaction of the stomach most commonly results from poor dentition or consumption of low-quality foodstuffs (e.g., straw). Dilatation occurs as a primary event as a result of ingestion of excessive amounts of food (e.g., grain), water, or air. The most common cause of secondary dilatation is bowel obstruction (physical or functional), particularly diseases involving the small intestine, although gastric dilatation can occur with obstructions of the large bowel. Because horses are unable to vomit, rupture of the stomach is a frequent sequel to dilatation. Gastric rupture is avoided by rapid recognition of dilatation and repeated decompression.

History and Presenting Signs

- Evidence of dental abnormalities (e.g., "quidding")
- Rapid eating, a common characteristic of horses low in the social order
- Consumption of poor-quality feed or large volumes of feed or water, especially grain
- Vices (e.g., crib biting or "windsucking")
- Colic

Clinical Findings and Diagnosis

- Abdominal pain ranging from mild with impactions to severe with dilatation. Some horses "dog sit" to decrease pressure on the stomach.
- Increased cardinal signs, dehydration (injected mucous membranes), and shock are common in severe cases.
- Electrolyte deficits (e.g., hypokalemia, hypochloremia) may occur due to pooling of gastric fluids.
- Significant gastric reflux (5–15 L) is common.

KEY POINT ▶ A nasogastric tube must always be passed.

- It is important to use a nasogastric tube with a number of fenestrations on the side and to repeatedly backflush the tube with water with a large syringe or hose (500–1000 ml) to promote optimal reflux; otherwise, the tube will block with feed material (see Figs. 6-10 to 6-13). Repeated decompression is necessary. The tube can be removed and replaced or left in situ, being

taped to the headstall or sutured to the dorsolateral part of the nostril.
- Rectal examination may reveal distended loops of small or large bowel in cases of secondary gastric dilatation.
- Gastric rupture is often accompanied by an immediate reduction in pain, followed by a progressive deterioration of clinical signs (shock) as fulminant peritonitis progresses. In these cases, abdominocentesis will reveal evidence of ingesta and biochemical and cytologic changes consistent with peritonitis. Euthanasia is the only option if there is gastric rupture.

Differential Diagnosis

- Consumption of poor-quality feed
- Ingestion of large volumes of grain, other feeds, water, or air
- Anterior enteritis
- Bowel obstructions
- Other causes of colic (e.g., peritonitis, enteritis/colitis)

Treatment

KEY POINT ▶ Gastric decompression is imperative (see above). Lavage of the stomach with warm water also may assist in removal of grain and ingesta.

- Correction of the inciting cause is the key to therapy, and this may require referral for surgery if indicated.
- Symptomatic therapy. Intravenous fluids are required in dehydrated horses. Isotonic, polyionic fluids are usually indicated (see Chap. 17).
- Pain control may be necessary. Choices of analgesics include xylazine (0.3–0.7 mg/kg IV; Treatment No. 108) or detomidine (10–20 µg/kg IV; Treatment No. 28) and nonsteroidal anti-inflammatory drugs such as flunixin meglumine (0.25 mg/kg IV q6h; Treatment No. 52).

Pyloric Stenosis

Pyloric stenosis is a rare acquired disorder in horses occurring secondary to gastroduodenal ulcer disease or as a primary entity owing to growth of fibrous masses in the pylorus.

History and Presenting Signs

- Most common in horses less than 1 year old
- Possible previous history of ulcer disease
- Signs similar to those described for gastric dilatation
- Weight loss, colic, and possibly diarrhea

Clinical Findings and Diagnosis

- Signs of colic usually occur after eating.
- Bruxism (teeth grinding) and increased salivation are common.
- Poor body condition
- Positive gastric reflux may be found. Decompression often relieves colic signs.
- Nonspecific laboratory findings such as mild inflammatory changes in abdominal fluid may be identified.
- Diagnosis is made from the combination of recurrent clinical manifestations together with endoscopy, radiography, or necropsy.

Treatment

- Medical supportive therapy (e.g., fluids and electrolytes, pain control, and possibly antiulcer therapy; see Gastroduodenal Ulcers, p. 226) is indicated in the acute phase of the disorder.
- Surgical management of the stenosis is reported and may be possible in a referral surgical facility. Surgical correction is commonly done by performing a pyloroplasty.

Gastric Neoplasia

Gastric neoplasia is rare, with squamous cell carcinoma being the most common tumor in the stomach.

History and Presenting Signs

- Occurs in horses more than 2 years old
- Weight loss, anorexia, chronic diarrhea in some cases
- Recurrent low-grade colic related to eating
- Increased salivation or dysphagia in some cases

Clinical Findings and Diagnosis

- Signs are frequently nonspecific, with weight loss, colic, and dysphagia being found most commonly. In some cases, volumes of fluid (4–8 L) given by nasogastric tube, which would normally be well tolerated, result in signs of abdominal pain.
- In chronic cases, there may be mild anemia, and fecal examination may show presence of occult blood.
- Abdominocentesis may reveal increased nucleated cells and protein.
- Diagnosis can be assisted by radiographs or gastric endoscopy, although both techniques require sophisticated equipment and in most instances

are not practical except in a university teaching hospital. Most commonly, diagnosis is made at necropsy.

Treatment

There is no worthwhile treatment.

Gastroduodenal Ulcer Disease

Gastroduodenal ulceration in foals is discussed in Chapter 8. This section discusses ulcer disease in adult horses. Gastroduodenal ulceration has been recognized more commonly in adult horses in recent years, particularly since the advent of long, flexible fiberoptic endoscopes suitable for insertion into the stomach. As with ulcer disease in foals, stress appears to play an important role in the genesis of this disorder. As a result, the incidence of ulcers is reported to be much higher in horses undergoing training than in those living more sedentary, sedate lives. Ulcers occur with greatest frequency on the squamous gastric mucosa.

Nonsteroidal anti-inflammatory drugs promote gastric ulceration by inhibiting local mucoprotective mechanisms. Toxicity with these agents also results in large colon mucosal (and renal) lesions.

History and Presenting Signs

- Horses more than 6 months old
- In many cases ulcers are "silent," producing no overt signs of disease.
- Recurrent colic, weight loss, inappetence, and diarrhea
- Perforation frequently results in rapid deterioration due to fulminant peritonitis. This may be the first sign in some cases.
- Prior history of nonsteroidal anti-inflammatory medication

Clinical Findings and Diagnosis

- The signs may be nonspecific, mild recurrent colic being most common.
- Some horses show signs of depression, and there is often poor condition and a rough hair coat.
- Pain may occur following eating, although this sign is not found in every case.
- In younger horses (6 months to 2 years of age), bruxism (teeth grinding) and increased salivation may be indicators of disease.
- Moderate gastric reflux may be found.
- Abdominal fluid changes are mild and nonspecific but may indicate mild inflammation.
- Discolored "coffee grounds" appearance of gastric reflux occurs in some cases, which is due to hemorrhage from the ulcers.
- Tentative diagnosis is often based on suspicion and the clinical findings discussed above. Diagnosis is confirmed antemortem by gastroscopy. However, equipment to perform this procedure is currently only available in veterinary teaching

hospitals and referral practices. Contrast radiography may be of value, but results are difficult to interpret. It is worthwhile noting that gastroduodenal ulcers are commonly identified as an incidental finding at necropsy.

Treatment

- Decrease any factors producing stress, and eliminate nonsteroidal anti-inflammatory drugs, if possible. This is vital to optimize the effects of antiulcer medications.

KEY POINT ► Use of histamine (H₂) receptor antagonists such as cimetidine (Treatment No. 26) (6.6 mg/kg PO or IV q6h) or ranitidine (Treatment No. 99) (6.6 mg/kg PO or IV q8h) for 2 to 3 weeks is the principal method of medical therapy.

- New drugs designed to block the proton pump and therefore inhibit acid secretion (e.g., Omeprazole) are effective in horses and will become more widely used in the future.
- Antacids composed of aluminium/magnesium suspensions (Milanta II, Stewart Pharmaceuticals, Wilmington, Del.) also have been prescribed (250 ml/500 kg PO q8h) and may assist in ulcer therapy or reduce recurrence.
- The mucoprotectant sucralfate (Treatment No. 101) (2–4 g/500 kg PO q6–12h) is thought to adhere to damaged gastric mucosa and stimulate local blood flow and mucous secretion. There is divided opinion as to the efficacy of this preparation.

- If gastric emptying is delayed, use of bethanachol (Urecoline, Merck Sharp & Dohme, Rahway, N.J.) (0.25 mg/kg SC q4h for several doses) is of benefit in some cases.

Gastric Parasitism

Infection with *Gastrophilus* spp. ("bots") is the most common cause of gastritis in adult horses. Infection with *Habronema* spp., *Draschia megastoma,* and *Trichostrongylus axei* also occurs. Although infection with any or all of these parasites is common, clinical manifestations are rare.

History and Presenting Signs

KEY POINT ► Clinical effects are rare, although ill thrift, colic, and gastric dilatation/rupture have been ascribed to these parasites, particularly "bots."

- Bot eggs seen on horses legs or bot maggots in feces

Clinical Findings and Diagnosis

Generally asymptomatic. In some cases, nonspecific signs (e.g., poor condition) or signs of recurrent, low-grade colic may be seen.

Treatment

All gastric parasites are effectively treated with ivermectin at a dose rate of 0.2 mg/kg PO (Treatment No. 62).

Diseases of the Small Intestines

Anterior Enteritis (Duodenitis–Proximal Jejunitis, Proximal Enteritis)

Anterior enteritis is the result of a hemorrhagic/necrotic lesion in the duodenum and proximal jejunum. This significant inflammatory lesion allows for transudation and secretion of large volumes of electrolyte-rich fluid into the intestinal lumen. Severe pain, gastrointestinal reflux, dehydration, and electrolyte abnormalities are common features of the disorder. The cause of this disease is not known, although lesions are similar to a disease occurring in humans due to infection with *Clostridium perfringens*.

History and Presenting Signs

- Adult horses (>3 years old) are most frequently affected.
- Possible recent history of dietary change, particularly an increase in the energy content
- Sudden onset of acute, severe colic and depression

Clinical Findings and Diagnosis

- Clinical manifestations of the disease are related to the severity of the small intestinal lesions.

KEY POINT ▶ Severe pain is evident initially with large-volume, fetid, sanguinous nasogastric reflux. Pain often temporarily abates following gastric decompression.

- Fever, injected mucous membranes, tachycardia

KEY POINT ▶ Depression is often profound.

- Ileus
- Small intestinal distension due to intestinal inflammation may be detectable per rectum.
- Dehydration (often severe), hyponatremia, hypochloremia, hypokalemia, hypocalcemia, and mild metabolic acidosis resulting in prerenal azotemia and shock are classical features.
- Hematology commonly reveals the presence of neutrophilia.
- Mild peritonitis [total nucleated cell count 5000–10,000 × 10^6/L (5000–10,000/μl)] with an elevated protein concentration of 30 to 45 g/L (3–4.5 g/dl) is common.

KEY POINT ▶ Diagnosis of anterior enteritis is particularly difficult because the clinical signs are similar to those occurring with other forms of small intestinal obstructive disease.

- Response to repeated gastric reflux and medical support can be useful in assisting the clinician in making a tentative diagnosis.

KEY POINT ▶ Unlike strangulating obstructions of the small intestine, horses with anterior enteritis frequently have a significant reduction in pain following gastric decompression (strangulating obstructions do not) but still remain profoundly depressed.

- Definitive diagnosis can be made at surgery, although there is questionable benefit to affected animals if subjected to surgical intervention, and the prognosis may be worsened. However, given the similarity of signs to those occurring with obstructive small bowel diseases, many horses with anterior enteritis undergo exploratory surgery.

Differential Diagnosis

- Small intestinal obstruction/strangulation
- Undifferentiated enteritis/colitis
- Large intestinal diseases/obstructions
- Acute peritonitis
- Acute liver failure, cholelithiasis
- Other causes of abdominal pain (e.g., nephrolithiasis)

Treatment

- Rapid institution of aggressive supportive therapy is the key to a successful outcome. Therapy is often time-consuming and expensive, since many cases require treatment for more than 3 to 4 days and some as long as 8 to 10 days until damage to the intestine is sufficiently repaired to prevent transudation of fluid into the lumen.

KEY POINT ▶ Repeated gastric reflux (every 1–2 hours) is vital to assist in the control of pain and to reduce the risk of gastric rupture.

- In many cases, the nasogastric tube is left indwelling, being sutured into the nostril or taped to the halter. Volumes of 6 to 10 L can commonly be obtained during initial gastric decompression.

KEY POINT ► Massive intravenous fluid administration is indicated using polyionic sodium-containing fluids (see Fluid Therapy, Chap. 17) at initial rates of 10 to 15 L/hour for a 500-kg horse, later reduced to 2 to 5 L/hour after hydration is restored.

- Addition of potassium to the fluids at a rate of 15 to 20 mmol/L (mEq/L) is indicated to assist in partially replacing deficits. *Note:* Reflux will often become more severe following induction of fluid therapy. Calcium supplementation is also often indicated. Appropriate clinical response is reflected by improved demeanor, decreased heart rate, increased pulse pressure, and a return of serum electrolyte, urea, creatinine, and acid–base values toward normal.
- Low dose nonsteroidal anti-inflammatory therapy such as flunixin meglumine (0.25 mg/kg IV q6–8h; Treatment No. 52) is useful to reduce pain, ameliorate the effects of endotoxemia, and as a prophylactic measure for laminitis, which is a common sequel to the enteritis.
- Intravenous administration of DMSO (0.5–0.9 g/kg IV slowly as a 10% to 20% solution; Treatment No. 34) has been suggested to assist in reducing the inflammatory bowel lesion and decrease complications such as thromboembolism and laminitis.
- Antimicrobial therapy with procaine penicillin [15,000–20,000 IU/kg (15–20 mg/kg) IM q12h; Treatment No. 83] has been prescribed on the basis that the disease may be the result of infection with *Clostridium* spp.
- With aggressive medical therapy, greater than 80% of horses with anterior enteritis recover.

Small Intestinal Obstruction

Obstruction of the small intestine is categorized as *simple,* where there is intraluminal blockage without strangulation, or *strangulating,* where the intestine is twisted on its axis. Small intestinal obstructions commonly cause severe pain due to (1) accumulation of fluid proximal to the lesion and (2) the discomfort of the obstructive lesion itself. In the case of strangulating lesions, the signs of discomfort are frequently magnified, because compromise of circulation to the bowel and liberation of toxins increases the sensitivity of pain receptors in the affected region. Following complete obstruction, there is a cascade of events, including pain, toxemia, dehydration, cardiovascular compromise, and "shock," that is often irreversible if untreated.

KEY POINT ► As a general rule, simple obstructions have a slower progression of signs and may be amenable to medical therapy, whereas strangulating obstructions are likely to be fatal without surgical correction.

Causes of Small Intestinal Obstruction

1. *Simple*
   a. *Intestinal stricture*
   b. *Adhesions due to previous surgery or peritonitis*
   c. *Ileal impaction*
   d. *Thickened ileocecal valve*
   e. *Intussusception*
   f. *Foreign bodies*
2. *Strangulating*
   a. *Volvulus*
   b. *Herniation through the epiploic foramen*
   c. *Mesenteric herniation*
   d. *Strangulating umbilical hernia*
   e. *Inguinal hernia*
   f. *Pedunculated lipoma*

History and Presenting Signs

- Inappetence/anorexia
- Pain varying from mild with depression to severe and uncontrollable, depending on the lesion
- Sweating, rolling, pawing

Clinical Findings and Diagnosis

- Simple obstructions tend to cause the least severe manifestations and progress more slowly than strangulating lesions. Some simple obstructions correct spontaneously. However, if there is complete obstruction and no treatment, all cases will demonstrate a progressive increase in severity of pain and/or cardiovascular compromise.
- Physical examination may reveal abnormalities such as distended loops of bowel in umbilical or inguinal hernias.
- Elevation in heart rate is usual (>50 beats/min), although some horses with substantial areas of infarcted bowel can be found to have normal heart rates.
- Obstructions commonly result in decreased intestinal sounds. In contrast, an increase in gut sounds may be heard in early cases of enteritis.
- Rectal temperature is usually normal or slightly elevated if the horse has been overtly active in its response to pain. In contrast, horses suffering from acute colitis and likely to "break" with diarrhea are more likely to have elevations in rectal temperature.
- Evidence of dehydration and cardiovascular compromise is usually found. There is decreased skin elasticity, diminished pulse pressure, increased capillary refill time, dry gums, and increased hematocrit and total plasma protein (see Table 6-3

for a summary of alterations occurring in PCV and TPP and their severity). If the disease involves bowel compromise, there is usually progressive endotoxemia and fluid derangements resulting in "shock." This is reflected by injected mucous membranes, cold extremities, progressive increases in heart rate, weak pulse, and central nervous system depression.

■ Nasogastric reflux is usually positive (>3–5 L).

■ Rectal examination may reveal distended loops of small intestine.

KEY POINT ▶ However, failure to detect abnormalities per rectum does not preclude the possibility of small intestinal obstruction.

■ The technique for performing a thorough rectal examination is outlined in Figures 6-1 to 6-9. Horses with anterior enteritis have distended loops of bowel; however, these are not likely to be as tightly distended as those occurring with small intestinal obstruction. In horses afflicted with enteritis, distension temporarily abates with nasogastric reflux.

■ Abdominocentesis is useful in assisting in decision-making processes (see Table 6-1, outlining results of peritoneal fluid analyses). As a general rule, there will be progressive increases in the total nucleated cell count, protein content, and serosanguinous appearance of the fluid as bowel compromise becomes more severe.

Differential Diagnosis

■ Small intestinal simple or strangulating obstruction
■ Anterior enteritis
■ Peracute enteritis/colitis (i.e., diarrhea)
■ Large bowel obstruction, displacement, or strangulation
■ Peritonitis
■ Other causes of colic (e.g., urolithiasis, nephrolithiasis, liver disease/cholelithiasis)
■ Laminitis
■ Pleural effusion

Treatment

■ Mild or partial simple obstructions may respond to medical therapy, including nasogastric decompression, restoration of fluid balance, and pain control (see p. 210). This type of lesion is rare.

■ Complete obstructions (simple and strangulating) require surgical intervention or euthanasia if surgery is not an option. Affected horses should be referred or subjected to exploratory surgery as soon as possible to avoid prolonging the time that bowel is compromised, which, in turn, increases the potential for detrimental effects of endotoxemia, shock, and bowel rupture to occur. Medical stabilization of the patient with fluids and analgesics prior to surgery or shipment for surgery is often indicated.

Diseases of the Large Intestines

LARGE INTESTINAL OBSTRUCTION

Diseases of the large colon constitute one of the most common causes of abdominal pain, and it is fortunate for both the affected horse and the veterinarian that many of these disorders are responsive to medical management. The large colon is a relatively mobile organ which, on a volume basis, constitutes the major proportion of the gastrointestinal tract of the horse. Given its size, mobility, and role in fermentation and water absorption, disorders of the large colon can result in significant pain, alterations in fluid balance, and gas accumulation. Definitions are similar to those applied to the small intestine; that is, obstructive lesions are referred to as *simple* or *nonstrangulating obstructions,* caused by intraluminal blockages (e.g., feed or sand impactions, foreign bodies/fecoliths/enteroliths) and displacements (e.g., left or right dorsal displacement). *Strangulating obstructions* involve vascular compromise and are commonly due to volvulus.

Feed Impaction

Impaction of feed in the large colon constitutes the most common form of colonic obstruction and is therefore a frequent cause of colic. It is not well established what causes the impaction. Factors thought to contribute include motor dysfunction that disrupts bowel motility, stress, diet (e.g., poor-quality roughage) or dietary change, poor dentition, parasites, and possibly decreased water intake.

History and Presenting Signs

- Inadequate parasite management
- Feed spilling from mouth during eating ("quidding")
- Poor-quality feed
- Recent change in environment
- Mild to moderate abdominal pain
- Inappetence

Clinical Findings and Diagnosis

- Mild to moderate abdominal pain is usual. This progresses to severe pain if left untreated. However, this progression may be over several days, unlike the more rapid succession of events with small bowel obstruction.
- The heart rate may be low initially. There is a progressive increase in heart rate (≥50–65 beats/min) if the obstruction is not resolved.
- The degree of dehydration is variable.
- There is a moderate to severe decrease in gastrointestinal sounds, which progressively worsens over 1 to 2 days.
- Abdominal distension may be seen in association with gas accumulation.
- Abdominocentesis is usually unremarkable, although with impactions of longer duration there may be increases in total nucleated cell count and a mild increase in protein concentration.
- Rectal examination may reveal a firm mass in the transverse colon, although the anatomic location of the impaction (anterior abdomen) may preclude its detection. It is common to find a gas-filled large colon.
- Hematology and plasma biochemistry show few changes, apart from an increase in total protein. Acid–base status is usually normal.

Differential Diagnosis

- Other causes of large colon impaction (e.g., enteroliths, sand)
- Large colon displacement or torsion
- Small intestinal obstruction or strangulation
- Acute colitis
- Liver disease/cholelithiasis
- Peritonitis
- Pleuropneumonia

Treatment

- Analgesics to control pain (see Medical Management of Colic, p. 210).

KEY POINT ▶ Fluid therapy is essential to correct dehydration and to soften the impaction.

- If gastric reflux is not present and there is evidence of gut sounds, fluids can be given by nasogastric tube (see Medical Management of Colic, p. 210). Intravenous fluid therapy is also valuable. Isotonic polyionic fluids (65–100 ml/kg/day IV) are given (see Fluid Therapy, Chap. 17).
- Since foreign-body impactions are difficult to distinguish from food impactions, laxatives are frequently used. Mineral oil (Treatment No. 77) and dioctyl sodium sulfosuccinate (DSS) (Treatment No. 35) are good choices (see Medical Management of Colic, p. 210).
- Medical therapy can be continued for up to 5 to 7 days if (1) pain is limited or easily controlled, (2) the horse voluntarily consumes fluids, (3) there is no deterioration in the animal's metabolic status, and (4) there is no significant increase in abdominal fluid total nucleated cell count or protein concentration. Deterioration in any of these signs constitutes an indication for referral for surgery.

Foreign-Body Obstruction (Fecolith)

This is a problem that is most common in young horses because of their less discriminating eating habits. Ingestion of rope, baling twine, straw bedding, shavings, plastic, and feed bags are common causes. These materials combine with ingesta and often result in obstruction of the gastrointestinal tract. Because of the reduction in luminal size at the beginning of the small colon, obstruction at that site is common. However, obstructions at more proximal sites occur.

History and Presenting Signs

KEY POINT ▶ Moderate abdominal pain initially, progressively becoming more severe

- Inappetence/anorexia
- Often younger horses (<3 years old)
- Abdominal distension
- Decreased fecal output

Clinical Findings and Diagnosis

- See section on large colon feed impactions (p. 231), since the signs are often difficult to distinguish from that disorder.
- Diagnosis is usually based on the history of abdominal pain, physical examination findings (e.g., lesion palpable per rectum), and response to management. Specific diagnosis may not be possible without surgery.

Differential Diagnosis

- Other causes of large colon impaction (e.g., feed, enteroliths, sand)
- Large colon displacement or torsion
- Small intestinal obstruction or strangulation
- Acute colitis
- Liver disease/cholelithiasis
- Peritonitis
- Pleuropneumonia

Treatment

- Since foreign-body impactions are difficult to distinguish from food impactions, treatment with laxatives is used. Mineral oil (Treatment No. 77) and DSS (Treatment No. 35) are good choices (see Medical Management of Colic, p. 210). Fluid therapy often is indicated (see Chap. 17).
- Expulsion of the foreign body and resolution of signs will occur spontaneously in some cases or in response to medical management. In other cases there is a progressive deterioration in signs requiring referral for surgical correction.

Sand Impactions

Horses maintained in sandy locations and which eat from the ground inevitably ingest sand. Alternatively, sand may constitute part of what the horse eats because of its inclusion in hay. Younger animals with indiscriminant eating habits, at times, voluntarily consume sand. Consumption of sufficient sand results in accumulation in the ventral colon, pelvic flexure, and transverse colon. Sand induces a physical colitis. This inflammatory response, associated with accumulation of sufficient volume of sand, can result in colonic rupture.

History and Presenting Signs

- Living in a sandy environment (e.g., Arizona, California, Florida are common locations for horses with this disorder)
- Eating off the ground in sandy environments
- Pain and presenting signs similar to those described for feed impactions

Clinical Findings and Diagnosis

- Many signs similar to those referred to for obstructions of the large colon (pp. 230–231)
- Rectal examination may reveal sand impactions in the ventral colon, which in some cases can be massive (>30 kg). Failure to detect sand or an impaction on rectal examination does not preclude the possibility of sand accumulation, since it may be deposited in a cranial portion of the gastrointestinal tract and is therefore out of reach. "Grit" may be detected when palpating or may be found on the rectal sleeve following removal of the veterinarian's arm from the rectum.

KEY POINT ► Dissolving feces in water in a bucket or rectal sleeve and observing for sand on the bottom of the bucket or sleeve may provide evidence of the likelihood of sand impactions.

- Small amounts of sand are frequently found in feces and do not necessarily reflect sand impaction. However, large amounts of sand provide strong evidence for impaction. *Note:* If in doubt, compare the amount of sand in the affected horse's feces with that from other normal horses in the region.
- Abdominal radiography can reveal sand impaction in foals, ponies, and miniature horses. Similarly, ultrasound examination can provide images consistent with accumulations of coarse, sandy material in the large colon.

Differential Diagnosis

- Other causes of large colon impaction (e.g., feed impaction, enteroliths)
- Large colon displacement or torsion
- Small intestinal obstruction or strangulation
- Acute colitis (diarrhea)
- Liver disease/cholelithiasis
- Peritonitis
- Pleuropneumonia

Treatment

- Laxatives to lubricate the gastrointestinal tract and assist in the movement of sand (see Medical Management of Colic, p. 210). The laxative of choice is psyllium hydrophilic mucilloid (Treatment No. 97) (0.5–1.0 g/kg q6–24h; mixed in 4–8 L water and pumped *rapidly* into the stomach via nasogastric tube before the mucilloid turns to gel). This treatment is maintained for several days to a week depending on the severity of the case. Following initial therapy, the psyllium can be fed to the horse in sweet feed.

KEY POINT ► Feces should be monitored for the rate of expulsion of sand.

- Therapy may need to be continued for weeks to ensure that sand is fully removed from the colon.
- Severely affected and unresponsive cases may require referral for attempted surgical correction. Surgery involves a pelvic flexure enterotomy and flushing of sand out of the large colon.
- Prevention of recurrence is important. This requires ensuring that horses eat their feed from a manger or bucket to avoid ingestion of sand. Alternatively, eating food off rubber mats or out of troughs (tires cut in half make cheap troughs) is indicated. Removal of hay containing sand from the horse's diet is important. Intermittent administration (1 g/kg PO q24h) of psyllium mucilloid for several weeks to remove any accumulations of sand also may be indicated. Longer-term

administration is likely to result in an increased rate of degradation of the mucilloid by colonic microbes and a decrease in laxative effects. Feeding diets high in fiber (e.g., grass hay) is advisable.

Enteroliths

Enteroliths are mineral concretions that form in the large colon. They create partial or complete obstructions when passed into the small colon. Enteroliths are more common in horses in certain geographic regions (e.g., California and the southern states). Common anatomic sites for obstruction include the ampulla of the small colon and the transverse and small colons. Diets high in nitrogen, magnesium, and phosphorus result in the highest incidence of enteroliths, since these chemicals are integral components of mineraloliths. When alfalfa (lucerne) is a principal component of the diet, it is believed to predispose horses to the formation of enteroliths. This is thought to be the result of the high nitrogen and possibly magnesium contents of this feedstuff. Alfalfa also may allow intestinal pH to rise, thereby promoting the potential formation of the mineralolith.

History and Presenting Signs

- Adult/older horses
- Alfalfa diet
- Presenting signs are similar to those for feed impactions of the large colon.
- Pain may be intermittent as the enterolith temporarily lodges in the ampulla of the small colon, and then discomfort abates when the enterolith passes back into the right dorsal colon.
- If the enterolith causes complete obstruction and vascular compromise, pain may be more intense.

Clinical Findings and Diagnosis

- Abdominal pain occurs. This is low-grade and similar to that occurring in other obstructive diseases of the large colon.
- There are usually only small amounts or an absence of feces. If there is only partial luminal obstruction, limited amounts of feces, gas, and mineral oil can still be passed.
- Progressive abdominal distension is found in many cases.
- A progressive decrease in gut sounds occurs until there is an absence of gut sounds.
- Rectal examination may reveal gaseous distension of the large colon. Enteroliths are palpable in some cases. If the horse is palpated with its forequarters elevated, retrograde movement of the gastrointestinal tract may increase the chance of the mineralolith being palpated.
- Abdominocentesis is usually unremarkable. However, if there is vascular compromise at the site of obstruction, there will be progressive changes in abdominal fluid constituents, including increases in total nucleated cells, protein, red cells, and blood pigments.

Differential Diagnosis

- Other obstructive diseases of the large colon
- Large colon displacement or torsion
- Small intestinal obstruction or strangulation
- Acute colitis (diarrhea)
- Peritonitis
- Liver disease/cholelithiasis
- Pleuropneumonia

Treatment

- Following diagnosis of an enterolith, surgical removal is the therapy of choice. However, at times, enteroliths will not be diagnosed on the initial workup and an exploratory celiotomy is performed, at which time the mineralolith is identified.
- On farms or in areas with a high incidence of enteroliths, feeding of vinegar (250 ml PO in feed q12h) has been recommended. It is thought the vinegar decreases colonic pH and reduces the potential for formation of mineraloliths.

STRANGULATING OBSTRUCTIONS OF THE LARGE COLON

Colonic Volvulus

Severe torsion (≥270 degrees) of the large colon and vascular compromise and tissue devitalization are potent stimuli for induction of signs of abdominal pain in the horse. Although less severe torsions do occur, correction almost invariably requires surgical intervention. Survival following surgery remains low (approximately 30%). The etiology remains controversial. Some speculate that brood mares are more commonly affected related to parturition. However, this association is not proven.

History and Presenting Signs

- Variable abdominal pain with severe torsions, producing extreme, uncontrollable pain
- Most common in adult horses, particularly brood mares
- Highest incidence in summer
- Possibly related to parturition
- Inappetence/anorexia, depression
- Reduced fecal output

Clinical Findings and Diagnosis

- Variable, often severe abdominal pain
- Elevated heart rates are found, usually greater than 75 beats per minute.
- Progressive abdominal distension occurs over several hours.

- Dehydration is common, with signs of cardiovascular compromise and "shock."
- Rectal examination reveals a distended large colon. The colonic wall may feel thickened (edema).
- Abdominal fluid analysis results are variable. In some cases there is a profound increase in total nucleated cells, protein, and blood pigments. However, in others there are few changes, and those which exist do not reflect the extent of tissue devitalization that has occurred.
- Diagnosis may be confirmed on the basis of clinical signs and rectal examination in most cases. In others, diagnosis is not confirmed until an exploratory celiotomy or necropsy is performed.

Differential Diagnosis

- Other obstructive diseases of the large colon
- Large colon displacement
- Small intestinal obstruction or strangulation
- Acute colitis (diarrhea)
- Peritonitis

Treatment

- Initial therapy involves pain control, reconstitution of the circulating volume with intravenous fluid administration, and therapy for endotoxemia (see Medical Management of Colic, p. 210).
- Surgery is required to correct the torsion, and horses with suspected torsion should be referred to a surgical center as early in the course of the disease as practical.
- Euthanasia constitutes a rational alternative in cases where owners do not want surgical intervention.

Colonic Displacement

Displacement of the colon dorsally over the nephrosplenic ligament (left dorsal displacement) and right dorsal displacement, where the colon rotates around the cecum, are the most common types of colonic displacement. The cause of these displacements is not known, but it is thought to be the result of alterations in gut content (e.g., accumulation of gas or ingesta and alterations in motor activity of the colon).

Left Dorsal Displacement. In this disorder, the left portion of the large colon becomes lodged between the body wall and left kidney, with the nephrosplenic ligament supporting the colon in its displaced position. Two mechanisms are thought to contribute to colon entrapment at this site. One involves the pelvic flexure migrating over the top of the nephrosplenic ligament. The alternative mechanism requires splenic contraction or ventromedial movement allowing migration of the colon between the spleen and body wall. When the spleen subsequently expands or returns to its normal position, the colon is trapped in this dorsal location. Once

lodged in the nephrosplenic space, the colon rotates on its long axis, causing a partial obstruction.

Right Dorsal Displacement. Right dorsal displacement occurs when the large colon rotates (180 degrees) around the mesenteric attachment, resulting in the colon being located between the cecum and body wall on the right. The cause of this rotation is not known.

History and Presenting Signs

- Most common in large horses
- Mild to moderate abdominal pain
- Inappetence, decreased fecal output

Clinical Findings and Diagnosis

- Normal or slightly elevated heart rate. In severe cases the heart rate is often higher.
- Variable pain
- Variable degrees of abdominal distension are found, depending on the duration and degree of obstruction.
- Dehydration and cardiovascular compromise are mild in early cases. With progression, there is increased gas and fluid accumulation, tissue compromise, and potential for "shock."
- Rectal examination. With *left dorsal displacement,* there is gaseous distension of the large colon and displacement of the spleen away from the body wall and toward the medial part of the abdomen. In some cases, the colon lodging in the nephrosplenic ligament is palpable. Horses suffering from *right dorsal displacement* have a gas-distended colon with the pelvic flexure not palpable because it is relocated in the cranial abdominal region owing to the rotation of the colon on the mesenteric stalk.
- Abdominocentesis is unremarkable, except in severe cases where tissue devitalization has occurred, which would be reflected by increases in total nucleated cells and protein and, possibly, blood staining.

Differential Diagnosis

- Other obstructive diseases of the large colon
- Large colon displacement
- Small intestinal obstruction or strangulation
- Acute colitis (diarrhea)
- Peritonitis
- Liver disease/cholelithiasis
- Pleuropneumonia

Treatment

- Medical management involves symptomatic therapy to control pain and fluid derangements.
- In some mild cases of left or right dorsal displacement, correction will occur spontaneously if feed is withheld. The reduction in gut fill allows the colon to shrink and possibly relocate in a more normal anatomic location.

- Attempts to roll the horse have been described to correct *left dorsal displacement*. The horse is anesthetized, placed on its right side, and is then lifted into the air by the legs with a hoist. The horse is then lowered onto its left side and allowed to recover, hopefully with the colon replaced in its normal anatomic location. This is a worthwhile procedure where economic considerations prevent surgery as an option.
- In severe cases of left or right displacement, where conservative therapy fails or if the horse's condition deteriorates, referral for surgical exploration, confirmation of the diagnosis, and correction of the problem is indicated.

Other Gastrointestinal Diseases

Acute Diarrhea (Acute Colitis)

In most cases of acute diarrhea, substantial inflammatory involvement of the large colon and cecum occurs, with affected horses showing signs of abdominal pain, dehydration, and "shock." The diarrhea may be severe, and clinical progression of the disease may be rapid. Given these considerations, the clinician's main efforts are directed at maintaining fluid and electrolyte balance, treating shock, and preventing untoward sequelae. The etiology of individual cases of colitis frequently remains obscure despite vigorous diagnostic efforts. Even if a diagnosis is made, the cause of the diarrhea is rarely known at the time of onset of clinical signs. A number of causes for acute colitis have been described:

Salmonella spp. are frequently implicated in this syndrome. Salmonellosis most often occurs in horses living in crowded conditions and in association with concurrent disease or stress (e.g., following surgery). Salmonellosis has a much higher prevalance in hospital environments. Diarrhea results from increased fluid *secretion* due to a toxin released by the organism, *inflammation* of the bowel mucosa, and *malabsorption/maldigestion* due to villous destruction.

Clostridium perfringens type A ("colitis X," edematous bowel syndrome, peracute diarrhea syndrome) produces a syndrome that often resembles peracute salmonellosis, although horses may die of shock and complications before diarrhea occurs.

Equine monocytic ehrlichiosis ("Potomac horse fever") is caused by *Ehrlichia risticii*, resulting in typhlocolitis. *E. risticii* is likely to be spread by an insect vector, although none has been identified positively.

Other causes of acute diarrhea/colitis include excessive nonsteroidal anti-inflammatory therapy, antibiotic administration, heavy-metal toxicosis, plant toxicoses, cantharadin (blister beetle; *Epicauta* spp.) toxicosis, peritonitis, and parasites.

History and Presenting Signs

Salmonellosis

- All ages are affected, but it is most common in younger horses.
- Stress (e.g., training, transport, overcrowding, anesthesia, and/or surgery) and recent dietary change predispose horses to salmonellosis.
- Outbreaks may occur, with large numbers of horses affected.
- Depression, inappetence, and colic, often before the onset of diarrhea, are common.
- Acute, profuse, foul-smelling, and possibly bloody diarrhea

Clostridium perfringens Type A

- Profound depression and inappetence
- Severe pain frequently unresponsive to routine analgesia
- Death may occur before the onset of diarrhea.

Equine Monocytic Ehrlichiosis

- All ages of horses are affected.
- Sporadic cases or outbreaks can occur.
- Endemic areas exist. The disease is more com-

mon in, but not restricted to, horses living near large waterways.

■ Highest incidence in late spring, summer, and fall. Most cases occur in July through September.

■ Depression and inappetence are common.

Other Causes of Acute Colitis

■ Prior administration of antibiotics. Agents most commonly implicated include tetracyclines, trimethoprim–sulfamethoxazole, erythromycin, and lincomycin. However, administration of any antibiotic may result in diarrhea.

■ Administration of nonsteroidal anti-inflammatory agents

■ Exposure to heavy metals (e.g., arsenic, lead)

■ Ingestion of alfalfa contaminated with blister beetles

■ Ingestion of plants known to cause colitis (e.g., acorn or oak, oleander, Japanese yew)

■ Weight loss and other evidence of a heavy internal parasite burden

Clinical Signs and Diagnosis

Salmonellosis

■ Fever and depression together with abdominal pain are typical. After early colic-type signs, a profuse watery diarrhea develops.

■ Diarrhea may be voluminous, fetid, bloody, and contain mucosal tags.

■ Elevated cardinal signs (increased HR, RR, temperature) and injected mucous membranes. Gut sounds may be decreased or absent early in the course of the disease.

■ Septicemia and endotoxemia are features of the disease.

■ Dehydration is often profound and is accompanied by hyponatremia (in horses that are drinking), hypochloremia, hypokalemia, and azotemia.

■ Metabolic acidosis is found owing to bicarbonate loss and lactacidemia. In some severe cases, plasma bicarbonate concentrations may be as low as 10 mmol/L (mEq/L).

■ Leukopenia (with or without left shift) is often present before the onset of diarrhea.

■ Hypoproteinemia is a common finding in cases where diarrhea has been present for a few days. Early in the disease, an increase in total plasma protein may be found.

■ Proximal enteritis can accompany colitis.

■ Milder forms exist, and some cases show initial evidence of colonic impaction followed by diarrhea.

■ Complications associated with *Salmonella* septicemia include laminitis, thrombophlebitis (DIC), hepatitis, nephritis, and chronic colitis resulting in persistent diarrhea.

■ Diagnosis is based on clinical findings and isolation of organisms from feces (see Chap. 15). Three cultures using at least 10 g of fecal material

are advised. Concomitant culture of rectal mucosal biopsies improves the likelihood of a positive culture. Postmortem cultures of colonic mucosa and mesenteric lymph nodes also may yield organisms.

Clostridium perfringens Type A

■ Extreme, uncontrollable pain requiring euthanasia is often a feature of this disease.

■ Important findings are signs of toxemia, including fever, injected mucous membranes, and a weak, thready pulse.

■ Hemoconcentration is found, there being a very high hematocrit (often >60%) and rapidly progressive cardiovascular collapse.

■ Some horses are found dead with few prior signs.

■ Diagnosis is made by increased fecal concentrations of *Clostridium perfringens* type A being found on fecal culture.

Equine Monocytic Ehrlichiosis

■ A number of syndromes can be attributed to infection with *E. risticii.*

■ The most common form results in biphasic fever, depression, decreased borborygmi, and mild abdominal pain.

■ Moderate diarrhea lasting 24 to 72 hours may ensue.

■ Severely affected horses develop profuse watery diarrhea lasting up to a week if supportive treatment is provided.

■ Some horses develop ileus, profound toxemia, and disseminated intravascular coagulation and die.

■ Laminitis is a relatively common sequel to the disease (up to 25% of cases in some situations). The severity of laminitis can vary from mild to life-threatening.

■ Leukopenia often occurs early in the clinical course, commonly followed by a leukocytosis.

■ Diagnosis is tentatively based on clinical findings and evidence of seroconversion (useful in approximately 50% of cases). An indirect immunofluorescence antibody test is the current test of choice. Titers increase before the onset of signs or within a week of their occurrence.

KEY POINT ► To optimize effectiveness of serologic testing, an initial sample must be collected at the onset of signs.

■ Horses with titers greater than 1:160 (that have not been vaccinated) and with signs similar to those described above are likely to have the disease.

KEY POINT ► A fourfold increase or decrease in the titer is strongly suggestive of infection with *E. risticii.*

■ Unfortunately, more than 50% of cases remain undiagnosed.

- Serology to identify endemic areas is important, since horses showing early signs suggestive of equine monocytic ehrlichiosis can be treated aggressively.

Other Causes of Acute Colitis

- Antibiotic-induced colitis can result from overgrowth by *Salmonella* or *Clostridium* spp. There is variable severity of diarrhea and depression. Inappetence and initial abdominal pain are likely.
- Nonsteroidal anti-inflammatory drugs can cause depression, hypoproteinemia, anemia, diarrhea, and secondary septicemia.
- Heavy-metal intoxication produces colitis, depression, inappetence, diarrhea, possibly ileus in terminal stages, and circulatory failure.
- Cantharadin toxicosis produces signs referable to irritation in the gastrointestinal and urinary tracts. Signs include abdominal pain, depression, anorexia, frequent attempts to urinate, and shock. Pertinent laboratory findings include evidence of dehydration, hypocalcemia and hypomagnesemia, and evidence of renal failure.
- Acorn (*Quercus* spp.) toxicosis produces abdominal pain, depression, dysentery, shock, and possibly sudden death. Acorn husks may be found in the feces. Urinary dysfunction is also a feature of the disease.

Differential Diagnosis

- Salmonellosis
- Clostridiosis
- "Colitis X"
- Equine monocytic ehrlichiosis
- Nonsteroidal anti-inflammatory drug–induced diarrhea
- Diarrhea secondary to antibiotic therapy
- Plant toxicoses (e.g., acorn poisoning)
- Blister beetle poisoning
- Internal parasitism (strongylosis, cyathostomiasis)

- Heavy-metal intoxication
- Bowel obstruction/strangulation
- Peritonitis
- Liver disease

Treatment

Salmonellosis

KEY POINT ► Aggressive *fluid and electrolyte administration* is required. This involves attention to losses of total-body water, which may approach 8% to 12% of the body weight in severe cases.

- Electrolyte administration usually requires attention to losses of Na^+, Cl^-, K^+, and HCO_3^- (i.e., metabolic acidosis). Although fluid therapy is dealt with elsewhere (see Chap. 17), a subjective method for estimation of dehydration in horses with diarrhea is summarized in Table 6-8.
- From the information provided in Table 6-8, it can be estimated what the likely fluid deficit for a horse might be.
- It is important to provide the horse with sufficient fluids for ongoing maintenance and anticipated losses. For example, a 450-kg horse that has severe diarrhea and is about 10% dehydrated will require 45 L of fluid for replacement of the deficits. Maintenance is usually estimated to be 30 to 40 ml/kg per day, which amounts to an additional 15 to 20 L. If the diarrhea is severe, the ongoing losses could amount to 30 to 40 L per day. Thus, in this example, the horse may require more than 100 L of fluid during the first day of therapy.
- Balanced polyionic fluids such as Multisol-R (see Fluid Therapy, Chap. 17) are good choices in the early part of the disease, followed later by maintenance fluids containing lower concentrations of sodium.
- These fluids can be administered while awaiting results of laboratory data (e.g., PCV, TPP, SUN, SCr, electrolytes, bicarbonate).

TABLE 6–8. Degree of Dehydration, Clinical Findings, and Fluid Requirement in a 450-kg (1000-lb) Horse with Acute Diarrhea

Degree of Dehydration	Bodyweight Loss (%)	Fluid Deficit (L)	Clinical Findings	Fluids Required, Rate and Method of Administration (ml/kg/h)
Mild	5–7	23–32	↓ skin turgor, moist gums, PCV 45–50%	5–10, PO or IV
Moderate	8–10	36–45	Depressed, sunken eyes, tacky gums, ↑ HR CRT > 2 s, PCV 50–65%	10, IV
Severe	>10	>45	Cold extremities, ↑↑ HR, profound depression, CRT > 3 s ± recumbency, PCV > 65%	15–20 (up to 40 in the first 1–2 hours in cases of severe shock), IV

- Losses of sodium (2000–6000 mmol or mEq) and potassium (500–3000 mmol or mEq) occur, and the estimated deficits and likelihood of correction of these by the fluid therapy need calculating (see Fluid Therapy, Chapter 17).
- *Addition of potassium chloride* to replacement fluids such as Multisol-R or 0.9% NaCl at a rate of 20 to 40 mmol/L (mEq/L) is very helpful. Administration of potassium in the form of KCl via a nasogastric tube (30–60 g in 2L water q6–8h) also can be a useful way to replete potassium losses.
- Based on the measurement of the bicarbonate value or base deficit in the plasma, estimates for the bicarbonate requirements can be made using the formula

0.3 × body weight (kg) × base deficit

In cases where severe bicarbonate loss has occurred, bicarbonate can be replaced intravenously or via nasogastric tube. Oral administration is frequently the safest, with doses of 150 to 200 g/450 kg in 6–8L water being given q12h or q6h during the acute phase of the disease provided there are no signs of ileus.

- In extremely compromised patients, fluids can be administered by pump systems at rates of up to 1 L/min. Use of large-bore catheters (teflon and polypropylene are the least thrombogenic) in several sites and administration via gravity from fluid bags can be used to deliver fluids at rates of 20 to 25 L/h.
- Use of hypertonic fluids (1.8% NaCl or double-strength Ringer's) has become more popular for the treatment of horses with severe diarrhea, particularly those experiencing substantial sodium losses and significant falls in plasma osmolality. These fluids should be used judiciously.

KEY POINT ► Oral fluid administration may be of great value in horses with acute diarrhea.

- Fluids can be administered via nasogastric tube, and the horse also can be offered fluids by free choice with provision of supplemented water. Horses can be provided with a bucket (6–8 L) of fresh water and one containing 60 to 80 g KCl. A third bucket containing 1 to 5 g/L of bicarbonate also may be provided.

KEY POINT ► When offering supplementary electrolytes, it is vital that horses are always given free-choice water, since some animals *will not* drink electrolyte "spiked" fluids.

- *Plasma transfusions* are of value when plasma protein values become low [albumin <20 g/L (2 g/dl); total plasma protein <40g/L (4 g/dl)]. The requirement for plasma is usually 5 to 10 L for a 450- to 500-kg horse, although smaller amounts appear to have favorable clinical effects.

- Use of commercially available antisera (1.5–4.0 ml/kg IV once) is reputed to be of value (Polymune J, Veterinary Dynamics, Inc., Chino, Calif.; Endoserum, Immvac, Columbia, Mo.) in horses with acute colitis.
- Nonsteroidal anti-inflammatory drugs (e.g., flunixin meglumine; Treatment No. 52) are recommended to reduce pain and ameliorate some of the clinical effects of endotoxemia. The dose rate of flunixin used should not exceed 0.25 mg/kg q8h.
- *Antidiarrheals/protectants* such as bismuth subsalicylate [1–2 L (32–64 oz) q8–12h via nasogastric tube] are useful. These agents also may have a local anti-inflammatory effect and thereby decrease fluid secretion. Kaopectate and activated charcoal also have been recommended, although their efficacy is not proven.
- The *use of antibiotics* in acute diarrhea, although common, should be considered likely to be detrimental. In many cases of salmonellosis, antibiotic use precedes the onset of the disease. Foals or debilitated adults may benefit from the use of antibiotics, since these agents may reduce the chance of organisms seeding to other organs *if* the horse is septicemic.

KEY POINT ► Antibiotics do not appear to reduce the duration of salmonella diarrhea.

- Additional caution is indicated because several studies have shown rapid development of resistance to antibiotics by *Salmonella* organisms involved in hospital outbreaks.
- *DMSO* (0.5–0.9 g/kg IV q24h as a 10% to 20% solution IV; Treatment No. 34) is thought to be useful because of its purported extensive therapeutic effects, including anti-inflammatory, antibacterial, and oxygen free-radical-scavenging properties.

Clostridium perfringens Type A ("Colitis X")

KEY POINT ► Many of the principles of therapy are similar to those described for salmonellosis, particularly voluminous fluid replacement.

- Pain is often severe in "colitis X," requiring potent analgesics. Xylazine (0.3–0.5 mg/kg IV as required; Treatment No. 108) and detomidine (20 μg/kg IV as required; Treatment No. 28) are useful agents, although they do have some adverse cardiovascular effects, causing a decrease in arterial pressure (see Table 6-5). Butorphanol (0.03–0.06 mg/kg IV as required; Treatment No. 15) can be combined with xylazine or detomidine for more potent analgesia (see Table 6-5).
- *Clostridium* spp. are sensitive to penicillin; therefore, administration of Na or K benzyl penicillin (25,000 IU/kg IV q6h) (Treatment Nos. 84 and 85) may be of value.

Equine Monocytic Ehrlichiosis

- Clinical manifestations dictate the degree of therapy required. Mild cases require only symptomatic and nursing care.

KEY POINT ► Severe cases require aggressive therapy, particularly fluids (see Salmonellosis).

KEY POINT ► *E. risticii* is sensitive to a number of antibiotics, especially tetracyclines.

- Oxytetracycline (6.6 mg/kg IV q24h) (Treatment No. 80) is the antibiotic therapy of choice. Early cases show dramatic response to antibiotic and supportive therapy, whereas more established disease responds more slowly. Antibiotic therapy should be continued for 7 to 10 days.
- Complications (e.g., laminitis) may still occur despite apparent good early response to therapy.
- Recurrence of the disease in horses in a geographic region where the disease has been diagnosed is common.
- Prophylaxis with bacterins (Treatment No. 112) gives short-lived protection (3–6 months) requiring repeated vaccinations.
- Vaccination in the face of an outbreak is often of limited value.

Other Causes of Acute Colitis

- Remove the inciting cause (e.g., discontinue nonsteroidal anti-inflammatory drug therapy or treat for internal parasites).
- Provide appropriate supportive therapy as required (see Salmonellosis).

Chronic Diarrhea

Chronic diarrhea is defined as an increased fluidity of feces that has been present for 3 weeks or more. Affected horses usually have stools with a consistency more commonly associated with bovine feces. Although a wide variety of diseases can result in chronic diarrhea, a precise diagnosis is often elusive. However, the chances for successful diagnosis and therapy are greatly increased if a systematic approach is used combined with judicious use of appropriate investigative procedures and laboratory tests. Despite the advent of new and particularly effective anthelmintics, parasitic causes of diarrhea due to *Strongylus* spp. or Cyathostomes are encountered relatively frequently. We have found an approach used by Dr. Goetz at the University of Illinois to be useful.

Diagnostic Approach to the Horse with Chronic Diarrhea

- Complete history
- Thorough physical examination, including rectal examination
- Fecal examination for parasite ova, serial bacteriology (for *Salmonella*)*
- Hematology and serum or plasma biochemistry (e.g., full blood count and plasma fibrinogen concentration; serum AP, SDH, GGT, AST, and bile acids; serum protein electrophoresis*; and plasma Na^+, K^+, Cl^-, HCO_3^-, and pH*)
- Abdominocentesis
- Urinalysis*
- Carbohydrate absorption tests*
- Rectal biopsy*
- Liver ultrasound/biopsy*

History and Presenting Signs

- Increased fecal volume of more than 3 weeks' duration
- Affected horses may be reported to have loss of body condition.
- Appetite is often normal to increased.
- History of poor parasite management or repeated dosing with anthelmintics with limited or no response

Clinical Findings and Diagnosis

- Cardinal signs are usually normal.
- Diarrhea with possible excoriation of skin on perineum
- Loss of weight is common.
- Dehydration is *not common*, although some animals with more severe signs demonstrate significant fluid deficits.
- Total white blood cell counts are often normal.
- Hypoproteinemia (hypoalbuminemia) is a common finding and is indicative of protein loss or inflammation of the gut.
- Increased numbers of parasite ova in feces are associated with chronic diarrhea in horses with poor management, infrequent administration of anthelmintics, or lack of response following repeated antihelmintic administrations. Severe strongylosis causes anemia, hypoproteinemia, poor coat quality, weight loss, and diarrhea.

KEY POINT ► However, low egg counts do not rule out the possibility of strongylosis since the infection may be pre-patent or egg production may be suppressed by previous anthelmintic administration.

- Sand in the feces is often reflective of increased sand ingestion and a secondary colitis due to its irritant nature.
- Pertinent rectal examination findings may include thickening of the bowel, possibly reflective of inflammatory bowel disease; roughened peritoneal surfaces indicative of peritonitis; enlarged mes-

---

*If indicated.

enteric lymph nodes; abdominal abscessation; and abdominal masses.

■ Elevated liver enzyme activities can be found, and there may be increased concentrations of bile acids reflective of a hepatopathy. A liver biopsy may assist in confirming a hepatopathy.

■ Abdominocentesis is often normal but, depending on the cause of the diarrhea, may reveal inflammatory or neoplastic cells. Bacteria may be present in cases of chronic peritonitis.

■ D-Glucose and/or D-xylose absorption tests may show decreased absorption of D-xylose or D-glucose, indicating small intestinal malabsorption (see Figs. 6-20 and 6-21). However, definitive diagnosis requires histopathology, usually performed on bowel biopsy samples or samples obtained after euthanasia. If the bowel disease is generalized, a rectal mucosal biopsy may be useful.

Differential Diagnosis

■ Strongylosis (e.g., cyathostome or *Strongylus vulgaris* infestation)
■ Chronic salmonellosis
■ Inflammatory bowel disease/malabsorption syndromes (granulomatous enteritis)
■ Sand-induced colitis
■ Abdominal abscessation
■ Alimentary lymphosarcoma
■ Chronic liver disease/septic cholangitis
■ Gastric neoplasia
■ Idiopathic chronic diarrhea
■ Chronic peritonitis

Treatment

■ *Strongylosis* is best treated with ivermectin (0.2 mg/kg PO; Treatment No. 62), or if larval forms of strongylosis are suspected, fenbendazole (10 mg/kg PO for 5 consecutive days; Treatment No. 51) may be used. Fenbendazole is reputedly more effective against these forms of the parasite than ivermectin. Treatment regimens often need to be repeated because encysted larvae are resistant to the anthelmintic. Altering management to decrease exposure to parasite larvae is also important.

■ *Chronic salmonellosis* is difficult to treat regardless of the medication utilized. Antibiotic therapy is useless. Symptomatic therapy is required to maintain fluid and electrolyte balance.

■ *Inflammatory bowel disease* (e.g., granulomatous enteritis, malabsorption syndrome, protein-losing enteropathy), *alimentary lymphosarcoma,* and *gastric neoplasia* respond poorly to therapy. Some types of inflammatory bowel disease respond to systemic corticosteroid therapy, but the response tends to be only short term.

■ *Sand ingestion* is managed by reducing access to sand, feeding of laxatives and diets high in fiber (see Sand Impaction, p. 232).

■ *Chronic liver disease* may improve with good supportive care and dietary management (see Liver Disease, p. 245).

■ *Abdominal abscessation* is responsive to therapy on occasion. This is covered under the section dealing with peritonitis (p. 243).

KEY POINT ▶ Most cases of chronic diarrhea fall into the category where no specific diagnosis is made and are referred to as "idiopathic" chronic diarrhea.

■ These cases may show temporary response to iodochlorhydroxyquin (10 g/500 kg PO q24h) (Rheaform, Squibb, Princeton, N.J.). If there is response within 48 hours, the dosing should be continued for another 3 to 4 days, after which the dose is reduced to a level that controls the diarrhea. Those animals not responding in the first 48 hours should have the drug discontinued.

■ An additional treatment includes administration of a cecal contents liquor. Cecal contents are collected from a dead horse, and if they are not to be used immediately, they should be kept in a bucket covered with a 2- to 3-cm layer of mineral oil. The liquor is then diluted with water to a consistency that passes through a nasogastric tube, and 5 to 6 L of the preparation is administered via this method. Daily administration for a few days may be required. Response is quite variable but, in some cases, quite dramatic.

■ Change of diet to grass hay is also thought to be of value. Antibiotics have no place in the treatment of chronic diarrhea and are likely to worsen the clinical course.

Internal Parasites

Internal parasites are ubiquitous, with horses being continually exposed throughout their lives. Infestation with *Strongylus* spp. is the most common and is usually regarded as producing the most significant pathogenic effects. Administration of anthelmintic agents and management strategies designed to limit parasite burdens constitute one of the most important aspects of veterinary preventive medicine practiced today. Anthelmintics for the treatment of internal parasites are outlined in Chapter 17.

Strongyloides westeri

■ A parasite that lives in the small intestine, commonly affecting young foals. The most frequent method of transmission of the parasite is via consumption of milk from an infected mare. Ingestion of infective larvae when eating is also a potential source of infection

■ Infections reach peak patency by 3 to 6 weeks of age, after which fecal egg counts rapidly decline. In most cases, foals have developed sufficient resistance to maintain infections at minimal levels by 12 to 16 weeks.

■ Patent infections are diagnosed by fecal flotation.

Ascarids

- Infection with the roundworm, *Parascaris equorum,* is common in foals. This parasite has progressively less significance with increasing age and is almost clinically irrelevant in horses 2 years of age and older. Strong immunity to the parasite develops in the first year of life.
- Adult *Parascaris equorum* live in the small intestine. Eggs are passed in the feces with foals ingesting embryonated eggs from the previous foal crop. After hatching in the intestine, larvae migrate through the liver and lungs for 17 days and then return to the small intestine. Patent infections occur by 3 months of age.
- Clinical manifestations include intestinal blockage and rupture, intussusception, ill thrift, diarrhea, and possibly respiratory signs.
- Diagnosis is confirmed by demonstration of characteristic thick-shelled eggs in the feces.

Pinworms

- *Oxyuris equi* are regarded as the most common pinworms, with adults living in the large and small colons. Females migrate to the anus, rupture, and deposit their eggs on the perineum, in the feces, or on surrounding bedding. Infective eggs are ingested, molt, and develop into adults in the colon.
- Primary clinical manifestations relate to perineal irritation from rupture of the females, resulting in tail rubbing and a "rat-tailed" appearance.
- Diagnosis is based on examination of transparent tape that is briefly adhered to the perineum and then examined under a microscope.

Stomach Worms

- *Habronema* spp. and *Draschia megastoma* are spiurids who live in the stomach. Larvae may invade skin wounds, causing "summer sores," and the eyes, inducing conjunctivitis. Flies act as intermediate hosts and transfer the larvae to these sites. Adult worms may cause gastric inflammation.
- Diagnosis of gastric infection is difficult. Cutaneous infestations are confirmed by demonstration of larvae in scrapings or biopsies.

Tapeworms

- *Anoplocephala perfoliata* and *Anoplocephala magna* are the tapeworms of the horse. *A. perfoliata* lives in clusters around the ileocecal valve and are the most common tapeworm. In contrast, *A. magna* is a bigger parasite that is less frequently encountered.
- Clinical signs are not common, although in some cases mucosal ulceration, weight loss, colic, diarrhea, and rupture of the gut has been ascribed to *A. perfoliata.*

- The life cycle involves orbatid mites who live in pasture as intermediate hosts.
- Diagnosis is based on the demonstration of typical angular eggs in fecal flotation preparations.

Bots

- Infestation with *Gastrophilus* spp. (stomach bots) is almost routine for horses living in temperate climates. Bots live in the stomach over winter and are then passed in the feces. Adult botflies deposit eggs on body hairs. These hatch following an increase in moisture, temperature, and the action of the lips of the horse. Larvae hatch and then progressively develop as they progress from the mouth to the stomach.
- Larvae produce deep pits in the stomach mucosa and may at times penetrate the gut wall, resulting in peritonitis. Ulceration of the stomach is common.
- Diagnosis is difficult, although the presence of bot eggs on the hair coat provides strong circumstantial evidence of infection.

Small Strongyles (Cyathostomes)

- Over 50 species of small strongyles affecting horses exist.
- The life cycle is direct, with females laying eggs that are passed in the feces. Here they develop into infective larvae and are eaten by grazing horses. Once in the gut, infective larvae invade the wall of the cecum and large colon, develop into the next larval stage, and remain in the gut wall for 1 to 2 months. Larvae then emerge into the gut and mature into adults.
- Cyathostomes induce pathology by larvae directly damaging the gut wall. In addition, the rapid emergence of encysted larvae in the spring can result in clinical signs of disease, including colic and diarrhea. Adult parasites produce decreased colonic motility, appetite, and weight gain. Encysted larvae have increased refractivity to anthelmintic therapy.
- Resistance by cyathostomes to anthelmintics is an emerging problem in horse populations and warrants careful attention by equine practitioners.
- Diagnosis of infection is made by the presence of strongyle eggs in the feces; however, the extent of infection is not necessarily reflected by this procedure because of a variety of factors, including prepatency and previous anthelmintic administration limiting fecal egg shedding.

Large Strongyles

- This group of parasites is composed of *Strongylus vulgaris, Strongylus edentatus,* and *Strongylus equinus,* with the latter having few significant clinical effects. Large strongyles are regarded as the most pathogenic of all equine internal parasites, with *S. vulgaris* being regarded as the most injurious.

■ The life cycle of large strongyles is similar to that described for small strongyles. Adults attach to the cecum and ventral colon. *S. vulgaris* larvae migrate from the gut, through the submucosal arterioles, to the cecal and colic arteries, reaching the cranial mesenteric artery within 4 months. They then return to the gut via the lumina of the arteries. The prepatent period is about 6 to 7 months.

■ Larvae of *S. edentatus* have a broad migratory path, progressing via the portal veins, liver, peritoneum, and gut wall. The prepatent period is 11 to 12 months. As with small strongyles, migrating larvae of *S. vulgaris* and *S. edentatus* have increased resistance to anthelmintic therapy.

■ *S. vulgaris* exerts its injurious effects by promoting inflammation in blood vessels along the course of migration. Vascular occlusion and aneurism of affected blood vessels, particularly the cranial mesenteric artery, can occur, resulting in inflammation, ischemia, and infarction, particularly of the distal small colon, cecum, and ventral colon.

KEY POINT ► This process often results in thromboembolic colic, ill thrift, diarrhea, and possibly death in affected horses.

■ *S. edentatus* larvae can damage the liver and produce peritonitis. Low-grade fever, depression, inappetence, colic, constipation, and diarrhea may all be features.

■ Diagnosis of large strongyle infections can be assumed if eggs are found in the feces. However, owing to the prolonged prepatent period of all species in this group, eggs will not be present in the feces in animals less than 9 to 12 months old. Clinical signs also may be useful indicators of infection.

■ Management practices to reduce the potential for transmission of the parasites are important. Such practices are based on routine anthelmintic administration and management strategies to reduce pasture contamination.

Rectal Perforation

Rectal tears are most commonly iatrogenic, occurring as a complication of rectal palpation. There is often little warning, with the veterinarian only suspicious that a tear has occurred after seeing blood on the sleeve following the examination. On occasion, rectal tears may result from breeding accidents when the stallion's penis enters the rectum. Idiopathic, spontaneous occurrence of rectal perforation also has been reported. Most rectal tears occur in the dorsal region near the mesenteric attachment.

KEY POINT ► All rectal tears should be regarded as an emergency.

Classification

Rectal tears are classified according to the number of tissue layers disrupted:

Grade 1—Involves the mucosa and submucosa.

Grade 2—Only the muscularis is disrupted, resulting in a mucosal–submucosal diverticulum. Rupture is rare.

Grade 3—Perforation of the mucosa, submucosa, and muscularis layers. The serosa remains intact and is the only layer between the rectum and peritoneal and pelvic cavities.

Grade 4—All layers are perforated, with direct communication between the rectum and pelvic and peritoneal cavities.

History and Presenting Signs

■ Prior rectal examination
■ Blood on the sleeve following examination
■ Sweating and signs of abdominal pain
■ Following breeding

Clinical Findings and Diagnosis

■ Blood on the sleeve is common following a tear. A few flecks of blood are likely to reflect mucosal irritation and possibly a grade 1 or 2 tear. More substantial hemorrhage is common with grade 3 and 4 tears.

■ The most dramatic clinical signs occur in horses with grade 4 tears. These can include progressive elevations in heart rate, signs of pain and sweating, and endotoxemia and subsequent shock. Signs are most profound when rupture into the abdominal cavity occurs and peritonitis ensues.

■ Tears greater than 15 cm (6 in) cranial to the anus are likely to be craniad to the peritoneal reflection and are more likely to result in peritonitis.

■ Grade 3 tears will often produce similar signs to those occurring with grade 4 tears; however, they may be more slowly progressive.

■ Some indication of the severity of tears and the degree of abdominal contamination can be obtained by repeated analyses of abdominal fluid (see Table 6-1).

■ Clinical manifestations are usually less acute if fecal material enters the pelvic (retroperitoneal) cavity. However, horses with retroperitoneal cellulitis can become extremely debilitated.

■ Horses with grade 2 tears may show no overt clinical signs. In this case, the mucosal–submucosal diverticulum may only be identified at a subsequent rectal examination that is performed for another reason. Other horses with grade 2 tears may be presented because of signs consistent with mild peritonitis or related to straining and fecal impaction.

■ Clinical signs are often limited in association with grade 1 tears. Those which do show systemic manifestations may show inappetence and mild depression for a few days.

- Diagnosis is confirmed by careful manual examination of the rectum. Some veterinarians perform this examination using a nongloved hand to improve digital sensitivity. This examination can be augmented by the use of tranquilization with acepromazine (Treatment No. 1), xylazine (Treatment No. 108), or detomidine (Treatment No. 28). If the horse continues to show evidence of straining, propantheline bromide (Treatment No. 95) can be administered in an attempt to reduce tenesmus. Alternatively, 25 to 50 ml of lidocaine (Treatment No. 67) mixed with an equal volume of lubricant or saline administered as an enema is also useful. In horses that still do not cease straining sufficiently to allow a thorough examination, epidural anaesthesia using xylazine (Treatment No. 108) is indicated (see Chap. 7).
- A speculum or endoscope also can be used to examine the rectum.
- Once a tear is identified, its size, position, depth, and distance from the anus should be assessed.

Treatment

- Grade 1 and 2 tears will often heal spontaneously. Regular monitoring for deterioration in condition should be undertaken. Systemic antibiotics, such as procaine penicillin G (Treatment No. 83) and gentamicin (Treatment No. 56) and possibly metronidazole (Treatment No. 75), are also indicated to assist with control of any pelvic or peritoneal contamination that may have occurred. Reduction in pain and signs of mild systemic toxemia may be provided by administration of flunixin (Treatment No. 52) and/or intravenous fluids. The feeding of lush green grass or high-quality alfalfa hay helps keep stools loose and will assist in allowing mucosal healing to occur more rapidly.

KEY POINT ▶ Grade 3 and 4 tears are to be regarded as emergencies and life-threatening if not treated rapidly and aggressively.

- The plan should involve rapid transport to a surgical referral facility. Epidural analgesia should be induced. Xylazine (Treatment No. 108) is the best choice for this because it produces less ataxia and weakness than does lidocaine or the other local anesthetics.
- The rectum should be carefully evacuated of remaining fecal material, and it should be packed craniad to the tear with cotton soaked in povidone-iodine.
- A number of surgical procedures have been described for treatment of rectal tears. The choice of procedure depends on the extent and size of the tear and the experience of the surgeon. Regardless of technique used, attempted correction of rectal tears is expensive, with the prognosis for grade 3 and 4 tears being poor.

Peritonitis

Peritonitis is relatively common in the horse and is classified relative to the origin of the inciting cause (*primary* or *secondary*), degree of involvement of the peritoneum (*diffuse* or *localized*), and in terms of the onset, severity, and duration of signs (*peracute, acute,* or *chronic*). The terms *septic* and *nonseptic* describe the presence or absence of bacteria, respectively. Most commonly, peritonitis occurs secondary to bowel compromise (e.g., colic), parasitism, and abdominal abscessation.

History and Presenting Signs

- Poor management consistent with parasitism
- Trauma (direct to abdominal wall, known history of rectal perforation, previous surgery)
- Parturition or coitus resulting in uterine or vaginal perforation
- Colic with evidence of compromised bowel

KEY POINT ▶ Depression, inappetence

- Weight loss in chronic cases
- Diarrhea

Clinical Findings and Diagnosis

- Variable, ranging from almost no signs to severe systemic manifestations
- Evidence of vaginal discharge or perforation, metritis, or a uterine tear in the mare postpartum or postcoitus
- Rectal tear is a frequent cause, usually the result of rectal examinations, and is determined by history and careful manual or speculum examination.
- Fever and elevated heart and respiratory rates are commonly present.
- Other signs include abdominal "splinting" and ileus.
- Dehydration is common, with mild electrolyte derangements (especially hypocalcemia) being present. Shock is found in severe cases.
- Diagnosis is based on history, clinical findings, and laboratory findings.
- Rectal examination may indicate roughened (gritty) peritoneal surfaces, thickened serosal surfaces on bowel, pain, or evidence of an abdominal mass.
- Hematology shows leukocytosis (neutrophilia), together with an elevated fibrinogen concentration. There may be anemia due to bone marrow depression in chronic cases.
- An increase in total plasma protein is found in some more chronic cases, which may be due to dehydration and/or hypergammaglobulinemia. *Note:* Hypoproteinemia occurs in some acute diffuse cases owing to protein effusion into the peritoneal cavity.

KEY POINT ▶ Abdominocentesis is vital for diagnosis.

- Changes in abdominal fluid may include increased total nucleated cell count (>50,000 × 10^6/L or 50,000/µl), increased protein concentration (>45 g/L or 4.5 g/dl), and increased turbidity (see Table 6-1).

KEY POINT ▶ In addition to cytologic and biochemical analyses, samples should be subjected to Gram staining and bacterial culture and sensitivity testing.

- More than 60% of septic peritonitis cases are due to mixed bacterial infections.

Differential Diagnosis

- Causes of peritonitis include abdominal abscessation associated with *Streptococcus* spp., *Rhodococcus* or *Corynebacterium* spp., *E. coli*, or anaerobes (e.g., *Bacteroides* spp.); neoplasia; parasitism; uterine perforation; gastrointestinal impaction/strangulation/rupture; enteritis; trauma to abdominal cavity or foreign body; rectal perforation; postoperative, e.g., complication of castration or abdominal surgery; ruptured bladder, foals; associated with urachal infection, foals; and secondary to septicemia, foals.
- Laminitis
- Myopathies
- Pyelonephritis
- Pleuritis
- Colic

Treatment

- In secondary peritonitis, treatment of the primary disease is vital (e.g., management of internal parasites, rectal/vaginal tears, etc.).
- In acute cases, initial management includes *fluid therapy* to rehydrate the animal, control cardiovascular compromise, and correct electrolyte and acid–base abnormalities. Isotonic polyionic fluids (see Fluid Therapy, Chap. 17) should be given intravenously (10–20 ml/kg/h initially) as required. *Nonsteroidal anti-inflammatory drugs* (e.g., flunixin meglumine 0.25–0.5 mg/kg IV q6h; Treatment No. 52) are given to control some of the effects of endotoxin production and provide mild analgesia. Endotoxin antiserum (1.5–4.0 ml/kg IV once) (Endoserum, Immvac, Columbia, Mo.; Polymune J, Veterinary Dynamics, Inc., Chino, Calif.) is indicated in cases where endotoxemia exists.
- *Nasogastric intubation* for gastric decompression should be performed when required in cases with ileus or colic (see Figs. 6-10 to 6-13).
- *Mineral oil* (5–10 ml/kg PO q12–24h) (Treatment No. 77) can be administered when no gastric reflux occurs and feces are dry or rectal findings are suggestive of an impaction.

KEY POINT ▶ Appropriate antimicrobial therapy should be given based on results of culture and sensitivity.

- Initial introduction of antibiotic coverage directed against the most common pathogens implicated in peritonitis is indicated while awaiting culture results. Procaine penicillin at a dose rate of 15,000 IU/kg (15 mg/kg) IM q12h (Treatment No. 83) or ampicillin sodium at a dose rate of 11 mg/kg IV q6–8h (Treatment No. 6) in combination with gentamicin (2–3 mg/kg IV q6–8h) (Treatment No. 56) are good choices. In cases where anaerobes (e.g., *Bacteroides fragilis*, implicated in approximately 10% of septic peritonitis cases) are suspected, addition of metronidazole (15 mg/kg PO q6h) (Treatment No. 75) is indicated because penicillin is not active against this bacteria. Antimicrobial therapy often needs to be prolonged (>3 weeks), and the decision to discontinue therapy is based on clinical response and return of the leukogram, fibrinogen, and abdominal fluid constituents to normal or near normal. In cases where bacteria are susceptible to trimethoprim–sulfadiazine (15–20 mg/kg of the combined drug PO q12h; Treatment No. 107), this combination provides a useful alternative therapy. Advantages include (1) the horse does not have to receive injectable antibiotics, (2) owners can administer these agents for the long periods frequently required, and (3) the combination is relatively cost-effective.
- *Abdominal drainage* through a teat cannula or abdominal drain may be beneficial in some cases of acute septic peritonitis to assist in removal of offending bacteria and residual debris.
- *Peritoneal lavage* is advocated by some, particularly in cases of generalized peritonitis. Several liters of warm isotonic polyionic fluid are infused through a catheter in the paralumbar fossa, with the fluid drained from the ventral abdomen with an abdominal drain. Multisol-R and lactated Ringer's (see Fluid Therapy, Chap. 17) are good choices because they are less irritant than many other fluids.
- *Heparin* (20–40 IU/kg diluted in several liters of isotonic polyionic fluid IP or 10–50 IU/kg q8–12h IV; Treatment No. 59) has been advocated to reduce abdominal adhesions. This treatment is controversial.
- *DMSO* (0.5–0.9 g/kg IV q24h as a 10% to 20% solution IV; Treatment No. 34) is thought to be useful because of its purported extensive therapeutic effects, including anti-inflammatory, antibacterial, and oxygen free-radical-scavenging properties, all of which are thought to decrease the incidence of abdominal adhesions.
- Referral of the horse for exploratory celiotomy can be considered, with the aim being to assist in defining the cause of the peritonitis or to physically remove debris/necrotic material from the peritoneal cavity.

Liver Diseases

Compromise of hepatic function in horses is probably more common than realized. However, such is the compensatory capacity of the liver that clinical manifestations of hepatic disease are uncommon. Hepatic failure/insufficiency only occurs when more than two-thirds of liver function is compromised.

KEY POINT ▶ Manifestations of hepatic failure include alterations in appetite, weight loss, icterus, dermatitis of unpigmented areas, derangements of CNS function, low serum protein concentration, ascites, coagulopathies, hemolytic crises, colic, and pruritus.

The usual reason horses with liver failure are presented to the veterinarian for examination are icterus, weight loss, and deranged CNS function. Signs of CNS dysfunction may be very subtle, ranging from very mild behavioral alterations that may only be noted by those familiar with the horse to depression, incoordination, aimless wandering, yawning, and head pressing. The cause of the hepatoencephalopathy is not clear, but it may be the result of low blood glucose concentrations, elevated blood ammonia values, or alterations in the ratios of amino acids in the central nervous system. This imbalance may lead to a failure of homeostasis in neurotransmitters or the production of false neurotransmitters. Accumulation of other toxic products that have not been cleared by the liver also may contribute to alterations in CNS function.

Acute Liver Failure

KEY POINT ▶ The most common cause of acute hepatic failure is Theiler's disease (serum hepatitis).

Theiler's disease occurs only in adult horses and can involve an individual animal or there may be sporadic "outbreaks" over a matter of weeks. Most cases are reported in the fall. Administration of equine-derived biologic products has been the most frequently reported activity associated with the onset of this disease, hence the common name "serum hepatitis." The frequency of this disease has declined, probably as a result of a reduction in the use of these products. However, cases still occur where horses succumb to acute hepatic failure with no prior history of administration of biologics. Despite the epidemiology of this disease, no infectious agent has been identified. Affected horses are seronegative for human serum hepatitis antibodies. Other rare causes of acute hepatic failure include acute toxicosis with mycotoxins, pyrrolizidine alkaloids, rubratoxins, liver abscessation, suppurative cholangitis, and cholelithiasis. Hyperlipidemia and subsequent hyperlipemia with fatty infiltration of the liver in ponies also may result in fulminant acute hepatic failure.

History and Presenting Signs

- Depression
- Inappetence/anorexia
- Central nervous system derangements (hepatoencephalopathy)
- Possibly a history of administration of equine-derived biologic products (e.g., tetanus antitoxin)
- Pruritus/photosensitization
- Colic

Clinical Findings and Diagnosis

- Depression and inappetence are common.
- Icterus is normally a feature of acute hepatic failure
- CNS derangements (e.g., head pressing, aimless wandering, and yawning) due to hepatoencephalopathy may occur.
- Coagulopathies are rarely a feature of acute liver failure.
- Diagnosis is usually based on the history, clinical signs, and clinicopathologic derangements.

KEY POINT ▶ The most common alterations in serum biochemistry values include elevations in the activities of AST, GGT, SDH, AP, LDH, and the concentrations of bilirubin and bile acids.

- Hypoglycemia is also a common feature of this disorder.
- In cases where hepatic failure occurs secondary to septic cholangitis or liver abscessation, there may be an indication of a systemic inflammatory response reflected by leukocytosis and hyperfibrinogenemia.
- A liver biopsy (Figs. 6-18 and 6-19) is valuable in confirming the diagnosis and assists with deter-

mination of the prognosis. There is usually evidence of acute hepatocellular degeneration. We have found that ultrasound examination greatly facilitates the collection of liver biopsies.

Differential Diagnosis

- Central nervous system diseases causing depression/abnormal behavior (e.g., trauma)
- Gastrointestinal tract colic
- Systemic diseases causing inappetence/anorexia (e.g., endotoxemia)
- Primary photosensitization
- Chronic liver failure
- Chronic active hepatitis

Treatment

KEY POINT ▶ Therapy for acute hepatic insufficiency should be directed at control of the abnormal behavior and support of liver function until hepatic compensation can occur. A low-protein, high-energy diet should be fed.

- If the horse is anorexic, nasogastric intubation and provision of high-energy foods are recommended. Infusions with 5% dextrose (2 L/h IV) may provide some of the caloric needs of affected horses and boost blood glucose concentrations.
- Beet pulp (a good source of branched-chain amino acids) is a suitable supplement. Mixing beet pulp with molasses will improve palatability and the energy content of this supplement. The administration of branched-chain amino acids appears to reduce the severity of neurologic signs.
- Drugs such as xylazine (Treatment No. 108), detomidine (Treatment No. 28), and chloral hydrate (all to effect) are useful for the control of manic behavior.
- Parenteral administration of B-complex vitamins is indicated.
- Efficacy of the supportive therapy is demonstrated by a rapid improvement of the horse's condition, a desire to drink and eat, and a substantial reduction in signs of CNS impairment.

Chronic Liver Failure

KEY POINT ▶ Horses with this disorder are usually presented because of chronic weight loss or the onset of signs consistent with hepatic insufficiency.

Hepatic insufficiency occurs because hepatocellular compromise is such that the functional reserve capacity of the organ is surpassed.

KEY POINT ▶ The most common cause of chronic hepatic failure is exposure to hepatotoxic plants, particularly those containing pyrrolizidine alkaloids.

Exposure to these toxins can occur directly by the ingestion of toxin-containing plants in the field or via the ingestion of contaminated hay. Recent studies show that horses need to consume more than 200 mg of the alkaloid per kilogram of body weight before severe (usually fatal) liver disease is induced. Chronic liver failure also may result from cholangitis, liver abscesses, or biliary obstructions.

Clinical Findings and Diagnosis

KEY POINT ▶ Weight loss is often the most prominent feature of chronic liver failure.

- Anorexia or inappetence is common.
- A variety of behavioral changes can occur in severe cases, including yawning, head pressing, somnolence, dysphagia, dysphonia, and ataxia.
- Decreased gut sounds, colic, and watery feces occur in some cases.
- Dependent edema can occur if the plasma protein concentration becomes sufficiently low.
- Skin lesions (photosensitization/pruritus) may be seen.
- Some horses also demonstrate polydipsia and polyuria.
- Profound icterus *need not* be a feature of chronic liver disease, although some degree of icterus is usually found.
- Diagnosis is based on the same principles as those described for acute hepatic insufficiency.
- Elevations in the activity of liver enzymes (AST, GGT, SDH, AP, and LDH) and the concentrations of bilirubin and bile acids in the plasma are all good indicators of liver disease. However, in long-standing chronic liver disease, liver enzymes may be normal because there is no longer active damage.
- Hypoproteinemia (hypoalbuminemia) and low blood urea nitrogen concentrations may be a feature of chronic liver disease.
- A liver biopsy (Figs. 6-18 and 6-19) will confirm the diagnosis of pyrrolizidine alkaloid toxicosis. Pathognomonic histopathologic changes include hepatomegalocytosis and biliary hyperplasia.
- A response to therapy/rest and a downward trend in the enzyme activities and bile acids probably provide the best information regarding the prognosis.

Treatment

- Strategies similar to those described for acute hepatic insufficiency are prescribed (see p. 000). Plasma transfusions (6–10 ml/kg IV) may help by promoting temporary increases in plasma protein concentration and oncotic pressure.

KEY POINT ▶ Horses with chronic liver failure have a poor prognosis, and most therapies are designed to be supportive in nature while awaiting results and hoping that hepatic function returns to adequate levels. This does not often occur.

Chronic Active Hepatitis

Chronic active hepatitis describes a group of diseases that appear to involve a relatively active and progressive liver disease. Based on empirical observations, most cases seem to have an infectious or immune basis.

History and Presenting Signs

- Depression, weight loss, and variable icterus
- Signs present for weeks to months

Clinical Findings and Diagnosis

KEY POINT ▶ Febrile episodes often accompany the clinical manifestations of liver disease.

- Physical examination usually reveals elevated cardinal signs, depression, and a variety of other neurologic signs. Signs consistent with abdominal disease also may be noted.

KEY POINT ▶ Some affected horses have an exfoliative dermatitis. This is thought to be the result of an immune-mediated vasculitis.

- Diagnosis is based on the clinical findings and laboratory procedures. Affected horses often have substantial elevations in serum GGT and AP activities, serum bilirubin concentration, and bile acid concentrations.
- An increase in TPP due to *hypergammaglobulinemia* occurs in some cases.

KEY POINT ▶ Diagnosis is confirmed by liver biopsy revealing periportal cholangiohepatitis and in some cases, septic cholangitis.

Treatment

- Successful treatment requires intensive efforts involving fluids, antibiotics, corticosteroids, and aggressive supportive care.
- Support includes control of abnormal behavior (e.g., xylazine; Treatment No. 108), provision of high-energy diets, intravenous fluids (5% dextrose in water, 2 L/h IV), and systemic antibiotics. Trimethoprim–sulfonamide (15–20 mg/kg of the combination IV or PO q12h; Treatment No. 107) or procaine penicillin G [15,000 IU/kg (15 mg/kg) IM q12h; Treatment No. 83] and gentamicin (2–3 mg/kg IV or IM q8–12h; Treatment No. 56) empirically provide relief of signs in some cases.

- Favorable response to corticosteroid administration also has been reported. Prednisolone (1.5 mg/kg PO q12h for 3 days, then 1.0 mg/kg PO q12h for 3 days, followed by 1.0 mg/kg PO q24h for 5 days and then 0.5 mg/kg PO q24h for 5 days) has been a successful treatment in our experience (Treatment No. 56).
- Improved mental status, appetite, and behavior are signs consistent with response to treatment. Some horses have shown a slow response to therapy and have taken several weeks to return to normal. Others do not respond to therapy or the costs become prohibitive and require euthanasia.

Cholelithiasis

Calculi in the common bile duct are thought to be the result of ascending or hematogenous infection from the duodenum. Calculi can be single or multiple, and if biliary stasis occurs, clinical manifestations will usually result. The condition can occur without clinical signs being evident.

History and Presenting Signs

- Usually in horses more than 5 years old
- Mild colic, often with repeated bouts
- Inappetence
- Depression

Clinical Findings and Diagnosis

- Depression and alterations in behavior (hepatoencephalopathy) may be apparent
- Signs of colic (e.g., pain, increased cardinal signs)
- Fever in some cases

KEY POINT ▶ Diagnosis may be assisted by clinical pathology findings, including hyperproteinemia, hyperfibrinogenemia, and leukocytosis, which are common.

- Marked increases in the activity of GGT and AP and in total bilirubin and bile acids are common. The ratio of direct-to-total bilirubin is usually greater than 0.25. Increases in the activity of AST and SDH and in blood ammonia also occur.
- Coagulopathies can be present.
- Abdominocentesis may reveal an increased volume of yellow–orange fluid with an increase in protein and nucleated cells consistent with chronic inflammation.
- Bilirubinuria, as detected by dipstick examination, is common.
- Ultrasonography is of value in revealing an enlarged liver, dilated bile ducts, and hyperechoic areas in ducts.
- A liver biopsy (Figs. 6-18 and 6-19) may provide evidence of the histologic changes and bacterial organisms involved. A liver biopsy should not be performed if the horse has evidence of coagulop-

athy. Results of the biopsy will not confirm the diagnosis but provide important prognostic information. Common histopathologic changes occurring in association with cholelithiasis indicating a poor prognosis include periportal fibrosis, bile duct proliferation, accumulations of bile pigment, and hepatocellular necrosis.

Treatment

- Therapy is often unrewarding and should be tempered based on the findings of clinicopathology, biopsy, and ultrasound examinations.
- Antibiotic therapy is prescribed in an attempt to reduce biliary infection. Trimethoprim–sulfonamide combinations (15–20 mg/kg of the combination PO q12h; Treatment No. 107) or procaine penicillin G [15,000 IU/kg (15 mg/kg) IM q12h; Treatment No. 83] and gentamicin (1–2 mg/kg IV or IM q8–12h; Treatment No. 56) for several weeks are good choices.
- Dietary manipulation and fluid therapy as described for horses with hepatic failure (p. 246) are useful, particularly in animals showing signs of depression or behavioral abnormalities
- Referral to a university or large clinic for potential surgery is indicated in valuable animals.

Hyperlipemia/Hyperlipidemia

Hyperlipidemia is common in horses and ponies and is the result of exercise or reduced caloric intake (e.g., colic, surgery, etc.). *Hyperlipidemia* is usually readily reversible following resumption of normal ingestion of food. In contrast, *hyperlipemia* is a more severe metabolic disorder that is common in ponies. It is characterized by depression, inappetence, fatty liver, and cloudy serum. *Hyperlipemia* is often secondary to a primary disorder that induces decreased caloric intake (e.g., pregnancy, lactation, colic). This section addresses *hyperlipemia*.

History and Presenting Signs

- Common in ponies, although horses can be affected
- Pregnancy or lactation
- Depression
- Anorexia/inappetence
- Most common in winter

Clinical Findings and Diagnosis

- Affected ponies are often fat. Examination reveals depression and lack of interest in food.
- Diarrhea is common.
- Central nervous system abnormalities can occur and may be manifest by incoordination and weakness.

KEY POINT ▶ Clinical pathology changes include cloudy serum with triglyceride

concentrations of 5.7 mmol/L (500 mg/dl) or more and elevations in liver enzyme activities (AST, AP, GGT, SDH), bilirubin, and bile acid concentrations.

- Azotemia is common.
- Metabolic acidosis may occur in the terminal stages of the disease.
- Liver biopsy reveals massive fatty infiltration.
- Postmortem examination reveals cloudy serum and pale, swollen liver and kidneys as a result of fatty infiltration. When cut, these organs have a greasy texture. In some cases the liver may rupture, resulting in death.

Treatment

- Remove or treat the primary disease in an attempt to promote an increase in intake of feed.
- Constant slow infusion of glucose (dextrose 5% in water 1 L/h IV) is the usual first line of therapy. Protamine zinc insulin (30 IU IM q12h) with glucose (0.5 g/kg PO q12h) on the first and subsequent odd days, followed by insulin (15 IU/kg IM q12h) and galactose (0.5 g/kg PO q12h) on even days, to provide energy has been recommended.
- Heparin (100–250 IU/kg SC q12h; Treatment No. 59) is also prescribed in an attempt to assist in reducing plasma triglyceride concentrations. This dose rate of heparin and the effects of liver dysfunction may result in alterations in hemostasis.
- The prognosis for ponies with hyperlipemia is poor.

References

Adams, S. B. Diseases of the alimentary system. In: *Equine Medicine and Surgery—4th edition.* Colahan P. T., Mayhew I. G., Merritt A. M. and Moore J. N. (eds), Goleta, Calif.: American Veterinary Publications, 1991, pp. 473–489.

Bramlage, L. R.: Examination in acute abdominal crisis. In: *Equine Medicine and Surgery—3rd edition.* Mansmann R. A. and McAllister E. S. (eds), Santa Barbara: American Veterinary Publications, 1982, pp. 548–559.

Campbell Thompson, M., and Merritt, A.: Diagnosis and treatment of gastroduodenal ulceration and gastric outflow obstruction in foals and adult horses. *Proc. 35th Annu. Conv. Am. Assoc. Equine Pract.,* 1989, p. 57.

Divers, T. J., and Palmer, J. E.: Antimicrobial therapy in equine gastrointestinal disease. *Proc. 32d Annu. Conv. Am. Assoc. Equine Pract.,* 1986, p. 223.

Hoffmann, W. E., Baker, G., Rieser, S., and Dorner, J. L.: Alterations in selected serum biochemical constituents in equids after induced hepatic disease. *Am. J. Vet. Res.* 48:1343, 1987.

Morris, D. D., and Henry, M. M.: Hepatic encephalopathy. *Compend. Contin. Educ. Pract. Vet.* 13:1153, 1991.

Murray, M. J.: Therapeutic procedures for horses with colitis. *Vet. Med.* 85:510, 1990.

Palmer, J. E., Benson, C. E., and Whitlock, R. H.: Resistance to development of equine ehrlichial colitis in experimentally inoculated horses and ponies. *Am. J. Vet. Res.* 51:763, 1990.

Palmer, J. E., Whitlock, R. H., and Benson, C. E.: Equine ehrlichial colitis: Effect of oxytetracycline treatment during the incubation period of *Ehrlichia risticii* infection in ponies. *J. Am. Vet. Med. Assoc.* 192:343, 1988.

Prescott, J. F., Staempfli, H. R., Barker, I. K., et al.: A method for reproducing fatal idiopathic colitis (colitis X) in ponies and isolation of a clostridium as a possible agent. *Equine Vet. J.* 20:417, 1988.

Schneider, R. K., Meyer, D. J., Embertson, R. M., et al.: Response of pony peritoneum to four peritoneal lavage solutions. *Am. J. Vet. Res.* 49:889, 1988.

Schumacher, J.: Peritonitis following castration in 3 horses. *J. Equine Vet. Sci.* 7:220, 1987.

Taylor, T.: Equine colic: Referral considerations and presurgical management. *Proc. 35th Annu. Conv. Am. Assoc. Equine Pract.,* 1989, p. 95.

Uhlinger, C. A.: Equine small strongyles: Epidemiology, pathology, and control. *Compend. Contin. Educ. Pract. Vet.* 13:863, 1991.

Uhlinger, C.: New information on parasite control and the incidence of colic: Anthelmintic protocol for prevention of colic. *Proc. 35th Annu. Conv. Am. Assoc. Equine Pract.,* 1989, p. 99.

White, N., II: Medical management of the colic patient. *Proc. 34th Annu. Conv. Am. Assoc. Equine Pract.,* 1988, p. 81.

White, N. A.: Examination and diagnosis of the acute abdomen. In: *The Equine Acute Abdomen,* N. A. White (ed.), Philadelphia: Lea and Febiger, 1990, pp. 102–142.

Whitlock, R. H.: Colitis: Differential diagnosis and treatment. *Equine Vet. J.* 18:278, 1986.

Ziemer, E. L., Whitlock, R. H., Palmer, J. E., and Spencer, P. A.: Clinical and hematologic variables in ponies with experimentally induced equine ehrlichial colitis (Potomac horse fever). *Am. J. Vet. Res.* 48:63, 1987.

CHAPTER 7

Reproduction

Reproductive problems and general reproductive examinations for pregnancy diagnosis form an important part of clinical practice for many equine practitioners. While the rectal examination glove still forms the basis for much equine stud farm practice, the availability of ultrasound equipment and a variety of hormonal assays has permitted much greater diagnostic accuracy than previously possible. It is important for the veterinary surgeon involved in breeding work to fully evaluate the mare before any treatment. Part of the knowledge base involves a good understanding of reproductive physiology. Some of the key aspects of reproductive physiology as they relate to the broader considerations of reproduction problems in mares and stallions will be discussed in the section on reproductive physiology and management in this chapter.

Much time and effort are expended by veterinary surgeons in the treatment of various genital problems in mares and in attempts to improve reproductive efficiency. While significant improvements have been made in individual stud farms, there have been few changes in overall foaling rates in the last 50 years. Throughout the world, the average foaling rate for thoroughbred mares of 60% to 70% has remained reasonably constant. It is therefore important to carefully evaluate various treatments and management strategies to ensure that progress is being made.

KEY POINT ▶ In many cases, mares may have a wide range of routine procedures performed, such as rectal examinations, cervical and uterine swabs, and ultrasound examination, without any clinical indication.

Worse than this, situations can arise where mares receive costly hormonal and/or antibiotic therapy for a nonexistent clinical problem. We saw one case where a maiden mare was diagnosed as having bacterial endometritis on the basis of a routine cervical bacteriologic swab. The diagnosis of endometritis was followed by several courses of antibiotic ther-

apy, with the mare being presented for further investigations because of infertility. In taking the history, we found that one of the main reasons for infertility was that the mare had not been served. This case highlights the potential problems in broodmare practice of overservicing and overtreatment.

In this section we will discuss important aspects of reproductive physiology, approach to examination and diagnosis of reproductive disorders, and aspects of therapy that can be applied in a nonspecialized practice setting.

EXAMINATION OF THE REPRODUCTIVE SYSTEM

The Mare

A logical series of steps in examination of the reproductive system should be undertaken. The degree to which specialized diagnostic aids are required will depend on the history and initial findings.

History

While specific aspects of reproductive history are often given careful attention by veterinarians, other details such as vaccination history, diet, and medical problems are relevant to reproductive performance.

KEY POINT ▶ At the start of the breeding season, it is important to know details of the previous year's reproductive performance.

The following details are relevant:

- Number of foals successfully delivered
- Number of previous pregnancies
- History of any dystocias
- Details of previous estrous cycles
- Duration of estrus

- Number of breedings before mare failed to return to estrus
- History of early embryonic loss following a confirmed pregnancy
- History of foaling injuries
- History of discharge from vulva
- Details of previous investigations and treatment

If the history suggests difficulties in the mare conceiving the previous year, a full medical history should be obtained that includes details of all investigations and therapy. In some cases this will be readily available if the mare is on a stud farm attended by the practice in previous years. However, if the mare is new to the particular stud farm, it may be necessary to obtain records from the veterinary practice previously attending the mare.

Equine stud-farm practice is a demanding life with long hours and a busy workload for 4 to 5 months of the year. Because of this, many veterinarians keep inadequate records. It is important to institute a record system that is simple but allows quick referral to features such as state of the ovaries, size of follicles, appearance of the cervix, color of discharge, and so on. Mares that are difficult to get into foal may require examination many times during the course of a breeding season. In these cases, it is essential that accurate records be kept to allow comparisons to be made between examinations.

Examination of the External Genitalia

It is best to examine the external genitalia during estrus, although this option is obviously not always available.

KEY POINT ▶ One of the single most important steps in a reproductive examination is assessment of the conformation of the vulva.

The vulva and the anus normally should be in the same plane; when the anus has a "sunken" appearance and the vulva is sloping forward, the mare is prone to infection through pneumovagina and fecal contamination. The vulval lips are examined for any signs of previous lacerations or evidence of Caslick's surgery. Using disposable gloves, the vulval lips should be separated and the entrance to the vagina examined for discharge, scarring, or inflammation.

KEY POINT ▶ Of importance is observation of the relationship of the pelvic floor to the orientation of the vulva.

If the pelvic floor is palpated and much of the vulva lies dorsal, contamination of the vagina is possible because of pneumovagina. The clitoris can then be examined, and although it is seldom affected by clinical disease, it is of importance because it can act as a reservoir for the contagious equine metritis (CEM) organism. The clitoral fossa

and clitoral sinuses are sites that have been shown to harbor the CEM organism, and these areas can be cultured if infection is suspected. The clitoral fossa and sinuses also may be the primary areas for harboring organisms that cause endometritis.

Visual Examination of Vagina and Cervix

Integrity of the cervix is vital for pregnancy to be sustained. Examination not only allows assessment of any abnormalities but also permits evaluation of changes associated with various stages of the estrous cycle. Prior to internal examination, the vulva should be cleaned with disinfectant so that infection is not introduced at the time of examination.

KEY POINT ▶ It is important to remember that all disinfectants are potentially irritant, and therefore, care should be taken to make up an accurate concentration.

The commonly used technique of splashing disinfectant into a bucket of water until the correct color appears is inaccurate and may lead to a concentration of disinfectant that is damaging to the sensitive mucous membranes.

Cervical examination is best undertaken using a disposable cardboard speculum system that can be connected to a light source. The danger of using the duck-billed speculum, immersed in disinfectant between mares, was shown when it was proven that some veterinarians using this technique were instrumental in the transmission of CEM. In the initial examination, as the speculum is inserted, note should be taken of any purulent discharges, cervical lesions, or urine pooling in the anterior vagina. Urine pooling is a common cause of reproductive failure.

During the breeding season, the cervix changes in appearance from the pale-colored, tight structure that does not permit insertion of a finger to a pink, loose structure under the influence of estrogens. Near ovulation, the cervix can appear congested and sometimes edematous. It is also moist and lies ventrally in the vagina. At this stage, the cervix will readily admit two to three fingers. Direct palpation of the cervix, after thorough cleansing and disinfection of the perineal region, permits assessment of the tone of the cervix and whether any adhesions exist.

Rectal Examination

Preparation for the Rectal Examination. Rectal examination provides a technique whereby the uterus and ovaries can be assessed and pregnancy either ruled out or diagnosed. Rectal examination is not a technique without some risk, since rupture of the rectum can occur, particularly in nervous or fractious horses. The examination should be performed with the mare adequately restrained and with a generous amount of obstetrical lubricant.

KEY POINT ▶ If the mare strains excessively, the use of propantheline bromide (Treatment No. 95) at a dose rate of 0.1 to 0.2 mg/kg IV will significantly reduce the risk of a rectal tear.

Propantheline should be administered approximately 5 minutes before a rectal examination is performed. Some veterinarians have reported colic after propantheline use.

KEY POINT ▶ Some rectal examination gloves have a sharp edge along the seam. For this reason, we find that there is less likelihood of damage to the rectum if the glove is turned inside out prior to its use.

The hand should be introduced with plenty of lubricant, and the fingers should be pushed closely together in a cone shape. Once the hand is in the rectum, a brief period should be given for the mare to relax. The arm should initially be advanced further into the rectum than the level required and then withdrawn, since this usually provokes less discomfort and straining. The feces present in the rectum are then removed with the palm of the hand facing dorsally. After application of further lubricant, the hand is reinserted, and any additional feces are removed. The arm is moved cranially, and if resistance or straining is encountered, the arm should not be advanced further. Most cases of rectal rupture occur when the hand is advanced cranially as the mare strains.

Systematic Rectal Exploration of the Reproductive Tract. A systematic examination should be adopted, commencing with one ovary (usually the side opposite the particular arm used) and proceeding along the uterus to the opposite ovary.

Ovarian Examination. The ovaries are attached to the sublumbar region by the broad ligament and can be located by using the ilium as a reference point. The only structure that can be confused with an ovary is a fecal ball in the small colon.

KEY POINT ▶ The size of the ovaries varies with the breeding season.

During winter to early spring, when mares are in anestrus, the ovaries are small, being approximately 3 cm in diameter. During spring, with the mare cycling, the ovaries approximately double in size. An ovary can be held between the thumb and index finger to determine follicle size (range 2–6 cm) and changes in contour. Accurate determination of follicle size is important to enable determination of the imminence of ovulation. Examination of follicle size ("follicle testing") is extensively used by some stud farms to reduce the number of matings for individual stallions.

With experience, the corpus luteum can be discriminated, but this is somewhat difficult because it does not protrude from the ovarian surface, unlike follicles. The ovulation fossa can be located ventromedially.

Uterine Examination. The uterus is palpated to determine tone, which is important in the early stages of pregnancy. The nonpregnant uterus of the mare is much more flaccid than that of the cow and can be difficult to locate if the examiner is inexperienced. The arm should be introduced deep into the rectum so that the hand, with the palm facing ventrally, comes to lie past the rim of the pelvis. If the arm is then slowly withdrawn, the body of the uterus will come to rest within slightly flexed fingers. If the mare is pregnant, there will be gradual enlargement of one of the uterine horns, close to the body of the uterus.

KEY POINT ▶ The presence of increased uterine tone and evidence of slight bulging on the anterior and ventral surfaces of the uterus can indicate early pregnancy.

Once the body of the uterus has been examined, the hand should sweep up either side to examine the uterine horns.

Cervical Examination. The cervix lies further caudal to the body of the uterus on the pelvic floor. In the anestrus mare, the cervix is soft and has little or no tone. It is sometimes possible to pass the speculum straight into the uterus in a mare in anestrus. In diestrus, the cervix is firm and hard, being approximately 6 cm long and 2 cm wide. With the mare in anestrus or estrus, the cervix may be more difficult to distinguish as a distinct structure. More information about the state of the cervix can be gained by direct palpation via the vagina.

Bacteriologic Examination

Taking a cervical or uterine swab is one of the most common procedures carried out in equine stud-farm practice. However, this technique has been abused in that bacteriologic results have not been evaluated to assess whether a clinical infection exists.

KEY POINT ▶ It should be remembered that there is a normal flora of bacteria in the caudal genital tract and the presence of bacteria per se does not constitute infection.

It is important when cervical or uterine swabs are taken that smears onto glass slides are made for cytology. Thus, if there is clinical infection, neutrophils (>5 per high-power field) should be present on cytologic examination.

The most common technique for taking a swab for bacteriologic examination involves the use of a long, guarded swab stick. Several types of swabs are available commercially that are double guarded and have a distal cap which is removed once the swab is in position (Harford Veterinary Supply, 9100 Persimmon Tree Rd., Potomac, MD 20854).

With direct visualization or introducing the swab using a sterile-gloved hand, the guarded swab is pushed deep into the cervix. Clearly, effective bacteriologic swabs are best collected with the mare in estrus, since a swab cannot be introduced readily into the cervix when the mare is in diestrus. Once the swab is in position, well into the cervix or, preferably, within the uterus, the guarded end of the swab is displaced by pushing the swab stick cranially within the guarded outer tube. Once the cotton tip of the swab has been exposed, it is withdrawn into the guarded outer tube before the device is withdrawn from the cervix and vagina. If there is to be a delay in processing of the swab, the cotton end can be broken off and placed in suitable transport media (see Chap. 15). For cytologic examination, cells can be taken from the cap of the first culture swab. Alternatively, a second swab can be taken, and the collected material can be smeared onto a clean glass slide. Various commercial products are available (Diff Quick) to permit rapid fixation so that the cytology can be examined later in the laboratory. Alternatively, the slides can be air-dried and stained using new methylene blue. A single drop of dye is used followed by application of a coverslip.

KEY POINT ▶ It is important to note that obstetrical lubricant inadvertently applied to the slide can stain in a manner similar to fungi.

Care should be taken to ensure that fungal endometritis is not mistakenly diagnosed in such circumstances.

KEY POINT ▶ In the interpretation of cytologic findings, there should be sheets of epithelial cells, and infection is likely when there are greater than 5 inflammatory cells per high-power field.

Another important point in examining bacteriologic swabs is that direct sensitivity testing of antimicrobial agents should never be performed. In such cases, wrong information for treatment can be gained because the bacteria were not identified prior to sensitivity testing. The bacterial growth should be examined initially, followed by Kirby-Bauer sensitivity testing of the isolates. Further details are given in Chapter 15.

Endometrial Biopsy

Endometrial biopsy has been found to be a valuable diagnostic tool for the problem mare. Changes in the endometrium sometimes may be found on histologic examination when gross examination has not revealed any abnormalities. Experienced pathologists and veterinarians who do broodmare work are able to effectively classify endometrial changes into various grades, which permits a prognosis to be given for future reproductive performance. The biopsy should be collected during estrus or diestrus.

KEY POINT ▶ The major evaluation is the assessment of glandular activity and degree of fibrosis and inflammation present.

A small sample of the endometrium may be collected easily from a mare using alligator-jaw biopsy forceps approximately 60 cm long (Pillings biopsy punch). The forceps have basket-type jaws that are 2 cm long and 4 to 5 mm wide (Fig. 7-1). While the size of the sample to be collected looks rather horrific, problems associated with endometrial biopsy are seldom encountered. If the sample size is too small, accurate interpretation is not possible. A useful method for sterilization of the forceps between mares is immersion in dialdehyde (Cidex; Treatment No. 31) for 10 minutes prior to use. If Cidex is used, the forceps should be rinsed carefully with sterile saline, because the chemical is very irritating to tissue. After thorough cleansing of the perineum and evacuation of the rectum, the sterile biopsy forceps are introduced into the vagina with a sterile-gloved hand. It is usual to do this with the left hand so that the right hand can be used to operate the jaws of the biopsy forceps. The index finger of the left hand is passed into the uterus via the cervix, and the biopsy forceps is passed along the finger into the uterus. The left arm is then withdrawn and placed in the rectum, where the uterus and forceps can be palpated. Using the hand in the rectum to guide the forceps, a piece of endometrium is pressed into the side of the open jaws of the biopsy forceps. This is easier and less risky than attempting to push the endometrium through the front of the open jaws of the biopsy forceps. The jaws are closed and the biopsy taken, after which it is placed in Bouin's solution for fixation prior to submission for histology. Within 24 hours, the fixative should be changed to alcohol or the tissue sample will become too friable for good sections to be cut.

Because of the changes in endometrial appearance that occur with ovarian activity, it is important to identify the stage of the estrus cycle during which the biopsy is collected. Most reliable results are found in the middle part of the breeding season. During the early part of the breeding season, mares may be still in anestrus, and interpretation of the findings may be difficult.

Classification of the histologic findings has been suggested by Kenney and Doig (1986), since such a system has been found useful in predicting future reproductive performance. The crucial histologic assessments include the following:

1. Evaluation of the inflammatory response, particularly in the stratum compactum and luminal epithelium. Acute changes are characterized by polymorphs, whereas in chronic endometritis there

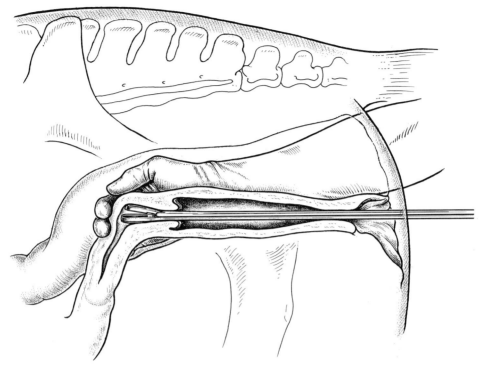

Figure 7–1. Uterine biopsy forceps shown being inserted into the uterus of a mare.

are lymphocytes and a variety of other cells, including plasma cells.

2. Determination of endometrial fibrosis. Endometrial fibrosis is of particular significance because the findings indicate the likelihood of long-term problems in either conception or carrying a pregnancy to term.

The classification scheme suggested by Kenney and Doig is as follows:

Category I—Essentially normal endometrium. Mares within this classification can be anticipated to have a foaling rate of up to 90%.

Category IIA—Moderate inflammatory changes that involve the superficial endometrial layers. Minor fibrotic changes associated with some of the glands also would allow classification. The anticipated foaling rate for mares within this classification is in the range 50% to 80%.

Category IIB—Inflammatory changes are more widespread and involve deeper tissue. This also applies to any fibrosis that is more widespread and severe than in mares in category IIA. The anticipated foaling rate for mares in this category ranges from 10% to 50%.

Category III—Inflammatory or fibrotic changes are very severe and diffuse. There is usually considerable fibrosis that involves the gland branches. Mares within this category have a very poor prognosis for future breeding, with foaling rates varying from 0% to 10%.

Endometrial biopsy is an exceptionally useful clinical tool for examination of problem mares. However, the prognosis given only provides a population index, and care must be taken when giving a prognosis for an individual mare. There are plenty of cases where mares placed in category III have conceived and had foals. Where there are extensive inflammatory changes and the mare undergoes therapy for endometritis, repeating the biopsy may be of value.

Ultrasonography

Over the past few years, ultrasound examination of the reproductive tract of mares has become a widely used technique in stud-farm practice. A 5-MHz linear-array probe is used most commonly. It is introduced via the rectum after removing the feces. Pregnancy can be diagnosed as early as 12 days after ovulation by ultrasound examination.

KEY POINT ▶ The most important application of ultrasonography for pregnancy diagnosis is the early determination of twin pregnancy so that termination of one of the two pregnancies can be performed.

Twin or double ovulations are common in mares, with some reports suggesting that up to 40% of ovulations are involved. Despite this, the incidence of twin births is less than 1%, indicating a high incidence of embryonic loss.

Most ultrasound units used in practice allow real-time linear-array scanning and should have a printer for hard-copy information. With these units, the ultrasound probe lies perpendicular to the axis of the uterus. Fluid-filled structures (e.g., a vesicle) are anechoic, or dark, in appearance. The uterine tissue will show up as gray in color. While a vesicle is often easily identified by ultrasonography, it is important to thoroughly examine the uterine horns and body to ensure that there is only a single conceptus. The most common problem encountered in pregnancies less than 18 days after ovulation is confusing the presence of a vesicle with uterine cysts.

KEY POINT ► Diagnosis of pregnancy is possible as early as 12 days, but the embryonic vesicle is most easily and reliably visualized from 20 to 25 days after ovulation, when it may be somewhat irregular in appearance.

After day 25, the presence of more fluid in the vesicle permits the circular form of the vesicle to be clearly identified, and around 30 days, a fetal heart beat may be detectable. Most observations are undertaken between 30 and 45 days after ovulation, and the embryo is clearly visible at this stage.

Because the endometrial cups form around day 36, diagnosis of twinning must be established prior to this so that termination of one of the pregnancies or complete termination may be performed. Once the endometrial cups are established, because of the high concentrations of pregnant mare serum gonadotropin (PMSG) produced, the mare will not return to ovarian cyclical activity for 3 to 4 months, even if the pregnancy is terminated.

The crucial aspect of ultrasound examination is recognizing the unusual. Ultrasound is useful for detecting ovarian follicles, the presence of a corpus luteum, and the presence of fluid in the uterus. We have found that it is essential to repeat the examination several times if unusual findings are seen or if there is doubt about the possibility of the ultrasound findings indicating twin pregnancies. The first examination should be performed around 15 to 18 days after ovulation, with follow-up examinations completed by day 34 to ensure that termination of pregnancy can take place, if necessary, before formation of the endometrial cups.

Examination of the Uterus Using Endoscopy

Flexible fiberoptiscopes have proven useful in examination of the uterus. We use a flexible colonoscope to view the endometrium directly. The colonoscope is prepared by immersion of the viewing end and 60 cm of the distal end of the scope in dialdehyde (Cidex; Treatment No. 31) for 10 minutes. After the endoscope is removed from the Cidex, it is rinsed carefully with sterile saline before being inserted in a manner similar to the insertion of endometrial biopsy forceps. The perineum

of the mare should be cleansed and disinfected prior to insertion of the endoscope, which is passed using sterile gloves to protect the tip of the endoscope. Once the endoscope is in position, the air-insufflation channel can be used to inflate the uterus to allow the endometrial surface to be visualized. Alternatively, saline can be used to inflate the uterus because it is less irritating than air. Endoscopic examination can sometimes be useful to delineate problems identified on rectal examination or to clarify the results of ultrasound findings. However, endoscopic examination is used less commonly these days because real-time ultrasound machines have allowed better indirect visualization of the reproductive tract.

Epidural Anesthesia

Epidural anesthesia is simply performed and is of great assistance in correction of some dystocias as well as for perineal surgery.

KEY POINT ► The technique must be undertaken with the mare standing evenly on both hindlegs.

If the mare is resting one of the hindlegs, there will be uneven analgesia because more of the local anesthetic will run to one side of the epidural space. Following clipping and routine surgical disinfection, the space between the first and second coccygeal vertebrae is palpated by lifting the tail. This usually coincides with the level at which the coarse tail hairs begin. A bleb of local anesthetic (1 ml of 2% lidocaine or mepivacaine; Treatment Nos. 67 and 72) is injected subcutaneously. After sterile gloves are applied, a 19-gauge, 3.75-cm (1.5-in) needle is inserted to a depth of 2.5 cm (1 in) (Fig. 7-2). The amount of 2% lidocaine or mepivacaine needed for epidural anesthesia varies, but no more than 5 ml/500 kg should be used initially to assess the effects. The needle is left in place and after a period of 5 minutes, additional local anesthetic can be injected into the epidural space. More than 8 ml of local anesthetic should not be used because instability of the hindlegs can occur. More recently, xylazine (Treatment No. 108) has been used in epidural analgesia. A dose rate of 0.17 mg/kg (100 mg/450 kg) xylazine diluted in 10 ml saline is used. It has the advantage of a longer duration of action, and mares do not become as incoordinated as when local anesthetics are used. Some practitioners have reported less effective analgesia with xylazine as compared with lidocaine.

The Stallion

Examination of the genital system of the stallion is conducted primarily to evaluate infertility. Most stud farms will have good records concerning the pregnancy rates of particular stallions. In conducting an examination, the veterinarian needs to take a complete history that details medical problems

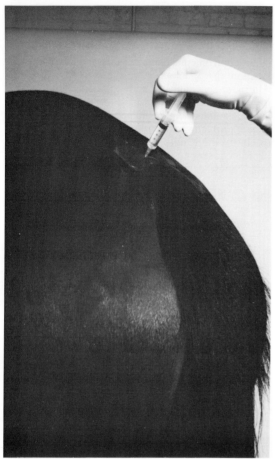

Figure 7–2. Epidural anesthesia. A needle (19-gauge, 1.5-in or 3.75-cm) is inserted into the epidural space between the last sacral and first coccygeal vertebrae. The space is located by moving the tail up and down and palpating for the space between the two vertebrae. After desensitizing the skin over the site with local anesthetic, the needle is inserted in the dorsal midline and directed in a slightly cranial direction into the epidural space. An initial volume of 1 ml/100 kg of 2% lidocaine or mepivicaine is injected slowly, and there should be no resistance to injection. Alternatively, xylazine (100 mg/450 kg), diluted to a volume of 10 ml with saline, may be used.

and any drug therapy the stallion has been receiving over the past 2 months.

General Examination

The physical condition of the stallion is important in the initial evaluation. There may be problems with management, nutrition, or a medical disorder that could lead secondarily to deterioration in semen quality. One of the key aspects of the initial examination is observation of the stallion in a small yard or at pasture so that any musculoskeletal or other physical problems can be observed. Problems that should be noted include chronic degenerative joint problems, chronic laminitis, and back disorders.

Examination of the Penis. Most stud farms wash the penis of the stallion prior to service, and this is a convenient time for examination.

KEY POINT ▶ It should be noted that the use of disinfectants and even water may favor the colonization of specific bacteria and may lead to infection with bacteria such as *Pseudomonas.*

Use of the promazine tranquilizers (e.g., acepromazine, promazine, chlorpromazine) should be avoided because of the risk of penile paralysis. Examination of the testicles can be performed following breeding because the stallion will be more easily handled. In examination of the penis, considerable care must be taken by the examining veterinarian, first, to avoid damage to the penis and, second (and probably most important), to avoid personal injury from a stallion that can kick in any direction. The penis can be grasped proximal to the glans, and the distal part of the penis, particularly the urethral process, can be examined for *Habronema* infection and evidence of trauma or neoplasia (squamous cell carcinoma). Examination further proximal allows assessment of scarring or injuries. While injuries to the penis are not common, trauma can occur because of a kick from the mare or lacerations from barbed wire on fences.

Examination of the Scrotum, Testicles, and Epididymides. Examination of the scrotum and testicles is most easily performed after breeding. The scrotum itself is rarely affected by disease, and therefore, examination is directed at the testicles and epididymides. The testicles and epididymides should be palpated carefully to assess tone as well as for abnormalities in size, consistency, or symmetry. Both testicles should be of similar size and consistency, although it is common to find that one testicle is slightly smaller than the other.

KEY POINT ▶ Because there is a correlation between the width of the scrotum across the greatest diameter of both testicles and sperm output, measurement with calipers may be useful.

The normal range in mature stallions is from 9 to 12.5 cm. While the head and body of the epididymides are often difficult to palpate, the tail of each epididymis is easily palpated at the caudal pole of the testicle.

The accessory sex glands (vesicular glands, prostate, and bulbourethral glands) can be palpated during rectal examination at the level of the neck of the bladder. Most of these structures are difficult to palpate, although the prostate can be palpated routinely approximately one hand's length in from the anal sphincter. There have been few reported pathologic changes involving the accessory sex glands.

Bacteriologic Culture

If swabs are taken for suspected infections of the penis and prepuce, it must be remembered that large numbers of bacteria (including organisms such as *Pseudomonas, E. coli, Staphylococcus,* and *Streptococcus*) will be found in normal horses. However, if a single organism is isolated together with the presence of inflammatory cells and evidence of poor semen quality, an infection can be considered. For bacteriologic swabs to be collected from the urethra, more consistent results are obtained if the swabs are taken after mating. The only organism that can be universally regarded as a significant pathogen is the CEM organism *Taylorella equigentalis.* This is a microaerophilic organism that requires special culture conditions, and swabs should be handled appropriately (see Chap. 15).

Breeding Soundness Examination

Semen examination for breeding soundness is an important part of stud-farm practice.

KEY POINT ► Apart from the semen evaluation, note should be taken of the stallion's libido, manners, ease of ejaculation, and ability to mount a mare.

Two semen samples must be collected about 1 hour apart. The second sample should contain between 1.8 and 2.2×10^9 live motile sperm. Because sperm output drops in winter, semen samples collected during winter months require less sperm to qualify as being normal.

Determination of live motile sperm cells is based on the percentage of morphologically normal sperm times the percentage of motile sperm times concentration (volume times number of sperm per milliliter).

SOME ASPECTS OF MARE AND STALLION MANAGEMENT AND REPRODUCTIVE PHYSIOLOGY

Artificial Lighting

It has been well established for some years that in both the northern and southern hemispheres, the breeding season is not coincident with optimal ovarian activity of the mare. This is so because mares are long-day breeders with endocrinologic changes determined by the day length. The peak of ovarian activity takes place late in the breeding season, and in the early part of the season, many mares are still in anestrus. During the early season, many mares also may be in a transition period in which there may be follicular activity but not ovulation because of low levels of luteinizing hormone (LH). For this reason, various treatments have been tried to induce regular estrus activity in the early part of the breeding season.

KEY POINT ► Artificial lighting is now widely used on stud farms throughout the world to induce earlier onset of regular ovarian activity.

The pineal gland has been shown to be actively involved in the mechanism of action of photoperiod, although the exact mechanisms are still not clear. From a practical point of view, the following points are important: The light wavelength and intensity are critical, as is the duration of exposure. While the exact wavelength and intensity of light to produce an effect are not known, either incandescent or fluorescent light bulbs are satisfactory with an intensity of light greater than 10 footcandles. While this is usually done indoors, outdoor lighting also has been shown to be effective. Studies from the University of Florida have shown that extension of day length by 2 to 3 hours is effective in advancing the breeding period. However, this should be done by delaying effective sunset rather than providing an earlier sunrise. Most stud farms use 16 hours of lighting a day in the late winter months (December 1 to March 1 or June 1 to September 1 in the southern hemisphere) to advance the breeding season.

KEY POINT ► Because of the somewhat long period of transitional estrus early in the breeding season, synthetic progestogens may be used to induce estrus and regular cyclical activity.

The agent of choice is allyl trenbolone (Treatment No. 3) given orally for 10 days at a dose rate of 27.5 mg per mare. Best results are found when there are at least 25-mm-diameter follicles on the ovaries and when the drug is used in combination with additional lighting. Use of this synthetic progestogen in this way blocks gonadotropin release and after the trenbolone is stopped, regular cyclical activity may result. Estrus behavior and ovulation can be anticipated following withdrawal of trenbolone in 80% to 90% of mares in transitional estrus.

Endocrinology of the Estrous Cycle

The hormonal events of the estrous cycle are of major importance because endocrine therapy is required in some reproductive disorders.

- As detailed earlier, increasing day length is a key trigger to the release of adequate quantities of gonadotropin-releasing hormone (GnRH), which is a prerequisite for luteinizing hormone (LH) release and ovulation.
- Follicle-stimulating hormone (FSH) is released from the anterior pituitary. FSH results in development of ovarian follicles, which secrete estrogen. Estrogen release is responsible for the behavioral changes during estrus, as well as the physical changes involving the vagina and cervix that are seen via a speculum examination.

- The high levels of estrogen act via a feedback effect to stimulate luteinizing hormone (LH) release from the anterior pituitary. The result of this is ovulation.
- Following ovulation, the corpus luteum forms and produces progesterone. The progesterone level is maintained past day 18 if the mare becomes pregnant. Otherwise, prostaglandin release terminates diestrus by causing luteolysis, and the mare returns to estrus around 18 to 20 days after ovulation. The result of this is that the blood levels of progesterone decreases to zero.
- With the abrupt decrease in progesterone, the anterior pituitary secretes further FSH, and the pattern of hormonal cyclical activity recommences.

While the description given is highly simplified, it is clear that a variety of hormonal aberrations can give rise to certain clinical problems. Prolonged diestrus may be the result of a persistent corpus luteum. Prostaglandin therapy (Treatment No. 53) may be indicated in such cases. Many mares will demonstrate prolonged estrus due to high levels of FSH and an apparent lack of feedback of the high estrogen concentrations to cause LH release. The use of human chorionic gonadotropin (hCG) (Treatment No. 25) is often effective in inducing ovulation in these circumstances.

Pregnancy Diagnosis

Most stud-farm managers will maintain records of service dates and number of services and indicate when estrus ceased, denoted by a lack of response to teasing. While ultrasound examination has replaced the manual detection of pregnancy on larger stud farms, an experienced veterinarian can detect pregnancy via a rectal examination after 20 to 25 days. However, it is possible to be most accurate with rectal palpation after 30 days of gestation. Details regarding care that is necessary when performing a rectal examination are outlined on p. 251. The earliest sign of pregnancy is the appearance of increased cervical and uterine tone. The uterus is normally quite flaccid, and the presence of increased tone is one indicator of pregnancy. At around 30 days, the characteristic enlargement or bulge in one of the uterine horns can be palpated. This enlargement continues so that at 42 days, when many mares are certified as being pregnant or nonpregnant, there may be some dorsal enlargement of the horn; the disparity in size between the pregnant and nonpregnant horns is quite apparent.

Ultrasound examination has permitted earlier establishment of a diagnosis of pregnancy. However, because of early embryonic loss, many mares that are pregnant at 20 days gestation may not be pregnant at 42 days. For this reason, repeat examinations are required to establish normal growth of the embryonic vesicle. If twin conceptuses are diagnosed, it is possible to manually crush one of the vesicles at around days 14 to 25 of gestation. This can be followed up with further ultrasound examinations to confirm the viability of the remaining embryonic vesicle.

In some smaller pony mares, rectal or ultrasound examination may not be possible. In these cases, tests to determine the presence of PMSG may be used to establish the diagnosis of pregnancy. The simplest and most readily available of these tests is the mare immunologic pregnancy (MIP) test, which is based on hemagglutination inhibition. The test is quite accurate between 40 and 120 days, but the main problem is false-positive results. These can occur as a result of early embryonic death, in which PMSG levels can still be elevated despite death of the fetus.

Induction of Parturition
Indications

Foaling induction should be approached with great caution because of the possible complications. The most obvious problem is induction of the foal prior to full term. Rossdale also has shown that while some pregnancies may be at full term in gestational length, the foal may be still not be ready to be born. In such cases, induction of parturition at 340 days, for example, may lead to a foal that is not physiologically prepared for birth and therefore may suffer adaptation problems. The normal gestational length in the mare is an average of 340 days and ranges from 320 to 360 days. In pony mares, the gestational length is shorter.

KEY POINT ▶ Mares that are candidates for induction are those which have experienced previous foaling problems or foaling injuries or those with injuries, increased gestational length, or medical problems. If gestational length is known accurately, it is preferable that induction be delayed until the mare is at least 335 days.

Colostral Electrolyte Concentrations

If an accurate service date is not available, some reliance can be placed on udder development and mammary secretion electrolyte concentrations to assess the proximity to foaling. In mares with known and unknown service dates, precolostral and colostral electrolyte concentrations are valuable in predicting if foaling is imminent.

KEY POINT ▶ Colostral electrolyte concentrations are an accurate indicator that the foal is ready for birth, and we have found them to be extremely useful in making a decision for or against induction of parturition.

The mammary secretions in the weeks prior to foaling have concentrations of sodium and potassium similar to those of serum or plasma. The sodium values are usually in the range 125 to 135 mmol/L (mEq/L) and potassium 7 to 12 mmol/L (mEq/L). Calcium values remain low and are usually less than 2 mmol/L (8 mg/dl) until the mare is within 12 to 24 hours of foaling. Sodium values in the mammary secretions decrease to less than 30 mmol/L and potassium concentrations increase to greater than 30 mmol/L within 24 to 48 hours prior to foaling. Calcium values increase more precipitously in the 24 hours prior to foaling, and values greater than 10 mmol/L (40 mg/dl) indicate that foaling is imminent. Therefore, if there is udder enlargement and evidence of "waxing" of the teats, the mare should have a sample of mammary secretion submitted for electrolyte analysis prior to a decision being made for or against induction. A commercial kit is available that assesses calcium concentration in mammary secretions by a color change (Predict-A-Foal, Animal Healthcare Products, Vernon, Calif.).

KEY POINT ► While it is useful to examine the cervix using a speculum, we have found that the cervical changes are not of great use in indicating whether induction should take place. A decision for induction should therefore be made on the basis of changes in the appearance of the udder and electrolyte alterations in the mammary secretions.

Various agents can be used for induction, but the ones that we have found to be the safest are fluprostenol and oxytocin. Fluprostenol (Treatment No. 53) will not induce parturition if the mare is not at full-term gestation. A dose of 500 µg given intramuscularly will usually result in induction of parturition within 1 to 4 hours. In some cases, separation of the placenta can occur immediately prior to presentation of the amnion. Placental separation can result in adaptation problems in the immediate neonatal period. For this reason, we prefer the use of oxytocin (Treatment No. 81). Although large doses of oxytocin have been recommended, we have found these to produce adverse reactions, including signs of colic and excessive straining.

KEY POINT ► For induction, doses of oxytocin should not exceed 5 to 10 IU given intravenously every 30 minutes, and the total dose should not be greater than 30 IU.

In most cases, only one to two doses are necessary before the onset of stage II labor, and the amnion is presented in the majority of cases within 40 to 60 minutes of the initial oxytocin injection. We have found this regimen to give reliable results, and viable full-term foals have been delivered successfully.

Breeding Soundness Examination and Artificial Insemination

While thoroughbred societies throughout the world do not permit the use of artificial insemination (AI), it is possible in most other breeds, including standardbreds. The breed societies that do permit AI require fresh semen to be used, although some do allow transported semen. The greatest advantage is that the stallion can be used more efficiently, with more mares being mated each breeding season, and there is a decreased risk of disease.

Semen collection for breeding soundness assessment and for AI is performed using a mare in estrus or a phantom mare, which is suitable for experienced stallions. An artificial vagina is used, and we prefer the Missouri model. The sleeve of the artificial vagina is filled with warm water so that the temperature is between 42 and 45°C. The inside of the artificial vagina is lubricated before use with a nonspermicidal lubricant such as K-Y jelly, and the collection bottle is warmed to body temperature and attached to the end of the device just before use.

The stallion should be restrained from mounting the mare or phantom until it has a full erection. Once mounted, the penis is diverted to the side of the mare or phantom and into the artificial vagina. The artificial vagina is kept in place until the stallion dismounts and the water is removed from the device so that all the semen is collected in the collecting bottle. It is essential to ensure that the semen is kept away from sunlight, air, or water because it is susceptible to cold shock. The semen should be stored at 37°C until it is assessed for concentration, motility, and morphology. The volume of the ejaculate also should be recorded.

For AI, most stud farms use a semen extender, and the following has been reported to be effective: powdered milk, 2.4 g; glucose, 4.9 g; sodium bicarbonate, 2 ml of 7.5% solution; gentamicin sulfate, 100 mg; and distilled water, added to make up a volume of 100 ml. Commercially available extenders are now available, and Easy Mix Semen Extender is one that is useful. The extender should be kept in a water bath at a temperature of 37°C and added to the semen to be used in a 1:1 ratio depending on the sperm concentration. Insemination of at least 250 million normal motile sperm is required, and mares should be inseminated every second day during estrus until ovulation occurs. The alternative is to base insemination on findings on ovarian palpation so that insemination is timed to occur around the time of ovulation.

Reproductive Disease in the Mare

Abortion

KEY POINT ▶ Abortion is one of the most common problems afflicting the mare, and losses have been placed as high as 15%.

There are a wide range of causes for abortion in the mare, but in general, older mares have a higher incidence of abortion. Various bacteria can cause an endometritis and lead to abortion or may have produced chronic fibrosis with subsequent inability to maintain a pregnancy.

Apart from bacterial endometritis, other causes of abortion include viral or fungal infections, twinning, and endocrine abnormalities.

KEY POINT ▶ The most common viral cause of abortion is equine herpesvirus 1 (EHV-1) infection, which generally causes abortion in the last trimester of pregnancy.

The other major viral infection that can cause abortion is equine viral arteritis.

There is still considerable controversy as to whether endocrine factors can play a role in abortion. In particular, debate has raged over the validity of exogenous progesterone administration.

KEY POINT ▶ Most studies have not shown any beneficial effects of progesterone therapy in a mare with a history of an inability to carry the foal to term.

History and Presenting Signs

- Return of the mare to estrus
- Discharge from the vulva
- Fetus found
- Retention of fetal membranes
- Dripping milk prematurely

Clinical Findings and Diagnosis

- If the abortion occurs in the early stages of pregnancy, the only sign can be that the mare returns to estrus. In the later stages, a fetus may be found, and on occasions, the placenta may be retained.
- If the fetus is found, an autopsy should be performed, and if infection is suspected, samples should be collected for microbiology.
- Early embryonic loss after establishment of the endometrial cups may not be recognized for some time because the high PMSG concentrations prevent a return to estrus.

Differential Diagnosis

- Bacterial abortion, caused by *Streptococcus, E. coli, Salmonella, Klebsiella, Actinobacillus,* and others
- Twinning
- Endometrial fibrosis
- Nutritional deficiencies, including malnutrition
- Viral abortion, caused by equine herpesvirus 1 (EHV-1), arteritis virus, and infectious anemia
- Fungal abortion, caused by *Aspergillus fumigatus* and other species

Treatment

- If endometritis has been the cause of the abortion, intrauterine irrigation with saline and an appropriate antibiotic (following results of culture and sensitivity tests) should be undertaken (see Endometritis).
- If inadequate progesterone levels are thought to be the cause of previous abortion, progesterone therapy may be given. Although no research work has been able to show a beneficial effect of progesterone, there is anecdotal evidence for its use. To maintain effective blood levels (>1 ng/ml plasma), progesterone in oil can be administered at a dose rate of 200 mg every 48 hours, or daily oral allyl trenbelone (Treatment No. 3) can be given at a dose rate of 27.5 mg per mare.

Contagious Equine Metritis (CEM)

CEM was first recognized in Ireland and England during the 1977 breeding season.

KEY POINT ▶ It is a highly contagious, venereally transmitted disease that produces a copious mucopurulent vulvar discharge in infected mares.

The disease subsequently spread throughout the world. The organism involved was found to require microaerophilic culture conditions, which is why normal culture methods were not satisfactory. Subsequent work established the organism to be a new bacteria, which was named *Taylorella equigenitalis*.

History and Presenting Signs

- Copious discharge from the vulva
- Infertility

Clinical Findings and Diagnosis

- The signs are those of an acute endometritis, there being a profuse mucopurulent discharge from the vulva of the mare. However, some mares show no signs of the infection while carrying the disease.
- In most mares with CEM, the discharge ceases within 5 to 7 days whether treatment is given or not.
- Although the stallion carries the organism, it usually produces no pathogenic effects.
- Diagnosis is by bacteriologic culture, and special chocolate agar media and microaerophilic culture techniques have to be used.

KEY POINT ▶ It is important that swabs are taken from the clitoral fossa and sinuses when doing bacteriologic swabs to check for the presence of the CEM organism.

- The clitoral fossa seems to be a favorite site for localization of the organism, which can often be recovered even in pregnant mares.

Differential Diagnosis

- Bacterial endometritis
- Vaginal injuries

Treatment

- The organism is sensitive to a wide range of antibiotics, but the cheapest and most appropriate is penicillin (see Antibiotic Therapy, Chap. 17). However, whether or not treatment is instituted, the carrier rate in mares remains high.
- In stallions, washing the penis with chlorhexidine (see Disinfectants, Chap. 17; Treatment No. 23) is quite successful in eliminating the organism. Care must be taken because overgrowth of other bacteria can occur.

Dystocia

Second-stage labor in the mare is an explosive event and is quickly completed, usually in 15 to 20 minutes. Because of this, unlike the situation in the cow, there is little time to correct dystocias (difficult births). During first-stage labor, the foal moves into anterior and dorsosacral presentation. When labor is prolonged or there is a lack of progress of first- or second-stage labor, dystocia should be suspected. Early examination is essential if a live foal is to be delivered.

History and Presenting Signs

- Prolonged discomfort and sweating
- Straining without appearance of the amnion
- Appearance of the amnion or a limb without further progress

Clinical Findings and Diagnosis

- When there is lack of progress of delivery, careful examination of the position of the foal is essential. In some mares this can be performed with minimal restraint, whereas in others the use of minimum doses (0.2–0.4 mg/kg) of xylazine (Treatment No. 108) is necessary. It is often useful to combine the xylazine with butorphanol (0.05–0.1 mg/kg) (Treatment No. 15) or an opiate to produce more effective analgesia. If initial examination indicates that extensive manipulation is required, general anesthesia may be necessary.
- Epidural anesthesia (see Fig. 7-2) may be helpful to prevent straining and allow the foal to be manipulated more easily.
- After good lubrication of the arms of the operator, the position of the foal should be assessed and decisions made concerning attempted correction of the dystocia.

Differential Diagnosis

- Malposition of the limbs
- Incorrect presentation
- Oversize foal
- Large colon torsion

Treatment

Correction of Presentation

KEY POINT ▶ If the foal is not lying in a dorsosacral position, attempts can be made to turn the foal, with the aid of several liters of obstetrical lubricant.

This is a difficult job that requires considerable strength and persistence. Most commonly, one or both of the forelimbs are positioned incorrectly, and therefore, the foal must be repelled out of the pelvic cavity back into the uterus. This must be done carefully to avoid damage to the uterus. Following repulsion, the malposition can be corrected and the foal delivered using an obstetrical chain or rope.

Fetotomy. If the foal is malpositioned and this cannot be corrected, fetotomy is one of the options when no other treatment appears possible to save the foal. Fetotomy is usually required when labor has been in progress for some hours and the foal cannot be repelled or correction of the malposition is not possible. At this stage, the foal is usually dead, and the use of a fetotome to perform a partial fetotomy will allow delivery of the foal. Epidural anesthesia may be required but is usually not necessary prior to the fetotomy. Some sedation also may be necessary. In some mares, general anesthesia must be used to allow the fetotomy to proceed. The fetotomy should never employ more than three cuts, and it is essential that the fetotome be placed in the uterus, not the cervix.

Cesarean Section. Cesarean section is infrequently required but may be indicated where there is uterine torsion or malposition that cannot be corrected rapidly or in a mare with previous pelvic injuries with resultant narrowing of the birth canal. While standing cesarean section has been reported, we have found that this is impractical, and general anesthesia should be used. A number of surgical sites have been used, but a midline laparotomy provides the best exposure and enables the foal to be extracted more easily than the flank approach.

Endometritis

Endometritis, or infection of the endometrium, is the most common disease necessitating treatment in the mare.

KEY POINT ► A wide range of factors can predispose to infection, including vulval conformation and local endometrial factors, particularly local immunity.

A mare with a normal endometrium appears to be able to overcome infection even when a large number of pathogenic microorganisms are inoculated into the uterus. A great range of bacterial species may be found in mares with endometritis, but the most common ones are *Streptococcus equi* var. *zooepidemicus*, *E. coli*, *Psedomonas*, *Klebsiella*, and *Staphylococcus* species.

The reason why infection becomes established is critical to the outcome of treatment, because treatment with antibiotics alone will not resolve the underlying problem.

History and Presenting Signs

- Failure to conceive
- Mucopurulent discharge from the vulva
- Early embryonic loss
- Short estrous cycles (<14 days)

Clinical Findings and Diagnosis

- There may or may not be signs of vulval discharge, and in some cases, failure to conceive or maintain pregnancy may be the only signs.
- Definitive diagnosis is by collection of bacteriologic swabs from the cervix or endometrium, which should be undertaken under strict aseptic conditions. The use of guarded swabs limits the possibility of contamination from other sites. It is important to interpret bacteriologic findings in

the light of cytology (see Chap. 15) to ensure that a clinically significant infection is present.
- The mere presence of bacteria is not enough to diagnose infection. It must be remembered that the reproductive tracts of the mare and stallion have a normal flora of bacteria.

KEY POINT ► The combination of bacteriologic and cytological findings is important because the presence of neutrophils on cytologic examination of smears from the cervix and/or uterus is of more significance than the presence of bacteria.

- Examination with a speculum is an important part of the workup and can be performed when the bacteriologic and cytologic swabs are collected. Note should be taken of any inflammatory changes to the mucosa, presence of purulent exudate, pooling of urine, and indications of trauma to the vagina or cervix.

KEY POINT ► Endometrial biopsy is useful to grade the severity of the changes to the endometrium and may assist in assessing the prognosis for future breeding, based on the degree of gland atrophy and/or fibrosis present.

Treatment

- It is important to correct any anatomic abnormalities, such as perineal abnormalities, using Caslick's episioplasty or Pouret's operations. This is combined with treatment of the infection with a suitable antimicrobial agent based on the bacteria isolated.

KEY POINT ► Intrauterine therapy is the technique used most consistently, although systemic antibiotic treatment also may be worthwhile.

- If intrauterine antibiotic therapy is to be used, the antibiotic used will depend on the sensitivity pattern of the bacteria that were isolated.
- One technique involves using a disposable plastic uterine pipette to infuse the antimicrobial agent of choice in a volume of 60 to 200 ml of polyionic electrolyte solution.
- The usual dose of antibiotic per treatment is as follows: Na or K penicillin, 3 g (5 million units); Na ampicillin, 3 g; ticarcillin, 6 g; chloramphenicol, 3 g; gentamicin sulfate, 2 g; neomycin, 2 g; amikacin, 2 g. The antimicrobial agent selected will depend on the sensitivity pattern found on bacteriology.

KEY POINT ► However, it should be noted that many of the antibiotics irritate the endometrium, and this is particularly so for the tetracyclines, which should not be used in a local infusion.

- For this reason, systemic antibiotics may be of more value.
- Some practitioners use antiseptics (notably povidone-iodine) in a saline infusion, and good results have been reported. It should be noted, however, that these agents are nonspecific and are also extremely irritating. Antiseptic solutions should only be used as a last resort. The antiseptic of choice is povidone-iodine (Treatment No. 91), diluted 1:10. This infusion is repeated daily for 3 to 5 days, and after being left in place for 5 to 10 minutes, it should be drained and a saline solution used to decrease the irritant effects of the iodine.
- To help in combating the local breakdown in uterine defenses, Asbury has suggested the use of uterine lavage with 3 to 6 liters of a balanced polyionic electrolyte solution such as Ringer's lactate. This is followed up by infusion of 100 ml of plasma harvested from blood collected from the mare. The blood is collected in normal blood donor packs that have plasma transfer packs attached. If facilities are not available for centrifuging these packs, the blood packs can be allowed to stand so that the red cells settle out. Asbury also recommends plasma infusion within 1 to 2 days of breeding.
- In cases of chronic endometritis with evidence of glandular atrophy and fibrosis, there have been reports of the beneficial effects of uterine currettage.

Metritis–Laminitis Syndrome

If there is retention of the placenta or other factors leading to infection postfoaling, metritis may occur, followed by septicaemia and laminitis due to endotoxemia.

KEY POINT ► Metritis–laminitis is a very common sequela to retention of fetal membranes (see Retained Placenta, p. 266).

History and Presenting Signs

- Obstetrical interference during delivery
- Retention of the placenta
- Vulval discharge
- Dull, depressed, anorexic

Clinical Findings and Diagnosis

- Signs of ill health are usually noted 12 to 24 hours after foaling.
- There may be a discharge from the vulva, and the mare will have elevated heart rate, respiratory rate, and temperature.
- Signs of laminitis may be found (see Chap. 3).
- Diagnosis is possible by a combination of history and clinical signs.

- Bacteriologic swabs from the uterus are useful to enable correct antibiotic selection.

Differential Diagnosis

- Pleuritis
- Peritonitis
- Cystitis
- Colic due to various causes (e.g., large colon rupture, necrotic small colon)

Treatment

KEY POINT ► Aggressive therapy is required and, if possible, is aimed at prophylaxis.

- Any mare with retained placenta or signs of metritis should be treated with antibiotics, both systemically and intrauterine (see Retained Placenta, p. 266).
- If sensitivity results are not available, then the use of systemic penicillin and gentamicin or amikacin (see Antibiotic Therapy, Chap. 17) for up to 5 days are probably the best choices.
- If culture results indicate the presence of anaerobic bacteria and *Bacteroides fragilis* is present (which is not sensitive to penicillin), metronidazole (Treatment No. 75) can be administered orally at a dose rate of 15 mg/kg q6h.
- If there is accumulation of purulent exudate in the uterus, attempts should be made to drain the fluid or to irrigate the uterus.
- It also may be useful to administer flunixin meglumine (Treatment No. 52) at a dose rate of 0.2 mg/kg to aid in preventing laminitis.
- If there are signs of laminitis, a range of treatment options is available, depending on the duration and severity of signs (see Laminitis, Chap. 3).

Ovarian Disorders

Ovarian abnormalities are usually found on rectal and/or ultrasound examination. The history is quite variable depending on the hormonal alterations induced by the ovarian disease. The major ovarian disorders include

- Tumors, most commonly granulosa cell tumors
- Gonadal dysgenesis (e.g., chromosomal abnormalities, particularly XO genotype)
- Persistent corpus luteum, resulting in prolonged diestrus (see Hormonal Events, p. 257)
- Follicular atresia, causing failure of ovulation
- Ovarian atrophy (i.e., decrease or absence of ovarian activity in older mares)
- Ovarian hematoma. Hemorrhage can occur during ovulation and may result in quite dramatic ovarian enlargement.
- Large follicles with mares showing persistent estrus
- Mares in persistent anestrus (i.e., no signs of estrus behavior during breeding season)

History and Presenting Signs

- Prolonged diestrus
- Persistent estrus
- Changes in behavior
- Anestrus

Clinical Findings and Diagnosis

- Mares with granulosa cell tumors present because of changes in behavior, with most mares becoming aggressive. There is also irregular or even absent cyclic activity, with affected mares not coming into estrus.
- Most other ovarian abnormalities present because of irregular estrus or anestrus. In some cases, there is prolonged estrus.

KEY POINT ▶ Diagnosis is by rectal examination, where the enlarged or abnormal ovary can be palpated.

- In some cases, it may be useful to examine the ovary using ultrasound.
- In some cases, the ovarian enlargement is remarkable, with granulosa cell tumors the size of soccer balls being reported.

Treatment

Granulosa Cell Tumors. Although other ovarian tumors, notably teratomas, have been reported, granulosa cell tumors are the most common.

KEY POINT ▶ Because these tumors are unilateral, ovariectomy may be undertaken to remove the affected ovary.

Unless the ovary is larger than a big orange, we have found that a flank approach provides the best access. However, it should be noted that subcutaneous seromas are common after flank laparotomy. In larger tumors, a midline laparatomy is required because the ovary cannot be removed through the flank. The fertility of mares after surgery is good, although it may be some time before normal cyclic activity becomes reestablished.

Persistent Corpus Luteum. Failure of normal luteolysis will result from persistent corpus luteum.

KEY POINT ▶ Once persistent corpus luteum has been differentiated from early pregnancy, treatment with fluprostenol (Treatment No. 53) will result in luteolysis.

The normal dose rate is 500 µg/450 kg of body weight. This will usually result in ovulation, where there are follicles present, within 5 to 10 days.

Follicular Atresia. While the exact cause of follicular atresia is unknown, the characteristic rectal finding is a small, firm follicle that does not enlarge and become softer with maturation. Diagnosis is usually made on the basis of a lack of follicle enlargement on regular examinations. If this is the

case, treatment with a GnRH pump may give positive results.

Large or Cystic Follicles. Characteristic behavior in mares with large follicles is prolonged or irregular estrus. The problem is most often found during transitional estrus.

KEY POINT ▶ In such cases, the use of human chorionic gonadotrophin (Treatment No. 25) at 2000 IU given IV on consecutive days may result in reestablishment of regular estrus cycles.

If the main signs relate to irregular estrus, administration of daily oral allyl trenbelone (Treatment No. 3) given at a dose rate of 27.5 mg per mare is effective.

Chromosomal Abnormalities and Ovarian Atrophy. In both these conditions, there is no effective treatment. Mares with chromosomal disorders usually will have very small ovaries and a small uterus. Ovarian atrophy or senility usually occurs in mares older than 20 years of age.

Ovarian Hematomas. Ovarian hematomas usually follow ovulation and may reach quite large dimensions. In most cases, the finding is incidental, since there are usually no abnormal behavioral signs. While some hematomas may be persistent, there are usually no adverse effects, and no treatment is required.

Ovulation Failure. Failure of ovulation is a relatively common event, particularly in the early part of the breeding season. It is the result of inadequate or failure of production of luteinizing hormone (LH). Rectal examination will reveal well-developed follicles.

KEY POINT ▶ The intravenous administration of 1000 to 4500 IU of hCG (Treatment No. 25) IV usually will result in ovulation within 24 to 48 hours of injection.

This treatment is only effective if the follicle is mature and the mare is in late transitional estrus. Nothing appears to be useful for the mare in early transition.

Anestrus. Failure of mares to enter estrus is a common problem during the early part of the breeding season. As detailed in the section on management, the use of artificial lighting for 2 months prior to the start of the breeding season is useful to hasten the onset of regular estrus. More recently, GnRH pumps also have been found to be valuable in bringing mares out of anestrus. Lactational anestrus is quite common after foaling, with mares showing estrus at the time of the "foal heat," after which there is no further activity. The cause is unknown, and the problem is unrelated to prolactin release. Removing the foal does not appear to aid in resolving the problem. Many mares will resume cyclicity after 60 to 120 days. The characteristic feature of the ovaries in mares with anestrus is that they are small and firm.

Perineal Lacerations

Because of the explosive nature of a second-stage labor in the mare, if a foal's limb is positioned slightly abnormally, it may result in a tear in the dorsal vagina and through into the rectum. In some cases this tear is a localized communication (rectovaginal fistula), whereas in others a complete defect may result (third-degree perineal laceration). These injuries may be difficult to repair and can require one or more follow-up repairs after the original surgery.

History and Presenting Signs

- History of dystocia
- Feces appearing at vulva
- Obvious communication between rectum and vagina

Clinical Findings and Diagnosis

- The signs are obvious, and diagnosis is by visual examination to determine the type and extent of the perineal laceration.

KEY POINT ▶ Note should be taken of the cranial extent of the injury because of the difficulty in repairing lacerations that are some distance away from the vulva.

- Injuries are classified into three grades:

   First Degree—Superficial injuries to vaginal mucous membrane and rupture of the dorsal commissure of the vulva

   Second Degree—Rupture of the perineal body

   Third Degree—Penetration of the vaginal wall and rectum

- In addition, rectovaginal fistula, a fistulous tract allowing direct communication between the rectum and the vagina, is possible. In this case the perineal body is intact.

Differential Diagnosis

- Uterine rupture

Treatment

- First- and second-degree lacerations do not require major treatment and can be repaired without surgical intervention.
- Surgical repair should be performed with third-degree lacerations, although there is some debate as to whether immediate or delayed surgery is best.
- It appears that immediate surgery produces a higher rate of wound breakdown, although repair may be easier at this stage.
- If surgery is to be delayed, at least 3 to 4 weeks should elapse before reconstruction is attempted

so that swelling and localized infection are under control.
- For localized rectovaginal fistulas, repair may be more easily accomplished under general anesthesia with the mare positioned in dorsal recumbency than with the mare standing. However, this is a matter of individual surgical preference.
- For third-degree perineal lacerations, where there is a common opening between the rectum and vagina for some distance, we have found that standing repair using epidural anesthesia (see Fig. 7-2) is the technique of choice. In such cases, it is important that the mare be kept at pasture or fecal softening agents are used so that excessive tension on the suture lines does not occur. Feed should also be restricted for 24 hours prior to surgery.

Perineal Conformation Problems

For more than 50 years, veterinarians in stud-farm practice have been aware of the role of perineal abnormalities in the genesis of infertility.

KEY POINT ▶ A sloping vulva, together with a sunken anus, allows pneumovagina with resulting endometritis in many cases.

The other major conformational problem is cranial displacement of the vestibule and urethral opening. This results in urovagina, which is commonly called "urine pooling."

History and Presenting Signs

- Infertility
- Discharge from the vulva

Clinical Findings and Diagnosis

- The normal position of the pelvic brim should be at the level of the dorsal commissure of the vulva. By manual palpation, it can be determined whether more of the vulval opening than normal lies above the level of the pelvic brim.
- The normal position of the vulva should be vertical. If the vulva slopes forward, this predisposes to fecal contamination and, combined with pneumovagina, may lead to cervicitis and endometritis.
- Examination with a speculum will indicate whether there is evidence of urine pooling in the anterior vagina.

Differential Diagnosis

- Rectovaginal fistulas
- Perineal lacerations

Treatment

Caslick Operation. The Caslick operation is widely used, and probably overused, in stud-farm veterinary practice. It is the procedure of choice in mares that have a sloping vulva or those in which the dorsal commissure of the vulva is displaced dorsally above the pelvic brim.

Local infiltration of 2% lidocaine (Treatment No. 67) is used at the mucocutaneous junction of the vulva. The anesthetic is placed so that the vulva can be sutured to the level of the pelvic brim. This requires a total of approximately 10 ml of local anesthetic in most mares. Using a pair of sharp, curved scissors, a thin strip (2–3 mm) of the mucocutaneous junction is removed from the left and right sides, extending from the level of the pelvic brim to the dorsal commissure. Some clinicians prefer to make an incision at the mucocutaneous junction rather than removing the epithelium. The advantage of the incision technique is that less scarring and resultant skin thickening occur at the vulval edges. Suturing is performed using an absorbable suture such as 2-0 polyglactin (Vicryl, Johnson & Johnson) in a continuous interlocking pattern. If some tissue is excised, it is important that as little as possible be removed so that severe scarring does not result. Deformation of the vulva may occur in mares that require a Caslick operation each breeding season.

An episiotomy is required prior to foaling and also may be necessary prior to mating. In these cases, the episiotomy opening should be resutured as soon as practical.

Pouret's Operation. Because of the vulval damage that occurs and the reduction in the vulval opening, Pouret described an alternative operation that is useful to correct pneumovagina and also may be of value in correcting urine pooling. Pouret proposed that in older mares, the cranial displacement of the rectum and anus leads to similar displacement of the vagina and vulva because of the intimate soft-tissue connections between these structures.

KEY POINT ► Surgery involves separation of the soft-tissue connections between the rectum and caudal vagina so that the vagina can move into a more normal caudal position.

This is done with the mare in a standing position utilizing an epidural anesthetic. The surgery involves a horizontal incision midway between the anus and the vulva, followed by blunt dissection for 10 to 12 cm cranial to the perineum. This frees up the attachments between the rectum and vagina so that the rectum can move cranially.

Retained Placenta

Retention of the placenta in the mare is far less common than in the cow. The placenta is normally expelled rapidly, and if it is still present for longer than 3 hours after foaling, steps should be taken to consider removal. The cause of retention of the placenta is not always clear, and it is interesting that the majority of placentas are retained in the nonpregnant horn. Retention of the placenta is a common sequela to induction of parturition or abortion.

History and Presenting Signs

- Foaling induction
- Premature delivery of foal
- Dystocia

Clinical Findings and Diagnosis

- The clinical signs are obvious, but if the membranes have been present for longer than 6 to 8 hours, the possibility of infection should be seriously considered.
- Careful clinical examination should be performed to determine whether there are signs of infection or laminitis.
- Determination of heart rate, respiratory rate, temperature, and capillary refill time will provide an indication as to systemic involvement or endotoxemia.

Differential Diagnosis

- Uterine prolapse

Treatment

Oxytocin

- The first line of therapy is oxytocin (Treatment No. 81).
- A dose of 40 IU given IM may be used. This regimen is often sufficient to cause expulsion of the placenta within 30 minutes.
- If the oxytocin has not had a result within 60 minutes, a further 40 IU may be given safely.
- A problem with bolus administration of oxytocin is that it often causes abdominal discomfort, pain, and sweating.

KEY POINT ► An alternative to intramuscular injection is to administer the oxytocin as an infusion.

- A 1-L polyionic IV solution is used, into which is placed 150 IU of oxytocin. This is infused slowly, and if the mare shows any signs of discomfort, the flow rate is decreased. A total of 500 to 750 ml usually is required.

Manual Removal

- If oxytocin is unsuccessful, local antibiotics may be used, and the extent of attachment can be evaluated by internal exploration.
- Manual removal of the membranes may be contraindicated because hemorrhage, endometrial scarring, and tags of placenta may be the result.

Antimicrobial and Anti-Inflammatory Therapy

- When the placenta is retained for only a short period after foaling, antibiotic therapy is not required in most cases. However, if there has been obstetrical intervention or prolonged (>6 hours) retention of placenta, local and systemic antibiotics are obligatory.
- A range of bacteria is cultured if uterine swabs are collected. However, in some cases, pure bacterial growth may be obtained, and it may be worthwhile to have sensitivity patterns if there is a lack of response to the therapy that has been initiated.

KEY POINT ► Antibiotic infusions administered in saline (see Endometritis, p. 262, for dosages) should be combined with systemic antibiotics.

- The agents of choice, while awaiting culture results, are procaine penicillin (Treatment No. 83) at a dose rate of 15 mg/kg q12h and gentamicin (Treatment No. 56) at a dose rate of 2–3 mg/kg q8h.
- The use of flunixin meglumine (Treatment No. 52) at dose rates of 0.2 mg/kg q6h may be useful to aid in prevention of endotoxemia and laminitis.

Twinning

Twinning is a common problem in mares because of the high incidence of abortion associated with it and the lack of commercial viability of foals that are delivered. The incidence of twin pregnancies is as high as 10% of conceptions. The availability of ultrasound examination has improved the potential for early diagnosis of twinning and the possibility of elimination of one of the conceptuses or termination of the pregnancy prior to formation of the endometrial cups.

History and Presenting Signs

- There may be a history of double ovulations.
- There may be little in the history or early signs of pregnancy to indicate that twin pregnancies are present.

Clinical Findings and Diagnosis

- Rectal palpation is extremely inaccurate for diagnosis of twins in the early stages of pregnancy and therefore is of little diagnostic use.
- Ultrasound examination provides the possibility of a definitive confirmation of the presence of twins, although care must be taken not to confuse fetal sacs with endometrial cysts.

KEY POINT ► Diagnosis of twin pregnancy via ultrasound is best undertaken around 15 days after ovulation.

- If there is any doubt about the appearance of the fetal sac, a follow-up examination must be performed prior to a decision about elimination of one or both fetuses.
- It is important to note that the fetal sacs may be together in one horn or separated so that there is a separate fetus in each uterine horn.

Differential Diagnosis

- Endometrial cyst

Treatment

- Most clinicians attempt to eliminate one of the fetal sacs, and this is most easily accomplished if the fetuses are in separate horns. The manual elimination of one of the fetal sacs is best undertaken before 20 days' gestation.

KEY POINT ► The smaller of the sacs is usually eliminated, and this is done by squeezing the sac or applying pressure against the brim of the pelvis until rupture of the sac is felt.

- Ultrasound examination at this stage will confirm the result of the intervention.
- If the twin pregnancies occur in the same horn, the use of a synthetic prostaglandin such as fluprostenol (Treatment No. 53) to cause luteolysis will result in the mare returning to estrus. Thus the mare can be mated again before the breeding season concludes.

Uterine Prolapse

Uterine prolapse is uncommon in the mare, which is fortunate because it can be a difficult condition to correct. It usually occurs soon after foaling and is more common in mares that have had complicated deliveries.

History and Presenting Signs

- Recently foaled mare
- Tissue mass protruding from the vulval lips

Clinical Findings and Diagnosis

- Diagnosis is not difficult because the prolapsed uterus appears as a red, soft mass with a wrinkled surface. Depending on the duration of the exposure, there may be ulceration and the exposed surface may be desiccated.
- The other possible diagnoses that can be mistaken for uterine prolapse include rectal prolapse and prolapse of the bladder.

Differential Diagnosis

- Prolapse of the bladder
- Prolapse of the vagina
- Prolapse of the rectum

Treatment

- Prompt treatment is essential if the uterine prolapse can be corrected soon after it occurs and there has been minimal trauma.
- First aid measures include keeping the prolapsed mass moistened with warm saline and preventing the mare from lying down.
- Epidural anesthesia (see Fig. 7-2) should be carried out to prevent straining and to ease replacement of the uterus.
- Medication to be administered should include tetanus prophylaxis, systemic antibiotics (see Antibiotic Therapy, Chap. 17), and intramuscular oxytocin (40–50 IU given intramuscularly) (Treatment No. 81) to aid in uterine contraction.

- The uterus is rinsed with warmed normal saline containing Na or K penicillin (1 million units per liter of saline). Massage of the uterus will permit replacement, but care must be taken that the endometrium is not torn because it can become extremely friable. Once the uterus is replaced, it is useful to administer a further 40 to 50 IU of oxytocin intramuscularly.
- Vulval retention sutures can be used to prevent the uterus from prolapsing again, although this procedure is not as effective as it is in the cow. If the mare shows signs of straining, it may be worthwhile to give a tranquilizing drug that is of longer duration of action, such as acepromazine (Treatment No. 1) at a dose rate of 15 to 20 mg/500 kg.

Reproductive Disease in the Stallion

Castration

Castration is the most common surgical procedure performed by veterinarians in equine practice. Castration is performed mainly as a management strategy for horses that have no breeding future. In most cases, horses are presented for castration around 2 years of age. The main options are whether to perform the surgery with the horse standing or under general anesthesia.

Surgical Technique

Standing Castration

- Standing castration is preferred by practitioners who work with thoroughbred and standardbred racehorses. These horses are usually well handled, and with adequate restraint, the technique is simple and has few complications. The standing technique for castration is most useful in horses less than 3 years of age. The main complication is injury to the operator from a kick by the horse due to insufficient desensitization.
- We prefer the horse to be tranquilized with 0.5 mg/kg xylazine (Treatment No. 108) and 0.05 to 0.1 mg/kg butorphanol (Treatment No. 15) given intravenously. An alternative to xylazine is de-

tomidine (Treatment No. 28) at a dose rate of 10 to 20 μg/kg given IV. This will result in profound sedation of the horse, at which time local anesthetic (10–15 ml of 2% lidocaine; Treatment No. 67) may be injected subcutaneously along the median raphe of the scrotum using a 23-gauge needle (Fig. 7-3). After allowing 2 to 3 minutes for the local anesthetic to take effect, 50 ml of 2% lidocaine is injected through the desensitized scrotal skin into the body of each testicle using a 19-gauge, 3.75-cm (1.5-in) needle. The alternative is to use an 18-gauge, 8.75-cm (3.5-in) spinal needle inserted up through the testicle into the spermatic cord (Fig. 7-4) and injecting 20 ml of 2% lidocaine. Local anesthetic injected into the testicle will diffuse into the spermatic cord and block local sensation.
- Surgery commences after appropriate skin disinfection of the scrotum, with a right-handed operator standing on the right side of the horse, although some veterinarians prefer to stand on the horse's left side. The scrotum and testicles should be held in such a way that the incision is made away from the operator. The left testicle should be removed first, and the incision is begun at the cranial pole of the testicle, about 5 mm (0.2 in) from and parallel to the median raphe of the

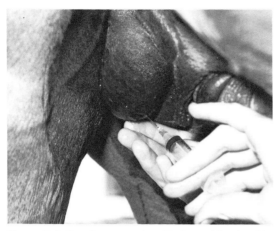

Figure 7–3. Standing castration. To desensitize the skin prior to desensitizing the spermatic cord, a 23-gauge needle is used to inject about 10 ml of 2% lidocaine along the median raphe of the scrotum.

scrotum. The incision should be at least 12 to 15 cm (5 to 6 in) long.

KEY POINT ▶ The most common complication from standing castration is excessive swelling around the penis and prepuce because the incision in the scrotum is too small and does not permit adequate drainage.

- It is usual for the scrotum and parietal tunic to be incised together so that the testicle falls through the scrotal opening.
- For emasculation of the testicle, we prefer the use of a triple-crush emasculator and initial emasculation of the fibrous components (including the tunic) of the spermatic cord. This is followed by

emasculation of the vascular pedicle, and the emasculators should be left in situ for at least 1 minute (Fig. 7-5).
- Before the emasculators are removed, a large hemostat is applied to the cord proximal to the emasculators. Thus, if there is hemorrhage when the emasculators are removed, the cord can be retrieved. A separate incision is made similar to the first, 5 mm (0.2 in) from the median raphe on the right side, and the right testicle is similarly removed.
- To ensure that there is adequate drainage, we prefer to remove the median raphe between the two incisions.

Castration under General Anesthesia

- The combination of 1.1 mg/kg xylazine (Treatment No. 108) IV followed 3 to 5 minutes later by 2.2 mg/kg ketamine (Treatment No. 64) IV (see section on General Anesthesia in Chap. 17) is a simple combination that provides adequate time for castration.

KEY POINT ▶ For right-handed operators, castration is most easily performed with the horse lying on its left side.

- A rope approximately 4 m (12 to 14 ft) long is tied around the pastern of the right hindleg and taken between the front legs and underneath the left side of the neck. The free end is then taken to form a half hitch around the right hind pastern so that the leg is flexed up and the foot is pulled cranially.
- Surgery is performed similarly to that described above, except that the lower (left) testicle is removed before the upper (right) testicle.
- Stallions older than 3 years should only be castrated under general anesthesia and the vascular pedicle ligated rather than emasculated.

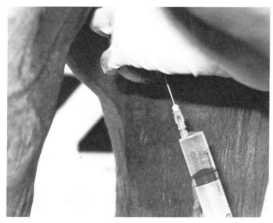

Figure 7–4. Standing castration. Desensitizing the spermatic cord can be done using an 18-gauge, 7.5-cm (3-in) spinal needle directed through the desensitized skin of the scrotum into the spermatic cord. Prior to injection of the local anesthetic, the operator should ensure that the needle is not in a vessel.

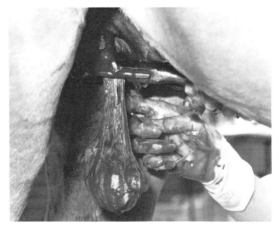

Figure 7–5. Standing castration. After incising through the scrotum and tunics, the testicle is removed using a triple-crush emasculator.

Postoperative Care

- Procaine penicillin (15–20 mg/kg or 15,000–20,000 IU/kg) (Treatment No. 83) is given IM prior to surgery. In a series of cases we did not administer penicillin and had an unacceptably high rate of local wound infections with *Streptococcus* species. A single dose appears to be adequate in controlling problems with postoperative infection.
- Administration of 4–6 mg/kg phenylbutazone (Treatment No. 88) is helpful in preventing excessive swelling at the castration site in the immediate postoperative period.
- If the horse has not been vaccinated for tetanus, tetanus antitoxin (3000 IU) is given subcutaneously.
- The horse should be observed carefully for signs of hemorrhage in the first few hours after surgery. Exercise is important in preventing excessive swelling and aiding in local drainage. Horses should be exercised twice daily for the first 5 to 7 days after surgery. Usually this involves lunging the horse for 10 to 15 minutes, followed by hosing the scrotal area with cold water, avoiding the wound.

Complications

Although castration is a simple operation, there are a range of complications that can cause problems for both the horse owner and the veterinarian.

Excessive Hemorrhage. Emasculation is a technique that is not foolproof for hemostasis. After most castrations, there will be minor degrees of hemorrhage, with blood dripping from the castration wound. In most cases, this stops within 30 to 60 minutes. However, if there is more severe hemorrhage, with blood coming from the wound in a steady stream, it is more serious and may require exploration of the site if the hemorrhage has not stopped within 30 minutes. To find the offending vessel, the horse is anesthetized and placed on its back. After appropriate skin disinfection and draping, the side where hemorrhage is evident is investigated to find the spermatic cord and ligate the particular vessel. In most cases it is not difficult to find the site of the hemorrhage, although it is usually necessary to explore some distance down the inguinal canal. If the source of the hemorrhage cannot be found, sterile gauze packing may be used to pack the region and apply pressure for hemostasis.

Excessive Local Swelling. This is the most common complication of castrations. It is more common after standing castrations, because when a castration is performed standing, it is more difficult to ensure that the scrotal skin incision is of adequate length. If the incision is too small, there will not be adequate drainage, and therefore, excessive local swelling is the result. Under these circumstances, it may be necessary to enlarge the original incision so that drainage is effective.

KEY POINT ► In most cases, the problem will resolve with 10 to 15 minutes of daily exercise, nonsteroidal anti-inflammatory drugs such as phenylbutazone (Treatment No. 88) at a dose rate of 2.2 mg/kg orally q12h, and local hosing.

Local Infection. This is another common complication of castrations because in most circumstances the technique is carried out under conditions where sterility cannot be ensured. We have found that most local infections are due to *Streptococcus* species, and therefore, IM procaine penicillin (Treatment No. 83) at a dose rate of 15 mg/kg q12h is the treatment of choice. If sufficient drainage is ensured, most cases will respond to simple treatment. However, in some cases infection can ascend in the spermatic cord and result in scirrhous cord.

Scirrhous Cord. Scirrhous cord is a serious problem that results from infection ascending the spermatic cord. In some cases this is manifested as local swelling and purulent discharge from the scrotal wound. However, in some cases the infection may ascend and spread to the intraperitoneal part of the cord.

KEY POINT ► Such cases may present many months after castration with signs such as hindlimb swelling and colic.

Cases of scirrhous cord must be treated by surgery, with removal of all infected cord. This can be very difficult when the infected cord extends through the internal inguinal ring. In these cases, marsupialization may be necessary so that the infection can drain externally. Appropriate samples (tissue and/or pus) should be taken at the time of surgery and appropriate antimicrobial therapy instituted.

Eventration. Eventration, with abdominal contents, usually small intestine, descending through the inguinal canal and out through the scrotum, is a rare but disastrous complication of castration. It usually occurs immediately after or within a few hours of surgery but in rare cases may occur several days later.

KEY POINT ► Eventration is more common in standardbreds than other breeds and should be anticipated in any colt that has had a history of a scrotal hernia as a foal.

If eventration does occur, early treatment is essential before contamination is severe and irreversible. To replace the intestine, a flank laparotomy is usually necessary.

Cryptorchidism

A *cryptorchid* is a colt or stallion with one or both testicles retained somewhere between the original embryologic site near the kidney and the scrotum. Cryptorchids are usually discovered when presented for castration, and many veterinarians have been embarrassed to discover that the horse they have anesthetized for a routine castration is a cryptorchid. For this reason, it is obviously essential to carefully examine any horse presented for castration prior to surgery. The most difficult situation is the horse presented with no testicles evident, no history available, but stallion-like behavior. If a testicle is retained, it is most commonly found somewhere in the inguinal canal. However, the testicle also can be intraabdominal.

History and Presenting Signs

- Presence of only one testicle
- No testicles present but stallion-like behavior

Clinical Findings and Diagnosis

- One or no testicles apparent on palpation of the scrotum.
- In some cases, deep palpation of the external inguinal ring with the horse under tranquilization will result in the testicle or epididymis being palpable.
- Rectal examination should be performed to determine whether some of the cord structures can be palpated traversing the internal inguinal ring. While this is often difficult, in some cases of a retained intraabdominal testicle, the testicle can be palpated close to the internal inguinal ring.

KEY POINT ► If there is doubt about the presence of one or both testicles in a horse showing stallion-like behavior, it is possible to perform plasma hormone analyses to aid in diagnosis.

- In horses older than 3 years of age, measurement of plasma estrone sulfate concentrations is useful, with cryptorchid horses having values greater than 400 pg/ml. In younger horses, a hCG response test is used, with plasma being collected for testosterone concentrations before and 24 hours after the administration of 6000 IU of hCG. Cryptorchid horses will show a substantial rise in testosterone concentrations after hCG. It also should be noted that basal testosterone levels are also higher than in geldings.

Differential Diagnosis

- Castrated horse with adrenal production of testosterone
- Castrated horse with epididymis removed and mistaken for testicle

Treatment

- Because of the likely hereditary nature of cryptorchidism, the horse should be castrated rather than attempts made to relocate the testicle.

- The majority of cryptorchid cases are unilateral, and the affected testicle is removed via an inguinal approach.
- In cases where the testicle is enlarged, the testicle may not be capable of being removed via the inguinal canal, and a paramedian laparotomy is the technique of choice.

Habronema Infestation

Larvae from *Habronema muscae* can burrow into the urethral process, which is attractive to the flies because of the moist surfaces. The resulting lesion can resemble a squamous cell carcinoma, and histopathology may be necessary to confirm the diagnosis.

History and Presenting Signs

- Swelling around the prepuce
- Discharge from the prepuce
- Hemospermia

Clinical Findings and Diagnosis

- In early cases there may be little to be found on clinical examination. Longer-standing cases usually demonstrate localized edema involving the urethral process, and there may be a granulomatous reaction.

KEY POINT ► Lesions can occur on the prepuce but are more common on the urethral process.

- In chronic cases there is usually some degree of ulceration, and typical caseous lesions are spread throughout the affected site.
- If there is doubt about the diagnosis, a biopsy of material may be necessary at the time of treatment.

Differential Diagnosis

- Neoplasia
- Viral papillomatosis
- Balanoposthitis
- Trauma

Treatment

- Ivermectin administration may cure some cases of habronemiasis.
- Treatment with organophosphates and dimethylsulfoxide (DMSO) (Treatment No. 34) applied topically has been reported to be successful in some cases.
- In chronic cases of infestation of the urethral process, amputation of the process may be necessary. To prevent constriction, the urethral mucosa is then sutured to the skin around the process.

Neoplasia of the Penis

Neoplasia of the penis and/or prepuce is rare in the horse. Squamous cell carcinomas are by far the most common tumors affecting the penis. Early diagnosis is important because metastasis to regional lymph nodes can occur. Other tumors that can affect the penis include melanomas, sarcoids, and hemangiomas.

History and Presenting Signs

- Discharge from the prepuce
- Hemospermia
- Swelling around the preputial area

Clinical Findings and Diagnosis

- Horses will vary in presenting signs, but many cases are presented because of discharge from the prepuce.
- Examination should be done under the influence of a tranquilizing agent such as acepromazine (Treatment No. 1) at a dose rate of 15 to 20 mg/500 kg of body weight. While there are some dangers associated with the use of this drug (see Penile Paralysis), it enables the penis to be examined easily.
- Squamous cell carcinomas appear usually on unpigmented skin and have an erosive appearance. Melanomas are most common in gray horses and may be found in the preputial area without causing any adverse clinical signs.
- If the lesion is localized, it should be biopsied to enable histopathology to be performed and a definitive diagnosis made.
- In more extensive lesions, it may be necessary to amputate the penis. This technique is obviously more useful in geldings than in stallions.

KEY POINT ▶ In some cases where there is a squamous cell carcinoma that has been present for some time without causing adverse clinical signs, there may have been metastasis to regional lymph nodes. It is important to palpate the inguinal lymph nodes and to also palpate abdominal lymph nodes by a rectal examination.

- In cases where metastasis has occurred, there may be obstruction of local lymphatic drainage, resulting in local swelling around the prepuce; there also may be swelling of one or both hindlegs.

Differential Diagnosis

- Habronemiasis
- Trauma
- Balanoposthitis
- Viral papillomatosis

Treatment

- Where the lesions are found early in the course of the problem, local excision using cryosurgery appears to provide the best results.
- In some cases, radiation therapy using implants of ^{222}Rn has been found to be effective in treating localized lesions.

KEY POINT ▶ Where the tumor is more extensive, amputation of the penis is required.

- This is a salvage procedure in a stallion and is used most commonly in geldings. Where there is more extensive disease, it may be necessary to ablate the prepuce and divert the penis caudally so that the urethra opens ventral to the ischium.
- If there is evidence of metastasis, the prognosis is very poor, and euthanasia is the only real option.

Penile Paralysis

KEY POINT ▶ Penile paralysis is most common in stallions after receiving one of the phenothiazine-derivative tranquilizers, such as promazine (Treatment No. 94) or acepromazine (Treatment No. 1).

Since the advent of xylazine, the phenothiazine tranquilizers are used less commonly, and the incidence of penile paralysis has become less.

History and Presenting Signs

- Administration of a phenothiazine-derivative tranquilizer
- Prolonged protrusion of the penis

Clinical Findings and Diagnosis

- Diagnosis is not a difficulty, but an accurate history should be taken to determine whether other neurologic problems have contributed to the problem.
- The penis appears to be engorged and partially erect, and edema usually develops early in the course of the problem.
- There is congestion and stagnation of blood in the corpus cavernosum, which accentuates and aggravates the condition.

Differential Diagnosis

- Neurogenic paralysis
- Traumatic paralysis
- Phenothiazine-induced paralysis

Treatment

- If the injury is the result of a kick or other trauma, local anti-inflammatory measures, including the application of ice packs, are useful.
- If the problem is drug-induced, early support may prevent passive congestion and edema. Suc-

cessful treatment of an acepromazine-associated penile paralysis has been reported using benz-tropine mesylate (Cogentin, Merck Sharp & Dohme, West Point, PA) given IV at a dose rate of 8 mg for a 500-kg horse.

- Local massage and support of the penis are essential to reduce the edema and congestion. Supporting the penis in some type of sling prevents the stasis and congestion of blood that occurs by virtue of the dependency. It is useful if the sling is made of a mesh material (usually nylon), which enables the stallion to urinate without restriction.
- If the penis can be returned to its position in the prepuce, using some type of skin emollient to prevent local trauma, the prognosis is improved.
- If there is marked inflammation and swelling, the use of systemic phenylbutazone at initial dose rates of 4.4 mg/kg bid for 2 days, followed by 2.2 mg/kg bid for 4 to 7 days, may be of assistance.
- If there are doubts about the horse's ability to pass urine, catheterization of the urinary bladder may be required.
- In cases that are nonresponsive to medical management, the reefing operation or, in more severe cases, amputation of the penis is required.

Venereal Diseases

While a variety of viral, bacterial, and protozoal venereal diseases occur in the stallion, most of these are uncommon and unlikely to be encountered in clinical situations. However, many of the diseases have significance in relation to quarantine concerns. Some diseases no longer occur in North America, and many are unknown in the southern hemisphere.

History and Presenting Signs

- Preputial discharge
- Infertility
- Anorexia
- No presenting signs

Clinical Findings and Diagnosis

Dourine. This protozoal disease has been eradicated from North America and is found only in Africa, the Middle East, and South America. It has a slow incubation period of several weeks, and the horse may have a urethral discharge. Systemic involvement is evident, with elevated body temperature and plaques developing on the lower body. Later in the course of the disease, penile paralysis may occur, and neurologic signs such as ataxia and, in extreme cases, paralysis are found. Diagnosis is best made using a serum sample for a complement fixation test.

Herpesvirus. Herpesvirus 3 infection is known as *coital exanthema*. It is a self-limiting disease, but in the acute stages it can produce vesicles on the penis, which can ulcerate and become secondarily infected with local bacteria.

Equine Viral Arteritis. This disease is very commonly carried by stallions, which may be asymptomatic. It is particularly common in standardbred stallions. Only a small number of horses in an affected group may show clinical signs, and the signs can vary from ocular to abdominal. In mares, abortion is the most significant sign of viral arteritis. Confirmation of infection is best done using a viral neutralization test on blood.

Equine Infectious Anemia. This viral infection has important economic consequences and is spread by biting flies. However, because the virus has been found in semen, a venereal mode of transmission has been proposed. Diagnosis is made on serum samples using a Coggins test.

Bacterial Diseases. Contagious equine metritis was the most important bacterial venereal disease in recent years and resulted in outbreaks of infection in both the northern and southern hemispheres. Due to rigorous bacteriologic testing, the disease has now been brought under control. Other bacterial venereal diseases of sporadic significance include those caused by *Klebsiella* and *Pseudomonas*. These infections are usually diagnosed because of endometritis in a number of mares that have been mated with the affected stallion.

Differential Diagnosis

- Contagious equine metritis organism
- Other bacterial venereal diseases
- Herpesvirus 3
- Equine viral arteritis

Treatment

- Most of the venereal infections are not responsive to treatment and must be controlled by sexual rest.
- Many of the viral diseases are self-limiting and will resolve with time.
- Bacterial venereal infections are particularly difficult to treat and control. Local washing and disinfection of the penis may lead to worsening of the infection. Local treatment with antibiotics, particularly gentamicin, may be worthwhile in some cases.

References

Adams, G. P., and Ginther, O. J.: Efficacy of intrauterine infusion of plasma for treatment of infertility and endometritis in mares. *J. Am. Vet. Med. Assoc.* 194:372, 1989.

Arighi, M., and Bosu, T. K.: Comparison of hormonal methods for diagnosis of cryptorchidism in horses. *J. Equine Vet. Sci.* 9:20, 1989.

Asbury, A. C.: Infectious and immunologic considerations in mare infertility. *Compend. Contin. Educ. Pract. Vet.* 9:585, 1987.

Caudle, A. B., and Fayrer Hosken, R. A.: Stallion fertility evaluation I. *Equine Pract.* 11:26, 1989.

Hyland, J. H.: Reproductive endocrinology: Its role in fertility and infertility in the horse. *Br. Vet. J.* 146:1, 1990.

Kenney, R. M., and Doig, P. A.: Equine endometrial biopsy. In D. A. Morrow (Ed.), *Current Therapy in Theriogenology,* Vol. 2. Philadelphia: W. B. Saunders, 1986, pp. 723–729.

LeBlanc, M. M.: Treatment protocols and preventative practices for mares with endometritis. *Vet. Med.* 84:906, 1989.

LeBlanc, M. M.: Diseases of the Reproductive System: The Mare. In P. T. Colahan, I. G. Mayhew, A. M. Merritt, and J. N. Moore (Eds.), *Equine Medicine and Surgery,* 4th ed. Goleta, Calif.: American Veterinary Publications, 1991, p. 949.

McKinnon, A. O., Voss, J. L., Trotter, G. W., et al.: Hemospermia of the stallion. *Equine Pract.* 10: 17, 1988.

Pickett, B. W., and Amann, R. P.: Extension and storage of spermatozoa: A review. *J. Equine Vet. Sci.* 7:289, 1987.

Ricketts, S. W.: Reproduction. In N. E. Robinson (Ed.), *Current Therapy in Equine Medicine,* Vol. 2. Philadelphia: W.B. Saunders, 1987, pp. 491–573.

Rossdale, P. D., and Ricketts, S. W.: *Equine Stud Farm Medicine,* 2d Ed. London: Balliere Tindall, 1980.

Shires, G. M., and Kanepts, A. J.: A practical and simple surgical technique for repair of urine pooling in the mare. *Proc. 32nd Annu. Conv. Am. Assoc. Equine Pract.,* 1986, p. 51.

Slusher, S. H., Freeman, K. P., and Roszel, J. F.: Infertility diagnosis in mares using endometrial biopsy, culture and aspirate cytology. *Proc. 31st Annu. Conv. Am. Assoc. Equine Pract.,* 1985, p. 165.

Squires, E. L., Voss, J. L., Villahoz, M. D., and Shideler, R. K.: Use of ultrasound in broodmare reproduction. *Proc. 29th Annu. Conv. Am. Assoc. Equine Pract.,* 1983, p. 27.

Varner, D. D., and Schumacher, J.: Diseases of the Reproductive System: The Stallion. In P. T. Colahan, I. G. Mayhew, A. M. Merritt, and J. N. Moore (Eds.), *Equine Medicine and Surgery,* 4th Ed. Goleta, Calif.: American Veterinary Publications, 1991, p. 847.

Youngquist, R. S.: Equine. In D. A. Morrow (Ed.), *Current Therapy in Theriogenology,* Vol. 2. Philadelphia: W.B. Saunders, 1986, pp. 635–786.

CHAPTER 8

Pediatrics

CLINICAL ASPECTS OF NEONATAL PHYSIOLOGY

In the change from intrauterine to extrauterine existence, remarkable adaptations occur as the foal moves from a fluid to a gaseous environment. If these adaptations do not follow in proper sequence or some fetal circulatory pathways remain open (e.g., ductus arteriosus, foramen ovale), signs of maladaptation may appear.

In the period immediately following delivery, gasping respiration occurs, and the alveoli open, with absorption of pulmonary fluid. Arterial blood gases reflect the changes in gas exchange across the lung, and over the first few days of life they show a pattern of decreasing tensions of carbon dioxide ($PaCO_2$) and increasing tensions of oxygen (PaO_2), as demonstrated in Figure 8-1. The respiratory rate is high during the first 4 to 6 hours after birth, with values in the range 50 to 90 breaths per minute. This rate will be influenced by environmental temperature, with higher respiration rates in colder conditions.

KEY POINT ▶ Body position has a major influence on pulmonary gas exchange and is of major significance when managing the sick foal.

Even in healthy, normal foals, the PaO_2 may be 10 to 30 torr (mmHg) lower when the foal lies in lateral recumbency as compared with sternal recumbency. Therefore, when there are signs of maladaptation or cardiorespiratory problems, foals should be placed in sternal recumbency to ensure that the arterial oxygenation is optimized.

In the immediate neonatal period, there may be extensive right-to-left shunting of blood because the various fetal circulatory pathways do not close immediately.

KEY POINT ▶ The major fetal circulatory pathway of clinical importance is the ductus arteriosus, which usually closes within 12 hours of birth.

Most foals older than 24 hours do not have a patent ductus arteriosus, although it has been reported in normal foals for up to 5 to 6 days after birth.

KEY POINT ▶ A systolic heart murmur is a normal finding in foals for up to 3 to 4 months after birth and should not be confused with the continuous "machinery" murmur of a foal with patent ductus arteriosus.

Immediately after delivery, the foal obtains up to 1.5 L of blood from the placenta, which is important for establishing normal blood volume.

KEY POINT ▶ In some mares that foal standing or when the mare stands quickly after delivery, the umbilical cord may rupture and deprive the foal of vital blood.

This may result in hypovolemia and shock, which may be manifest in an affected foal as maladaptation, there being a prolonged period before the foal gets to its feet and sucks. Acid–base measurements in these foals has shown quite a profound metabolic acidosis because of reduced peripheral perfusion and lactate production. Normally, there are no metabolic acid–base disturbances in newborn foals, the values for base excess and standard bicarbonate being within the normal adult range.

KEY POINT ▶ Most foals will stand within the first hour after birth and should suck from the mare by 2 hours after birth.

Foals that do not conform to these criteria should be examined carefully, because a range of congenital abnormalities and metabolic derangements can lead to the presenting sign of maladaptation.

During the first week after birth, there are gradual increases in the PaO_2 and improvements in cardiac function. This first week is the period when foals are most susceptible to any problems that result in cardiorespiratory dysfunction. The most common causes of cardiorespiratory abnormalities are bacterial infections that result in septicemia.

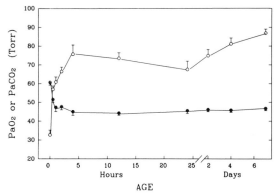

Figure 8–1. Arterial oxygen (PaO₂) (○) and carbon dioxide (PaCO₂) (●) tensions in foals from birth to 7 days of age. (From Stewart, J.H., Rose, R.J., and Barko, A.M.: Respiratory studies in foals from birth to one week of age. *Equine Vet. J.* 16:323, 1984, with permission.)

CLINICAL EXAMINATION OF THE FOAL

In Chapter 1 we discussed details of the general clinical examination, particularly related to adult horses. This approach also applies to examination of the foal, but there are some specific aspects of foal examination that need to be emphasized.

General Examination

History. Collection of the history is important with any condition, but in the case of newborn foals, it should also include questions relating to the health of the mare. Prior to foaling, details such as the presence of milk dripping from the teats, vulval discharge, and previous foaling difficulties (including foals born dead or dying shortly after birth) should be obtained.

Demeanor. The demeanor of the foal provides important clues to its state of health. Most sick foals look sick.

KEY POINT ▶ Foals with metabolic derangements, sepsis, respiratory distress, and maladaptation usually stop sucking the mare, so the mare's udder becomes engorged and the mare may drip milk.

Mucous Membranes and Pulse. In taking the vital signs, attention should be paid to the mucous membranes, capillary refill, and peripheral pulses. The extremities should be warm, and a pulse should be palpable in the great metatarsal and brachial arteries.

Auscultation of the Heart. The normal heart rate in foals from 24 hours to 7 days of age is usually in the range 60 to 110 beats per minute. A systolic

heart murmur can be heard in a high percentage of foals for up to 2 to 3 months after birth. In most cases, the murmur is grades I to III (see Chap. 5) and is a normal finding.

Respiratory System. The respiratory rate is highest in the first hour after birth. The range of respiratory rates in foals up to 1 week varies from 25 to 60 breaths per minute. Rates in the range 70 to 90 breaths per minute may be found during the first hour after birth. Because respiratory rate is affected by the state of excitement of the foal, care should be taken when recording the rate.

KEY POINT ▶ Auscultation of the chest can be misleading in some foals with severe respiratory disease, there being no abnormal lung sounds despite severe pneumonia and atelectasis.

Foals with suspected pulmonary disease should have chest radiographs taken and, if possible, arterial blood gas analysis performed (see Diagnostic Aids, p. 277).

Gastrointestinal System. Auscultation of the abdomen is important to detect ileus, and palpation may help to determine some impactions. Foals will often show signs of severe abdominal pain, which may be difficult to localize. In general, a conservative approach to management is indicated, and exploratory laparotomy is seldom required. The major problem of the newborn foal is retained meconium, which is found more commonly in colts than in fillies.

Rectal Temperature. Rectal temperature is usually in the range 38 to 39°C (100–102.5°F). The temperature increases from birth to 4 days of age and thereafter plateaus. Newborn foals that have subnormal temperatures have a worse prognosis than those with normal or elevated temperatures. In foals that are active or have been out in the sun, the temperature may be transiently elevated to greater than 39°C. However, temperatures greater than 39°C should be regarded with suspicion.

Urinary System. While urine may not be passed until the foal is 6 to 10 hours of age, frequent urination of dilute urine is normal in newborn foals.

KEY POINT ▶ The most important area to examine is the umbilicus, which may be infected or more commonly involved in a patent urachus.

In this condition, there is a communication between the urinary bladder and the umbilicus so that urine dribbles from the umbilicus.

Musculoskeletal System. Examination of the musculoskeletal system of the newborn foal can provide useful clues about the foal's maturity.

KEY POINT ▶ In premature foals, there is often overextension of the fetlocks, and the foals will be weak and have difficulty in standing.

Radiographs of the carpus and tarsus may be useful to assess the degree of ossification. Evaluation for evidence of joint effusion is also important because localization of bacterial infection in joints ("joint ill") and epiphyses is a common problem.

Placenta. Where problems are found very soon after birth, examination of the placenta for abnormalities should be done. Weighing the placenta also can provide an indication of possible placental insufficiency. Normal weights for placentas in thoroughbred horses are in the range 4.5 to 7.0 kg.

Uterine Bacteriology. If a bacterial infection is suspected in a newborn foal, it may be valuable to obtain uterine swabs from the mare (see Chap. 7) to determine whether infection is present.

RESTRAINT OF FOALS

In neonatal foals, restraint in lateral or sternal recumbency usually is required for venous catheterization, arterial blood collection, or intranasal oxygen administration. However, when nasogastric tubing, intravenous or intramuscular injections, or venous blood collection is necessary, foals can be restrained while standing. For injections and venous blood collection, it can be helpful to back the foal into a corner of a box stall and grasp both ears, as shown in Figure 8-2. Figure 8-3 shows restraint by holding one arm around the chest and the other arm pulling the tail up over the rump.

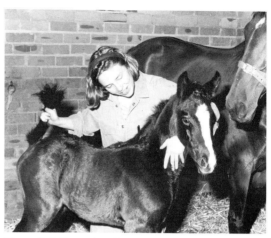

Figure 8–3. Restraint of the foal. For minor procedures, the foal can be restrained by holding one arm around the chest and pulling the tail up over the back.

DIAGNOSTIC AIDS

A range of diagnostic aids will be useful to assess various diseases in newborn foals. Many of these (e.g., transtracheal aspiration, bronchoalveolar lavage, abdominocentesis, CSF collection) have the same indications and technique as in adult horses, and the particular diagnostic aid is discussed under the appropriate body system. However, some techniques may be of more importance in the foal or may be somewhat different from those in the adult horse. The most commonly used of these techniques are discussed below.

Blood Culture

KEY POINT ▶ The use of blood culture is a vital part of the workup in any foal with suspected septicemia.

In some cases, bacteria may even be seen on a blood smear and can provide useful information for commencing antimicrobial therapy. Details of blood culture methodology are given in Chapter 15. Particular care must be taken to avoid contamination with skin microorganisms, and therefore, attention must be paid to appropriate skin disinfection.

Arterial Blood Gas Analysis

KEY POINT ▶ Arterial blood gas and acid–base analyses are essential aspects of the evaluation of newborn foals showing maladaptation or signs of dyspnea.

Venous blood may be used to assess acid–base status, but only arterial blood samples may be used to evaluate gas exchange. More specialized practices may have a blood gas machine in the practice laboratory. However, in most cases, arrangements

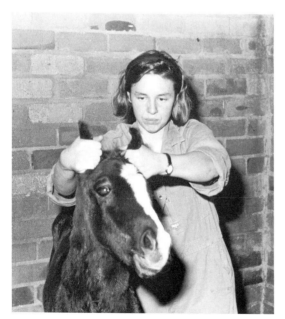

Figure 8–2. Restraint of the foal. The foal is restrained by backing it into a corner of a box stall and grasping both ears.

can be made with a local hospital to process the occasional blood gas sample. Special blood gas syringes are available containing powdered heparin, but it is just as easy to use 2-ml syringes and fill the dead space of the syringe with sodium heparin (1000 IU/ml). It is important to ensure that there are no air bubbles in the syringe because the blood gas values obtained will be erroneous. Approximately 1.5 to 2 ml of blood should be collected and immediately capped by bending the needle over or inserting the needle into a rubber stopper such as the top from a Vacutainer tube. The sample should be placed in ice or an ice water bath prior to analysis, which should be completed within 4 hours of collection. Because the blood gas measurements are made at 37°C, it is important to note the foal's body temperature at the time of collection. Temperatures above 37°C will result in upward correction of the blood gas measurements. Most machines perform the correction automatically if the patient's temperature is programmed in during the sample processing.

In foals up to 2 weeks of age, arterial blood samples are most easily collected with the foal restrained in lateral recumbency. Following collection, digital pressure should be applied for 2 minutes to the site of needle penetration. The following sites may be used for arterial blood collection:

Great Metatarsal Artery—On the lateral aspect of the third metatarsal bone, the great metatarsal artery is easily palpated and is relatively fixed in position. We find that either 23- or 25-gauge, 15-mm (5/8-in) needles can be used for blood collection. Most foals will struggle briefly when the needle is inserted, and therefore, the hindleg should be restrained and the needle inserted quickly through the skin prior to connection of the heparinized syringe (Fig. 8-4). In foals showing signs of shock, it may not be possible to palpate a pulse in the great metatarsal artery.

Palmar (Digital) Artery—The palmar arteries are readily palpable on the abaxial surface of the fetlock. Sometimes a pulse will not be detected, but it is possible to insert a 25-gauge, 15-mm (5/8-in) needle into the artery, as shown in Figure 8-5.

Brachial Artery—In newborn foals that have weak or absent peripheral pulses, usually it is possible to palpate a pulse in the brachial artery as it crosses the medial aspect of the proximal forearm near the insertion of the pectoralis descendens muscle. A blood sample can be collected using a 23-gauge, 25-mm (1-in) needle.

Intranasal Oxygen Administration

Intranasal oxygen is used therapeutically in foals with respiratory distress if there is hypoxemia.

KEY POINT ► Intranasal oxygen administration is also useful as a diagnostic tool to assess cardiopulmonary function.

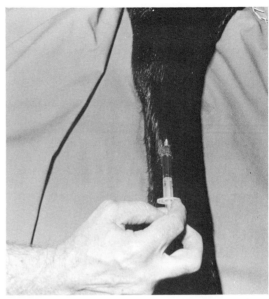

Figure 8–4. Arterial blood gas collection from the great metatarsal artery on the right hindleg. The artery runs along the lateral aspect of the metatarsus and is relatively immobile.

With the foal restrained in lateral recumbency, a soft infant nasogastric catheter is placed via the ventral nasal meatus into the nasopharynx. An oxygen cylinder with a rotameter capable of delivering 10 L/min of oxygen is used, and the oxygen is bubbled through a container of water to humidify

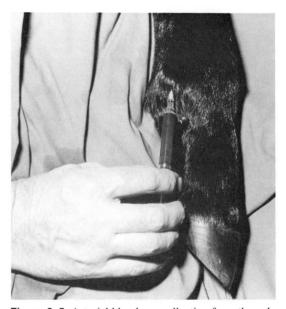

Figure 8–5. Arterial blood gas collection from the palmar (digital) artery. The artery is easily palpable over the abaxial surface of the sesamoids. However, the artery is much more mobile and therefore slightly more difficult to penetrate than the great metatarsal artery.

the gas (Fig. 8-6). In foals up to 1 week of age, a flow rate of 10 L/min is equivalent to administering 100% oxygen using a mask and valve system. Foals with normal cardiopulmonary function should at least double the arterial oxygen tension. The normal response of foals administered oxygen in lateral recumbency is shown in Figure 8-7, and it is apparent that 5 minutes of intranasal oxygen is sufficient to evaluate the capability of elevating the arterial oxygen tension.

Thoracic Radiography

While thoracic radiographs will not allow specific disease diagnosis, radiographs are essential to determine the degree of lung pathology.

KEY POINT ► Using portable x-ray machines, satisfactory films can be obtained, particularly using rare earth screens.

The most common abnormality in infectious respiratory disease is an interstitial pattern or pulmo-

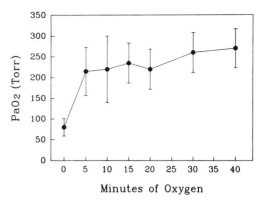

Figure 8–7. Administration of intranasal oxygen at a flow rate of 10 L/min to normal thoroughbred foals in the first week of life. Note that 5 minutes of intranasal oxygen is sufficient to produce a maximum elevation in arterial oxygen tension (PaO₂). (From Rose, R.J., Hodgson, D.R., Leadon, D.P., and Rossdale, P.D.: The effect of intranasal oxygen administration on arterial blood gases and acid–base parameters in spontaneously delivered, term induced and induced premature foals. *Res. Vet. Sci.* 34:159, 1983, with permission.)

nary infiltrate. In some cases, the infiltrate may be localized to certain regions of the lung fields (e.g., cranioventral or caudodorsal), suggesting inhalation or aspiration pneumonia. Some pulmonary diseases produce a typical radiographic appearance, for example, *Rhodococcus equi* pneumonia with large abscesses.

Hematology and Biochemistry

The normal hemogram of the newborn foal is similar in many regards to that of the adult. Foals do not have fetal hemoglobin, and the red cell indices decrease rapidly after birth. The hemoglobin decreases from values in the range 140 to 180 g/L (14 to 18 g/dl) at birth to 120 to 160 g/L (12 to 16 g/dl) at 24 hours of age. Thereafter there are few changes in mean values, the red cell indices being a little lower than those in adult horses. Red cell size is smaller than in adult horses, with MCV values around 35 to 40 fl. Leukocyte values are also similar to adult values, there being a predominance of neutrophils. The number of neutrophils gradually diminishes with age, and at about 6 months, foals have similar numbers of neutrophils and lymphocytes. During the first few days of life, the neutrophil-to-lymphocyte ratio is greater than 1.5, and values less than this may be found in foals with prematurity associated with low levels of plasma cortisol. Studies in Newmarket, U.K., have shown that premature foals with neutrophil-to-lymphocyte ratios of less than 1.5 have a poorer chance of survival than those with higher ratios.

Enzymes in foal plasma or serum are often considerably higher than in adults, and little significance can be attached to elevations until the foal is

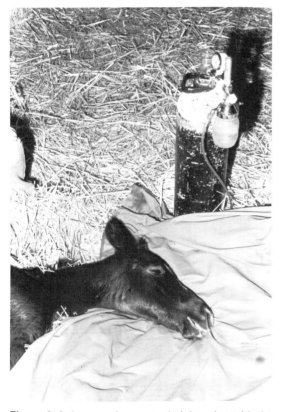

Figure 8–6. Intranasal oxygen administration with the foal lying in a box stall. This may be used diagnostically to determine the elevation in arterial oxygen tensions or therapeutically to correct hypoxemia associated with pulmonary problems. Flow rates around 10 L/min of oxygen are used, and the gas is humidified. In foals with pulmonary disease, sternal recumbency is preferred to lateral recumbency.

more than 3 months of age. The most notable change is in alkaline phosphatase, where values in the first few days of life may be greater than 1000 IU/L. However, elevations in muscle-derived enzymes are of clinical significance. Plasma or serum electrolytes are similar to values in adult horses except that values for potassium are slightly higher.

NEONATAL INTENSIVE CARE IN PRACTICE

Most equine practices will not have the range of sophisticated equipment necessary for full intensive care, such as may be found in human neonatal intensive care units. Such facilities will probably never be possible for foal intensive care, although many university clinics offer sophisticated intensive care services. The key to the success of even the most basic intensive care is the availability of personnel with some nursing skills. In many diseases, foals require support for 1 to 3 days without a great degree of sophistication in resources. The important aspects of low-level intensive care in a practice environment are as follows.

Temperature Control of Environment. It is metabolically costly for a sick foal to expend energy in thermoregulation. On many stud farms, foals are kept in cold environments. The simple process of warming the foal and ensuring that environmental temperatures are in the range 25 to 30°C (77 to 86°F) will be beneficial.

Feeding the Foal. Nursing care to assist the foal to suck from the mare, bottle feeding, or, in some sick foals, nasogastric intubation is an important component of intensive care. Some of the important points in feeding a sick foal are discussed later in this chapter.

Assessment of Passive Immunity and Plasma Transfusion. Failure of passive transfer with resulting low IgG levels in the serum or plasma of newborn foals is one of the most common predisposing factors to infectious diseases in foals. For this reason, measurement of the IgG concentration in the plasma of foals admitted to a critical-care facility is essential. Where the IgG concentration is low (<8 g/L, or <800 mg/dl), plasma transfusion is the treatment of choice. For this reason, a bank of frozen plasma should be maintained.

A Simple Facility for Oxygen Administration. Intranasal oxygen administration (see Diagnostic Aids, p. 278) is easily performed with a cylinder of oxygen and a water bottle for humidification of the gas, as shown in Figure 8-6. In foals with respiratory distress, where the oxygen tension is critical, positioning in sternal rather than lateral recumbency should be done. This will optimize the arterial oxygen tensions. Premature foals often will have hypoxemia (Fig. 8-8), and intranasal oxygen administration at flow rates of 5–10 L/min will be beneficial in elevating arterial oxygen tensions (Fig. 8-9).

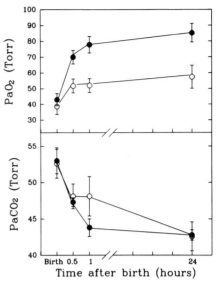

Figure 8–8. Arterial oxygen (PaO₂) and carbon dioxide (PaCO₂) tensions in full-term (●) and premature (○) foals in the first 24 hours after birth. Note the lower arterial oxygen tensions in the premature foals. (From Rose, R.J., Rossdale, P.D., and Leadon, D.P.: Blood gas and acid–base status in spontaneously delivered, term induced and induced premature foals. *J. Reprod. Fertil. Suppl.* 32:521, 1982, with permission.)

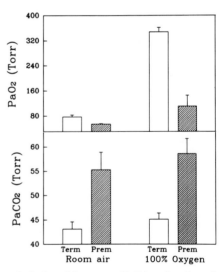

Figure 8–9. Arterial oxygen (PaO₂) and carbon dioxide (PaO₂) tensions in term and premature foals breathing either room air or 100% oxygen. (From Rose, R.J., Hodgson, D.R., Leadon, D.P., and Rossdale, P.D.: The effect of intranasal oxygen administration on arterial blood gases and acid–base parameters in spontaneously delivered, term induced and induced premature foals. *Res. Vet. Sci.* 34:159, 1983, with permission.)

Basic Blood Chemistry. Because foals require attention over a 24-hour period, usually at inconvenient hours, it is important for the practice that is involved in neonatal intensive care to be able to perform the following measurements: total protein (refractometer) and hematocrit (microhematocrit). Additional measurements that are useful during intensive care of foals include plasma glucose, plasma or serum electrolytes, blood gases, and acid–base measurements. Some of the equipment necessary, for example, for glucose and bicarbonate measurements is not expensive and could be cost-effective within a practice.

NEONATAL THERAPEUTICS

Foals are not simply little horses, and appropriate adjustments to therapy need to be made when considering drug selection and dosage regimens. This is particularly important during the first week of life. It is best to avoid the anti-inflammatory drugs in young foals (<2 weeks of age), which carry the risk of gastrointestinal ulceration. There are a few important general considerations that will affect the approach to drug therapy in foals:

- Foals have a larger extracellular fluid volume than older horses and less body fat.
- There may be an increase in the permeability of the blood–brain barrier.
- The consequences are a larger volume of distribution of some drugs and prolongation of action of drugs that require redistribution to fat. For these reasons, barbiturate anesthetics may be best avoided and inhalation anesthetic induction used.
- Alterations in hepatic and renal function may affect the metabolism and distribution of a number

of drugs, particularly during the first few days of life. However, most studies have shown that in the case of renal function, the glomerular filtration rate is similar to that in adults within a few days of birth.

In this section on neonatal therapeutics, we will consider two main areas: antibiotic and fluid therapy.

Antibiotic Therapy

The broad principles of antibiotic therapy, as applied to the adult horse, are also true for the foal. However, the use of oral antibiotics is possible in foals, and the mouth is often a convenient route of administration. Important aspects of the major antibiotics used in foals are discussed below. Details of dose rates, frequency, and routes of administration are given in Table 8-1.

Penicillin G—The drug of choice to treat infections caused by Gram-positive bacteria and the majority of anaerobes. It is bactericidal and relatively inexpensive. Penicillin is available in a short-acting form as the sodium or potassium salt, which may be given IV or IM (Treatment Nos. 84 and 85). Alternatively, procaine penicillin can be used to obtain more prolonged blood and tissue concentrations. For details of brand names, see Treatment No. 83. Dose rates are given in Table 8-1.

Semisynthetic Penicillins—Ampicillin and Amoxycillin—The "broad-spectrum" penicillins have a similar range of activity against Gram-positive pathogens but are less effective than penicillin G. These antibiotics are effective against some Gram-negative foal pathogens, but the range is quite limited. Therefore, if a Gram-negative infection is suspected, ampicillin or amoxycillin are not the drugs of choice.

TABLE 8–1. Dose Rates of Commonly Used Antibiotics in Foals

Antibiotic	Dose Rate	Route	Frequency
Penicillin—Na or K	20,000 IU/kg	IV, IM	6 hourly
Penicillin—procaine	15,000 IU/kg or 15 mg/kg	IM only	12 hourly
Ampicillin—sodium	15 mg/kg	IV, IM	6 hourly
Amoxycillin—trihydrate	25 mg/kg	PO only	8 hourly
Cloxacillin—sodium	25 mg/kg	IV only	6 hourly
Gentamicin—sulfate	2–3 mg/kg	IV, IM	12 hourly
Kanamycin—sulfate	7–10 mg/kg	IV, IM	12 hourly
Neomycin—sulfate	5–10 mg/kg	IM	12 hourly
Amikacin—sulfate	7–10 mg/kg	IV, IM	12 hourly
Erythromycin—ethylsuccinate	25 mg/kg	PO only	8 hourly
Erythromycin—gluceptate	5 mg/kg	IV only	6 hourly
Trimethoprim—sulfonamide	15–20 mg/kg of combined drugs	IV, PO (higher dose for PO)	12 hourly
Rifampin	5–10 mg/kg	PO only	12 hourly
Cephalothin	18 mg/kg	IV, IM	8 hourly
Cefazolin	12 mg/kg	IV only	8 hourly
Cefotaxime	30 mg/kg	IV only	8 hourly
Ceftiofur	4 mg/kg	IV, IM	12 hourly

KEY POINT ▶ The greatest value of amoxycillin is that it can be administered orally in syrup form, and therefore, injections can be avoided.

This is advantageous if clients administer the antibiotic treatment. Details of dose rate and route of administration are given in Table 8-1.

Beta-Lactamase–Resistant Penicillins—These include cloxacillin, flucloxacillin, and oxacillin. The main indication for these antibiotics, which are very expensive, is treatment of beta-lactamase–producing *Staphylococcus aureus*. Details of dose rate and route of administration are given in Table 8-1.

Aminoglycosides—Gentamicin, Amikacin, Kanamycin, and Neomycin—These antibiotics are effective mainly against gram-negative bacteria.

KEY POINT ▶ Because gram-negative septicemia is relatively common in foals, the aminoglycosides are important in therapy.

Streptomycin was one of the most commonly used aminoglycosides and is still incorporated into many commercial preparations in combination with penicillin. However, streptomycin is active against few, if any, equine pathogens.

KEY POINT ▶ The main aminoglycosides used are gentamicin and amikacin, which are often effective against *Pseudomonas, Klebsiella,* and various bacteria from the Enterobacteriacae family.

Details of dose rate and route of administration are given in Table 8-1.

Trimethoprim–Sulfonamide Combinations—Useful against a range of gram-positive and gram-negative bacteria. At higher dose rates (25–30 mg/kg of the combined ingredients), the combination is bactericidal, but care should be taken because severe toxic enteritis has been reported. Trimethoprim–sulfonamide preparations are well absorbed after oral administration and are available in both powder and paste forms. Details of dose rate and route of administration are given in Table 8-1.

Erythromycin and Rifampin—Used to treat *Rhodococcus equi* infections. The combination is quite expensive to use and is of limited usefulness with other infections. However, the combination of rifampin and other antibiotics may be of value in the treatment of infections of the growth plate because of good bone penetration and effectiveness against intracellular organisms. *Rhodococcus equi* treatment often has to be continued for several months. The advantage of erythromycin and rifampin is that they can be administered orally. Details of dose rate and route of administration are given in Table 8-1.

Fluid Therapy

The major reason for intravenous fluid therapy in neonatal foals is diarrhea. Diarrhea can produce severe fluid and electrolyte disturbances in a short time period in foals.

KEY POINT ▶ In the adult horse, approximately two-thirds of the total body weight is water, whereas in the first 1 to 2 weeks of life, the percentage of body weight as water approaches 80%.

This is mainly because of the relatively larger extracellular fluid volume, which can account for more than 40% of the body weight.

KEY POINT ▶ While the fluid requirements of the neonatal foal approximate 100 ml/kg per day (5–6 liters for a 50-kg foal), milk consumption is approximately double this.

This volume of milk is necessary for the foal to ingest adequate calories, which have been estimated at 150 to 200 kcal/kg per day depending on the state of the foal's health. Therefore, in the case of maladjustment, infection, or any condition that results in the foal being unable to suck the mare, maintenance fluid requirements are approximately 100 ml/kg per day. If there is diarrhea, an additional 200 to 300 ml/kg per day of electrolyte solution may be required to maintain hydration.

While oral fluids or fluids administered by stomach tube may be useful in certain circumstances, the great majority of clinical conditions require intravenous fluid administration. The site that we find most useful for intravenous catheterization of newborn foals is the cephalic vein (see Chap. 17).

KEY POINT ▶ Where prolonged catheterization is required for fluid administration, great care must be taken in aseptic technique for catheter insertion, and catheters should be replaced every 48 to 72 hours.

Some of the major theoretical considerations in fluid therapy are discussed in Chapter 17.

Assessment of Fluid Losses

■ Clinical examination, taking into account skin turgor, mucous membranes, capillary refill time, heart rate, and pulse quality, will allow broad classification of the dehydration as mild (around 5%), moderate (around 8%), or severe (above 10%).

KEY POINT ▶ Regular body weight measurements permit accurate assessment of acute changes in fluid balance. It is also worthwhile remembering that during the first month of life, foals will gain weight at about 1 kg per day.

■ Laboratory analyses that are useful in evaluating the extent of dehydration as well as in assessing the response to therapy include measurement of total plasma protein (TPP), hematocrit (PCV), osmolality, and serum or plasma electrolytes. Measurement of plasma bicarbonate concentration provides valuable information concerning the nonrespiratory component of any acid–base disturbance. Simple and inexpensive equipment is available to measure the total carbon dioxide (95% of which is bicarbonate) by titration and this measurement is performed by most autoanalyzers in commercial laboratories.

KEY POINT ▶ Because foals under metabolic stress can become hypoglycemic, it is important to measure plasma glucose concentrations.

KEY POINT ▶ Care should be taken when interpreting changes in TPP and PCV. Changes in concentrations of the globulins may be the principal reason for a lower or higher than expected TPP, and the PCV may have a wide normal range, similar to the adult horse.

Choice of Fluid

KEY POINT ▶ In most circumstances, replacement fluid is the fluid of choice where there have been losses of fluid and electrolytes such as in diarrhea. Replacement fluids (see Chap. 17) have a similar electrolyte composition to plasma.

■ *Maintenance fluids* should be used where the sodium losses do not continue, since the sodium requirements are lower and potassium requirements are higher than in acute volume depletion. This is typically the case after the acute volume deficits have been replaced. Maintenance fluids (see Chap. 17) have sodium and chloride concentrations in the range 40 to 50 mmol/L (mEq/L) and potassium in the range 15 to 20 mmol/L, with 2.5% to 5% dextrose used to make up the osmotic balance.

■ *Bicarbonate* often is overused in neonates and should only be given where there is loss of base, such as in severe diarrhea. In many other situations, the acidosis is due to lactate accumulation because of poor tissue perfusion.

KEY POINT ▶ The treatment of choice in this situation is the intravenous administration of replacement fluids to increase peripheral perfusion.

■ The lactate will then be metabolized in the liver. If bicarbonate is required, it can be calculated using the formula

HCO_3^- requirement in mmol (mEq) = $0.4 \times (27 - \text{measured } HCO_3^-) \times$ body weight (kg)

Because bicarbonate solutions are hypertonic, it is useful to add bicarbonate to hypotonic fluids, such as 0.45% sodium chloride.

■ *Hypertonic fluids* should be avoided in foals.
■ *Plasma administration* may be necessary, particularly where there is substantial protein loss, such as in diarrhea. The use of normal electrolyte solutions in these circumstances will result in further hypoproteinemia with resulting movement of fluid out of the vascular compartment. The use of plasma avoids these problems and is also useful for increasing IgG levels in foals with failure of passive transfer of immunity.
■ *Oral fluids* have been used with success in the treatment of diarrhea in calves. We have found that the administration of fluid and electrolyte mixtures by stomach tube is useful in foals in which the diarrhea is mild and there are no signs of hypovolemia.

KEY POINT ▶ To enhance absorption in the small intestine, the combination of glucose, glycine, and electrolytes is useful, and commercial preparations are available (Treatment No. 57).

Volume and Rate of Fluid Administration

■ Maintenance requirements are around 100 ml/kg per day, and this volume should be administered over a period of 24 hours.

KEY POINT ▶ In cases of severe hypovolemia, initial flow rates can be in the range 10 to 20 ml/kg per hour to restore the central circulation. Following improvements in signs of hypovolemia, the flow rate can be slowed.

■ It is particularly important in cold climates to warm fluids to body temperature prior to administration because there is a significant energy cost to the foal, which may already be in a critical energy state.
■ The volume of plasma used is in the range 20 to 40 ml/kg. These volumes are usually sufficient to correct IgG deficiencies due to failure of passive transfer.

KEY POINT ▶ If frozen plasma is used, it can be administered after partial thawing because the protein fraction is available during the first part of thawing. This enables the globulins to be increased without administering a large volume of fluid.

■ Monitoring the flow rate is important during intravenous fluid administration. Apart from hypovolemic shock, fluid should be given over a prolonged period; otherwise, it may be rapidly excreted via the urinary tract.

Diseases of Foals

Abdominal Pain

KEY POINT ▶ The most common cause of abdominal discomfort or pain in the first few days of life is retained meconium.

A variety of other problems may give rise to abdominal pain, however. It is important to examine foals with abdominal pain carefully and to note whether there is any abdominal distension.

History and Presenting Signs

- Age of foal when first presented
- Presence/absence of abdominal distension
- Change in fecal consistency
- Change in demeanor
- Passage of urine

Clinical Findings and Diagnosis

- A good general examination is critical for determining the cause of the pain.
- As with adult horses, determination of the vital signs (heart rate, respiratory rate, temperature, capillary refill time) and gut sounds is essential in making an assessment of the extent of the problem.

KEY POINT ▶ If the foal is straining, it should be determined whether it is straining to urinate (legs spread) or straining to defecate (arching of the back).

- Digital rectal examination should be performed to determine if there is retention of meconium.
- Passage of a nasogastric tube should be done to determine whether there is gastric reflux, which may indicate an upper intestinal obstruction.
- Abdominocentesis will assist in determining whether there is a problem that is likely to require surgery (see Chap. 6 for further details). This is most easily done in newborn foals with the foal in lateral recumbency, but it also may be carried out with the foal standing. A 19-gauge, 3.75-cm (1.5-in) needle is inserted through the midline of the abdominal wall.
- Determination of the acid–base status is essential if compromise of bowel is thought to have occurred. Metabolic acidosis (decreased bicarbon-ate concentrations) may indicate decreased perfusion of intestine in conditions such as volvulus and intussusception.
- The hemogram and serum or plasma electrolytes may be useful in assessing the requirements for fluids and electrolytes (see Fluid Therapy, p. 282).
- In more specialized practices, techniques such as endoscopic examination of the stomach, abdominal radiography, and ultrasound are now becoming more widely used. These techniques do require considerable experience before accurate interpretation can be made.

KEY POINT ▶ Cases that undoubtedly require surgery are those with persistent abdominal pain where there is increasing abdominal distension. The degree of abdominal distension can be assessed by sequential recordings of abdominal circumference.

Differential Diagnosis

- Impaction with meconium
- Atresia ani or coli
- Ruptured urinary bladder
- Obstruction to intestine
- Peritonitis
- Gastric ulceration

Treatment

- Because of the wide range of possible conditions that can give rise to abdominal pain, it is essential to narrow the diagnostic possibilities.

KEY POINT ▶ Retained meconium can be treated by the use of enemas, and most cases resolve without complicated treatment.

- Soapy water is quite satisfactory as an enema solution, but there are commercial products available. This can be supplemented by the use of mineral oil (500 ml) given by nasogastric tube.
- Exploratory laparotomy is not often necessary in newborn foals but should be considered if there is severe, unremitting pain together with increasing abdominal distension.
- Analgesics should be used judiciously.

KEY POINT ► The nonsteroidal anti-inflammatory drugs have considerable potential to cause gastrointestinal ulceration. They should be used at low dose rates and for short periods.

- Flunixin (Treatment No. 52) is the anti-inflammatory drug of choice, and the dose rate should be in the range of 0.2 to 0.5 mg/kg. Although some adverse effects have been reported with xylazine (particularly hypotension), we have had good results from dose rates in the range of 0.1 to 0.2 mg/kg given IV (Treatment No. 108).

Angular Limb Deformities

See Chapter 3.

Combined Immunodeficiency

Combined immunodeficiency (CID) is a hereditary disorder principally of Arabian foals.

KEY POINT ► The condition results in failure of production of both T- and B-lymphocytes.

It is an autosomal recessive trait, and therefore, the incidence of clinical disease is low, but the incidence of carriers may be quite high.

History and Presenting Signs

- Presented usually around 1 to 3 months of age
- Nasal discharge and/or cough
- Recurring respiratory infections

Clinical Findings and Diagnosis

- Because foals have passive immunity from colostrum, it is not until the IgG levels decline around 2 to 3 months of age that signs of the problem appear.
- The most common presenting problems are respiratory infections that may be viral or bacterial. Adenovirus infections, which are nonpathogenic in normal foals, will cause a severe pneumonia in foals with CID. A range of other bacterial and viral infections also can be found in foals with CID.
- Combined immunodeficiency should be one of the differential diagnoses in any Arabian foal presented with signs of infection.

KEY POINT ► Hematology is helpful diagnostically, and the principal finding is severe lymphopenia.

- A persistently low lymphocyte count of less than $1.0 \times 10^9/L$ (1000/μl) is usually considered strongly supportive of a diagnosis of CID. However, in some normal foals with severe infections, the lymphocyte count also may be low. Therefore, serial hemograms are useful, and in most

foals with CID, the lymphocyte counts may be less than $0.5 \times 10^9/L$ (500/μl).
- Determination of IgM concentrations after 1 month of age also supports a diagnosis of CID because foals with the disorder will have no or very little IgM. IgM will be absent from the serum of affected foals prior to drinking colostrum.
- A positive diagnosis of CID can only be made at necropsy after histopathologic examination of the thymus, lymph nodes, and spleen.

Differential Diagnosis

- Septicemia
- Severe bacterial or viral infections

Treatment

- While bone marrow transplantation has been performed experimentally, there is no other treatment that is worthwhile.
- Identification of carrier animals is important. Unfortunately, under most circumstances, this is only possible from the results of matings.

Diarrhea

KEY POINT ► Diarrhea is a very common problem in foals and in most cases is self-limiting.

This is important because many cases are treated with a variety of medications that are unnecessary. Because substantial fluid and electrolyte deficits can develop quickly, it is important to assess the hydration state and administer appropriate fluids. Diarrhea is a common finding in foals with septicemia as well as in local enteritis.

KEY POINT ► "Foal heat" diarrhea is a transient problem usually found between 5 and 10 days of age and seems to represent changes in intestinal function and bacterial flora.

History and Presenting Signs

- Signs of systemic disease or not
- Diarrhea, volume and fecal consistency

Clinical Findings and Diagnosis

- Careful clinical examination is important to determine whether there is systemic disease or metabolic derangements associated with the diarrhea. Factors such as temperature change, prolongation of capillary refill time, poor pulse quality, and elevated heart rate may indicate not only substantial fluid loss but also septicemia.

KEY POINT ► Routine hematology and fibrinogen and electrolyte measurements should be performed to assess the possibility of systemic disease and to determine electrolyte alterations.

- Because diarrhea is a common presenting sign in foals with septicemia, blood cultures may be indicated.
- Fecal culture may be indicated if there is suspicion or a bacterial enteritis. It is necessary to specify to the laboratory the range of likely pathogenic bacteria.
- If rotavirus is suspected, commercial testing kits are available (Rotazyme, Abbott Laboratories, Abbott Park, Ill.; Rotatest, Wampole Laboratories, Cranbury, N.J.).

Differential Diagnosis

- "Foal heat" diarrhea—foals usually healthy with a "pasty" diarrhea
- Rotavirus diarrhea—watery diarrhea with mild systemic signs and a number of foals affected
- Bacterial diarrhea (e.g., *E. coli*, *Clostridia*, *R. equi*, and *Salmonella* spp.)
- Nutritional diarrhea—overfeeding, orphaned foals
- Antibiotic-related diarrhea—usually from broad-spectrum oral antibiotics
- Parasitic diarrhea—confirm by fecal flotation

Treatment

KEY POINT ► Maintenance of hydration is the critical factor in management of foal diarrhea.

- In cases where foals are not systemically ill, provision of adequate milk or, in older foals, drinking water may be all that is required.
- As with calves, oral rehydration fluids (see Fluid Therapy, Chap. 17) may be used, administered by nasogastric tube. Combinations of glucose–glycine and electrolyte (Treatment No. 57) are most effective in enhancing electrolyte and fluid uptake in the small intestine. Volumes up to 15 to 20 ml/kg may be administered in a single dose by nasogastric tube.
- Intravenous fluids are necessary in foals that are assessed at more than 8% dehydrated. These foals usually have lost large amounts of bicarbonate and may have a severe metabolic acidosis. Bicarbonate solutions should be considered when the blood bicarbonate concentrations decrease to less than 15 mmol/L (mEq/L). For prolonged IV fluid therapy, we find the best site for catheter placement is the cephalic vein. With the use of flexible tubing suspended in the stall, the foal can have unrestricted movement and access to the mare.

KEY POINT ► Antibiotics should be avoided unless there are systemic signs or a strong suspicion that septicemia may be a problem.

- The use of antibiotics may produce diarrhea. However, because of the possibility of septicemia (Gram-negative organisms in particular), it may be necessary to cover this possibility after a blood culture has been taken. The combination of Na or K penicillin (Treatment Nos. 84 and 85) (20,000 IU/kg) and gentamicin (Treatment No. 56) (2–3 mg/kg) or amikacin (Treatment No. 4) (7–10 mg/kg) is the first choice.
- In foals with severe diarrhea, there is also hypoproteinemia, and therefore, plasma transfusions may be useful. Intravenous plasma at 20 to 40 ml/kg will help to restore plasma oncotic pressure as well as boosting the immunoglobulin concentrations.
- In most foals with diarrhea, there is no need to remove the foal from the mare. However, if the diarrhea does not respond to standard treatments, it may be useful to restrict milk intake for a 24-hour period and only allow clear fluids.

Failure of Passive Transfer of Immunoglobulins

While the foal has some immunologic function as a fetus, immunity is essentially a passive transfer of colostral immunoglobulins during the first 6 to 12 hours after birth. Failure of passive transfer of immunoglobulins is quite common in newborn foals, and therefore, assessment of IgG concentrations in plasma is important in management.

KEY POINT ► The volume of colostrum normally consumed by newborn foals in the first 8 to 12 hours has been estimated at between 1 and 2 L.

It also should be noted that alveolar macrophage function is substantially reduced in foals compared with adults.

KEY POINT ► The optimal levels of IgG in foal plasma 24 hours after birth are greater than 8 g/L (800 mg/dl).

Values less than 4 g/L are considered to reflect failure of passive transfer, and those between 4 and 8 g/L are suboptimal concentrations. Foals with low IgG concentrations are more likely to be predisposed to a variety of bacterial infections.

History and Presenting Signs

- Mare with a very distended udder, indicating foal has not sucked
- Foal with suspected septicemia
- Foal presented with "joint ill"
- Maladaption

Clinical Findings and Diagnosis

- The availability of quick, reliable measurements of IgG concentrations in foal plasma has enabled early diagnosis of failure of passive transfer, before a foal is presented with an infection.

KEY POINT ► A number of techniques are available for measuring immunoglobulin concentrations.

- These vary from the least expensive and nonspecific (zinc sulfate turbidity and glutaraldehyde coagulation tests) to the more recent CITE test (Idexx, Portland, ME), which enables classification of IgG levels into several ranges, from 2 to 8 g/L (200 to 800 mg/dl). The latter measurement is the technique of choice for assessment of IgG concentrations, although the test is relatively expensive.
- Measurement of the colostral specific gravity in mares provides a good guide to the likely IgG concentrations in their foals. Colostral specific gravities greater than 1.06 generally indicate adequate antibody concentrations.

Differential Diagnosis

- Neonatal maladjustment syndrome

Treatment

- Maintenance of a colostral bank is vital on a large stud farm so that foals with failure of passive transfer or which are likely to have inadequate IgG concentrations can be given supplementation of colostrum. In most cases, around 1 L of colostrum should be given within the first 8 to 12 hours after birth.
- If colostrum is not available or if the foal is older than 24 hours, plasma transfusions are required to increase the IgG concentrations. Normally, 20 to 40 ml/kg is required to increase the IgG levels to around 8 g/L (800 mg/dl). Further details are provided in the section entitled Fluid Therapy (p. 282).

Gastroduodenal Ulcers

KEY POINT ► This appears to be a relatively new disease for which stress plays an important role in the pathogenesis.

The precise etiology is unknown, with some investigators proposing a role for various bacteria and viruses such as rotavirus. Where there is primary gastric ulceration, the clinical signs are not as severe as those involving both the stomach and duodenum.

History and Presenting Signs

- Teeth grinding
- Excessive salivation
- Pain manifested by the foal lying in dorsal recumbency
- Decreased appetite
- Pain after feeding

Clinical Findings and Diagnosis

- Clinicians are alerted to the possibility of gastroduodenal ulcers by the classical presenting signs, detailed above.
- Examination of gastric reflux is helpful to determine the presence of blood. Many foals will show considerable discomfort when the nasogastric tube is passed through the distal esophagus.
- If an appropriate endoscope is available (8–10 mm diameter, 180 cm long), direct examination of the stomach is useful. This is done after 3 to 4 hours of feed restriction by passing the endoscope via the ventral nasal meatus into the stomach and slightly distending it with air.
- In severe cases of gastric ulceration, there may be gastric rupture. In such cases, the foal will show signs of severe colic and shock, and its condition will deteriorate rapidly.

Differential Diagnosis

- Septicemia
- Peritonitis
- Intestinal obstruction

Treatment

- If there is gastric distension, refluxing via a nasogastric tube should be done.

KEY POINT ► A number of H₂ antagonists have been used and found to be clinically useful, although no double-blind trials of efficacy have been undertaken.

- The two most widely used H_2 antagonists are cimetidine (Treatment No. 26) at dose rates of 6 to 8 mg/kg orally every 6 to 8 hours or ranitidine (Treatment No. 99) given orally at dose rates of 6 to 8 mg/kg every 8 hours. Both these drugs also may be administered IV, at dose rates similar to those used for oral treatment.

KEY POINT ► A variety of gastric protectants have been found to be useful, and the most commonly used is sucralfate (Treatment No. 101) at a dose of 30 mg/kg given orally every 6 to 8 hours.

- In some foals, there may be partial or complete obstruction at the level of the pylorus due to stricture. In such cases, surgical treatment is necessary to bypass the stricture. This type of procedure is best done at a specialist clinic.

Infection/Septicemia/Pneumonia

Bacterial infection is probably the most important clinical disorder in foals. Infection may be localized, but in the majority of cases it is generalized, with subsequent localization to areas such as the lung, joints, and physes. Infections may be acquired in utero but in most cases are acquired after birth. The most important predisposing cause of infection in failure of passive transfer of immunity (see p. 286).

KEY POINT ► It is an important part of management on stud farms to screen the colostrum IgG concentrations and/or IgG level in the foal in the first 6 to 12 hours after birth.

History and Presenting Signs

- Previous history of abortion or death of foals
- Overcrowding/poor management
- Chronic long-standing infectious disease (e.g., *Rhodococcus equi, Salmonella*)
- Dystocia
- Premature foal
- Depressed, sick foal presented

Clinical Findings and Diagnosis

KEY POINT ► The most important signs of septicaemia are behavioral.

- Affected foals will appear depressed and stop sucking. The first thing noticed by the stud-farm manager or owner may be that the mare has a distended udder. Because foals infected in utero may show signs similar to those with neonatal maladjustment syndrome, it is important to investigate sepsis as a possible cause of any foal with maladaptation.
- Body temperature provides no accurate guide to the presence or absence of infection, with normal, increased, and decreased temperatures being reported.
- There may be an increase in respiratory rate, but even in cases of pneumonia, abnormal lung sounds may not be heard, unlike the situation in adult horses.
- Diarrhea is a common finding in foals with septicemia.
- Sudden onset of lameness is an important sign, which may suggest localization of infection in a joint or physis.

KEY POINT ► Hematology is a vital diagnostic aid, but total white cell count does not appear to be a good indicator of infection.

- The most consistent findings are increased band forms of neutrophils (normally not present or in very low numbers in normal foals) and toxic changes within the neutrophils.
- Fibrinogen is often increased in foals with septicemia, and values are usually greater than 5 g/L (500 mg/dl). However, there is usually a delay of 48 hours before the fibrinogen increases.
- Hypoglycemia is a common finding in septicemia, with values less than 5 mmol/L (90 mg/dl).
- Because many foals with septicemia have pneumonia, hypoxemia is common and should be anticipated even if access to a blood gas machine is not possible.

KEY POINT ► Blood cultures are essential (see Diagnostic Aids, p. 277, and Chap. 15), and blood samples should be collected using impeccable sterile technique.

- It is vital to take blood for blood culture prior to beginning antibiotic therapy. It also should be noted that because some bacteria take up to 5 to 6 days to grow, a negative blood culture result should not be given too quickly.
- Transtracheal aspirates for bacteriology and cytology also may be indicated because a high percentage of cases will have pneumonia.
- Chest radiographs are also useful in assessing the degree of pulmonary compromise. Atelectasis is common in foals with pneumonia, and the lung fields will have an increase in density.

Differential Diagnosis

- Combined immunodeficiency
- Neonatal maladjustment syndrome

Treatment

KEY POINT ► The combination of penicillin (sodium or potassium) (Treatment Nos. 84 and 85) given IV at a dose rate of 20,000 IU/kg and IV gentamicin (2–3 mg/kg) (Treatment No. 56) or amikacin (7–10 mg/kg) (Treatment No. 4) (see the section entitled Antibiotic Therapy, p. 281) appears to be the treatment of choice while culture results are awaited.

- The duration of antibiotic treatment should be based on clinical response and subsequent hemograms. In some cases, 5 to 7 days is adequate, while others may require up to 2 weeks of treatment.
- The most common sequelae of septicemia are septic arthritis or septic physitis, enteritis, and in foals that are recumbent for some time, corneal ulceration.

"Joint Ill" (Polyarticular Septic Arthritis/Osteomyelitis)

"Joint ill" is a common term used for polyarticular septic arthritis in foals, usually following a systemic bacterial infection/septicemia. Most commonly, infection involves multiple larger joints and/or the physes, but in some cases it may involve the metaphysis adjacent to the physis. "Joint ill" is a serious condition that carries a poor prognosis for future athletic function.

History and Presenting Signs

- Prematurity
- Failure of passive transfer
- Mare with uterine infection
- Poor hygiene at foaling

Clinical Findings and Diagnosis

- Foals with "joint ill" are often clinically ill and will show signs of systemic infection, with depression, inappetence, and fever.

KEY POINT ▶ However, it should not be assumed that a foal does not have joint ill just because it has no signs of systemic disease.

- Foals are often reluctant to move and will show variable signs of lameness.
- Careful examination will usually reveal joint effusion, with one or more joints being distended with fluid and showing thickening of the dorsal joint capsule.
- Radiographs may not show changes in the early stage of disease but are useful to help in assessing the prognosis. One of the difficulties in radiographic interpretation of bone infection is that the bone around the physes often has a similar appearance to infected bone.

KEY POINT ▶ Synovial fluid collection is essential for diagnosis and should be performed prior to any antibiotic therapy.

- Details of collection and sample handling are given in Chapters 3 and 15. It is critical that the aspiration of synovial fluid be done in a sterile manner, with a cap, mask, and gloves worn by the operator and sterile drapes used around the site. We find it easy to collect samples with the foal given a gaseous anesthetic induction if the foal is less than 2 weeks old. Samples should be collected into tubes containing EDTA for a total and differential nucleated cell count. Synovial fluid nucleated cell counts greater than 10,000 × 10^6/L (10,000/μl) with a predominance of neutrophils and an elevated total protein (normal range 15–25 g/L, 1.5–2.5 mg/dl) suggest that there is infection. For bacteriology, it is best if samples are collected and submitted in a brand-new, sterile disposable syringe, after which the sample is centrifuged and the deposit placed into enrichment media.
- It may be worthwhile to take blood for blood culture early in the course of the disease.

Differential Diagnosis

- Trauma
- Nonseptic joint effusion

Treatment

- It is important to obtain samples for bacteriology prior to beginning any therapy.
- If a Gram stain of the synovial fluid deposit reveals bacteria, antibiotic therapy can be based on the result of the Gram stain.
- If there are no Gram stain results, the use of a bactericidal combination of drugs such as IM penicillin (15,000 IU/kg, or 15 mg/kg) (Treatment No. 83) and IV gentamicin (2 mg/kg) (Treatment No. 56) given twice daily is appropriate.
- Irrigation of infected joints by joint lavage (see Septic Arthritis, Chap. 3) is worthwhile using polyionic fluid. This should be done with the foal under general anesthesia.

Neonatal Isoerythrolysis

Neonatal isoerythrolysis is a condition found most commonly in thoroughbreds when during pregnancy the mare manufactures antibodies against the foal's red cells. After birth, ingestion of colostrum by the foal results in absorption of the anti–red cell antibodies which destroy the foal's red cells.

KEY POINT ▶ The condition is found mainly in multiparous mares and is associated with specific antibodies, usually Aa and Qa.

History and Presenting Signs

- Multiparous mare
- Foal shows weakness within first few days of birth

Clinical Findings and Diagnosis

- Foals are normal at birth and for the first 12 to 72 hours after birth.
- The onset of clinical signs is variable and depends on the amount of antibody ingested and absorbed.
- Foals usually show signs of listlessness and decreased appetite.

KEY POINT ▶ Clinical examination reveals severe jaundice of the mucous membranes and elevated heart and respiratory rates. The temperature is normal.

- Blood for hematology shows very low red cell values, with the hematocrit usually in the range 0.10 to 0.20 L/L (10%–20%), and icteric plasma. An increase in the white cell count is also common and may be a stress-related response. In most foals that show clinical signs, the hematocrit is usually below 0.10 L/L (10%).
- Urine samples will demonstrate hemoglobinuria.

Differential Diagnosis

- Equine herpesvirus
- Neonatal septicemia
- Tyzzer's disease
- Rupture of the bladder

Treatment

- Prevention is the most important aspect of management, and mares that have lost foals within a few days of birth should be suspected. Blood samples can be taken for determining the presence of Qa and Aa antibodies. If the mare does not have these red cell antigens (Qa or Aa negative), the risk of producing antibodies likely to cause neonatal isoerythrolysis is increased.
- If there is a likelihood of neonatal isoerythrolysis, colostrum from the mare should be discarded and colostrum from a colostrum bank administered. The foal can be muzzled for at least 48 hours to prevent anti–red cell antibodies.

KEY POINT ▶ Treatment of an affected foal involves a blood transfusion with administration of the mare's blood which has had the red cells washed three or four times.

- We have had good cooperation from local blood banks. Alternatively, cross-matching may be carried out and a suitable donor found. If facilities are not available to do this, a transfusion from a gelding is unlikely to cause a transfusion reaction. Usually 20 to 30 ml/kg of packed red cells is adequate to produce a hematocrit in the range 0.15 to 0.20 L/L (15%–20%), and this is satisfactory for the foal to survive until further red cells are manufactured. If the mare's red cells have been washed, packed red cells are returned after centrifugation. If a gelding's plasma is to be used, most of the plasma can be removed prior to the transfusion.
- It is important to perform an IgG evaluation to determine whether there has been failure of passive transfer of immunity. Many foals with neonatal isoerythrolysis survive only because they absorb inadequate IgG. Therefore, plasma transfusion may be necessary, and the foal should be covered for 3 to 5 days with a bactericidal broad-spectrum antibiotic combination such as procaine penicillin (Treatment No. 83) (15,000 IU/kg, or 15 mg/kg q12h) IM and gentamicin (Treatment No. 56) (2–3 mg/kg q12h) IV.

Neonatal Maladjustment Syndrome

KEY POINT ▶ Neonatal maladjustment syndrome is really a descriptive term that may encompass a number of conditions resulting in maladaptation in the newborn foal.

The condition appears to be related to central nervous system dysfunction and may be induced by birth asphyxia or intracranial hemorrhage. It is important to distinguish maladjusted from septicemic foals.

History and Presenting Signs

- Dystocia in some cases
- Most foals affected are not premature.
- Signs usually noticed within 24 hours of birth

Clinical Findings and Diagnosis

- Foals will stop sucking and show a progression of disease from depression and weakness through to wandering behavior, loss of recognition of the mother, and finally recumbency.
- Foals may have a grunting respiration and make an abnormal sound. For this reason, they have been termed "barker foals" by some clinicians.
- Neurologic signs can include rigidity of fore- and hindlegs, apparent blindness, and convulsions.
- Most foals will demonstrate some degree of dyspnea, and it is important to eliminate a primary respiratory complaint.
- Blood cultures may be necessary to eliminate the possibility of septicemia.

Differential Diagnosis

- Septicemia
- Blood loss (via umbilical rupture during birth)
- Metabolic disorders

Treatment

- Nursing care is the key to management, ensuring that metabolic and hydration status is normal.
- Some foals will be hypoxemic and may require intranasal oxygen administration.
- No specific treatment is useful, although it is essential to ensure that foals are not septicemic.
- Foals that have reversible disease usually show improvement within the first 3 to 5 days.
- Benefit may also be gained from administration of IV DMSO (Treatment No. 34) at a dose rate of 0.5g/kg as a 10% solution.

Prematurity

While premature foals are usually considered to be those born at less than 325 days of gestation, Dr. Peter Rossdale, in Newmarket, U.K., has highlighted the importance of "readiness for birth." That is, a foal may be full term in gestational length but still unready to be born and show some of the signs of prematurity. Premature foals may have dysfunction in a number of body systems and require careful management. For a successful outcome, many of these foals require full-time intensive care for several weeks, and economic factors are of major importance in decisions about treatment.

History and Presenting Signs

- Mare with vulval discharge
- Mare showing signs of dripping milk from the udder
- Weak foal, unable to stand and suck within 1 to 2 hours of birth

Clinical Findings and Diagnosis

KEY POINT ► Premature foals are usually small and are generally weak, being unable to get to their feet and suck within a few hours of birth.

- The hair coat is often short and may have a silky appearance, particularly over the rump.

KEY POINT ► The majority of premature foals will have an exaggerated range of fetlock movement, there being overextension of the joints. This results in the fetlocks sinking toward the ground.

- Many premature foals are delivered because of placental insufficiency. These foals have a better prognosis for survival than those delivered prematurely because of infection.
- A number of body systems may not be functioning normally:

Adrenal Dysfunction—Can be recognized on routine hematology because the neutrophil-to-lymphocyte ratio is less than 1.5:1. A low white cell count ($<5.0 \times 10^9$/L, i.e., 5000 cells/μl) is an unfavorable sign.

Pulmonary Problems—Resulting in some cases from surfactant deficiency and in others because of in utero infection will cause hypoxemia and hypercapnia.

Musculoskeletal Immaturity—Is often the major reason why these foals are not viable in the long term. Tarsal and carpal collapse and angular deviations are common, particularly if foals are not restricted and their limbs supported. Radiographs should be taken of the carpi and tarsi to evaluate skeletal maturity.

Infection—Is a common problem in premature foals, and blood cultures and transtracheal aspirates should be considered. Plasma fibrinogen concentrations should be measured, and values over 5g/L (500 mg/dl) indicate an inflammatory focus.

Differential Diagnosis

- Neonatal maladjustment syndrome
- Septicemia

Treatment

- Complete evaluation of the main body systems is necessary to identify the problem areas. Infection should not be ruled out until there is supporting hematologic evidence and negative blood cultures.
- Antibiotic prophylaxis may be worthwhile, and a combination of penicillin and an aminoglycoside is most appropriate while waiting for culture results. For dose rates, see the section entitled Antibiotic Therapy (p. 281).

KEY POINT ► Hypoxemia and hypercapnia are common in premature foals, indicating ventilation–perfusion mismatch and alveolar hypoventilation.

- It is important for premature foals to be positioned in sternal recumbency, and intranasal oxygen administration is often worthwhile if the hypoxemia is severe ($PaO_2 < 60$ mmHg).
- Exercise and weight bearing should be restricted because of the excessive loads on the immature skeleton. Taping wooden tongue depressors to the heels as extensions to the foot may be useful in preventing overextension of the fetlocks.

Rhodococcus Equi Infection ("Rattles")

Rhodococcus equi (formerly *Corynebacterium equi*) is an important cause of infection in foals aged from 1 to 3 months.

KEY POINT ► Infection may be acquired via the alimentary or respiratory routes, and there may be localization of infection in several sites, including joints.

The exact factors that lead to infection in foals (but not adults) are incompletely understood. Reduced activity of the alveolar macrophages has been reported, and there may be factors in local gut immunity that give rise to infection. *Rhodococcus equi* infections can cause extensive morbidity and mortality on some stud farms, although the problem tends to be found only in dry climates and where there are sandy soils. The infection is common in California, the southern part of the United States, and Australia.

History and Presenting Signs

- Foal aged 1 to 3 months
- Signs of respiratory or alimentary disease

Clinical Findings and Diagnosis

- Foals usually appear depressed and have a decreased appetite. The mare will often have a distended udder.
- Involvement of the respiratory tract is the most common form of the disease, and foals will often have a productive cough.

- Dyspnea is usually evident, and auscultation of the chest will reveal gurgling sounds over the hilar region.
- Variable degrees of fever are found, and there are typically exacerbations and remissions.
- Diarrhea is often a feature of the gastrointestinal form of the disease.
- Most stud-farm owners are adept at recognizing *Rhodococcus equi* infections, but positive confirmation is only possible by demonstration of the typical appearance of the organism on a Gram stain from a transtracheal aspirate. However, in very ill foals a transtracheal aspirate may result in further debility or death. Blood cultures may be useful if there are systemic signs, although it often requires up to 5 days of incubation for the bacteria to grow.
- Chest radiographs can be valuable in assessing the extent of abscessation. *Rhodococcus equi* typically causes multiple abscesses throughout the lungs and various abdominal lymph nodes.

Differential Diagnosis

- Bacterial pneumonia
- "Foal heat" diarrhea
- Bacterial diarrhea
- Septicemia

Treatment

KEY POINT ► Prolonged antibiotic treatment for 2 to 3 months is essential, and even in cases with severe pulmonary abscessation, complete recovery is possible.

- The antibiotics of choice are erythromycin (Treatment Nos. 38 and 39) and rifampin (Treatment No. 100). These are available in forms that can be administered orally. Erythromycin ethylsuccinate is given orally at 25 mg/kg q8h, and rifampin is administered at a dose rate of 5 to 10 mg/kg q12h. This treatment should be continued for 2 to 3 months to enable complete resolution of the infection. Obviously, this treatment is very costly and only worthwhile in valuable foals.
- In foals in which cost precludes the use of erythromycin and rifampin, we have had some good response to the use of neomycin at 5 mg/kg q12h given IV or IM. Neomycin is slightly more nephrotoxic than the other aminoglycosides but does not cause major renal dysfunction in most foals if administered over 10 to 14 days.
- Some experimental studies have shown the protective effects of hyperimmune plasma administered prophylactically to foals. The hyperimmune plasma is prepared by administering a *Rhodococcus equi* vaccine to horses that will be used as plasma donors to obtain an increase in

specific antibodies. Plasma is then administered prophylactically to foals after birth. On stud farms where *Rhodococcus equi* is endemic, such a program may be worthwhile.

Seizures

See Chapter 13.

Urachal Problems

The urachus is the normal communication pathway between the bladder and the allantois during fetal life. After the umbilical cord ruptures, the urachus may remain open or reopen several days after birth. It also may be the site of infection, and some cases develop abscessation.

History and Presenting Signs

- Foal usually less than 1 week of age
- Swelling around the umbilicus
- Urine dribbling from umbilicus

Clinical Findings and Diagnosis

- Infection around the urachus will usually be manifested as swelling around the umbilicus.
- Patent urachus is simple to diagnose, since there will be obvious urine leakage from the umbilical stump.

Differential Diagnosis

- Rupture of the urinary bladder or intraabdominal urachus

Treatment

- Many cases of patent urachus will resolve without any treatment.

KEY POINT ► If the urachal opening does not close within 2 to 3 days, we have found that a caustic agent such as phenol or strong tincture of iodine, applied carefully around the opening with a cotton bud, will result in closure or the urachus.

- If there is infection, surgical treatment is necessary to remove the infected umbilical stump.

Urinary Tract Disruption

Urinary tract disruptions occur relatively frequently in newborn foals. Rupture of the urinary bladder and the abdominal urachus can occur, resulting in uroperitoneum. Mostly this occurs during delivery, and the signs are manifested within a few days of birth. A small percentage of cases can occur from an infected umbilical stump.

History and Presenting Signs

- More common in male foals
- Small amounts of urine passed
- Abdominal distension
- Foal 2 to 3 days of age

Clinical Findings and Diagnosis

- Foals usually become depressed and stop sucking.
- By the time signs of depression are seen, there is usually significant abdominal distension.

KEY POINT ► Straining to urinate is often a sign, together with passage of small volumes of urine and progressive distension of the abdomen.

- Serum biochemistry profiles often show lower Na^+ and Cl^- values together with increased K^+ and urea. A mild metabolic acidosis is commonly found on acid–base assessment.

KEY POINT ► Abdominocentesis is the critical technique for the diagnosis of uroperitoneum.

- With the foal standing or in lateral recumbency, a 19-gauge, 25-mm (1-in) needle is inserted through the abdominal midline just caudal to the umbilicus.

KEY POINT ► The sample may smell like urine, and the creatinine concentration will be elevated to more than twice the concentration in the serum or plasma.

- It is worthwhile measuring the leukocyte count and the total protein in case there is urinary tract infection.
- If a sterile dye is available (methylene blue is the dye of choice), a small amount (5–10 ml) can be injected into the bladder via a urinary catheter and abdominal fluid later taken to determine if the dye is present. This technique is rarely used, and in most cases, abdominocentesis will yield diagnostic results.

Differential Diagnosis

- Rupture of the ureter
- Trauma to the urethra (from catheterization)
- Septicemia
- Gastrointestinal problems

Treatment

KEY POINT ► Surgery is necessary, but the foal should be stabilized prior to the surgery.

- This usually involves drainage of fluid from the abdomen while administering potassium-free polyionic fluid intravenously. A urinary catheter is placed to facilitate removal of urine. If the foal has a plasma or serum potassium value greater than 6 mmol/L (mEq/L), bicarbonate also should be given intravenously at a dose rate of 5 mmol/kg (5 mEq/kg).
- A midline laparotomy is necessary to repair the defect, and the usual approach is to make an elliptical incision around the umbilicus. After the abdomen is entered, it is important to determine if there are infected foci along the course of the urachus. The area of leakage in the urinary bladder is then identified and repaired.

References

Bernard, W. V., and Becht, J.: Antimicrobial therapy in neonatal septicemia. *Proc. 36th Annu. Conv. Am. Assoc. Equine Pract.*, 1990, p. 91.

Brewer, B. D.: Neonatal foal evaluation: Sepsis and survival scoring in private practice. *Proc. 33rd Annu. Conv. Am. Assoc. Equine Pract.*, 1987, p. 817.

Carter, G. K.: Supplemental feeding of the normal foal. *Proc. 36th Annu. Conv. Am. Assoc. Equine Pract.*, 1990, p. 95.

Clement, S. F.: Behavioral alterations and neonatal maladjustment syndrome in the foal. *Proc. 31st Annu. Conv. Am. Assoc. Equine Pract.*, 1985, p. 145.

Cudd, T. A., Toal, R. L., and Embertson, R. M.: The use of clinical findings, abdominocentesis and abdominal radiographs to assess surgical versus nonsurgical abdominal disease in the foal. *Proc. 33rd Annu. Conv. Am. Assoc. Equine Pract.*, 1987, p. 41.

Firth, E. C.: Hematogenous osteomyelitis in the foal. *Proc. 33rd Annu. Conv. Am. Assoc. Equine Pract.*, 1987, p. 795.

Fischer, A. T., Kerr, L. Y., and O'Brien, T. R.: Radiographic diagnosis of gastrointestinal disorders in the foal. *Vet. Radiol.* 28:42, 1987.

Koterba, A. M.: Respiratory insufficiency in the foal: Recognition and treatment. *Equine Pract.*, 13:24, 1991.

Koterba, A. M., Drummond, W. H., and Kosch, P. C.: *Equine Clinical Neonatology.* Philadelphia: Lea & Febiger, 1990.

Madigan, J. E.: Management of the newborn foal. *Proc. 36th Annu. Conv. Am. Assoc. Equine Pract.*, 1990, p. 99.

Madigan, J. E., and Goetzman, B. W.: Use of an acetylcysteine solution enema for meconium retention in the neonatal foal. *Proc. 36th Annu. Conv. Am. Assoc. Equine Pract.*, 1990, p. 117.

Martens, R. J., Martens, J. G., Fiske, R. A., and Hietala, S. K.: *Rhodococcus equi* foal pneumonia: Protective effects of immune plasma in experimentally infected foals. *Equine Vet. J.* 21:248, 1989.

McIlwraith, C. W., and Turner, A. S.: *Equine Surgery: Advanced Techniques.* Philadelphia: Lea & Febiger, 1987.

Rose, R. J., Rossdale, P. D., and Leadon, D. P.: Blood gas and acid–base status in spontaneously delivered, term induced and induced premature foals. *J. Reprod. Fertil. Suppl.* 32:521, 1982.

Rose, R. J., Hodgson, D. R., Leadon, D. P., and Rossdale, P. D.: The effect of intranasal oxygen administration on arterial blood gas and acid–base parameters in spontaneously delivered, term induced and induced premature foals. *Res. Vet. Sci.* 34:159, 1983.

Rossdale, P. D., and Ricketts, S. W. *Equine Stud Farm Medicine,* 2d Ed. London: Balliere Tindall, 1980.

Stewart, J. H., Rose, R. J., and Barko, A. M.: Respiratory studies in foals from birth to one week of age. *Equine Vet. J.* 16:323, 1984.

White, S. L., and Pugh, D. G.: Passive immunoglobulin protection for the colostrum-deprived foal. *Equine Pract.* 10:24, 1988.

CHAPTER 9

Urinary System

EXAMINATION OF THE URINARY TRACT

As with diseases in other body systems, the key to diagnosis when approaching a horse with suspected urinary tract disease is a thorough investigation following a logical sequence. Factors to be considered are the signalment, history, duration of signs, and physical examination findings so that a judicious selection can be made of appropriate tests (see Chaps. 1 and 2).

History

Some pertinent questions when approaching a horse with suspected urinary tract dysfunction include:

- Is the urine normal or discolored? Are there blood clots? Is the urine abnormal only at certain times during micturition (i.e., beginning, middle, or end)?
- Does the horse strain or adopt unusual postures when attempting to urinate?
- Does the horse make frequent attempts to urinate?
- Does urine flow in a normal stream, or is the horse incontinent?
- What volume of urine is passed?
- Does the horse drink large volumes of water?
- Is there a history of colic?
- Has the horse lost weight?
- Has the horse been exposed to toxic plants (e.g., fast-growing sorghum or Sudan grass) or other toxins (e.g., blister beetles in alfalfa, heavy metals, red maple leaves, bracken fern, wild onion)?
- Has the horse been administered potentially toxic products (e.g., aminoglycosides, vitamin K_3, high doses of nonsteroidal anti-inflammatory drugs)?
- Has the horse had a Coggins test recently? If so, what was the result?
- Are other horses on the farm affected?
- Is there a history of respiratory disease or abortion on the farm?

Physical Examination

After an appropriate history, a physical examination is performed. Particular attention should be focused on the following:

- Examination of the penis and prepuce in geldings and stallions looking for swellings, wounds, discharges, and obstructions due to smegma, tumors, or habronemiasis. Sedation with xylazine (Treatment No. 108) or acepromazine (Treatment No. 1) may be required to encourage the horse to extend its penis out of the prepuce. Examination of the vulva and perineum of mares also should be performed.
- Visual and manual inspection of the vulva and vagina should be considered in mares with the aim of determining whether perineal urine scalding, vaginal urine pooling, or pneumovagina is present.

KEY POINT ▶ A rectal examination is an important part of the physical examination.

- Care should be taken to examine the bladder (the bladder may require emptying by normal voiding or catheterization to facilitate thorough examination) for degree of filling, thickness of the bladder wall, and presence of abnormal masses (e.g., calculi). A check should be made to identify the ureters, which are only palpable if dilated or thickened. The pole of the left kidney should be located, taking note of size and the presence of pain. The pelvis should be palpated to detect any evidence of trauma (e.g., fractures).
- A neurologic examination may be indicated. Abnormalities can include paralytic bladder and hypotonia and hypalgesia of the tail, perineum, and anus. Retention of feces and dilatation of the anus also may be noted and are reflective of neurologic dysfunction. Care also should be taken to identify the presence of cranial nerve deficits, since these may occur in association with a lesion causing urinary tract dysfunction.

DIAGNOSTIC AIDS

Urinalysis

KEY POINT ▶ Urinalysis is utilized to assess the functional capacity of the kidneys and to reveal the presence of abnormal cells, pigments or bacteria in the urine.

- Urine is collected by (1) free catch into a sterile container or (2) catheterization of the urinary bladder using a sterile, lubricated urinary catheter or foal stomach tube (see Fig. 9-1). Geldings and stallions usually require sedation with xylazine (Treatment No. 108) or detomidine (Treatment No. 28) to ensure patient compliance and induce eversion of the penis out of the prepuce. Following collection, urine is subjected to the following analyses.
- *Specific gravity,* using a refractometer. Normal values are 1.008 to 1.040 for adult horses (1.001–1.025 in foals). Increases in specific gravity normally occur in response to decreased water intake. A failure to concentrate urine (>1.020) in the face of water deprivation may indicate renal tubular dysfunction.
- *"Dipstick" methods* can be used to measure urine pH and protein, glucose, and bilirubin concentrations. Normal values for pH are 7.5 to 8.5 in adults (5.5–8.0 in foals). Urine pH decreases with metabolic acidosis and following prolonged starvation. Normal urine should not contain protein, glucose, or bilirubin.

KEY POINT ▶ Since horse urine is normally alkaline, false-positive results for protein are common with the "dipstick" procedure.

- Highly concentrated urine also has the potential to produce false-positive results for protein. To overcome this, urine protein should be measured with the *sulfosalicylic acid procedure.* Glucose commonly spills into the urine after the renal threshold is reached. This value is thought to be greater than 10 mmol/L (180 mg/dl) for blood glucose. If blood glucose is not elevated and urine glucose is positive, the most likely cause is renal tubular dysfunction. Bilirubin in the urine occurs in response to cholestatic diseases, where the concentration of direct bilirubin in plasma increases to high values.
- *Pigments*—"dipsticks" give positive results for blood, hemoglobin, and myoglobin in urine. When positive results occur for pigments, proteinuria also will be present. Hemoglobinuria results from excretion of heme pigments in the blood secondary to hemolysis. Urine also may be hemoglobin-positive when there is hemorrhage within the urinary tract. Myoglobin is excreted in urine subsequent to myolysis.
- *Cytology* should be performed on urine sediment after centrifugation, looking for abnormal cells or bacteria. When examined by light microscopy, up to 5 red cells or leukocytes per high-power field are considered normal. Increases in the number of erythrocytes reflect hemorrhage. Elevations in urinary leukocytes indicate inflammation in the urinary tract and when combined with a bacteriuria are reflective of infection. Increased numbers of transitional cells in the urine may be indicative of neoplasia.
- *Casts* are the accumulation of protein and cellular material that form in the renal tubules. Their presence in urine is an indication of renal dysfunction, particularly tubular disease.
- *Crystals* are common in alkaline horse urine. Calcium carbonate crystals are the most common, particularly in horses eating alfalfa hay, and are considered a normal finding.

Bacteriologic Examination

Bacteria in small numbers are common in free-catch urine samples and are probably surface contaminants. In contrast, infections in the urinary tract are usually associated with a significant pyuria. When any doubt exists as to the presence of pyuria, a sample of urine collected aseptically by catheter is indicated. Urine sediment (following centrifugation at 5000 × *g* for 5 minutes) is examined by Gram stain and subjected to bacterial culture and antibiotic sensitivity testing (see Chap. 15). Quantitative bacterial colony counts provide some indication of infection severity.

Serum Biochemistry Values

Serum urea nitrogen (SUN) and creatinine (SCr) concentrations provide a crude indication of renal function in the horse. These variables should always be measured when investigating a horse with suspected urinary tract disease. They are, however, not particularly sensitive indicators of renal function.

KEY POINT ▶ Serum urea nitrogen and creatinine concentrations can be elevated in response to prerenal, renal, and postrenal disorders.

A common cause of prerenal azotemia is dehydration with a decrease in circulating blood volume. Renal tubular damage (acute or chronic renal failure) produces renal azotemia, whereas obstructive urinary tract disease (urolithiasis) and ruptured bladder are postrenal inducers of azotemia.

KEY POINT ▶ Total plasma protein and albumin concentrations may be altered in horses with renal disease.

Elevations are commonly seen in horses with plasma volume contraction and prerenal azotemia, whereas decreases can occur due to protein loss in response to glomerulotubular disease. In these latter cases, the urine commonly has elevated protein concentrations.

Electrolyte Determinations and Fractional Excretion Values

Serum electrolyte concentrations (Na^+, K^+, Cl^-, Ca^{++}, PO_4^-) also may be reflective of renal dysfunction.

KEY POINT ▶ Hypochloremia is the most common electrolyte abnormality in acute and chronic renal disease, and hyperkalemia, hyponatremia, hypercalcemia and hypophosphatemia have all been reported in adult horses with renal failure.

However, these derangements are variable depending on hydration status, diet, and age of the horse. Younger animals (<1 year old) respond similarly to other species and develop hyperphosphatemia and hypocalcemia with renal failure.

The excretion of electrolytes in urine is often altered in response to changes in the diet, renal function, water intake, and the activity of hormones that influence fluid and electrolyte balance. To overcome the effects of these influences and determine whether the kidney is controlling electrolyte homeostasis in an effective manner, the clearance of electrolytes in urine relative to creatinine can be determined. These are referred to as *fractional excretion (FE) values* and are calculated using the formula

$$FE_x\% = \frac{[\text{urine}]_x}{[\text{serum}]_x} \times \frac{[\text{serum}]_{Cr}}{[\text{urine}]_{Cr}} \times 100$$

where FE_x = fractional excretion of electrolyte x

$[\text{urine}]_x$ = urinary concentration of electrolyte x

$[\text{serum}]_x$ = serum concentration of electrolyte x

$[\text{urine}]_{Cr}$ = urinary creatinine concentration

$[\text{serum}]_{Cr}$ = serum creatinine concentration

Normal FE values for adult horses and foals are presented in Table 9-1.

KEY POINT ▶ Decreases in the FE of various electrolytes (e.g., sodium and chloride) may reflect dietary salt deficiency. In contrast, elevated FE_{Na} (>1.5%) in a horse with azotemia often reflects renal tubular damage with sodium wasting, whereas a low value for FE_{Na} (<1.0%) is supportive of prerenal azotemia.

Urinary GGT:Urinary Cr Ratio

Assessment of the activity of the enzyme gamma-glutamyltranspeptidase (GGT) activity in the urine and expressing it in terms of its ratio with the urinary creatinine (Cr) concentration has been advocated as a useful means of assessing tubular dysfunction. GGT is an enzyme found in the brush border of tubular epithelial cells and theoretically is liberated into the urine in response to damage. Activity of the enzyme in urine is compared with the concentration of creatinine, thereby normalizing for alterations in urine flow. A urinary GGT:Cr ratio of 25:1 has been suggested to be the upper limit for normal tubular function, with values above this indicating renal tubular damage. However, in our experience, this may not be the case, since some animals have normal values greater than 25:1 and simple adjustments such as alterations in the diet also may result in elevations of the ratio to above this level. In addition, this ratio has been suggested to be a good marker for the toxic effects of aminoglycoside antibiotic administration. If the ratio of 25:1 is used as an indication of when to discontinue aminoglycoside therapy, we have found that this will often result in premature discontinuation of therapy without any concomitant evidence of significant renal damage (e.g., casts).

KEY POINT ▶ We therefore recommend that caution be exercised when interpreting the results of urinary GGT:Cr ratios and suggest that a baseline value should be determined prior to the introduction of therapy.

The effects of potentially toxic medications can then be compared with this baseline value.

Catheterization of the Urinary Bladder

KEY POINT ▶ Bladder catheterization is a useful and easy technique for collection of urine samples, particularly when bacterial culture is to be attempted or to check the patency of the lower urinary tract.

Prior to insertion of the catheter, the horse should be placed in stocks. In males, sedation with xylazine (Treatment No. 108) or detomidine (Treatment No. 28) facilitates introduction of the catheter and relaxation of the penis. Sedation is optional in mares. After sedation in the male, the penis is grasped with one hand, and the glans penis is washed with an appropriate dilute disinfectant (e.g., povidone-iodine; Treatment No. 91). A sterile flexible urinary catheter or foal stomach tube is then picked up with the other surgically gloved

TABLE 9–1. Fractional Excretion Values for Various Electrolytes

	Fractional Excretion Value (%)	
Electrolyte	*Foal (Neonate)*	*Adult*
Sodium	0.15–0.45	0.02–1.0
Potassium	9–18	15–65
Chloride	0.10–0.75	0.04–1.6
Phosphate	0–7	0–9

hand, prepared with sterile surgical lubricant (K-Y Jelly, Johnson & Johnson), and inserted into the urethra (Fig. 9-1). The catheter is passed approximately 60 cm into the urethra until it reaches the bladder. Urine does not always flow freely initially, and suction on the catheter or injection of air with a sterile 60-ml catheter-tip syringe often promotes flow of urine. Samples are then placed in sterile containers and submitted for urinalysis and/or bacteriologic examination. Catheterization in mares is generally easier. The mare is placed in stocks, and the perineum is prepared with dilute disinfectant. A lubricated gloved hand is inserted into the vagina, and the urethral opening is identified on the floor of the vagina about 10 cm from the vulval opening. The lubricated sterile catheter (flexible or a rigid Chambers catheter) is then guided into the urethra using the index finger. After insertion, the procedure is similar to that described for stallions and geldings.

Endoscopy of the Lower Urinary Tract

Insertion of a flexible endoscope into the urethra and bladder is possible in adult horses of both sexes.

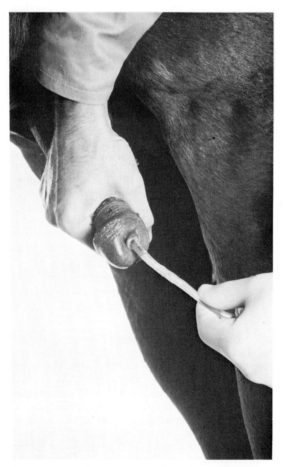

Figure 9–1. Catheterization of the urinary bladder in a gelding.

KEY POINT ► Indications for the procedure include identification of calculi; inflammation, hemorrhage, or tumors of the bladder and/or urethra; and the presence of abnormal urine discharging from a ureter.

In addition, the endoscope can be used to guide a catheter into a ureter in order to collect urine samples from that kidney or to collect biopsies from sites within the lower urinary tract.

A flexible endoscope, 60 cm long and 7 mm or less in diameter, is suitable for males, whereas a shorter or larger-diameter instrument can be used in the mare. The endoscope should be sterilized in an appropriate disinfectant (e.g., Cidex; Treatment No. 31) and rinsed with sterile water. Preparation of the horse is similar to that described for urinary catheterization, but general anesthesia may be required. The bladder is initially catheterized (see p. 297) and emptied of urine. Infusion of 50 ml sterile lidocaine (Treatment No. 67) into the bladder and urethra (done as the catheter is withdrawn) reduces the potential for discomfort during endoscopy. The tip of the endoscope is prepared with sterile surgical lubricant and then inserted into the urethra. Once in the bladder, any remaining urine can be evacuated with the suction apparatus of the endoscope.

Inspection of the bladder is then begun. If the clinician wishes to examine the trigonal region, it is necessary to turn the tip of the endoscope through 180 degrees. Biopsy of masses within the bladder can be performed through the biopsy port, or alternatively, a small-diameter catheter can be passed through the port and inserted into a ureter. Samples of urine can then be aspirated. In the mare, the procedure for endoscopy is similar to that described for catheterization. After insertion of a sterile gloved hand into the urethral orifice, the lubricated tip of the endoscope is passed into the urethra. Subsequent to this, the procedure is the same as that described for stallions or geldings.

Diagnostic Ultrasound

Ultrasound may be used to assess the shape, size, and structure of the kidneys and bladder.

KEY POINT ► Using this technique, it is possible to identify calculi in the pelvis of the kidney, renal neoplasia, and the presence of hydronephrosis.

In addition, ultrasound-guided biopsy of the kidney is possible.

Because penetration of the ultrasound beam is usually about 20 cm or less, interpretation of renal structures using transcutaneous techniques is possible. Transrectal examination of the caudal part of the left kidney and bladder may be done. Under most circumstances, sector scanners, which give superior resolution to that provided by linear-array machines, are the scan heads of choice for these examinations. Of course, if a sector scanner is not available, a linear-array scanner with a 3-MHz head can still provide quite useful images. Ultrasound-guided biopsy of the kidneys can be undertaken with greater potential for collection of diagnostic samples and decreased risk to the patient.

Renal Biopsy

Renal biopsy may be indicated in cases in which renal disease is suspected from findings such as profound proteinuria, or has been diagnosed.

KEY POINT ▶ Biopsy is performed to gain an indication of the site, extent, and prognosis of the disease. Two techniques are described: a percutaneous "blind" technique and an ultrasound-guided technique.

Prior to any renal biopsy, the horse's hemostatic status should be evaluated, and the procedure should be forgone in patients with evidence of a co-agulopathy. For the "blind" procedure, the horse is restrained in stocks and sedated with xylazine (Treatment No. 108) or detomidine (Treatment No. 28). The left paralumbar fossa is clipped, shaved, and aseptically prepared. An assistant then performs a rectal examination and identifies the left kidney and the site for infusion of local anesthetic. Then 10 ml of local anesthetic is infused at the site on the flank. A stab incision is made with a no. 11 or 15 scalpel blade. With the assistant stabilizing the left kidney, a Tru-Cut (Travenol Laboratories, Inc., Deerfield, Ill.) biopsy needle is advanced slowly through the body wall until the tip is either felt by the hand of the assistant in the rectum or it is introduced into the renal parenchyma with the assistant feeling the kidney move (Fig. 9-2). It is best if the kidney is guided to the point of the needle rather than trying to do the reverse. It is important to attempt to collect a biopsy from the caudal pole of the kidney to ensure (1) that a diagnostically useful sample is collected and (2) that major renal vessels are avoided. After the biopsy needle is inserted into the renal parenchyma, the biopsy is collected. *Note:* It is important that the kidney is well immobilized during the procedure to decrease the potential for hemorrhage. Following collection, the sample is placed in formalin and submitted for histopathologic examination. The horse should be kept quiet for 24 to 48 hours following the procedure and observed for clinical signs of blood loss (e.g., pale mucous membranes, tachycardia, anxiety or evidence of pain, decreasing PCV and TPP).

KEY POINT ▶ Ultrasound-guided biopsy of the kidney is now the most common method for collection of samples.

Biopsies can be obtained from the left or right kidney. The kidney is imaged, and precise identification is made of the site from which the biopsy is to be collected. Sedation of the horse, skin preparation, and infusion of local anesthetic are performed. With the scan head encased in a sterile surgical glove filled with coupling gel and sterile gel on the skin surface, the kidney is identified and the biopsy needle is passed into the renal parenchyma. Postoperative observation is the same as that described for the "blind" technique.

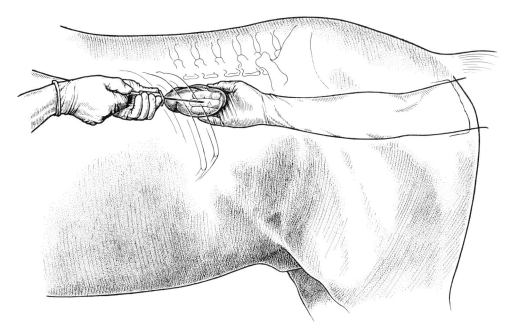

Figure 9–2. Renal biopsy. The drawing demonstrates the "blind" technique for renal biopsy. The left kidney is stabilized against the abdominal wall by an assistant. Following skin preparation, local anesthestic infiltration, and a stab incision in the skin, a Tru-Cut biopsy needle is inserted into the renal parenchyma.

Water Deprivation Test

KEY POINT ► This test is useful to determine if normal renal mechanisms exist to concentrate urine.

This test is particularly useful in assisting to differentiate between first-degree diabetes insipidus, nephrogenic diabetes insipidus, and psychogenic polydipsia (p. 301).

KEY POINT ► This test is contraindicated in horses with azotemia.

The test is initiated by collection of urine and blood samples. Urine may have to be collected by catheter. Urine specific gravity, PCV, and TPP are measured. If possible, body weight is also measured. Water is withheld, and urine and blood samples are collected at 12-hour intervals for 48 to 72 hours. This assumes that there is no dramatic increase in urine specific gravity or change in metabolic status of the animal (e.g., azotemia, dehydration, or dramatic reduction in body weight). If any of these events occur, the test is terminated. The maximal response is indicated by an increase in urine specific gravity to approximately 1.050, a 12% to 15% reduction in body weight, and a 12 g/L (1.2-mg/dl) increase in TPP after approximately 48 hours. Obviously, the test can be terminated well before this point is reached, particularly if the urine specific gravity is elevated to greater than 1.030, a level indicating appropriate renal concentrating capacity.

Diseases of the Urinary Tract

Cystitis

KEY POINT ► Primary cystitis is uncommon in horses, whereas cystitis secondary to conditions inducing urine stasis or bladder injury is more frequently diagnosed.

Most cases of cystitis are thought to be the result of ascending rather than descending urinary tract infections.

History and Presenting Signs

- More common in mares
- Frequent attempts to urinate
- Problems leading to urine stasis or bladder injury (e.g., urolithiasis and urinary obstruction)
- Ataxia/paralytic bladder
- Late-gestation or postpartum mare
- Repeated urinary catheterization

Clinical Findings and Diagnosis

- Pollakiuria (frequent passage of urine), dribbling urine, and urine scalding may be evident. Pain (grunting) may be obvious during urination, and the position adopted for micturition may be held for extended periods.
- Penile relaxation may be obvious in males.
- Increases in cardinal signs (heart rate, rectal temperature) may occur in more severe cases.
- In diseases where cystitis occurs unrelated to neurogenic causes, rectal examination often reveals a small bladder with a thickened wall. In contrast, neurogenic disorders resulting in secondary cystitis may have a distended, tense atonic bladder (see p. 308). Animals in the latter group also will often demonstrate other neurologic deficits (e.g., ataxia, weakness).
- Urinalysis shows proteinuria, pyuria, hematuria, desquamated epithelial cells, and debris. Bacteria will often be present in free-catch samples, but these are often contaminated with environmental bacteria and are not suitable for bacterial culture and sensitivity testing.

KEY POINT ► Samples for bacterial culture and sensitivity should be collected via catheterization (p. 297) using aseptic technique prior to the institution of antimicrobial therapy (see Chap. 15).

- Quantitative bacterial colony counts provide the most effective way of assessing the severity of the infection.
- Bacteria commonly implicated in the induction of cystitis in horses include *E. coli*, *Proteus mira-*

bilis, Enterobacter spp., *Klebsiella* spp., *Pseudomonas* spp., *Streptococcus* spp., and *Corynebacterium* spp.
- Cystoscopy reveals congested bladder mucosa, which may appear roughened, hemorrhagic, and ulcerated.
- Hematology may provide a nonspecific indication of inflammation (e.g., leukocytosis, hyperfibrinogenemia, hypergammaglobulinemia). However, these alterations are not present in all cases.

Differential Diagnosis

- Urolithiasis
- Urinary incontinence
- Pyelonephritis
- Neoplasia
- Prolapse of the bladder
- Ectopic ureter
- Renal failure
- Urethritis

Treatment

- Treatment of the primary disease is imperative. Consideration of hydration and metabolic status is also important, with administration of fluids being important if indicated. Maintenance of urine flow is important to ensure optimal removal of debris and infectious organisms from the bladder.
- Specific therapy directed at elimination of bacterial infection from the bladder also should be instituted. In mild cases of cystitis, resolution of the primary predisposing problem is often sufficient to allow local defense mechanisms to eradicate the infection.
- Initial therapy involves irrigation of the bladder with sterile isotonic fluids to remove sediment and debris from the bladder lumen.
- Selection of antimicrobial therapy should be based on the results of culture and sensitivity testing. Antimicrobial agents that are useful for treatment of bacterial cystitis include trimethoprim–sulfadiazine (Treatment No. 107), penicillin (Treatment Nos. 83–85), gentamicin (Treatment No. 56), amikacin (Treatment No. 4), ampicillin (Treatment No. 6), cephalosporins (Treatment Nos. 16, 18, 19, 20 and 21), and tetracyclines (Treatment No. 80). In chronic cases, antimicrobial therapy may need to be continued for 2 to 3 weeks or more, because bacteria localize in the bladder wall.

KEY POINT ► Urinalysis and urine culture should be repeated 3 to 4 days following completion of antibiotic therapy to ensure success of treatment.

- On occasion, cystitis will be resistant to therapy, and additional antibiotic therapy is necessary.

Polyuria/Polydipsia

Polyuria is an increase in urine output, whereas *polydipsia* describes an increase in water consumption. In general, a 500-kg adult horse will produce 12 to 17 L of urine per day, with an average urine specific gravity of 1.020 to 1.030. These values may vary slightly depending on diet and ambient conditions. However, under most conditions, daily urine production of more than 20 to 25 L is regarded as being indicative of polyuria.

Renal, hormonal, and psychogenic causes of polyuria have been reported. There are two common disease states that produce polyuria. Chronic renal failure, the most common cause, produces polyuria because there are an insufficient number of functional nephrons to concentrate urine. Tumors of the pars intermedia (pituitary) associated with secondary hyperadrenocorticism is a less common cause of polyuria found mainly in older horses.

History and Presenting Signs

- Increased water consumption (polydipsia)
- Abnormal behavior (e.g., restlessness, frequent searching for water, drinking of urine)
- Concurrent fluid therapy or administration of osmotic diuretics (e.g., glucose, DMSO, mannitol)
- Weight loss

Clinical Findings and Diagnosis

- Polyuria can result from an increased solute concentration of the urine (e.g., glucose), referred to as *solute diuresis,* or can be due to an increase in water content of urine, known as *water diuresis.* With solute diuresis, there is polyuria with urine having a specific gravity in the 1.008 to 1.012 range. In contrast, water diuresis results in urine with a specific gravity of less than 1.008.
- With solute diuresis, other frequently detected abnormalities may include glucosuria, proteinuria, or dramatically increased FE_{Na}.
- More common causes, lesions involved, and diagnostic procedures indicated in horses with polyuria are outlined in Table 9-2.

Treatment

- If there is chronic renal failure, treatment strategies for this disorder (p. 306) may be used.
- Tumors of the pars intermedia producing Cushing's disease, although often benign, are usually slowly progressive. However, given the severity of signs and age of the horses affected, treatment rarely is undertaken. Use of cyproheptadine (Periactin, Merck Sharp and Dohme, West Point, PA) has been suggested. The recommended dosage schedule is 60 mg/450 kg PO q24h in the morning for 1 to 2 weeks, with the dosage slowly increased to 120 mg/kg PO q12–24h. Response, if it occurs, should be present in 6 to 8 weeks. After 3 months of therapy, reduction to alternate-day

TABLE 9–2. Causes of Polyuria and Methods for Diagnosis

Disorder	Pathogenesis	Clinical Manifestations	Diagnosis/Diagnostic Tests
Chronic renal failure* (loss of nephrons)	Loss of > 75% of functional nephrons	Weight loss, isothenuria (SG 1.008–1.012), ± proteinura, urinary casts, ↑ SUN & SCr	Serum biochemistry, urinalysis, renal biopsy (see p. 299)
Hyperadrenocorticism* (Cushing's disease, tumors of the pars intermedia)	Increased production adrenocorticosteroids (usually due to pituitary tumors in older horses)	Weight loss, hirsutism, ↑ sweating, urine SG (1.008–1.012), persistent hyperglycemia and glucosuria, ± laminitis and ↑ susceptibility to infection.	Urinalysis; determination of ↑ plasma [cortisol], ↑ plasma [glucose]; ACTH stimulation (1 U/kg of gel IM) → <4X ↑ in serum [cortisol]. No response to dexamethazone suppression test
Exogenous isotonic fluid administration*	Parenteral fluids leading to volume diuresis	Increased plasma volume leading to ↑ GFR and diuresis, urine SG (1.008–1.012)	History of exogenous fluid administration; ↓ urine production and ↑ urine SG when fluid therapy reduced or terminated
First-degree diabetes insipidus	Decreased production of AVP by the hypothalamus	Very low urine SG (1.001–1.007)	Urinalysis; water deprivation test → inability to ↑ urine SG; exogenous ADH (40–80 units in oil IM) → ↑ urine SG > 1.025 in 24–36 hours
Nephrogenic (second-degree) diabetes insipidus	Decreased response of kidney to AVP	Very low urine SG (1.001–1.007)	Urinalysis; water deprivation test → inability to ↑ urine SG; no response to exogenous ADH (40–80 IU in oil IM)
Psychogenic water consumption	Psychological disorder producing compulsive water consumption	Maximally dilute urine (SG ≤ 1.001)	Urinalysis; water deprivation test → ↑ urine SG
Diabetes mellitus	Decreased insulin production	Weight loss; ↑ appetite; persistent hyperglycemia (300–500 mg/dl); urine SG (1.008–1.012); glucosuria; ketonuria.	Urinalysis, serum biochemistry
Psychogenic salt consumption	Behavioral abnormality → increased salt consumption → ↑ water consumption and diuresis	Urine SG (1.008–1.012)	History of ↑ desire to consume salt; urinalysis (increased FE_{Na})

*Most common causes.
AVP = arginine vasopressin (ADH)

treatment can be considered. Unfortunately, in our experience, responses have been quite disappointing.

- More recently, the use of bromocriptine mesylate at a dose rate of 0.1 mg/kg PO q12h (Parlodel, Sandoz, East Hanover, NJ) has been reported.
- Psychogenic water or salt consumption is rare, but when diagnosed, it is managed by reducing the animal's water or salt intake, respectively, to closer to daily needs.

KEY POINT ► It is important to ensure that water restriction does not produce continued polyuria and progressive dehydration. If this occurs, then the diagnosis of psychogenic water consumption or salt consumption is unlikely.

- Primary diabetes insipidus may respond to daily administration of exogenous arginine vasopressin (40–80 units in oil IM q24h).

- Only a few cases of diabetes mellitus have been reported in the horse. Often, tumors of the pars intermedia are confused with diabetes mellitus. Treatment of diabetes mellitus has been attempted using protamine zinc insulin. Dosages providing appropriate control of blood glucose concentrations are difficult to adjust, often making treatment unrewarding.

Prolapse of the Urinary Bladder (Displaced Bladder)

KEY POINT ► Bladder prolapse is unusual and occurs almost exclusively in mares after foaling.

Relaxation of the supporting pelvic muscles, regional edema, dilatation of sphincters in the urinary tract, and the straining associated with parturition all predispose to prolapse of the bladder.

History and Presenting Signs

- Mares
- Postpartum

Clinical Findings and Diagnosis

- The bladder is observed everting from the vulva in a postpartum mare. Edema of the bladder mucosa is common due to the restriction of venous drainage secondary to eversion.
- On rare occasions, the bladder may rupture, and intestines may prolapse out through the tear in the bladder wall.
- Affected mares commonly strain and show signs of abdominal pain.

Differential Diagnosis

- Eversion of the rectum
- Uterine prolapse
- Urolithiasis
- Cystitis

Treatment

- Affected mares are sedated with xylazine (Treatment No. 108) or detomidine (Treatment No. 28), and epidural anesthesia is induced with xylazine (see Chap. 7, p. 255) to control straining and reduce discomfort.
- The everted mucosal surface of the bladder is cleansed with saline or dilute povidone-iodine solution (Treatment No. 91).
- The bladder is replaced in its normal location via the urethra. In some cases a urethral sphincterotomy is required to allow replacement of the bladder. Once in its normal position, the sphincterotomy is sutured.
- Postoperatively, antibiotics should be administered (e.g., trimethoprim-sulfadiazine, 15–20 mg/

kg of the combination PO q12h; Treatment No. 107) for 5 to 7 days.
- In cases where bladder rupture has occurred and bowel has eventrated, induction of general anesthesia and a celiotomy are required. The affected bowel is cleansed with generous volumes of warm sterile saline. The integrity of the bowel is then assessed, and if it is in good condition, it is retracted into the abdomen. If the bowel is compromised, resection and anastomosis of offending bowel are undertaken. Following replacement of bowel into the abdomen, the rent in the bladder wall is sutured. Replacement of the bladder in the normal anatomic location then proceeds as described above.
- Complications of bladder prolapse include postoperative straining and reprolapse of the bladder.

Pyelonephritis

Pyelonephritis, a bacterial infection of the renal parenchyma, calyces, and pelvis, occurs most commonly in the adult horse as a result of ascending infection secondary to lower urinary tract infection and urine stasis. Embolic (hematogenous) pyelonephritis is rare.

History and Presenting Signs

- Inappetence, weight loss
- Abnormal urination
- Behavioral changes

Clinical Findings and Diagnosis

- Many of the clinical signs described for cystitis may be present (p. 300), since ascending infection from the lower urinary tract is the usual mechanism for induction of pyelonephritis.
- Systemic manifestations (e.g., fever and depression) may be present.
- Rectal examination may reveal evidence of cystitis and distended and thickened ureters or abnormalities of the kidneys (e.g., altered size, shape, or the presence of pain on palpation).
- Ultrasound examination of the kidneys is also useful to provide information relating to alterations in size, shape, or consistency of the kidneys.
- Urinalysis reveals pyuria, hematuria, epithelial cells, and possibly casts. Collection of urine using aseptic technique is necessary to ensure that appropriate samples are submitted for bacterial culture and sensitivity.
- Hematologic changes commonly occurring in chronic pyelonephritis include anemia, leukocytosis, hyperfibrinogenemia, and hypergammaglobulinemia. If there is sufficient renal involvement, elevations in SUN and SCr also may occur.

Differential Diagnosis

- Urolithiasis
- Urinary incontinence
- Neoplasia
- Ectopic ureter
- Renal failure
- Urethritis

Treatment

Many of the therapeutic strategies outlined for cystitis are suitable for pyelonephritis. In severe, unilateral cases, nephrectomy of the affected kidney is often a satisfactory means for providing resolution of the problem. In chronic bilateral cases, prolonged therapy is necessary but is often unrewarding. Horses showing evidence of renal failure (i.e., increased SUN and SCr) have the least favorable prognosis for successful treatment.

Renal Failure, Acute

Acute renal failure is characterized by a rapid fall in the glomerular filtration rate and clinical signs of uremia.

Causes of Acute Renal Failure

KEY POINT ▶ There are three major causes of acute renal failure: (1) toxic, (2) hemodynamic, and (3) obstructive.

Toxic—Acute renal failure is most commonly induced by aminoglycoside antibiotics and nonsteroidal antiinflammatory agents (NSAIDs) such as phenylbutazone. Aminoglycoside-induced acute renal failure is the most common resulting from a therapeutic drug and is more likely if the horse is concurrently suffering from a condition that limits renal blood flow (e.g., diarrhea, inadequate intake of fluids). Administration of high doses of NSAIDs, also in the face of decreased renal blood flow, is also a relatively common cause of acute renal failure. Other causes include heavy metals, acorn buds, blister beetle, and myoglobin/hemoglobin. A single severe bout or repeated episodes of rhabdomyolysis ("tying up") with liberation of muscle pigments into the circulation is also known to induce acute renal failure. This manifestation is more likely in association with significant reductions in the extracellular fluid volume. Acute renal failure should always be suspected in horses that remain depressed for 3 to 7 days after an episode of "tying up" or that have suffered from the "exhausted horse syndrome" at an endurance ride.

Hemodynamic—Acute renal failure also can result from hemodynamic causes. Diseases resulting in shock with secondary renal failure include acute diarrhea, endotoxemia, severe hemorrhage, and bacterial septicemia (e.g., pleuropneumonia). Hemodynamic acute renal failure usually results

from a combination of marked hypotension and release of vasoactive agents (e.g., endotoxin).

Obstructive—Obstruction of the urinary tract is likely to result in temporary renal failure. As described previously, obstruction to urine flow can be the result of urolithiasis, urethritis, paralysis of the bladder, neoplasia, trauma, or infection.

History and Presenting Signs

- Diseases causing cardiovascular compromise (e.g., acute diarrhea, colic, endotoxemia)
- Depression, inappetence
- History of exposure to known toxic substances (e.g., phenylbutazone, blister beetle, acorn buds)
- Signs of urinary tract obstruction (e.g., straining to urinate, discolored urine, frequent attempts to urinate)
- Reluctance to move (i.e., signs that may accompany laminitis, pleuritis, or a myopathy)

Clinical Findings and Diagnosis

- There will often be signs consistent with the primary cause of the disorder. For instance, horses with acute renal failure are commonly depressed, lethargic, and inappetent with variable fever. Other signs of shock such as increased heart rate, injected mucous membranes, and decreased skin turgor also may be present. Edema, laminitis, evidence of a severe myopathy or spontaneous hemorrhage, and colic also may be detected.
- Oliguria is relatively common, particularly when hemodynamic alterations predispose the horse to acute renal failure.
- Dysuria and discolored urine are apparent in some horses with acute renal failure.
- In addition to the history and clinical signs, diagnosis is often confirmed by ancillary tests, particularly laboratory analyses.

KEY POINT ▶ Horses with acute renal failure are azotemic and often hyponatremic and hypochloremic.

- The occurrence of alterations in serum potassium and calcium concentrations is variable. Metabolic acidosis is common due to bicarbonate loss in urine.
- Urinalysis reveals isosthenuria (urine specific gravity of 1.008–1.015), with casts, protein, and microscopic hematuria commonly identified. Values for the fractional excretion (FE) of sodium and phosphate are often elevated. Enzymuria (elevations in GGT and AP in the urine) also may be demonstrable.
- Routine assessment of the urine GGT:urine Cr ratio (p. 297) has been advocated by some when the potential for toxic nephropathy is high (e.g., protracted treatment with aminoglycosides). Ratios greater than 25:1 are considered to be abnormal. However, recent evidence suggests that this

technique is influenced by a variety of factors, not just the potentially nephrotoxic agent, and as such may be a less sensitive indicator of renal damage than previously suggested.

- Diagnosis in suspected cases of obstructive renal failure is assisted by rectal palpation and ultrasound examination of the kidneys and lower urinary tract. Aseptic collection of urine is indicated for the identification of pyuria, hematuria, epithelial cells, casts, and debris, the result of damage to the urinary tract.

Differential Diagnosis

- Colic
- Endotoxemia
- Hemorrhage
- Ingestion or administration of nephrotoxic substances (e.g., aminoglycosides, NSAIDs, acorn buds, blister beetles, etc.)
- Laminitis
- Pleuropneumonia
- Rhabdomyolysis
- Obstructive urolithiasis
- Pyelonephritis

Treatment

- Removal of the inciting cause (if known) is the primary aim of treatment.

KEY POINT ▶ Specific therapy also should be directed toward increasing the glomerular filtration rate. This usually involves intravenous fluid therapy with attention to volume deficits and correction of electrolyte and acid–base abnormalities.

- Normal saline or other polyionic isotonic fluid solutions are good choices (see Fluid Therapy, Chap. 17). If possible, regular monitoring of urine output, serum or plasma sodium, chloride, and potassium concentrations, and plasma bicarbonate concentration is of value. Fluids administered via nasogastric tube also should be considered.
- Following introduction of initial fluid therapy, it should be determined whether the renal failure has resulted in oliguria/anuria or polyuria. If oliguric renal failure is present despite the infusion of fluids, particular caution must be exercised to ensure that volume overload is avoided. Assessment for the presence of edema and regular monitoring of the body weight, PCV, and TPP are helpful in this process.
- When oliguric renal failure is present, administration of DMSO (Treatment No. 34) (0.5 to 0.9 g/kg IV as a 10–20% solution), mannitol (0.25–1 g/kg IV as a 20% solution once; Treatment No. 68) or furosemide (1.0 mg/kg IV q2h for two to three treatments; Treatment Nos. 54 and 55) is of value following the initial fluid and electrolyte therapy. To be effective, furosemide must be given early

in the course of the disease. It is hoped that with this combination of treatments the horse will begin producing increased amounts of urine.

KEY POINT ▶ Note: It is common for horses that initially have oliguric renal failure to subsequently develop polyuria as the disease progresses.

- Once urine flow is reestablished, continued infusion with isotonic polyionic fluids may result in marked reduction in the degree of azotemia. Initial therapy requires fluid administration at a rate of up to 50 to 100 ml/kg per day until the SCr level approaches the normal range.
- If endotoxemia or septicemia exists, treatment may include low doses of NSAIDs (flunixin meglumine 0.25 mg/kg IV q6h; Treatment No. 52) to assist in the maintenance of renal blood flow and systemic blood pressure.
- Treatment of acute renal failure, particularly fluids, should be continued IV or by nasogastric tube at rates of 20 to 50 ml/kg per day until the SCr returns to normal and the horse begins to eat and drink voluntarily.
- The prognosis for horses with acute renal failure is variable depending on the inciting cause.

KEY POINT ▶ In general, the following rules can be applied: (1) toxic nephropathies tend to have the best prognosis for return of appropriate renal function; (2) the shorter the time between onset of signs and induction of therapy, the better is the prognosis; and (3) a more rapid response to therapy (dramatic increase in urine output and fall in serum creatinine) is usually associated with a better prognosis.

Renal Failure, Chronic

Chronic renal failure is a problem that occurs most frequently in older horses and is the result of glomerular or tubulointerstitial disease. The most common cause of chronic renal failure is proliferative glomerulonephritis, which is thought to be the result of deposition of antigen–antibody complexes within the glomeruli. Other causes include renal glomerular hypoplasia, chronic interstitial nephritis, pyelonephritis, and a variety of other miscellaneous causes.

History and Presenting Signs

- Older horses

KEY POINT ▶ Weight loss is the most common sign associated with chronic renal failure.

- Inappetence and depression

Clinical Findings and Diagnosis

- Affected horses are often thin, and they may be depressed.

KEY POINT ▶ Polyuria and/or polydipsia are common features of chronic renal failure.

- Substantial plaques of ventral edema (anasarca) may be obvious in more advanced cases where protein loss has been substantial.
- Some horses have fetid breath and oral ulcerations. Dental calculus can be present.

KEY POINT ▶ Common clinicopathologic findings include anemia, azotemia, hypochloremia, and hyponatremia, as well as possibly hypercalcemia, hypophosphatemia, and hyperkalemia.

- Although hypercalcemia and hypophosphatemia have been suggested to be pathognomonic indicators of chronic renal failure, these changes only appear to occur in horses with chronic renal failure that are consuming diets rich in calcium (e.g., alfalfa hay). Variable hypoproteinemia may occur. In septic conditions, an inflammatory response may occur, as reflected by leukocytosis and hyperfibrinogenemia.

KEY POINT ▶ Urinalysis reveals isosthenuria (specific gravity 1.008–1.015), and proteinuria may be present.

- Pyuria, hematuria, and bacteriuria are possible, particularly if the chronic renal failure is secondary to pyelonephritis.
- Rectal examination should be performed to determine the size, shape, and consistency of the left kidney and ureters.
- Ultrasound examination of the kidneys also may be of value when attempting to assess the anatomy of structures within the urinary tract.
- Diagnosis is based on the history, presenting signs, physical examination findings, clinicopathology results, and possibly a renal biopsy. Certainly a renal biopsy is of value when attempting to determine the prognosis.

Differential Diagnosis

- Acute renal failure
- Obstructive urolithiasis
- Pyelonephritis
- Internal parasitism
- Neoplasia
- Abdominal abscessation/peritonitis
- Malabsorption syndromes (e.g., granulomatous enteritis)

Treatment

- Therapeutic principles are similar to those for acute renal failure (p. 304), with the aim to treat the primary inciting cause, if known, and to pro-

vide sufficient fluids, electrolytes, and nutrients for the horse. Supplementation with vitamin B complex and anabolic steroids also may be useful.

KEY POINT ▶ When considering prognosis, horses that are unable to increase their urine specific gravity to greater than 1.015 and have persistent elevations of SCr greater than 880 μmol/L (10 mg/dl), despite therapy, have substantial impairment of renal function, which is associated with a poor prognosis for prolonged life.

- Elevations of SCr greater than 1300 μmol/L (15 mg/dl) indicate a grave prognosis. In general, unless an easily treatable cause for the chronic renal failure is identified and removed (e.g., urolithiasis), the prognosis for long-term survival in most cases is poor.

Renal Tubular Acidosis

Renal tubular acidosis is a disorder of renal tubular function that is characterized clinically by metabolic acidosis and hyperchloremia. Renal tubular acidosis tends to occur for one of two reasons: (1) inability of the proximal tubule to resorb bicarbonate or (2) failure of the distal tubule to excrete hydrogen ions. Primary and secondary forms of renal tubular acidosis exist. Secondary renal tubular acidosis has been reported as a sequela to other systemic disorders such as endotoxemia and diarrhea.

History and Presenting Signs

- Depression, altered behavior
- Weakness, ataxia
- Weight loss
- Intermittent abdominal pain

Clinical Findings and Diagnosis

- Evidence of the presenting signs outlined above is usually sufficient to prompt further investigation of a metabolic derangement.

KEY POINT ▶ Clinicopathologic findings in horses with renal tubular acidosis are hyperchloremia (with values greater than 110 mmol/L being customary) and metabolic acidosis.

- In the latter case, plasma bicarbonate values may be less than 10 mmol/L (mEq/L) (normal ~27 mmol/L). This metabolic acidosis occurs in the absence of signs commonly associated with other causes of acidemia (e.g., colic, endotoxemia, diarrhea). Alkaline urine, in the presence of the systemic acidosis, is a recurrent finding. Hypokalemia may occur in some horses with renal tubular acidosis.

- Diagnosis is normally based on the clinical signs and clinicopathologic findings described and by ruling out other possible causes of these signs. In some cases, administration of ammonium chloride (100 mg/kg PO in 4–6 L of water) has been shown to result in urine acidification (pH < 6.5) by 4 hours after administration. *Note:* The bladder should be catheterized and emptied prior to administration of the ammonium chloride.

Differential Diagnosis

- Other forms of renal disease
- Neurologic diseases resulting in ataxia and weakness (e.g., spinal cord disease)
- Colic, endotoxemia
- Cardiac failure
- Rhabdomyolysis
- Pleuropneumonia
- Laminitis

Treatment

- Correction of low plasma bicarbonate is the major aim of therapy for renal tubular acidosis. The bicarbonate deficit can be calculated using the formula

  Body weight (kg) × 0.6 × base deficit (mmol)

Base deficit is calculated by subtracting the measured plasma bicarbonate value from the normal value of 27 mmol/L.

KEY POINT ▶   Initially, one-quarter of the bicarbonate deficit should be administered intravenously using isotonic sodium bicarbonate solution over 4 to 6 hours. The remainder of the calculated dose should be administered over the next 24 to 36 hours.

- Correction of the acid–base balance is usually associated with a worsening of the hypokalemia, particularly if the horse remains inappetent. Administration of potassium chloride [40–60 g (1.5–2 oz) in 4 L of water via nasogastric tube q8–12h] is effective. When the horse begins consuming feed voluntarily, the need for potassium supplementation diminishes.
- When the plasma bicarbonate values have been corrected, oral bicarbonate therapy is instituted (150 g/450 kg in feed q12h). This dose is usually sufficient for maintenance but should be modified in individual cases according to plasma bicarbonate values.
- Some cases will resolve spontaneously over 1 to 2 weeks, whereas others require protracted therapy to prevent recurrence of the renal tubular acidosis.

Rupture of the Urinary Bladder

KEY POINT ▶   Although relatively common in foals (see Chap. 8), rupture of the urinary bladder is an uncommon problem in adult horses. When it does occur, it is usually a sequela to foaling or urinary tract obstruction.

History and Presenting Signs

- Most common in mares, postpartum
- Depression and inappetence a few days after foaling
- Secondary to urolithiasis and obstruction in adult males

Clinical Findings and Diagnosis

- Depression and possibly a mild increase in heart rate and respiratory rate are found.
- Small amounts of urine may still be voided.
- Clinicopathology findings include azotemia, hyperkalemia, hyponatremia, and hypochloremia.
- Abdominocentesis reveals a large volume of yellow fluid. The presence of calcium carbonate crystals in the peritoneal fluid is strongly supportive of a diagnosis of uroperitoneum.

KEY POINT ▶   Diagnosis is confirmed by comparing serum creatinine concentration with that of the peritoneal fluid.

- In the presence of uroperitoneum, peritoneal fluid creatinine concentration is 1.5- to 2-fold greater than that in the serum.
- If obstructive urolithiasis has predisposed the bladder to rupture, many of the signs and diagnostic criteria outlined for urethral calculi (p. 309) are pertinent.
- Cystoscopy may assist in defining the presence of a urethral calculus or rent in the bladder wall. This procedure helps identify the extent and location of the tear.

Differential Diagnosis

- Other causes of colic
- Peritonitis
- Urolithiasis
- Renal failure
- Cystitis

Treatment

- Small tears with limited leakage of urine may be left to heal by second intention. Such tears are indicated by the ability of the horse to pass moderate amounts of urine and the presence of limited metabolic derangements.
- Horses with dehydration and other metabolic disorders benefit from the infusion of isotonic fluids

that *do not* contain potassium because of the presence of hyperkalemia. Good fluid choices include 0.9% sodium chloride or dextrose 5% in water (see Chap. 17).

■ Horses with more severe disruption to the bladder wall require surgery. In these cases, referral to a university or well-equipped surgical clinic should be considered.

Urethral Diverticular Concreiion ("Bean")

Urethral diverticular concretion is a disorder in which smegma accumulates in the urethral diverticulum.

KEY POINT ► In general, this process does not create any problems for the horse; however, on occasion, the size of the concretion and associated inflammatory response can result in adverse signs.

History and Presenting Signs

■ Adult males
■ Frequent attempts to urinate, penis extended
■ Urine spraying may occur

Clinical Findings and Diagnosis

■ Dysuria and urine spraying during micturition may be observed.
■ Urine staining or scalding on the legs is possible.
■ The region of the penis near the urethral opening may be swollen.
■ Diagnosis is based on examination of the penis, following sedation with xylazine (Treatment No. 108) or detomidine (Treatment No. 28) to encourage relaxation, revealing accumulation of a large amount of foul-smelling smegma in the urethral diverticulum.

Differential Diagnosis

■ Urethral calculi
■ Cystic calculi
■ Penile/urethral neoplasia (e.g., squamous cell carcinoma)
■ Habronemiasis of the penis
■ Penile injury (e.g., hematoma, lacerations)
■ Urethritis (stallion)

Treatment

Manual removal of the "bean" following sedation results in resolution of the problem.

Urethritis

Urethritis occurs most commonly in stallions and may be associated with hemospermia. The cause of the disorder is not known.

History and Presenting Signs

■ Stallions
■ Discolored discharge from the penis after mating
■ Difficulty urinating

Clinical Findings and Diagnosis

■ The penis may be extended from the prepuce, and there may be obvious swelling of the urethra.
■ Blood or serosanguinous discharge may be noted from the urethra after coitus, and hemospermia is common.
■ In severe cases, dysuria, pollakiuria (frequent passage of urine), stranguria (straining to urinate), and urinary retention can occur owing to a significant reduction in urethral lumen diameter.

KEY POINT ► Diagnosis is based on endoscopic examination of the urethra.

■ Bacterial culture and sensitivity of samples from the urethra can be useful when attempting to undertake treatment.

Differential Diagnosis

■ Hemospermia
■ Cystitis
■ Urolithiasis
■ Pyelonephritis
■ Trauma to the penis

Treatment

■ Sexual rest is advised.

KEY POINT ► Establishment of urethral patency is important, and in cases where urethral occlusion has occurred, a perineal urethrostomy is indicated (see p. 312).

■ Urethrostomy wounds are normally left to heal by second intention.
■ Systemic antibiotic therapy is useful using agents active against the bacteria involved and excreted in the urine. Local antibiotic therapy is possible, with drugs administered by a sterile catheter inserted through the urethral orifice or urethrostomy wound. Alternatively, suppositories can be inserted into the distal urethra.
■ Complications include poor response to therapy, urethral cicatrix formation with subsequent obstruction, and urethral fistula at the urethrostomy site.

Urinary Incontinence

Urinary incontinence results from a variety of disorders, including neurologic, bladder, and urethral causes. Neurologic causes of incontinence can result from those affecting the spinal cord above the sacral nerves (upper motor neuron) and those affecting the sacral nerves, detrusor muscle, and urethral sphincter (lower motor neuron).

KEY POINT ▶ The most common causes of urinary incontinence in the horse are herpesvirus myelitis, neuritis of the cauda equina, and the sorghum ataxia–cystitis syndrome.

Other causes include equine protozoal myeloencephalitis, trauma, urolithiasis, osteomyelitis, neoplasia, and ectopic ureter.

History and Presenting Signs

- Apparent difficulty urinating
- Small amounts of urine voided
- Recent history of consuming rapidly growing sorghum or Sudan grass
- Ataxia
- Respiratory disease
- More than one horse affected
- Possibly a young horse (ectopic ureter)

Clinical Findings and Diagnosis

- Intermittent passage of small amounts of urine.
- Exercise may induce an increase in the volume of urine voided.
- Horses with upper motor neuron signs may be ataxic and demonstrate no voluntary ability to urinate. Variable degrees of urine dribbling occur. Rectal examination reveals normal anal tone and a bladder of variable size. Resistance to emptying of the bladder by application of pressure during the rectal examination is often a significant finding. After a couple of weeks, a bladder voiding reflex is invoked, and spontaneous partial vesicular emptying occurs.
- With lower motor neuron disease, rectal examination reveals a large, tense, yet atonic bladder. Manual evacuation of the bladder is usually easy to achieve, unless the lesion involves the bladder wall or pelvic nerve. In the latter case, difficulty is encountered when attempting to manually empty the bladder. Anal hypotonia and hypalgesia are commonly associated with lower motor neuron dysfunction.
- With an ectopic ureter, the bladder will be normal on rectal examination; however, urine will constantly dribble from the urethra due to the discharge of urine into the proximal urethra.
- If an ectopic ureter is suspected in a young horse, referral for an excretory urogram is recommended.

Differential Diagnosis

- Equine herpesvirus myelitis
- Neuritis of the cauda equina
- Sorghum ataxia–cystitis syndrome
- Equine protozoal myeloencephalitis
- Osteomyelitis of the sacral vertebral column
- Trauma
- Neoplasia
- Urolithiasis
- Ectopic ureter
- Cystitis

Treatment

- There is no specific therapy for neurogenic incontinence.
- If primary disease predisposes the horse to incontinence (e.g., EHV-1 myelitis, equine protozoal myeloencephalitis, or urolithiasis), appropriate therapy should be undertaken. Of the primary diseases predisposing to urinary incontinence, EHV-1 myelitis has one of the best prognoses for return of appropriate bladder function.
- Symptomatic therapy involves manual expression of the bladder per rectum three to four times per day. Soft Foley catheters with inflatable cuffs can be inserted into the bladder, although the presence of the catheter is likely to be irritating and increase the chance of local infection.
- Empirical pharmacologic therapy involves phenoxybenzamine (0.6–1.0 mg/kg PO q6–8h) (Dibenzyline, Smith Kline Beecham, Philadelphia, PA) and bethanechol (0.02–0.08 mg/kg SC q8h, titrated for the patient) (Urecholine, Merck Sharp and Dohme, West Point, PA). These treatments appear to have most benefit in horses with EHV-1 myelitis and neuritis of the cauda equina. Possible, yet rare, side effects of treatment include penile relaxation, sedation, sweating, and abdominal pain.

KEY POINT ▶ Pharmacologic therapy must be instituted early in the syndrome to prevent the onset of severe bladder-wall contractile dysfunction.

Urolithiasis (Urinary Calculi)

Calculi can form at many levels of the urinary tract, including the kidneys, ureters, bladder, and urethra. Although urolithiasis is not common, when clinical manifestations occur, they are usually associated with urinary tract obstruction.

Factors Affecting the Incidence of Urolithiasis

KEY POINT ▶ Calculi in the bladder and urethra are more common causes of urinary tract obstruction in males, due to the narrow urethra, when compared with females.

- The short, large-diameter urethra of the mare generally allows natural evacuation of all but the largest cystic calculi.
- Stallions and geldings have a long urethra that narrows at the ischial arch.
- Many factors affect the formation of urinary calculi, including the following:

Urinary Constituents—Alkaline pH, high incidence of crystalluria, high concentration of mucoprotein, high mineral content (e.g., calcium carbonate), combination of desquamated epithelial cells and mucous clots may serve as a nidus for urolith formation.

Diet—Consumption of feed and water high in mineral content may predispose to cystic calculi.

Other Factors—Urine stasis, decreased water intake, bacterial infections.

Types of Calculi

The most common types of calculi are composed of calcium carbonate in various hydrated forms. At times calculi also will be composed of magnesium, ammonium, and phosphate. Calculi have two common appearances: (1) a rough spiculated type that is moderately friable, with a yellow-brown color, usually oval or irregularly shaped, and (2) smooth, round to oval, and white. Calculi range in size from 0.5 to more than 20 cm and in weight from a few grams to more than 5 kg.

Nephrolithiasis and Ureterolithiasis

The incidence of calculi in the kidney or ureter is low. When calculi do occur, there are often nonspecific clinical manifestations.

History and Presenting Signs

- Usually in adults (>3 years old)
- Weight loss may be reported.
- Poor performance
- Nonspecific hindlimb lameness
- Back pain
- Inappetence

Clinical Findings and Diagnosis

- The horse may be in relatively poor condition.
- Oral ulcerations and dental tartar may be present.
- Serum biochemistry often reveals azotemia (increased SUN and SCr), a reflection of renal failure. If chronic renal failure has occurred, hypochloremia, hyponatremia, alterations in calcium and phosphorus concentrations, and anemia may occur.
- Urinalysis demonstrates hematuria, proteinuria, and at times pyuria and cellular or protein casts.
- Rectal examination may reveal a dilated ureter or the presence of a calculus in the ureter.
- Ultrasound examination (transabdominal and per rectum) is useful to reveal the size and consistency of the kidney and also to indicate the presence of nephroliths in the renal pelvis.

KEY POINT ▶ If a nephrolith is identified, the contralateral kidney should always be examined.

- Cystoscopy may be used to indicate the patency of the upper urinary tract. The ureteral openings are visualized, and the normal pulsatile discharge of urine (1 to 2 times per minute) is looked for.
- Diagnosis is based on clinical signs and laboratory, ultrasound, and cystoscopic examination results.

Differential Diagnosis

- Cystic calculi
- Urethral calculi
- Other causes of urinary tract obstruction
- Other causes of colic
- Acute renal failure
- Chronic renal failure
- Bladder atony
- Other causes of weight loss (e.g., malabsorption syndromes, internal parasites)
- Pleural effusion
- Laminitis

Treatment

Treatment is difficult and often unrewarding. In cases where nephroliths are found as an incidental finding on ultrasound examination and the horse has no obvious evidence of renal dysfunction, continued observation is likely to be the best course of action. Techniques for the surgical removal of nephroliths are described. However, if chronic renal failure is present, removal of the urolith is unlikely to improve the long-term prognosis for the horse. In valuable animals or those with only limited evidence of impaired renal dysfunction, referral for surgery is an option.

▶ Cystic Calculi (Bladder Calculi)

KEY POINT ▶ Cystic calculus is the most common form of urolithiasis.

Clinical manifestations are more common in stallions and geldings than in mares for the reasons outlined above. Identification of cystic calculi can be an incidental finding during rectal examination. When clinical manifestations occur, they can be dramatic and consistent with urinary obstruction. These clinical signs are described below.

History and Presenting Signs

- More common in stallions and geldings
- Adult horses (>3 years old)
- Restlessness and evidence of colic
- Frequent attempts to urinate
- Small amounts or no urine passed
- Relaxation of the penis and adoption of an unusual stance when attempting to urinate.
- Discolored urine
- Lameness/stilted hindlimb gait

Clinical Findings and Diagnosis

- The signs are often nonspecific and similar to those demonstrated by horses with other causes of abdominal pain.

KEY POINT ► Dysuria, straining to urinate (stranguria), and increased frequency of urination (pollakiuria) are common.

- Urine scalding on the hindlimbs in the male and perineum in the mare may occur.
- Blood at the urethral orifice may be noticeable. At times, gross hematuria is evident, particularly after exercise and toward the end of urination. Microscopic hematuria is always present.
- Maintenance of the stance adopted for urination for protracted periods may be observed. The horse may strain, grunt, and appear anxious during these periods.

KEY POINT ► Diagnosis is based on rectal examination, which usually reveals a large, firm mass within the lumen of the bladder.

- If the bladder is distended with urine, it is necessary to pass a urinary catheter to evacuate the urine. Following catheterization, the bladder is again palpated per rectum.
- Ultrasound examination (per rectum) and cystoscopy will provide additional diagnostic information. Endoscopy helps define the size, shape, and number of calculi and the integrity of the bladder mucosa.
- Complications occurring with urethral calculi include persistent cystitis (p. 300), pyelonephritis (p. 303), rupture of the urinary bladder (p. 307), and bladder atony (p. 308).

Differential Diagnosis

- Nephrolithiasis, ureterolithiasis
- Urethral calculi
- Other causes of urinary tract obstruction (e.g., smegma accumulation)
- Other causes of colic
- Acute renal failure
- Chronic renal failure
- Bladder atony
- Other causes of weight loss (e.g., malabsorption syndromes, internal parasites)
- Pleural effusion
- Laminitis
- Myopathies

Treatment

- In the first instance, emptying of the bladder is important to reduce the possibility of rupture. This is done by the passage of a urinary catheter. This process may be difficult if the urolith is lodged in the outflow tract or urethra.
- In stallions or geldings, surgical correction by cystotomy under general anesthesia or pelvic urethrostomy subsequent to epidural anesthesia may be used. Referral to a university or well-equipped surgical referral clinic should always be considered an appropriate option. In mares, smaller calculi can, at times, be removed manually via the urethra. The mare is restrained in stocks, sedated with xylazine (Treatment No. 108) or detomidine (Treatment No. 28), and epidural anesthesia is induced with xylazine (see Chap. 7). The vagina is rinsed with appropriate disinfectant, and the surgeon's lubricated gloved hand is inserted into the urethra. The urethra is dilated sufficiently to allow the insertion of a lithotrite or grasping forceps. With large calculi, the lithotrite is used to break the calculus into small pieces to aid removal. The forceps can be better manipulated if the operator has his or her other hand in the rectum and on the bladder. If greater access is required, a dorsal urethral sphincterotomy can be performed. Following removal of the calculus, the bladder is rinsed using large volumes of saline to remove any residual fragments or debris, and the sphincterotomy is sutured (if performed).
- Postoperatively, the horse should be administered antibiotics (e.g., trimethoprim–sulfadiazine 15–20 mg/kg of the combination PO q12h; Treatment No. 107) for 5 to 7 days. Water intake and, therefore, urine output should be increased by feeding a diet rich in salt (30–60 g added to the feed morning and night) for approximately 2 weeks.

► Urethral Calculi

Urethral calculi are encountered almost exclusively in stallions and geldings owing to the long urethra that narrows near the ischial arch. The most common sites for obstruction are the pelvic or distal portions of the urethra.

History and Presenting Signs

- Males
- Adults (>3 years old)
- Similar signs to those described for cystic calculi

Clinical Findings and Diagnosis

- The signs are often nonspecific and similar to those seen in horses with cystic calculi (p. 310).

KEY POINT ► Dysuria, pollakiuria (frequent passage of urine), and stranguria (straining to urinate) are common.

- If the obstruction is complete, anuria will occur, but if it is partial, small amounts of urine may be voided. This urine is often discolored (red-brown) with obvious or microscopic hematuria.
- Blood draining from the external urethral orifice may be seen.

- Standing as if attempting to urinate for protracted periods. The horse may strain, grunt, and appear anxious during these periods.
- Rectal examination reveals a large, tense bladder (if it is not ruptured).

KEY POINT ▶ Diagnosis is based on the history, clinical signs, palpation of the urethra per rectum and percutaneously, by the passage of a urinary catheter (an obstruction to continued passage is met), and possibly by endoscopic examination.

- Complete obstruction eventually leads to rupture of the bladder (p. 307).

Differential Diagnosis

- Nephrolithiasis, ureterolithiasis
- Other causes of urinary tract obstruction (e.g., smegma accumulation)
- Other causes of colic
- Acute renal failure
- Chronic renal failure
- Bladder atony
- Other causes of weight loss (e.g., malabsorption syndromes, internal parasites)
- Pleural effusion
- Laminitis
- Myopathies

Treatment

- Given the risk of bladder rupture, correction of urethroliasis should be considered an emergency.
- Calculi in the distal urethra can often be expressed manually or by an incision through the median raphe over the calculus. This procedure is usually performed under general anesthesia and in dorsal recumbency to ensure patient compliance, to improve urethral relaxation, and to decrease the risk to the attending clinician. Following removal of the calculus, the wound is sutured or allowed to heal by second intention.
- Calculi lodged near the ischium can be removed via an ischial urethrostomy. This is performed in the standing horse following sedation with xylazine (Treatment No. 108) or detomidine (Treatment No. 28), and induction of epidural anesthesia with xylazine (see Chap. 7). A catheter is passed into the urethra to aid in location of the calculus and identification of the urethra. The skin over the urethra is prepared for surgery, and an incision into the urethral lumen is made. Once entered, the lumen is dilated to allow passage of a grasping forceps or lithotrite. The calculus is then removed while flushing saline into the urethra to assist with lubrication or is crushed with the lithotrite and the pieces removed. Care must be exercised during this procedure to avoid rupturing the urethra. Following removal of the cal-

culus, the bladder is emptied and flushed with water to remove fragments and debris. Endoscopy can then be performed to gain an estimate of any damage to the urethra and bladder.

- Following removal, the urethra is sutured or allowed to heal by second intention.
- Postoperative management is similar to that described for cystic calculi (p. 310).
- Acidification of the urine is indicated to prevent further formation of urinary calculi, but this is difficult to achieve.
- Complications include ruptured bladder or urethra, postobstruction urethral scar formation leading to subsequent obstruction, urethral diverticulum or fistula, persistent cystitis, and pyelonephritis.

References

Adams, R., and McClure, J. J.: Acute renal dysfunction: A review of 38 equine cases and discussion of diagnostic parameters. *Proc. 31st Annu. Conv. Am. Assoc. Equine Pract.*, 1985, p. 635.

Bayly, W.: A practitioner's approach to the diagnosis and treatment of renal failure in horses. *Vet. Med.* 86:632, 1991.

Behm, R. J., and Berg, I. E.: Hematuria caused by renal medullary crest necrosis in a horse. *Compend. Contin. Educ. Pract. Vet.* 9:698, 1987.

Crabbe, B. G., and Grant, B. D.: Complications secondary to a chronic urocystolith. *Equine Pract.* 13:8, 1991.

Crabbe, B. G., Bohn, A. A., and Grant, B. D.: Equine urocystoliths. *Equine Pract.* 13:12, 1991.

Divers, T. J.: Management of chronic renal failure in the horse. *Proc. 31st Annu. Conv. Am. Assoc. Equine Pract.*, 1985, p. 679.

Divers, T. J.: Treatment of acute renal failure in the horse. *Proc. 31st Annu. Conv. Am. Assoc. Equine Pract.*, 1985, p. 673.

Divers, T. J.: Nephrolithiasis and ureterolithiasis in horses and their association with renal disease and failure. *Equine Vet. J.* 21:161, 1989.

Divers, T. J., Whitlock, R. H., Byars, T. D., et al.: Acute renal failure in six horses resulting from hemodynamic causes. *Equine Vet. J.* 19:178, 1987.

Ehnen, S. J., Divers, T. J., Gillette, D., and Reef, V. B.: Obstructive nephrolithiasis and ureterolithiasis associated with chronic renal failure in horses: Eight cases (1981–1987). *J. Am. Vet. Med. Assoc.* 197:249, 1990.

Genetzky, R. M., Loparco, F. V., and Ledet, A. E.: Clinical pathologic alterations in horses during a water deprivation test. *Am. J. Vet. Res.* 48:1007, 1987.

Harris, P.: Collection of urine. *Equine Vet. J.* 20:86, 1988.

Kiper, M. L., Traub-Dargatz, J. L., and Wrigley, R. H.: Renal ultrasonography in horses. *Compend. Contin. Educ. Pract. Vet.* 12:993, 1990.

Mair, T. S., and Osborn, R. S.: The crystalline composition of normal equine urine deposits. *Equine Vet. J.* 22:364, 1990.

McCue, P. M., Brooks, P. A., and Wilson, W. D.: Urinary bladder rupture as a sequela to obstructive urethral calculi. *Vet. Med.* 84:912, 1989.

Penninck, D. G., Eisenberg, H. M., Teuscher, E. E., and Vrins, A.: Equine renal ultrasonography: Normal and abnormal. *Vet. Radiol.* 27:81, 1987.

Schmitz, D. G.: Toxic nephropathy in horses. *Compend. Contin. Educ. Pract. Vet.* 10:104, 1988.

Schmitz, D. G., and Green, R. A.: Effects of water deprivation and phenylbutazone administration on urinary enzyme concentrations in healthy horses. *Proc. 33d Annu. Conv. Am. Assoc. Equine Pract.,* 1987, p. 103.

Tennant, B., Dill, S. G., Rebhun, W. C., and King, J. M.: Pathophysiology of renal failure in the horse. *Proc. 31st Annu. Conv. Am. Assoc. Equine Pract.,* 1985, p. 627.

Weckman, T. J., Wood, T., Henry, P. A., et al.: Equine urine pH: Normal population distributions and methods of acidification. *Equine Vet. J.* 22:118, 1990.

Ziemer, E. L., Parker, H. R., Carlson, G. P., and Smith, B. P.: Clinical features and treatment of renal tubular acidosis in two horses. *J. Am. Vet. Med. Assoc.* 190:294, 1987.

Ophthalmology

Eye diseases are relatively common in equine practice, with traumatic and infectious problems being found most frequently. Many procedures and some of the diagnostic techniques are beyond the scope of the general equine practitioner, and there are increasing numbers of veterinary ophthalmologists available for the more complex problems. However, most common problems affecting the eye can be dealt with by the majority of practitioners. Once again, good history taking, a detailed physical examination, and use of appropriate diagnostic aids are the keys to successful diagnosis and therapy.

EXAMINATION OF THE EYE

History

The history collected will depend on the presenting problem. A presenting sign such as excessive lacrimation will tend to indicate the likelihood of trauma or infectious disease, whereas complaints about visual acuity may not allow easy classification of the disorder. Questions that can be useful in eye disease include

- Is there a problem with the horse's vision?
- Is the problem acute or insidious in onset?
- Is the problem improving or deteriorating?
- Is the problem unilateral or bilateral?
- Was there a specific incident (e.g., trauma) associated with the problem?
- Has there been any ocular discharge?
- Has the owner or trainer noticed any abnormalities in either eye?
- Is there evidence of pain (photophobia, blepharospasm)?

Physical Examination

KEY POINT ▶ While the initial part of the eye examination can be completed in normal light, a detailed eye examination is only possible in a darkened room.

Small changes in the eye may be significant, and a careful and detailed examination is important if the significance of minor abnormalities is to be accurately assessed.

Light Room: General Examination

This phase of the examination is important because it allows a rational decision to be made regarding special procedures needed to completely evaluate the problem. Evaluation of the eye and associated structures is enhanced if magnifying spectacles are used. The nature of the ocular tissues involved, severity, and clinical approach to the workup can be assessed quickly. If there is a history of any visual impairment, the pupillary light reflex and menace response should be tested. Signs to evaluate include the following:

Pupil Size. Look for abnormalities in size and shape. If doubt exists, compare with the opposite eye.

Presence of Periorbital Swelling. Detection of periorbital swelling is of considerable clinical relevance. Swelling can be caused by a wide variety of conditions, such as trauma, inflammation, and neoplasia. In some cases, the degree of periorbital swelling may be slight and easily missed without a careful examination.

Ocular Discharge. Is there epiphora, inflammatory transudate or exudate, or reflux nasolacrimal drainage?

Epiphora. Is the discharge of normal tears out of the palpebral fissure as a result of increased production and/or altered lid conformation preventing drainage.

KEY POINT ▶ Epiphora is quite common with most eye problems that produce pain and is not specific for a particular disease.

Inflammatory Transudate or Exudate. Indicates a nonspecific process that begins to develop within hours after an injury. Pain associated with blunt trauma to the adnexal tissues, corneal disease, or uveitis can result in this type of reaction. Cytologically, neutrophils will predominate, and microorganisms may not be present.

Reflux Nasolacrimal Drainage. Nasolacrimal duct obstruction is common and can mimic discharge associated with diseases of the eye and adnexa. This possibility should be evaluated prior to assuming that the problem is related to the globe or the conjunctiva.

Change in Size of the Globe. Globe size can often be evaluated by standing in front of the horse and noting the degree of protrusion of the globe of the eye and whether there is symmetry. The main disorder is:

Phthisis Bulbi (Shrunken Eye)—Is detected as a sunken appearance of the globe and is a common sequela to recurrent uveitis.

KEY POINT ► If there is evidence of eyelid trauma, tumors, conjunctivitis, corneal trauma, or inflammatory ocular discharge, always examine behind the third eyelid and in the conjunctival fornices for possible lesions. Topical anesthesia is required.

Dark Room: Detailed Examination

To conduct a detailed examination of the eyes, a pen light and focal light source is needed together with an ophthalmoscope to permit examination of structures deeper to the cornea.

KEY POINT ► It may be necessary to induce mydriasis using 1% tropicamide (Mydriacyl, Alcon, Fort Worth, TX) to enable examination of deeper parts of the eye.

A systematic examination is required, working from the anterior to the posterior part of the eye. Apart from the cornea, which can be examined using a pen light and/or magnifying spectacles to assess abnormalities, an ophthalmoscope is necessary.

Cornea—Corneal trauma is a very common clinical problem, and a pen light and/or magnifying spectacles can be used to illuminate the eye from the side, which aids observation. The superficial and deeper corneal layers should be evaluated for foreign bodies, punctures, ulcers, lacerations, stromal abscess formation, or edema (epithelial or endothelial origin).

Anterior Segment—The main structures to be examined are the anterior chamber and iris. Evaluation for foreign bodies, abnormal contents, evidence of uveitis or synechiae, should be made.

Posterior Segment—The lens can be assessed by detection of the Purkinje images by using a focal light and moving it from side to side so that images

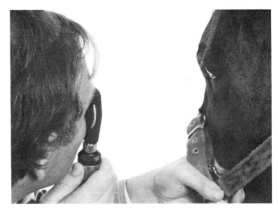

Figure 10–1. Position of the examiner for ophthalmoscopic examination of the eye.

can be seen from the cornea and lens. The lens images move in opposite directions, one image (from the convex surface) moving the same way as the corneal image and the other (from the concave surface) moving in the opposite direction. If there is cataract formation, there will be loss of one or both of the lens images, depending on the site of the cataract.

Fundus and Optic Disc—To assess the fundus, the direct ophthalmoscope is usually set on −3 diopters and the observer moves to within 12 to 15 cm (6 in) of the horse's eye (Fig. 10-1). The optic disc can be seen at the junction of the tapetal and nontapetal fundus (Fig. 10-2).

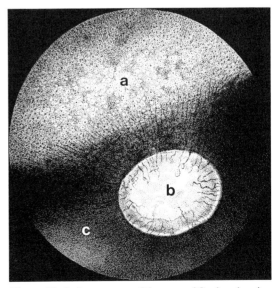

Figure 10–2. Appearance of the normal fundus showing the tapetal fundus (a), optic disk (b), and non-tapetal fundus (c).

DIAGNOSTIC AIDS

Chemical Restraint for Examination of the Eyes

If the horse is reluctant to allow adequate examination, some form of chemical restraint is essential, but it may be augmented with regional anesthetic blocks. A number of agents can be used (see Sedatives, Chap. 17), but we have found the following to be useful:

Xylazine—0.3 to 0.6 mg/kg IV is suitable for most nonpainful or minimally painful situations where minor restraint is required.

Xylazine + Butorphanol—0.2 to 0.5 mg/kg xylazine is given 2 to 3 minutes prior to administration of 0.03 to 0.08 mg/kg butorphanol. This combination provides excellent analgesia and may be useful for examination of the eye when there is significant pain.

Auriculopalpebral Nerve Block

KEY POINT ▶ Blepharospasm associated with ocular pain or examination can be reduced or eliminated by the use of an auriculopalpebral block.

While the block does not produce analgesia, the absence of motor movement of the upper eyelid is often of great assistance in enabling a detailed examination. The nerve block is performed using 4 to 6 ml of one of the local anesthetics (2% lidocaine, prilocaine, or mepivicaine). The nerve runs superficially and can be palpated over the highest point of the zygomatic arch, where the needle is inserted subcutaneously (Fig. 10-3). We use a 23-gauge, 15-mm (5/8-in) needle for the injection. Akinesia of the upper eyelid usually follows within 10 minutes of the local anesthetic injection.

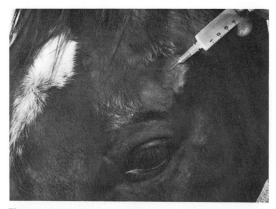

Figure 10–3. Auriculopalpebral nerve block. The needle is inserted at the highest point of the zygomatic arch, where the nerve can be palpated running subcutaneously. About 5 ml of 2% local anesthetic is injected to produce akinesia of the upper eyelid.

Frontal Nerve Block

The frontal nerve innervates the upper eyelid (which causes the most problems with examination interference). If desensitization is required (e.g., placing a subpalpebral lavage system), the nerve is easily blocked by infiltrating 3 to 4 ml of 2% local anesthetic into the supraorbital foramen (Fig. 10-4), into the supraorbital process of the frontal bone, or along the central portion of the dorsal orbital rim (this last location also will block a portion of the palpebral nerves).

Topical Anesthesia

Topical anesthesia is useful for some examinations, for collecting samples, for subpalpebral lavage, and for subconjunctival injections. The topical anesthetic of choice is 0.5% proxymetacaine (proparacaine) (Ophthaine HCl, Squibb, Princeton, NJ) applied as shown in Figure 10-5. Four to 5 drops of local anesthetic are applied to the eye, and after a period of 1 to 2 minutes, a further 2 to 3

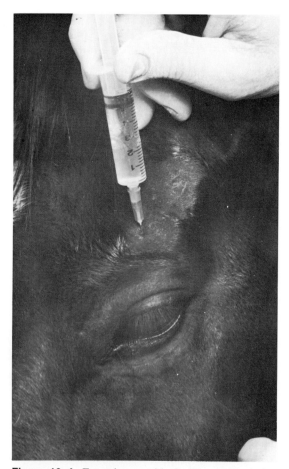

Figure 10–4. Frontal nerve block. The needle is inserted into the depression of the supraorbital foramen, which can be palpated at the dorsal aspect of the orbit.

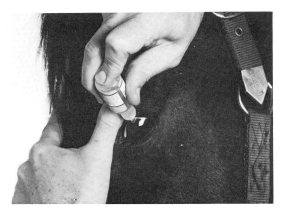

Figure 10–5. Application of topical local anesthetic drops for desensitizing the surface of the eye and conjunctiva.

drops are given. Analgesia occurs after approximately 5 minutes.

Culture and Sensitivity Testing

Corneal and Conjunctival Cultures and Cytology

While many equine practitioners do not routinely undertake cytology and bacterial cultures when there is suspected infectious eye disease, it is good clinical practice and will optimize therapy.

KEY POINT ▶ Cultures can be taken from the surfaces of the cornea, conjunctiva, and eyelid margins.

This is generally done by using a moist swab or a sterile scalpel blade and obtaining necrotic material from the edges of ulcers or from inflamed conjunctiva. In horses that have had prior antimicrobial therapy, fungal infection may be a possibility, and therefore, cytologic examination and fungal culture could be indicated.

Cytologic findings that are of significance include:

Eosinophils—These may indicate allergy or parasites (onchocerca, habronema).

Neutrophils—Usually signify acute or chronic inflammation.

Mononuclear Cells—Indicate antigenic stimulation or chronicity.

Bacteria—Large numbers are uncommon, but there could be a few scattered ones found on the normal eye. Large numbers of bacteria indicate infection.

Fungal Hyphae—A few may be present in the tear film, but they should not be found within the corneal tissue; hyphae often retain Giemsa stains poorly.

Anterior Chamber Paracentesis

The aqueous humor may be cultured by anterior chamber paracentesis, but this is seldom necessary and is indicated only in eye problems where the prognosis for vision is guarded. The procedure is usually reserved for deep-seated corneal infections or endophthalmitis. Good restraint or light anesthesia (xylazine + ketamine, see Chap. 17, General Anesthesia) is necessary for the procedure to be carried out. After heavy tranquilization, an auriculopalpebral block, and topical local anesthesia, a 25-gauge, 15-mm (5/8-in) needle attached to a 2-ml syringe is inserted into the cornea at the limbal region. Material is aspirated and subjected to cytologic and bacteriologic examination (see Chap. 15). After removal of the needle from the eye, pressure should be maintained at the puncture site for a few minutes to prevent leakage of aqueous humor.

Patency of the Nasolacrimal System

There are two methods for determination of nasolacrimal duct patency:

Fluorescein Passage—A normal fluorescein strip is used under the eyelid. About 15 to 30 minutes later, the distal punctum of the duct is examined for presence of dye. This test checks physiologic patency of the duct.

Mechanical Flushing—Is achieved using a small-gauge intravenous catheter (16- to 18-gauge) or tomcat catheter inserted into the distal punctum of the duct (Fig. 10-6). Topical anesthesia with lidocaine spray (4%) is useful for permitting introduction of the catheter so that saline can be flushed retrograde and the anatomic patency of the duct can be checked.

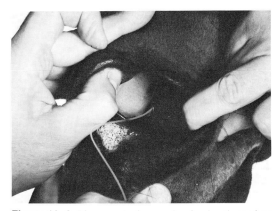

Figure 10–6. Placement of a nasolacrimal catheter into the distal punctum of the nasolacrimal duct of the left nostril.

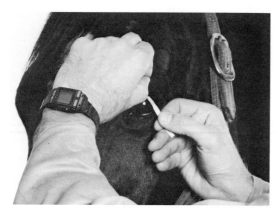

Figure 10–7. Application of a fluorescein strip for staining a corneal ulcer.

Fluorescein Staining

KEY POINT ► If there is a possibility of a corneal ulcer, fluorescein strips can be used to define the extent of the ulcer.

After moistening with local anesthetic, the strip is inserted under the eyelid, as shown in Figure 10-7. Excess dye is flushed from the eye using normal saline. If there is an interruption to the corneal epithelium, fluorescein stain is taken up by the ulcer, as is shown in Figure 10-8.

KEY POINT ► With some deep ulcers, dye may not be retained.

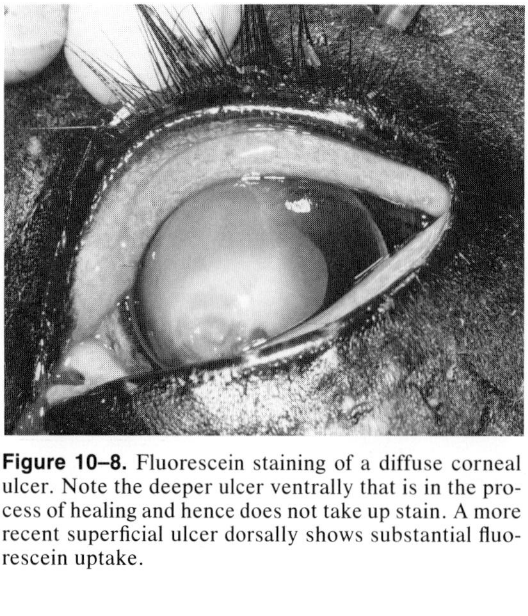

TECHNIQUES FOR OCULAR THERAPY
Subpalpebral Lavage

KEY POINT ► Because many eye conditions require frequent topical therapy, a subpalpebral system allows drugs to be administered without the need to put pressure on an already painful eye.

We find that the insertion of Silastic tubing (Dow Corning) for subpalpebral lavage results in less irritation to the eye than other materials. Subpalpebral lavage tubing can be placed under local anesthesia and tranquilization, but in our experience, it is best performed under general anesthesia. The tubing can be placed via a large-bore needle inserted as far dorsally as possible under the upper eyelid. A series of holes made in the tubing prior to placement lies underneath the eyelid, and the tubing emerges dorsal to the medial canthus. This end of the tubing is blocked, and the tubing is sutured in place (Fig. 10-9) or fixed in position using Superglue or Crazy-Glue. It is important that the tubing be placed as far dorsally as possible to prevent irritation to the cornea and further ulceration.

Nasolacrimal Lavage

KEY POINT ► An alternative to subpalpebral lavage is placement of a fine-gauge catheter (Equine Nasolacrimal Cannula, Jorgensen Laboratories, Loveland, CO) via the distal nasolacrimal punctum (see Fig. 10-6) to enable the frequent administration of medications.

Figure 10–8. Fluorescein staining of a diffuse corneal ulcer. Note the deeper ulcer ventrally that is in the process of healing and hence does not take up stain. A more recent superficial ulcer dorsally shows substantial fluorescein uptake.

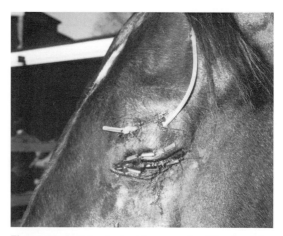

Figure 10–9. Subpalpebral lavage using Silastic tubing to enable medication to be administered for a corneal ulcer. Note that a tarsorrhaphy has been performed with bolster sutures placed over the eyelids.

To maintain it in position, we find it useful to take the nasolacrimal catheter through the false nostril prior to insertion into the distal punctum. The nasolacrimal lavage system is less easily maintained than the subpalpebral lavage system because it is more easily dislodged and may become blocked. However, it is more easily placed in the sedated horse.

Nasolacrimal lavage also may be required when the nasolacrimal duct becomes blocked. Mostly this occurs secondary to corneal and conjunctival inflammation and is characterized by excess lacrimation. The majority of cases can be treated by flushing the nasolacrimal duct via the distal punctum, as described above.

Subconjunctival Injection

KEY POINT ▶ The most common medications administered by subconjunctival injection are the long-acting corticosteroids such as betamethasone acetate (Treatment No. 12) and methylprednisolone acetate (Treatment No. 74).

After topical anesthesia and an auriculopalpebral nerve block, a 23- or 25-gauge, 15-mm (5/8-in) needle is introduced under the dorsal bulbar conjunctiva, and an appropriate dose of corticosteroids is injected. No more than 0.5 ml of the particular preparation should be used. The dorsal bulbar conjunctiva is the best site for subconjunctival injection, but this is often difficult to perform. We have found subpalpebral injection in the conjunctiva of

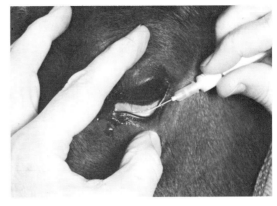

Figure 10–10. Subconjunctival injection of a long-acting corticosteroid. This site is not ideal but is simpler than injection into the dorsal bulbar conjunctiva.

the lower eyelid is a satisfactory alternative (Fig. 10-10).

KEY POINT ▶ Subconjunctival injection of corticosteroids is contraindicated unless corneal injury and infection have been ruled out.

On some occasions (keratitis), it may be useful to inject antibiotics subconjunctivally. The antibiotic selected should be based on initial cytology and culture results. Gentamicin sulfate (20–30 mg) is probably the first choice of the antibiotics that can be used. Cephalosporins also have been used at doses around 100 mg for a single treatment.

Diseases of the Eyelids

Entropion

KEY POINT ▶ Entropion is a relatively common and self-correcting disorder in foals.

It may be bilateral or unilateral and usually produces signs of ocular irritation within a few days of birth.

History and Presenting Signs

- Excess lacrimation
- Blepharospasm
- Photophobia

Clinical Findings and Diagnosis

- Any young foal with the presenting signs detailed above should be suspected of having entropion.
- Close examination of the eye will reveal inversion of the lower eyelid(s) margin.
- In some cases there may be corneal ulceration from abrasion due to the eyelashes.

Differential Diagnosis

- Keratitis
- Conjunctivitis
- Trauma

Treatment

KEY POINT ▶ Most cases resolve with conservative therapy, which may be as simple as eversion of the lower eyelid margin and use of antibacterial eye ointment if there is corneal ulceration.

- In more severe cases, mechanical eversion of the eyelid margin is required. This can be performed using saline or local anesthetic injected subcutaneously. Alternatively, skin staples may be used to evert the eyelid.
- Surgical correction of entropion is seldom required.

Eyelid Lacerations

Eyelid lacerations are very common because horses tend to rub their eyes on fences, feed bins, and other objects that result in trauma.

KEY POINT ▶ While many lacerations appear quite severe, because of the good blood supply, most will heal with appropriate treatment.

It is important that all vital tissue be preserved and that wound debridement be kept to a minimum to prevent distortion of the eyelid. The major objective is anatomic realignment of the tissues so that distortion of the eyelids does not occur.

History and Presenting Sign

- Obvious trauma

Clinical Findings and Diagnosis

- Diagnosis is not a problem with eyelid lacerations, but assessment of the extent of the laceration and decisions regarding treatment are critical to a cosmetic result.
- Profound sedation is required for assessment and treatment, and we often use a combination of xylazine (0.5 mg/kg) and butorphanol (0.05 mg/kg) given IV (see Chap. 17). If there is difficulty in restraint, xylazine + ketamine anesthesia or "triple-drip anesthesia" (see Chap. 17) may be required.

Differential Diagnosis

- Assessment of any corneal trauma

Treatment

Medication

- Systemic anti-inflammatory therapy is useful. The object is to promote wound healing, so corticosteroids are avoided. Nonsteroidal preparations given orally are helpful (e.g., phenylbutazone 4.4 mg/kg q12h for 3 to 5 days) to prevent extensive swelling.
- Systemic antibiotics are indicated, but probably are not entirely necessary. If antibiotics are needed, it would be preferred to treat systemically rather than topically because of the risk that the owner or trainer may injure the repaired tissue with their attempts to medicate.

- Topical antibiotics can be applied at the time of repair, but they should be used with caution.
- Tetanus prophylaxis is essential, as for any wound.

Repair
- Skin preparation is necessary because the skin is frequently contaminated but not actually infected. Saline lavage is the preparation of choice. All topical disinfectants should be avoided because of the tissue irritation they can cause.
- If there is evidence of local infection, it is possible to disinfect with dilute povidone-iodine (1 part povidone-iodine to 3 parts saline for the skin; 1 part povidone-iodine to 19 parts saline for the conjunctiva and cornea) (Treatment No. 91); irrigate and use a gentle rubbing action to clean the tissues for 2 to 3 minutes and then soak the tissues with a cotton or gauze pad for 2 to 3 minutes.
- Repair should involve minimal wound debridement; freshen the edges only.

KEY POINT ▶ Do not remove skin unless absolutely necessary.

- Close the wound precisely in at least two layers for greater strength than possible with only skin sutures. The conjunctiva does not require suturing, and 3-0 to 5-0 suture material should be used in the subcutaneous tissue (if necessary) and the skin. We prefer monofilament absorbable material such as polyglactin (PDS, Ethicon).
- If the wound is more than 24 hours old, local infection is usually present, along with substantial swelling. It is necessary in these cases to apply a topical water-soluble disinfectant under a bandage for 12 to 24 hours. When the bandage is removed, there is usually remarkable improvement in the appearance of the tissue, at which time surgical repair is possible.

Habronemiasis

Habronema infestation (see Chap. 12) is common around the eyelid margins, involving the eyelids and conjunctiva. Lesions are found most commonly near the medial canthus of the eye.

History and Presenting Signs
- Typical granulomatous lesions near eyelids
- Usually in summer

Clinical Findings and Diagnosis

KEY POINT ▶ Typical habronemiasis results in granulomatous reactions, with the lesions having a caseous appearance.

- It is quite common to find lesions in a number of sites, particularly the preputial area in geldings and stallions.

- Habronemiasis has a typical appearance, and biopsy samples are seldom required, unless there is concern about the possibility of neoplasia.

Differential Diagnosis
- Sarcoid
- Squamous cell carcinoma

Treatment

KEY POINT ▶ Ivermectin is effective in the treatment of most lesions when given orally at a dose rate of 0.2 mg/kg [10 ml Eqvalan (MSD-Agvet, Rahway, NJ) liquid or appropriate volume of paste per 500 kg of body weight].

- The host response to dying larvae is sometimes quite dramatic, with severe irritation being present. In these cases, topical ophthalmic corticosteroid drops should be used.
- Some chronic lesions with extensive fibrous tissue formation may require surgical excision to achieve a cosmetic result.

Sarcoid

KEY POINT ▶ Any mass around the eye should be suspected of being a sarcoid.

Further material on sarcoids is provided in Chapter 12.

History and Presenting Sign

Slowly progressive enlargement of a mass or masses close to the eye

Clinical Findings and Diagnosis
- Raised mass of tissue that is either covered with epithelium or appears similar to granulation tissue.
- Biopsy may be required to distinguish this tumor from squamous cell carcinoma. However, with most sarcoids, there is seldom any ulceration.

Differential Diagnosis
- Habronemiasis
- Squamous cell carcinoma
- Viral papillomatosis
- Trauma

Treatment
- Cryosurgery has been used with some success, but great care is required because of the possibility of damaging the cornea by freezing. Lesions should be frozen to −20°C, and three freeze–thaw cycles should be used.

KEY POINT ► Immunotherapy is most successful in our experience, and the injection of a mycobacterial cell-wall extract (Equimune, Vetrepharm, Athens, GA) into the base of the lesion has given excellent results.

- The dose that we have used is 1 ml/cm³ of tissue. The lesion is debulked prior to injection, and the volume of the tissue remaining is estimated so that an appropriate volume of solution is injected.
- Repeated injections every 2 to 3 weeks may be required for successful therapy. Subsequent injections tend to promote a more profound local inflammatory response 24 to 48 hours after injection. In these cases, systemic administration of flunixin (Treatment No. 52) at a dose rate of 1 mg/kg is indicated.

Squamous Cell Carcinoma

KEY POINT ► Squamous cell carcinoma is one of the two most common forms of neoplasia involving the eyelids, including the nictitating membrane, or third eyelid.

Horses most at risk are those with little or no pigment around the eyelids.

History and Presenting Signs

- Ulcerative lesion around the eyelid margins
- Nonpigmented skin at the eyelid margins

Clinical Findings and Diagnosis

- Ulcerative skin lesions close to the eyelid margins are suggestive of squamous cell carcinoma.
- In some cases there is involvement of the third eyelid, and this area should be examined closely by applying pressure on the eyeball through the upper lid to evert the third eyelid.
- A biopsy is essential for diagnosis.

Differential Diagnosis

- Habronemiasis
- Sarcoid
- Trauma

Treatment

- A combination of surgical excision and radiation therapy has proven to provide the best results, in our experience.
- Cryotherapy and immunotherapy with cell-wall extracts are reported to be of value in some cases.
- Removal of the third eyelid is indicated with lesions affecting this site.
- More extensive tumors may require removal of the entire eye.

Diseases of the Cornea and Conjunctiva

Conjunctivitis

Conjunctivitis may be the result of bacterial, viral, or occasionally parasitic infections.

KEY POINT ► Bacterial conjunctivitis is more common than other forms and is most commonly due to gram-positive cocci.

History and Presenting Signs

- Most common in summer with dusty conditions and flies

- Viral respiratory infection
- Enzootic outbreaks may occur.

Clinical Findings and Diagnosis

- Mucopurulent ocular discharge with evidence of inflamed and injected conjunctiva, which may be unilateral or bilateral
- Bacterial culture and sensitivity testing can be done on samples collected from the conjunctiva. There are frequently large numbers of neutrophils and bacteria on cytologic examination.

Fluorescein staining should be undertaken to determine whether there is corneal ulceration and is also helpful in determining whether there is obstruction of the nasolacrimal duct.

- Bacterial conjunctivitis secondary to a blocked nasolacrimal duct is common.

Differential Diagnosis

- Keratitis
- Uveitis
- Habronemiasis
- Squamous cell carcinoma

Treatment

Most cases respond quickly to an antibiotic eye ointment applied every 6 hours.

- The eye ointment of first choice is chloramphenicol 1% (Treatment No. 42) or a neomycin–polymyxin–bacitracin combination (Treatment No. 41).
- Local therapy is indicated with moistened gauze sponges to remove purulent material.
- If the conjunctivitis is secondary to viral respiratory disease, the discharge is usually serous, and no treatment is required.

Corneal Disease: Keratitis, Ulceration

Various forms of traumatic and infectious ocular diseases occur and result in similar clinical signs. Mild corneal abrasions usually heal quickly with minimal treatment. However, deeper abrasions and ulcerations that result from bacterial infection require accurate bacteriologic diagnosis and intensive therapy.

History and Presenting Signs

- Photophobia
- Blepharospasm
- Excess lacrimation
- Purulent ocular discharge

Clinical Findings and Diagnosis

- The presenting signs described are found in a range of ocular diseases and therefore are of no help in making a specific diagnosis.
- Important signs in assessing the extent of the problem and the prognosis include:

  Loss of Transparency—Due to corneal edema

  Vascularization—Is it deep or superficial? Deep vascularization suggests serious intraocular disease.

  Redness—Ciliary injection causes a deep red halo appearance of the perilimbal episclera; conjunctival injection is also very common.

Cellular Deposits—The anterior chamber and cornea are capable of accumulating a large number of neutrophils. Mostly this is a sterile leukotactic response, but it can be septic in some cases.

Ulceration—It is important to determine whether the ulceration is superficial or deep, progressive or static.

Auriculopalpebral and frontal blocks are required to permit examination of the cornea and desensitization for collection of scrapings for cytology as well as bacterial and fungal culture. In some cases, sedation also may be required.

- Fluorescein staining may be required to determine the extent of the ulcer.
- While a number of organisms are involved in corneal ulcers, the most dangerous are *Pseudomonas* spp. because of the rapid progress of the ulcer with ultimate corneal rupture. It is of critical importance to assess the depth of the ulcer, because deeper ulcers may quickly become full-thickness defects and lead to corneal rupture and iris prolapse.
- Examine behind the third eyelid if the presence of a foreign body in that site may be producing keratitis

Differential Diagnosis

- Corneal foreign bodies
- Stromal abscess
- Conjunctivitis
- Severe uveitis

Treatment

Corticosteroids should never be used in the treatment of acute-phase corneal ulcers because of the likelihood of worsening the ulcer and leading to rupture of the cornea.

► Bacterial Keratitis

- *Topical medical therapy* (q6h) is effective for superficial erosions. If complicated, then anticollagenase therapy should be added.
- Infection should be controlled using either gentamicin or tobramycin, unless there is an indication of fungal infection (see Mycotic Keratitis).
- Ocular pain can be managed using a cycloplegic such as atropine (q2h) until there is mydriasis, together with systemic nonsteroidal anti-inflammatory drugs. The agent of choice is flunixin (Treatment No. 52) administered at a dose rate of 1.1 mg/kg (0.5 mg/lb) IV daily.
- Anticollagenase therapy is essential in all serious ulcers due to the production of collagenases by bacteria and local inflammatory cells that can cause rapid corneal rupture, particularly in *Pseudomonas* infections. Agents such as 20% acetyl-

cysteine (Mucomist, Mead Johnson, Evansville, IN) and EDTA plasma have been used successfully in combination with the other parts of therapy. To use EDTA plasma, blood is collected from the horse into EDTA tubes, spun down, and the plasma harvested.

■ In treating corneal ulcers, a nasolacrimal or subpalpebral lavage system should be used to avoid irritation and pain associated with the administration of drops or ointments. In the early stages of treatment, the solution should be given every 2 hours.

KEY POINT ▶ The lavage solution consists of a mixture of the preceding ingredients, and a suggested composition is as follows: 2.6 ml gentamicin sulfate (50 mg/ml) or 3 ml tobramycin (40 mg/ml), 10 ml 20% acetylcysteine, 10 ml 1% atropine ophthalmic solution, and 17 ml artificial tears or hard contact lens wetting solution.

■ After making up this solution, it is stable for at least 1 month.
■ If there is necrotic debris associated with the ulcer, it may be necessary to debride the necrotic material, which can aid in stimulation of healing.
■ Systemic antibiotics may be indicated in severe ulcers or where there are corneal stromal infections.

KEY POINT ▶ In most corneal ulcers, tarsorrhaphy (suturing the eyelids) is

helpful to provide protection for the cornea.

■ However, in more extensive ulcers, either conjunctival or third eyelid flaps should be used. These flaps provide mechanical protection and also a local increase in vascularity.

▶ Mycotic Keratitis

■ Fungal keratitis is uncommon but sometimes is found after topical antibiotic therapy and corticosteroids that have allowed fungi to proliferate.
■ The common fungal species include *Aspergillus* spp., *Penicillium* spp., *Fusarium* spp., and *Alternataria* spp. Similar signs are found as with bacterial keratitis, and diagnosis is made on the basis of cytology (central and peripheral scrapings).
■ Loss of the eye is a common sequela to fungal infection if aggressive therapy is not instituted. Agents that can be considered include amphotericin B, which is quite irritating; natamycin ophthalmic preparation (Treatment No. 45); and miconazole (10 mg/ml) (Treatment No. 46).
■ The cyclopegic, anti-inflammatory, and anticollagenase therapies described above also should be instituted.

KEY POINT ▶ The prognosis for recovery in the case of fungal keratitis is quite poor.

■ Many cases are slow to respond, and rupture of the cornea may occur, often necessitating eye removal.

Uveal Diseases

Diseases of the uveal tract (iris, ciliary body, and choroid) may occur as primary or secondary disorders. Uveitis may occur secondary to severe keratitis but is most common as a primary immune-mediated disorder.

Immune-Mediated Uveitis (Recurrent Uveitis, Periodic Ophthalmia, Moon Blindness)

KEY POINT ▶ Immune-mediated uveitis is the most common uveal disease of horses,

and its recurrent nature can result in progressive loss of vision.

It is the most common cause of blindness, and inciting causes proposed include *Onchocerca* and *Leptospira* spp. In most cases, the cause of the uveitis cannot be determined, but symptomatic treatment is effective, at least in the short term.

History and Presenting Signs

■ Excessive lacrimation
■ Cloudy eye
■ Blepharospasm

Clinical Findings and Diagnosis

- In the acute phase of uveitis, there are signs of intense ocular pain with excessive lacrimation and photophobia.
- A cloudy eye (corneal edema) is a typical finding, and there is usually ciliary and conjunctival injection. In some cases there also may be aqueous flare or even hypopyon, but the latter is unusual. Peripheral corneal vascularization is common.

KEY POINT ▶ Miosis (constricted pupil) is a consistent clinical sign, and careful examination of the iris may show adhesions or synechiae, particularly when there have been several episodes of disease.

- Anterior synechiae are adhesions between the iris and cornea and are relatively easily seen with a light source and magnification. Posterior synechiae, adhesions between the anterior lens and the iris, are slightly more difficult to detect.
- A decrease in globe size is often the result of chronic, immune-mediated uveitis. This results from decreased aqueous humor production and may be detected in some cases by observation, because the eye has a sunken appearance. In other cases, palpation of the globe through the upper eyelid will reveal the decrease in intraocular pressure.
- Cataracts occur in some long-standing cases.

Differential Diagnosis

- Keratitis
- Conjunctivitis
- Septic uveitis
- Traumatic uveitis

Treatment

KEY POINT ▶ The aims of therapy are to reduce the inflammation and produce cyclopegia, which should be maintained until the clinical signs have abated.

- Subconjunctival corticosteroids (see preceding section) are usually given as well as topical corticosteroid eye drops (Treatment Nos. 47, 49 and 50). The topical corticosteroid eye drops should be maintained several times daily for up to 10 to 14 days to reduce the chance of recurrence of the uveitis.
- Systemic anti-inflammatory drugs may be used, and the nonsteroidal anti-inflammatories are the drugs of choice. Flunixin (Treatment No. 52) is given at 1 mg/kg q24h PO or IV, or phenylbutazone (Treatment No. 88) PO at a dose rate of 2.2 mg/kg q12h, for a period of 4 to 7 days. Aspirin (Treatment No. 9) also has been used at dose rates of 35 to 100 mg/kg (see Chap. 17) for treatment of immune-mediated uveitis.
- Cyclopegics should be applied to produce pupillary dilatation. They are useful to counter the pain associated with ciliary spasm and may prevent synechiae formation. Atropine (1%–2%) ophthalmic drops or ointment is effective but must be used at 2- to 4-hour intervals until there is pupillary dilatation. Note that this frequency of atropine administration may result in signs of colic, and therefore, care must be taken. After dilatation has been established, it may only be necessary to administer atropine once daily. Pupillary dilatation should be maintained until there are signs of lessening of pain and inflammation, therapy usually being necessary for 3 to 5 days.
- Owners should be warned of the likelihood of recurrence, and anti-inflammatory therapy should be restarted as soon as clinical signs are apparent.

Diseases of the Lens

Cataracts

Cataracts may be either congenital or acquired and focal or diffuse.

KEY POINT ► Congenital cataracts are more common and more amenable to surgical treatment than acquired cataracts.

There is some suspicion that cataracts may be heritable, particularly in the quarter horse and Appaloosa. Cataracts may occur unilaterally or bilaterally.

History and Presenting Signs

- Visual deficits
- Cloudy appearance of the lens

Clinical Findings and Diagnosis

- When the cataract is diffuse, there is little problem in diagnosis, the opaque lens being readily apparent. However, when the cataract is focal, a more careful examination is necessary.

- If there is diffuse disease, there will be disturbance to vision with absence of a menace response in the affected eye.
- Ophthalmoscopy can be undertaken to confirm the diagnosis. It is important to determine whether there are signs of uveitis and/or lens luxation, particularly in acquired cases.

Differential Diagnosis

- Synechiae
- Lens luxation
- Uveitis

Treatment

- Good results have been obtained with cataract surgery in foals. The surgery is best undertaken when the foal is a few months of age.
- Acquired cataracts in adult horses are best left untreated if unilateral. In the case of bilateral cataracts, surgery can be attempted, but the surgery is difficult and the results are often unsatisfactory.

Diseases of the Retina and Optic Nerve

Retinal Diseases

Retinal diseases are quite rare in the horse, although a number of congenital and acquired conditions can affect vision. Most present with little abnormality in the external appearance of the eye. Congenital retinal problems are probably more common than acquired problems.

History and Presenting Signs

■ Blindness
■ Problems with night vision

Clinical Findings and Diagnosis

■ Horses with retinal disease usually present with disturbances to vision, and initial inspection of the eye reveals no major abnormalities.
■ Detailed ophthalmoscopic examination is required, and it may be necessary to induce mydriasis with 1% tropicamide (Mydriacyl, Alcon, Fort Worth, TX).

Differential Diagnosis

■ Retinal detachment—congenital (standardbreds and thoroughbreds) or acquired (secondary to uveitis)
■ Night blindness—Appaloosas (normal ophthalmoscopic findings) with signs mainly during reduced lighting
■ Chorioretinitis—discrete lesions in the nontapetal zone with signs of visual deficit

Treatment

There is no effective treatment for any of the conditions described, but accurate diagnosis is necessary for accurate prognosis to be given.

Optic Nerve Disease

As with retinal problems, optic nerve disease does not produce external signs of ocular disease, but various degrees of disturbance to vision are found. There is no treatment for any optic nerve diseases.

History and Presenting Signs

■ Severe disturbances to vision
■ Normal external appearance of the eye

Clinical Findings and Diagnosis

Ophthalmoscopy is essential to determine changes in appearance of the optic disc. In some cases there may be atrophy and decreased vascular supply, whereas in other conditions where there is head trauma there will be edema of the optic disc and sometimes hemorrhage.

Differential Diagnosis

■ Hypoplasia of the optic nerve
■ Optic neuritis
■ Traumatic optic neuropathy

Treatment

There is no treatment for any of the problems involving the optic nerve, apart from lesions resulting from head trauma. Treatment in such cases is detailed in Chapter 13.

References

Abrams, K. L., and Brook, D. E.: Equine recurrent uveitis: Current concepts in diagnosis and treatment. *Equine Pract.* 12:27, 1990.

Brook, D.: Further development of an indwelling nasolacrimal cannula for the administration of medication to the equine eye. *Equine Pract.* 9:12, 1987.

Finocchio, E.: A practical approach to the treatment of corneal ulcers in horses. *Proc. 35th Annu. Conv. Am. Assoc. Equine Pract.,* 1989, p. 531.

Hakanson, N. E., and Merideth, R. E.: Ocular examination and diagnostic techniques in the horse: 2. Assessment of vision and examination of intraocular structures. *Equine Pract.* 9:6, 1987.

MacFadden, K. E., and Pace, L. W.: Clinical manifestations of squamous cell carcinoma in horses. *Compend. Contin. Educ. Pract. Vet.* 13:669, 1991.

Schoster, J. V.: Surgical repair of equine eyelid lacerations. *Vet. Med.* 83:1042, 1988.

Schoster, J. V.: Using conjunctival flaps to prevent rupture of deep corneal ulcers. *Vet. Med.* 84:307, 1989.

Schoster, J. V.: Revisiting ocular lavage systems for the horse. *Proc. 36th Annu. Conv. Am. Assoc. Equine Pract.,* 1990, p. 575.

Schwink, K.: Factors influencing morbidity and outcome of equine ocular squamous cell carcinoma. *Equine Vet. J.* 19:198, 1987.

Wolf, E. D.: Medical treatment for corneal ulcers. *Proc. 36th Annu. Conv. Am. Assoc. Equine Pract.,* 1990, p. 575.

Hemolymphatic System

Primary disease involving the hemolymphatic system is rare in the horse. However, the collection of blood samples for evaluation of systemic disease is perhaps the most common diagnostic procedure undertaken by equine practitioners. Where there is primary disease involving the hemolymphatic system, there may be a wide range of signs. Presenting complaints may vary from exercise intolerance to weight loss. A careful physical examination, concentrating on the mucous membranes, cardiovascular system, and peripheral lymph nodes, is important in suspected hemolymphatic disease.

EXAMINATION OF THE HEMOLYMPHATIC SYSTEM

History

The following questions may be pertinent to hemolymphatic disease:

- Has there been a change in attitude or demeanor, and if so, has it been sudden or insidious?
- Have there been recent changes in appetite?
- Are there signs of decreased exercise capacity?
- Has there been any change in urine color?
- Have any swellings been noticed in any region of the horse's body?
- If swellings have appeared, have these been related to episodes of minor trauma?
- Has there been weight loss or any signs of abdominal pain?
- Has the horse's breathing changed at all, either at rest or during or after exercise?

Physical Examination

A detailed physical examination is indicated, as in all the body systems. In hemolymphatic disease, the nonspecific nature of the problems emphasizes the importance of a careful physical examination.

KEY POINT ► The most common presenting signs in horses with hemolymphatic disease are inappetence, fever, and/or weight loss.

The following areas should be given careful attention in a physical examination:

Mucous Membranes—In a range of hemolymphatic diseases, abnormalities in the mucous membranes may be a key clinical feature. Normal mucous membranes vary in color from pale to darker pink, but anemia can exist without excessive pallor being evident. Other important findings include jaundice and petechial hemorrhage. The latter finding is particularly important if it occurs in the septicemic horse, because it may herald the onset of disseminated intravascular coagulation.

The Circulation—Should be carefully assessed, and particular note should be made of the large veins to assess the possibility of thrombosis. An elevation in heart rate may indicate compensation for decreased oxygen delivery as a result of anemia, as well as various systemic disorders such as septicemia, alterations in fluid balance, and pain. The presence of edema may indicate circulatory problems, decrease in plasma albumin concentrations, or localized lymphatic obstructions. The most common sites for edema are the ventral abdomen and the hindlegs, in the latter case usually where there is localized lymphatic obstruction.

The Lymphatics—Normally it is difficult to palpate lymph nodes in the horse, and those most frequently enlarged are around the head. Even with diseases such as lymphoma, it is unusual to find enlargement of superficial lymph nodes. More commonly, there will be signs of lymphatic obstruction resulting in local swelling or signs such as abdominal pain or dyspnea. These signs are the result of abdominal and/or thoracic lymph node enlargement.

Urinary System—Evaluation is important, particularly determination of whether there is hemoglobinuria.

Rectal Examination—Is an important part of the workup of many cases of suspected hemolymphatic disorders to determine the presence of internal abscesses or neoplasia. Further details on rectal examination are provided in Chapter 6.

DIAGNOSTIC AIDS
Venous Blood Collection

Blood samples are most easily collected in evacuated tubes (e.g., Vacutainer, Becton Dickinson, Rutherford, NJ) containing various anticoagulants. For most routine hematology determinations (e.g., complete blood count, or CBC), potassium EDTA is the anticoagulant of choice (purple-top Vacutainer tubes). For coagulation tests, sodium citrate tubes (blue-top Vacutainer tubes) are used. For plasma measurements, blood samples are usually taken in tubes containing lithium heparin as an anticoagulant (green-top Vacutainer tubes). For serum measurements, samples are collected in tubes containing no anticoagulant (red-top Vacutainer tubes).

Following collection of the blood sample, evaluation of cytology should be performed within 2 to 4 hours. Longer periods, particularly if the blood is kept at high temperatures, can result in changes in the morphology of cells, the most common being leukocyte vacuolation. Storage of the blood in ice or a refrigerator prolongs the time available for accurate total leukocyte counts. If a blood sample is taken in the late afternoon and cannot be processed until the next morning, a blood smear should be made prior to refrigeration of the sample.

The reference values for the hemogram of adult horses are presented in Table 11-1. One of the problems in interpreting the equine hemogram is that excitement and apprehension elevate the red cell indices because red cells are mobilized from the spleen under the influence of catecholamines. Thus care must be taken in interpreting results from a horse in which there has been apprehension during the sample collection. Such blood samples will usually have values at the high end of the normal range.

Some details of the hemogram in foals is given in Chapter 8.

Interpretation of the Leukogram
Neutrophils

Neutrophilia, even in acute infections, is not as dramatic as in some other species. Increases in neutrophils to more than 7×10^9/L (7000/µl) indicates neutrophilia. In some severe acute infections, neutrophil numbers can increase to more than $20 \times$

TABLE 11–1. Reference Range of Hematology Values in the Adult Horse

Hematology Value	Normal Range
Packed cell volume (PCV), L/L	0.30–0.48 (30%–48%)
Total plasma protein (TPP), g/L	55–75 (5.5–7.5 g/dl)
Fibrinogen, g/L	<4 g/L (<400 mg/dl)
Hemoglobin (Hb), g/L	110–160 (11–16 g/dl)
Erythrocytes (RBC), $\times 10^{12}$/L	7.5–11.0 (7–11 $\times 10^6$/µl)
Thrombocytes, $\times 10^9$/L	100–300 (100,000–300,000/µl)
Mean corpuscular volume (MCV), fl	41–49
Mean corpuscular hemoglobin concentration (MCHC), g/L	300–360 (30–36 g/dl)
Mean cell hemoglobin (MCH), pg	13–16
Erythrocyte sedimentation rate (ESR), mm/h	12–45
Leukocytes (WBC), $\times 10^9$/L	6.0–11.0 (6–11 $\times 10^3$/µl)
Neutrophils, $\times 10^9$/L	2.5–7.0 (2.5–7 $\times 10^3$/µl)
Lymphocytes, $\times 10^9$/L	1.6–5.4 (1.6–5.4 $\times 10^3$/µl)
Monocytes, $\times 10^9$/L	0.6–0.7 (0.6–0.7 $\times 10^3$/µl)
Eosinophils, $\times 10^9$/L	0.1–0.5 (0.1–0.5 $\times 10^3$/µl)
Basophils, $\times 10^9$/L	0–0.3 (0–0.3 $\times 10^3$/µl)

Note: Standardbreds usually have lower mean red cell indices than thoroughbreds, and horses used for endurance riding will tend to be at the low end of the normal range.

10^9/L (20,000/µl), but such changes are unusual. A physiologic neutrophilia is possible where there is catecholamine release, such as during excitement and apprehension, as well as during exercise. If blood is collected from an unexcited horse that has not been stressed, a neutrophilia generally indicates infection or a focus of inflammation. In severe disease there is usually a left shift (immature neutrophils present), and there are often toxic changes such as vacuolation in the neutrophils.

Neutropenia often is a sign of more serious disease than neutrophilia and can indicate the acute stages of severe infections such as salmonellosis. In the majority of cases, the neutropenia is due to inability of the bone marrow to replace neutrophils in the circulation resulting from the increased migration to the site of inflammation.

Lymphocytes

Lymphocytosis is found most commonly in blood samples collected from horses after fast exercise. Together with splenic release of erythrocytes, there is an increased number of lymphocytes released. A similar mechanism can be responsible for lymphocytosis in blood samples collected from excited horses. Diseases that can result in lymphocytosis include long-standing infections and leukemia.

Lymphopenia is commonly found in the early stages of some viral diseases, as well as with severe systemic infections.

Neutrophil–Lymphocyte (N:L) Ratio

Many practitioners use changes in the N:L ratio as an indication of disease in athletic horses. The normal N:L ratio is about 2:1, and if the ratio is inverted, this is taken as evidence for maladaptation to training. Changes in N:L ratio will mirror changes in plasma cortisol, which undergoes diurnal variation, the N:L ratio being higher with higher cortisol concentrations. Considerable care should be exercised in interpretation of the N:L ratio because various physiologic processes may result in temporary changes in the ratios of the two major cell types in the peripheral circulation.

Monocytes

Monocytes are present in relatively low numbers in the peripheral blood. An increase in monocytes usually indicates chronicity of some diseases, particularly when associated with neutrophilia.

Eosinophils

An increase in eosinophils is usually taken as indicative of significant internal parasite infestation, although care should be taken with such an interpretation. Eosinophil increases are also found in some allergic diseases. A decrease in eosinophil numbers is found as a normal stress response and in infectious disease. The appearance of eosinophils on sequential hemograms of horses with severe disease is often a good prognostic sign.

Bone Marrow Aspiration

Bone marrow aspiration is not a common diagnostic technique in practice and is usually reserved for cases where there is severe, unexplained anemia, persistent leukopenia or thrombocytopenia, or suspicion of leukemia. The usual sites for collection are the wing of the ilium, the ribs, or the sternum. In mature horses, it is often difficult to collect an adequate marrow sample from the ilium. We prefer to use the sternum because samples may be reliably collected. The site is on the ventral midline, just caudal to the olecranon when the horse is standing normally. A special bone marrow collection needle (Fig. 11-1) or an 18-gauge, 8.75-cm (3.5-inch) spinal needle may be used. After clipping of the hair and appropriate skin disinfection of the site, 3 to 4 ml

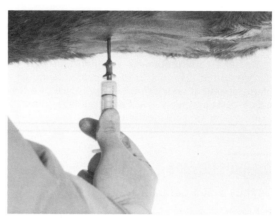

Figure 11–1. Bone marrow collection needle in position for collection of a bone marrow aspirate from the sternum.

of 2% lidocaine (Treatment No. 67) is infused subcutaneously, and the needle is inserted vertically. The needle is then inserted through the bleb of local anesthetic, and if a bone marrow collection needle is used, a prior stab incision in the skin is required. Once the needle reaches the sternum, increased resistance can be felt, and the needle is rotated with firm pressure against the needle hub. Once the tip of the needle is within the sternum, the stylet is removed and firm suction is applied using a 10- or 20-ml syringe (Fig. 11-1). To prevent clotting of the sample, it may be useful to aspirate a few drops of 15% tripotassium EDTA into the syringe prior to aspiration. Blood contamination of the sample is difficult to avoid; even if contamination does occur, however, the marrow sample can still be useful for interpretation. Alternatively, smears may be made immediately using glass slides.

Apart from determination of abnormal cell types, the myeloid–erythroid ratio (M:E) is determined by counting several hundred cells. The normal M:E ratio is in the range 0.5 to 1.5.

Lymph Node Biopsy

When there is generalized lymphadenopathy, lymph node biopsy may be indicated. Needle aspiration from enlarged lymph nodes seldom provide diagnostic information. The best technique is surgical removal of an affected node for histopathology. If this is not possible, use of a Tru-Cut biopsy needle (Travenol Laboratories Incorporated, Deerfield, IL) often will provide an adequate sample for diagnosis.

Hemolymphatic Diseases

Anemia

Anemia is one of the most commonly misdiagnosed disorders in horses. It can be defined as a decrease in the various erythrocyte indices below the lower end of the normal range. In athletic horses presented for reduced performance, a value below normal breed means for hematocrit, hemoglobin, or erythrocyte count is often a convenient explanation for the performance problem. However, the normal range for hematology in adult horses is quite wide (see Table 11-1), and a single blood sample taken from a horse that is normal on clinical examination will show values mostly within the normal range. A wide range of diseases (see Differential Diagnosis below) can cause anemia.

History and Presenting Signs

- Decreased exercise capacity
- Decreased appetite
- Depression
- Guttural pouch mycosis
- Trauma—acute blood loss
- After surgery

Clinical Findings and Diagnosis

▶ Acute Anemia

- Signs usually result from trauma or surgery. There may be signs of shock, with a weak pulse, prolonged capillary refill time, and elevated heart rate.
- In acute blood loss, there may be little change in hematocrit for 1 to 2 days. This is so because of the splenic red cell reserve acting under the influence of catecholamines to increase the circulating red cell pool. After a few days, there is expansion of the extracellular fluid volume and a dramatic decrease in hematocrit (values less than 0.20 L/ L, or 20%) may be found. It is common to find hypoproteinemia at this stage.
- Ingestion of red maple leaves results in methemoglobinemia and hemolysis with discolored urine due to methemoglobinuria and hemoglobinuria.

▶ Chronic Anemia

KEY POINT ▶ Anemia of chronic disease is the most common form of anemia in horses. A number of systemic infections, if prolonged, can result in decreased erythropoiesis.

- A careful clinical examination may indicate where the infection is localized, and blood should be collected for a CBC and fibrinogen estimation. This will often show a leukocytosis and an elevation in fibrinogen levels. A number of other diagnostic tests may be indicated if examination suggests infection involving the thoracic or abdominal cavities.
- In the case of intravascular hemolysis, there may be hemoglobinuria, and therefore, urinalysis should be performed.
- To evaluate erythropoiesis, bone marrow aspiration may be performed. Low M:E ratios (<0.5) usually indicate a suitable response to the anemia. Increased reticulocyte counts in bone marrow also can be used as an indication of a regenerative anemia.

KEY POINT ▶ Even when the bone marrow responds, reticulocytes do not appear in the peripheral circulation.

- Other tests that should be considered are Coombs (for autoimmune disorders) and Coggins (for infectious anemia) tests and evaluation of blood smears for blood parasites such as *Babesia* spp. Note that false-negative results are possible with a Coombs test.
- In infectious anemia there is often recurrent illness with nonspecific signs, such as inappetence, fever, and weight loss. In some cases there is also the presence of edema. Varying degrees of anemia are found, and icterus is usually one of the signs of disease.

KEY POINT ▶ Note that there are similar clinical findings in horses with babesiosis (piroplasmosis).

Differential Diagnosis

- Systemic infection
- Neoplasia

- Blood loss
- Hemolytic anemia
- Infectious anemia
- Babesiosis
- Ehrlichiosis
- Hemophilia
- Drug toxicity (particularly NSAIDs)
- Neonatal isoerythrolysis (see Chap. 8)

Treatment

▶ Acute Anemia

- If anemia is due to acute blood loss, the source of the hemorrhage should be controlled and consideration given to whether intravenous blood administration is necessary.

KEY POINT ▶ Blood administration is necessary if the hematocrit shows a sudden decrease to less than 0.15 L/L (<15%).

- Crossmatching should be performed, but if the facilities are not available, blood taken from any donor horse (20 ml/kg) may be administered with little likelihood of an adverse reaction. Blood is usually collected from a gelding into packs containing an appropriate volume of acid citrate dextrose and sodium citrate. These packs are commercially available for human use in 500-ml bags (Baxter Healthcare Corporation, Deerfield, IL).
- Blood administration should be performed initially at a slow rate (100–200 ml) over 10 to 15 minutes to determine if there is a transfusion reaction. This is usually manifest by sweating, restlessness, tachycardia, and dyspnea. If such signs occur, the transfusion should be stopped, and if there is further deterioration, epinephrine (Adrenalin chloride, Parke-Davis, Morris Plains, NJ) should be administered subcutaneously or intramuscularly at a dose rate of 1 to 1.5 ml/100 kg of a 1:1000 solution.
- Small volumes (1–2 L) of hypertonic saline (7%) will be useful for improving the central circulation by maintenance of cardiac output. This is only a temporary measure, and larger volumes (40–80 ml/kg) of isotonic replacement fluids should be administered (see Fluid Therapy, Chap. 17) for reestablishment of peripheral perfusion. Care should be taken to monitor the total plasma protein so that it does not fall below 45 g/L (4.5 g/dl), since this will allow fluid to move out of the circulation.
- Once the acute problems are resolved, with stabilization of the circulation and reestablishment of oxygen delivery, it is necessary to ensure a normal diet with adequate iron (see Chap. 16) so that normal erythropoiesis is possible.

▶ Chronic Anemia

- In cases of *immune-mediated hemolytic anemia,* corticosteroids are indicated at dose rates of dexamethasone (Treatment No. 29) up to 0.2 mg/

kg q12h for 1 to 3 days and maintenance with oral prednisolone (Treatment No. 92) at dose rates varying from 0.4 to 2 mg/kg per day. The aim is to reduce the dosage to around 0.4 to 0.6 mg/kg every other day.

- In areas such as Florida and Texas, as well as in many other countries where there is a hot, humid climate (Africa, Asia, South America), babesiosis (piroplasmosis) may be the cause of the anemia. Treatment is possible using imidocarb (Burroughs Wellcome, Research Triangle Park, NC). The dose rate is 2 mg/kg q24h for two treatments, but this is not effective against *B. equi.* Treatment with intravenous buparvaquone (Coopers Animal Health, Berkhamstead, UK) at 4 to 6 mg/kg is effective in the acute stages of disease.
- *Infectious anemia* is a viral disease with a worldwide distribution. Biting insects are the vector for the disease, which has a high incidence of carriers that do not show clinical signs. Apart from supportive therapy, there is little that can be done. It is important to identify carriers. Some states require that infected animals be slaughtered.
- Despite the widespread use of oral iron supplements by most horse trainers, iron-deficiency anemia is rare. Normal diets contain iron in excess of recommendations by nutritional authorities.

Disseminated Intravascular Coagulation

Disseminated intravascular coagulation (DIC) occurs secondary to various systemic disorders and results from the formation of excessive thrombin following depletion of coagulant factors.

KEY POINT ▶ The most common diseases producing DIC are laminitis, acute gastrointestinal problems, and septicemia.

The final common mediator in these conditions appears to be endotoxin production.

History and Presenting Signs

- There are few specific indications of DIC.
- Suspect in any severe systemic disorder
- Endotoxemia

Clinical Findings and Diagnosis

- The primary disorder will be the main presenting feature early to midway through the course of DIC. Microvascular thrombosis may occur early in the disease, and this can result in ischemia to vital organs such as the kidneys.
- In the later stages of DIC, coagulation systems may fail, resulting in hemorrhage and large-vein thrombosis.
- In any severe systemic disorder, DIC should at least be suspected, and as a screening measure,

platelet numbers can be measured. Normal platelet numbers are greater than 100×10^9/L (100,000/μl), and lower values could indicate DIC.

- If platelet numbers are decreased, a clotting profile should be undertaken. This involves measurement of prothrombin and partial thromboplastin times.

Differential Diagnosis

- Septicemia
- Shock
- Endotoxemia
- Infectious anemia
- Purpura hemorrhagica

Treatment

- Large volumes of intravenous fluids are useful to correct signs of shock and reduced tissue perfusion.
- Nonsteroidal anti-inflammatory drugs, particularly flunixin meglumine (Treatment No. 52) are useful to assist in combating the effects of endotoxemia (see Chap. 17). Aspirin (Treatment No. 9) has antithrombotic effects and may be given intravenously at a dose rate of 20 to 40 mg/kg.
- Administration of fresh plasma (6–8 ml/kg) may be of value to increase the antithrombin III levels, which may be reduced in cases of DIC.
- There is some evidence that administration of heparin at a dose rate of 5 to 10 IU/kg intravenously is of value in potentiating the action of antithrombin III.

Hemophilia

Hemophilia in horses is due to an inherited disorder of coagulation in which there is a deficiency of factor VIII coagulant activity. It is a rare condition and is the result of a recessive disorder described in a number of horse breeds.

KEY POINT ▶ Hemophilia is an X-linked chromosomal abnormality, and clinical signs are found only in males.

History and Presenting Signs

- Young horse (<6 months age)
- Presented following trauma or after injections
- Gross swelling around joints—due to hemarthrosis

Clinical Findings and Diagnosis

- Minor trauma may result in swelling due to a hematoma at the site. Joint trauma may result in hemarthrosis, whereas trauma at other sites will produce localized hematomas.
- Large-scale hemorrhage is also possible from a number of other sites.

- Routine clotting profiles show normal values apart from an increased activated partial thromboplastin time. An assay for factor VIII coagulant activity on blood collected into citrate should be performed to confirm suspected hemophilia.

Differential Diagnosis

- Trauma
- Abscesses
- Disseminated intravascular coagulation

Treatment

- Palliative treatment involving the administration of fresh plasma is possible to increase the levels of factor VIII coagulant activity. Unfortunately, this involves large volumes of plasma (20 L) given over several days and is seldom practical outside a university teaching hospital.
- Because it is an inherited disorder in which the mare is a carrier, it is important to ensure that the mare does not continue breeding because male offspring are likely to be affected and female offspring will act as carriers.

Leukemia

Leukemia is rarely found in horses and may involve one or more stem-cell types in the bone marrow. A younger population of horses is usually affected than with other forms of neoplasia.

History and Presenting Signs

- Acute or chronic course of disease
- Hindlimb edema
- Inappetence
- Depression

Clinical Findings and Diagnosis

KEY POINT ▶ Clinical signs are usually nonspecific. However, the presence of hindlimb edema is a typical feature in many reported cases of leukemia.

- In some cases there may be concurrent infections (often respiratory).
- Petechial hemorrhages of the mucous membranes have been reported in some cases.
- Routine hematology is usually what alerts the clinician to the diagnosis of leukemia. Abnormal cell types are found on a blood smear, but definitive diagnosis is possible only by a bone marrow aspirate (see p. 330) or biopsy. Anemia is often present, as with other lymphoproliferative and myeloproliferative disorders.

Differential Diagnosis

- Granulomatous enteritis
- Pleuritis
- Peritonitis

- Internal abscessation
- Infectious anemia
- Other neoplasia

Treatment

There is no treatment that is economically or practically feasible for leukemia in horses.

Lymphosarcoma

A range of neoplastic disorders may involve the hematopoietic system, but the most common is lymphosarcoma.

KEY POINT ► Lymphosarcoma is chiefly a disease of mature horses and may exist in localized forms (cutaneous, alimentary) as well as being generalized.

History and Presenting Signs

- Weight loss
- Depression
- Inappetence
- Localized edema
- Weight loss

Clinical Findings and Diagnosis

- The presenting signs detailed above are nonspecific but provide an indication that lymphosarcoma should be one of the differential diagnoses in a condition where there is an indication of chronic low-grade disease.
- Widespread lymph node enlargement is unusual in lymphosarcoma. While there may be involvement of specific lymph nodes, this is seldom apparent on clinical examination.
- Ventral edema is present in a high percentage of cases.
- Rectal examination is warranted to detect lymph node enlargement, particularly if there are signs referable to the abdominal cavity.
- It is common to find anemia when the disease is generalized.
- The forms of the disease that have been described include

  Generalized—Involving tissues such as the spleen, lymph nodes, liver, and kidney.

  Mediastinal—Enlargement of mediastinal lymph nodes may produce cardiorespiratory signs.

  Cutaneous—Results in multiple subcutaneous nodules, in some cases without systemic signs.

  Alimentary—Is a common presenting form of lymphosarcoma in horses. The small intestine is most frequently involved. Oral D-glucose and D-xylose absorption curves are usually flattened. Further details are given in Chapter 6.

- The presence of neoplastic lymphocytes in tissues or body fluids is the main criterion for diagnosis. However, such lymphocytes are rarely found in peripheral blood smears, even with generalized disease.
- The hemogram from affected horses often shows nonspecific changes, including increased fibrinogen, leukocytosis, hypoproteinemia, and anemia.
- Part of establishing a database in these cases (see Chap. 2, Weight Loss) involves urinalysis, abdominocentesis, and possibly thoracocentesis. Cytology of fluid samples obtained from the thoracic or abdominal cavities should be performed to determine whether neoplastic cells are present.
- If access is possible and there is enlargement of one or more superficial lymph nodes, a biopsy or excision is indicated (see above).
- Bone marrow aspirates may be required to make a diagnosis, and in some cases, we have needed to perform a bone marrow biopsy, which is relatively easily performed using a small trephine to collect a sample from the ileum.

Differential Diagnosis

- Nodular necrobiosis
- Granulomatous enteritis (inflammatory bowel disease)
- Pleuritis
- Peritonitis
- Internal abscessation
- Infectious anemia
- Other neoplasia

Treatment

There is no successful treatment for lymphosarcoma in horses.

Myeloma

Myelomas are unusual disorders characterized by proliferation of neoplastic plasma cells. The most common of the myelomas is multiple myeloma, involving the bone marrow.

History and Presenting Signs

- Inappetence
- Weight loss
- Depression

Clinical Findings and Diagnosis

- As with the lymphoproliferative disorders, the signs of disease are quite nonspecific.
- In some cases, the presentation has been for lameness or neurologic disease because of activation of osteoclastic activity resulting from the neoplastic cells.
- Anemia is common, and consistent findings on the hemogram include hyperproteinemia and hypercalcemia.

Differential Diagnosis

- Granulomatous enteritis
- Pleuritis
- Peritonitis
- Internal abscessation
- Infectious anemia
- Other neoplasia

Treatment

There is no successful treatment for plasma-cell myeloma in horses.

Thrombocytopenia

Platelet numbers less than 100×10^9/L (<100,000/μl) indicate thrombocytopenia. The majority of cases are associated with a decrease in the life span of platelets or when platelets are consumed, such as in disseminated intravascular coagulation. Idiopathic thrombocytopenia is an immune-mediated disorder in which platelets are destroyed. Idiopathic thrombocytopenia has been reported after a wide range of systemic diseases (bacterial and viral) as well as after administration of various drugs.

KEY POINT ▶ Because blood collected into EDTA can sometimes produce platelet aggregation, any low platelet counts should be repeated after collection of a second blood sample, preferably using citrate as an anticoagulant.

History and Presenting Signs

- Signs of severe systemic disease
- Idiopathic thrombocytopenia—few signs of disease

Clinical Findings and Diagnosis

- Petechial hemorrhage on the visible mucous membranes is typical of idiopathic thrombocytopenia. These are usually associated with platelet numbers below 40×10^9/L (40,000/μl).
- Gross hemorrhage is seldom found until platelet counts decrease to the range of 10 to 20×10^9/L (10,000–20,000/μl).
- Laboratory testing shows prolonged bleeding time together with a decrease in platelets. If the condition has been prolonged, there may be anemia and hypoproteinemia.
- Other tests of clotting function (e.g., prothrombin time, activated partial thromboplastin time) may be useful to eliminate other disorders of hemostasis.

Differential Diagnosis

- Disseminated intravascular coagulation
- Septicemia
- Viral arteritis
- Purpura hemorrhagica
- Infectious anemia
- Ehrlichiosis

Treatment

- If the cause of thrombocytopenia can be associated with drug administration, treatment should be stopped and in many cases there will be spontaneous recovery.
- If the thrombocytopenia is associated with DIC, appropriate therapy should be begun (see p. 332).
- Where platelet counts are particularly low and there is significant hemorrhage, blood administration is indicated, which, if fresh, will increase the platelet numbers.
- Idiopathic thrombocytopenia may respond to systemic corticosteroid treatment. Of the corticosteroids available, the best response is likely to be found from administration of dexamethasone (Treatment Nos. 29 and 30) at dose rates of 0.04 to 0.4 mg/kg given IV. Initially, higher dose rates (0.2 mg/kg) should be used once daily for up to 1 week to determine if the platelet numbers increase. Following this, the dose can be gradually reduced over a further 7 to 10 days. If the platelet counts have stabilized, therapy should be discontinued. However, if further treatment is required, oral prednisolone therapy (Treatment No. 92) may be given at dose rates of 0.5 to 1 mg/kg PO once daily in the morning, decreasing to an every-other-day dosage.

Vasculitis

Vasculitis is a syndrome usually resulting from hypersensitivity reactions secondary to systemic infections and occasionally as a result of drug reactions. In rare cases, the vasculitis may be due to direct damage to vessel walls associated with some viruses and toxins. Purpura hemorrhagica is the most common vasculitis and is thought to be associated with hypersensitivity to *Streptococcus equi* var. *equi* antigens. Other causes include influenza, infectious anemia, infection with *Ehrlichia equi,* and viral arteritis.

History and Presenting Signs

- Localized edema
- Skin necrosis

Clinical Findings and Diagnosis

- Localized areas of edema associated with the vasculitis can proceed to eventual sloughing of the affected skin. Areas around the limbs and face are often affected and occasionally regions on the trunk.
- The sudden appearance of localized subcutaneous edema is the main clinical sign that the problem may be due to vasculitis.
- Petechial hemorrhages associated with the mucosa are also common.

- While peripheral manifestations are most common, involvement of the alimentary and respiratory tracts, central nervous system, and muscles also may occur.
- Hematologic and biochemical findings are nonspecific. Because most cases are due to systemic disease, there is often leukocytosis and increased plasma fibrinogen levels.
- Histologic examination of skin punch biopsies (see Chap. 12) provides the opportunity for confirming the diagnosis. However, changes may not be found unless a large number of biopsies are collected.

Differential Diagnosis

- Disseminated intravascular coagulation
- Septicemia
- Viral arteritis
- Purpura hemorrhagica
- Infectious anemia
- Ehrlichiosis
- Thrombocytopenia

Treatment

- There is no specific treatment for vasculitis syndromes, but good supportive care is necessary together with appropriate anti-inflammatory therapy. Maintenance of electrolyte and fluid balance is essential, because with many of the diseases that produce vasculitis, there is a loss of appetite and depression.
- Some cases respond well to the therapy set out below, but a proportion of horses either do not respond or develop secondary complications, particularly laminitis and colitis.
- The nonsteroidal anti-inflammatory drugs that can be used include phenylbutazone (Treatment No. 88) at dose rates up to 2.2 mg/kg q12h, flunixin meglumine (Treatment No. 52) at dose rates up to 1 mg/kg q12h, and ketoprofen (Treatment No. 66) at 1 to 2 mg/kg, IV only, q24h.
- Procaine penicillin (Treatment No. 83) at a dose rate of 15 mg/kg (15,000 IU/kg) IM q12h may be used. This is particularly important if the streptococcal infection is still active.
- Clinical experience indicates response in many cases to systemic corticosteroid administration. Dexamethasone (Treatment Nos. 29 and 30) is the corticosteroid of choice and should be given at a dose rate of 0.1 to 0.2 mg/kg once daily, in the morning. With all corticosteroid therapy, the concept is to gradually reduce the dose rate once clinical response is found. Morning administration of dexamethasone results in less adrenal suppression than with afternoon treatment.

References

Adams, R., Calderwood Mays, M. B., and Peyton, L. C.: Malignant lymphoma in three horses with ulcerative pharyngitis. *J. Am. Vet. Med. Assoc.* 193:674, 1988.

Carlson, G. P., Harrold, D., and Ziemer, E. L.: Anemia in the horse: Diagnosis and treatment. *Proc. 29th Annu. Conv. Am. Assoc. Equine Pract.*, 1983, p. 279.

Clabough, D. L.: Equine infectious anemia: The clinical signs, transmission, and diagnostic procedures. *Vet. Med.* 85:1007, 1990.

Clabough, D. L.: The immunopathogenesis and control of equine infectious anemia. *Vet. Med.* 85:1020, 1990.

Loftin, M. K., Levine, J. F., McGinn, T., and Coggins, L: Distribution of equine infectious anemia in equids in southeastern United States. *J. Am. Vet. Med. Assoc.* 197:1018, 1990.

Morris, D. D.: Review of anemia in horses: I. Clinical signs, laboratory findings and diagnosis. *Equine Pract.* 11:27, 1989.

Morris, D. D.: Review of anemia in horses: II. Pathophysiologic mechanisms, specific diseases and treatment. *Equine Pract.* 11:34, 1989.

Morris, D. D.: Diseases of the hemolymphatic system. In P. T. Colahan, I. G. Mayhew, A. M. Merritt, and J. N. Moore (Eds.), *Equine Medicine and Surgery*, 4th Ed. Goleta, Calif.: American Veterinary Publications, 1991, p. 1753.

Morris, D. D.: Hematopoietic diseases. In N. E. Robinson (Ed.), *Current Therapy in Equine Medicine*, Vol. 3. Philadelphia: W.B. Saunders, 1992, p. 487.

Dermatology

Skin diseases in the horse are very common and present a diagnostic challenge for the clinician. The principal reason for this is that different skin problems can present with similar histories and clinical signs. For example, a number of conditions can cause pruritus and alopecia. Similarly, there is a wide range of conditions that can cause nodular skin disease. As with most other body systems, a thorough history and a careful examination to determine the extent of the skin disease followed by the appropriate use of various diagnostic aids are the important steps in making a diagnosis. In this section we will concentrate on the classification of skin disease via presenting signs.

EXAMINATION OF THE SKIN

History

After the signalment, that is, the breed, age, sex, and use of the horse is determined (see Chap. 2), the following questions are useful in a standardized workup of a horse presented because of skin disease:

- What is the main problem from the client's view point?
- Is the problem localized or generalized?
- Is the problem static or progressive?
- If there are other horses in contact, do they have similar signs?
- If there are other horses affected, is there any sharing of grooming equipment?
- Is there any evidence of itchiness?
- Is the horse showing any generalized signs of ill health?
- What treatment has been given for the condition to date?
- Important background information when considering the history and presenting signs is:

Geography—Location of the horse will have a big influence on the range of possible skin diseases.

In general, many skin diseases are more common in horses in hot and humid climates, as is found in the south of the United States.

Season—Some diseases are more common at different times of the year. For example, Queensland itch, or "sweet itch," is much more common in summer and in climates that are hot and humid and where sand flies are likely to cause this type of hypersensitivity. In contrast, dermatophilosis, or "rain scald," will be more common during the wetter winter periods.

Local Environment—If the horse is stabled, attention must be paid to the type of bedding and feed, the management of the horses in the stables, use of grooming brushes and cloths, and general care of the horse. If the horse is at pasture, then the pasture types, extent of shade, water and feeding facilities, and fencing should all be examined because of possible relevance to the presenting problem.

Physical Examination

The presenting signs with many skin problems often result in a lack of a detailed examination of the skin and a general physical being overlooked. When presented with a large lump on the limb or an area of alopecia on the thorax, it is easy to bypass a more detailed examination to determine other possible skin involvement, lymph node enlargement, evidence of anemia, or elevated body temperature. It is important to examine the whole animal with a general physical examination, as outlined in Chapter 1, as well as a physical examination of the skin starting at the head and ending at the tail. The general distribution of the lesions should be noted on a diagram of the horse that shows the animal from the left and right sides and from the front.

After noting the general distribution of the lesions, a systematic examination should be begun, working from the front to the back of the horse.

Apart from the obvious areas, regions such as the oral cavity, mucous membranes of the nose, and conjunctivae should be inspected.

Examination of the coronary band and hooves is also important because they may provide a guide to a more generalized problem. Note should be taken of particular lesions and whether there is any inflammatory response, loss of hair, change in the general hair coat, or change in the general character of the skin.

DIAGNOSTIC AIDS

For examination of skin problems, little sophistication is needed in the diagnostic aids that can be used. Nonetheless, our experience is that many clinicians, when faced with a skin disease, will opt for treatment rather than making a specific diagnosis.

Skin Scrapings

- Skin scrapings are always an important part of the diagnostic workup in a horse with skin disease. If possible, recent lesions should be scraped using a no. 10 or 12 scalpel blade, as shown in Figure 12-1.
- Samples can be collected into a Petri dish or directly onto glass slides that have had a few drops of mineral oil placed prior to the scraping.

KEY POINT ▶ If a fungal skin infection such as ringworm is suspected, some of the hairs obtained should be mixed with a 40% solution of potassium hydroxide. After a 15- to 30-minute incubation period with the coverslip in place, the slide can be examined for the presence of hyphae.

- If dermatophilosis is suspected, an impression smear can be taken from the surface of the raw wound underneath the scabs on the skin. This

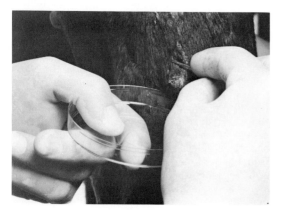

Figure 12–1. Skin scraping using a scalpel blade.

material is stained with either a Gram stain or methylene blue.
- It is also important to examine the collected material for the presence of ectoparasites.

Bacterial and Fungal Cultures

- Samples for bacterial culture should be collected from a nondischarging pustule. Swabs taken from purulent tracts are of little value for bacteriology because a mixed growth of secondary and invading organisms will be found.
- Prior to aspirating from a pustule, the area should be disinfected and aspirate collected into a sterile syringe.
- Samples for fungal culture should include hair scrapings and superficial keratin that has been scraped from the skin scrapings. Special media are available for fungal culture, and the laboratory should be informed of the provisional diagnosis. Fungal cultures may require up to 10 days before a positive finding is made. Because of this, the initial examination for the presence of hyphae on microscopic examination of hair shafts is very important.

Skin Biopsy

- Skin biopsy is a simple diagnostic aid that can be carried out easily with a minimum of equipment. Unfortunately, except in the case of skin tumors or diseases such as pemphigus foliaceus, the findings may be rather general and not enable a specific diagnosis to be made.
- In most cases, a punch biopsy is satisfactory, and disposable punch biopsy needles are best. A 6-mm-diameter biopsy punch is generally used, and after routine skin disinfection and injection of a small amount of local anesthetic, the biopsy punch is rotated with firm pressure to penetrate the skin down to the subcutaneous tissue (Fig. 12-2). The piece of skin is then removed using a pair of sterile forceps and a scalpel blade (Fig. 12-3). A single suture of nonabsorbable material such as 2-0 Prolene is placed.
- In cases where there are larger lesions, particularly cases involving vesicular and ulcerous lesions, a larger biopsy obtained by excision may be necessary. It is also useful to include some of the normal skin at the periphery of the lesion. The fixative most widely used for skin biopsies is 10% buffered formalin. If immunofluorescence is required, then a fixative such as Michel's medium should be used (see p. 339).

Allergy Testing

- Intradermal skin testing is becoming more widespread and may be useful for identifying allergens causing specific skin disease in horses.
- Testing is usually carried out after removal of any medication, in particular corticosteroids, for at least 7 to 10 days, and the side of the neck is usu-

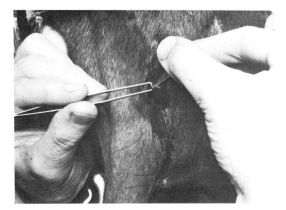

Figure 12–3. After the biopsy punch has been rotated through to the subcutaneous tissue, a scalpel blade and forceps are used to remove the piece of skin, after which a single interrupted suture is placed in the skin.

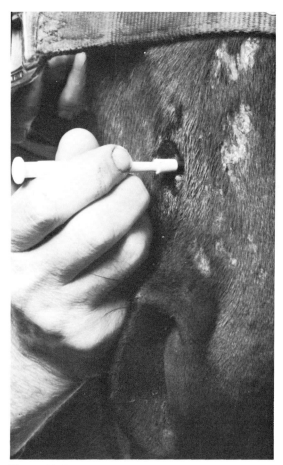

Figure 12–2. For collection of a skin biopsy, after injection of local anesthetic, a 6-mm biopsy punch is rotated through the skin to obtain the biopsy.

ally used. After clipping 2- to 3-cm (1-in) squares are marked for injection with specific antigens.

■ Most of the antigens used are present in concentrations of 1:1000 and are injected with a tuberculin syringe. The injection is given intradermally in a volume of approximately 0.1 ml. Subsequent swelling and local reaction in the skin are given a grading over the first 4 to 6 hours and then at 1 and 2 days after the intradermal injection. This type of testing is quite complicated and is best left to specialized clinics where the various antigens can be stocked.

Immunologic Testing

Autoimmune skin diseases are relatively common. Probably the most useful of the diagnostic tests is direct immunofluorescence, which is of value in confirming problems such as pemphigus foliaceus and systemic lupus erythematosus. Skin biopsies should be collected into Michel's solution, the details of which are given below.

Michel's Solution

Preparation of the Buffer. Add 2.5 ml of 1M potassium citrate buffer (pH 7.0) to 5 ml of 0.1 M magnesium sulfate and 5 ml of 0.1 M N-ethyl maleimide. Add this solution to 87.5 ml of distilled water, and adjust to pH 7.0 with 1 M potassium hydroxide.

Preparation of the Fixative. The fixative is prepared by dissolving 55 g diammonium sulfide in 100 ml of the buffer prepared above.

Skin Diseases

Skin diseases seldom fall into areas of neat diagnosis because of the similarities of many diseases as far as their appearance and presenting signs are concerned. To deal with the common skin diseases in this chapter, we will discuss the various major diseases under the following headings:

1. Traumatic skin disease
2. Granulomatous skin disease
3. Nodular skin disease
4. Pruritic and alopecic skin disease
5. Nonpruritic and alopecic skin disease

TRAUMATIC SKIN DISEASE

Skin Wounds

One of the most common reasons that clients present their horses to the veterinarian is trauma resulting in wounds to the skin. The most common wounds are those involving the distal limb and are the result of lacerations due to barbed wire, gates, or fences. Wounds to the distal limb of horses are a particular problem because of the poor wound contraction in this region. Wound contraction is accomplished by the myofibroblasts at the skin edges, which result in the skin being moved inward. The minimal wound contraction possible in the distal limb is the result of poor skin mobility, in contrast with areas such as the chest and neck where there is substantial loose skin. The result of the reduced wound contraction in the distal limb is the formation of excessive granulation tissue. This is probably the most common complication of wounds to the distal limbs of horses.

History and Presenting Signs

- Obvious skin wound
- May be a small puncture wound
- Determine the time since the wound occurred

Clinical Findings and Diagnosis

- While wounds are obvious, the extent of the wound, its depth, and the amount of soft-tissue damage may not be easy to determine, particularly if it is a puncture wound.
- Because of minimal soft-tissue covering of bone in the distal limb, inspection of the depth of the wound for any damage to the periosteum is important. Periosteal damage can lead to subsequent sequestrum formation with a discharging sinus.

KEY POINT ► Penetrating wounds in proximity to a joint in particular should be evaluated to determine whether there could be possible joint involvement.

- It is important to determine the extent of gross contamination of the wound with foreign matter.

Treatment

KEY POINT ► The major decisions in wound treatment are:
How much of the wound should I debride?
Should I suture the wound or not?
Should I use a drain or not?

- In areas such as the chest and neck, even extensive wounds may not require suturing because of the excellent wound contraction. This usually results in a good cosmetic appearance with minimal wound care within a period of 2 to 3 weeks.
- Distal limb wounds are the major problem for clinicians as far as achieving a cosmetic result and epithelial covering of the site.

KEY POINT ► We find the use of saline lavage of the wound to be of great value in achieving primary-intention healing of the wound.

- This is so because saline irrigation helps to decrease the degree of inevitable wound contamination. Some clinicians favor the use of povidone-iodine solutions, but even mild solutions irritate tissue. We find that the inclusion of an antiseptic in the lavage solution is of little value, and physiologic saline or a polyionic solution is preferable.
- While there are a large number of simple irrigation devices, the use of a Water Pik can be of great value in helping to remove gross contaminants prior to suturing.
- In some cases it may be necessary to remove some of the hair prior to suturing. However, our experience is that contamination of the wound with hair fibers occurs and is often hard to remove because they get trapped in tissue planes.

For this reason, unless there is a very thick hair coat, we prefer to suture the skin edges without removing the hair from the edges of the wound.

- If the wound is very deep and there are areas of dead space remaining, use of a Penrose drain, placed so that it exits distal to the most distal part of the wound, is helpful.

KEY POINT ▶ The use of local antibiotic solutions, ointments, and powders is to be avoided because they not only irritate wounds but also favor infection because of destruction of the normal bacterial flora.

- Skin sutures should be nonabsorbable and preferably monofilament. We prefer 0 polypropylene (Prolene, Ethicon). The suture pattern used is a matter of individual preference, but in wounds with excessive tension, vertical mattress sutures may be best.
- Debridement of the wound should be kept to a minimum. Blood clots should be removed and traumatized muscle trimmed. Skin flaps should be sutured in position, even if a deficiency in local blood supply is suspected. As a general guide to blood supply and viability of skin flaps, triangular flaps should have a base that is about twice the length of the vertical height of the flap.
- With all limb wounds below the elbow and stifle, effective bandaging to apply pressure to the wound should be used. We prefer paraffin gauze applied to the surface of the wound to prevent the bandage material from adhering to the wound. There is no advantage in using antibiotic-impregnated paraffin gauze over the normal paraffin gauze.

KEY POINT ▶ Wounds distal to the fetlock and other extensive wounds of the distal limb require support of the leg in a cast applied from the foot to just distal to the carpus or tarsus, respectively.

- This will result in a better cosmetic result and quicker overall healing time. While this is more expensive than normal treatment with bandaging, the decreased healing and convalescence time is a considerable advantage.

KEY POINT ▶ Tetanus prophylaxis is crucial in any horse that has a wound.

- Tetanus antitoxin should be given SC at a dose of 3000 IU.
- Use of antibiotics is debatable, but we find that better results are obtained in contaminated wounds when one or two doses of procaine penicillin are given at a dose rate of 15,000 IU/kg (15 mg/kg) (Treatment No. 83).
- A 4- to 5-day course of oral phenylbutazone, given at an initial dose rate of 4.4 mg/kg q12h for 24 hours, followed by 2.2 mg/kg q12h for 3 to 4 days, minimizes the degree of wound swelling

and the likelihood of wound dehiscence because sutures have pulled through the skin.

KEY POINT ▶ Where there is insufficient skin to cover the defect, a period of at least 3 months should elapse before consideration is given to grafting the wound.

- This is the maximum period that wound contraction is effective, and even large defects will be covered in this time if there is reasonable mobility of the surrounding skin. In cases where there is still not enough skin covering after 3 months, skin grafting can be considered. The most successful technique, though not the most cosmetic, in our hands, has been the use of punch grafts. We collect from the ventral abdomen or neck and put them into prepared sites in the granulation tissue bed. It is important to keep the site protected and immobile after the grafts are placed in position for at least 10 days. While the immediate results appear disappointing in many cases, after 4 to 6 weeks, many of the grafts are successful and provide good epithelial covering.

GRANULOMATOUS SKIN DISEASE
Exuberant Granulation Tissue ("Proud Flesh")

KEY POINT ▶ Exuberant granulation tissue is found most commonly in the distal limb, where poor skin mobility results in limited wound contraction.

The granulation tissue bed proliferates because of a lack of epithelial cover. This is a very common problem following wounds to the distal limbs in horses.

History and Presenting Signs

- Previous skin wound
- Proliferative granulomatous reaction at the wound site
- No local irritation, pruritus, or pain

Clinical Findings and Diagnosis

- Exuberant granulation tissue is self-evident and is usually associated with a nonhealing skin wound in the distal limb.
- If there is some doubt about the diagnosis, or if the granulation tissue appears to be slightly different in color to the pink, healthy appearance expected, a biopsy may be required. This should allow differentiation from some other abnormalities that may have a more serious prognosis.
- If there is a chronic wound with excessive granulation tissue and an intermittently discharging sinus, radiographs should be taken because osteomyelitis is a likely finding.

Differential Diagnosis

- Sarcoid
- Viral papillomas
- Habronemiasis
- Phycomycosis
- Bacterial and/or fungal granulomas
- Osteomyelitis

Treatment

- Wound contraction and epithelialization cannot proceed with the granulation tissue bed raised above the skin.

KEY POINT ► Treatment is directed toward excising the excessive granulation tissue down to just below skin level.

- Because there are no sensory nerves in the granulation tissue bed, this excision may be done without a local anesthetic using a scalpel blade. Although the hemorrhage is often quite dramatic immediately following excision, it can be controlled easily with pressure bandaging.
- A number of astringent-type preparations have been used to inhibit granulation tissue. The simplest of these is "white lotion," which is a mixture of 30 g lead acetate and 20 g zinc sulfate made up in 500 ml water. In the past, copper sulfate also has been used widely but is quite tissue toxic and can inhibit epithelialization around the margins of the granulation tissue. More recently, the use of metacresolsulfonic acid and formaldehyde (Lotagen, Boehringer Ingelheim, Germany) has provided good results.

KEY POINT ► A mild cleansing solution such as a combination of malic, benzoic, and salicylic acids (Derma-Clens, Smith Kline, Beecham, Philadelphia, PA) also may be useful in wounds that have some local necrotic reaction and low-grade infection.

- It is best to keep the wound bandaged, which helps to prevent exuberant granulation tissue from forming, and 3 months should elapse before further treatment is considered to allow for the full effect of wound contraction. At this stage, various types of skin grafts can be considered, and the most useful that we find are punch grafts.

Habronemiasis ("Summer Sores")

KEY POINT ► Habronemiasis is a common cause of skin disease, particularly in warmer, wet climates throughout the world, that results in ulcerative granulomas localized in moist regions of the body or in open wounds.

It is caused by various nematode species, particularly *Habronema muscae* and *Habronema majus*. Habronemiasis should be on the list of differential diagnoses when any chronic granulating wound is found.

History and Presenting Signs

- Nonhealing granulomatous wound—susceptible areas such as urethral process, conjunctiva, vulva
- Occurrence is mainly in spring and summer.

Clinical Findings and Diagnosis

- The classic appearance is similar to that of excessive granulation tissue with ulceration.
- In some cases caseous nodules may be present within the granulation tissue.
- In the majority of cases there is not extensive pruritus, but in a few the pruritus may be severe.

KEY POINT ► The appearance of the granulation tissue with the caseation is diagnostic.

- Confirmation of the finding may be made by a biopsy, which in some cases may reveal the presence of larvae but in most cases shows extensive eosinophil infiltration.

Differential Diagnosis

- Excessive granulation tissue
- Sarcoid
- Bacterial or fungal granuloma
- Squamous cell carcinoma (particularly for third eyelid lesions)

Treatment

- Organophosphates have been used systemically and topically in the past to treat habronemiasis, but oral or injectable ivermectin is now the treatment of choice.

KEY POINT ► Ivermectin (Treatment No. 62) treatment may have to be repeated several times, but usually two treatments at 10- to 14-day intervals is sufficient to give resolution.

- The dose rate used should be 0.2 mg/kg (10 ml Eqvalan liquid per 500 kg of body weight or Eqvalan paste, MSD-Agvet, Rahway, NJ).
- Where there is pruritus, to reduce the local reaction to dead larvae, the use of corticosteroids is of value. Oral prednisolone (Treatment No. 92) is the least expensive and most effective therapy. The initial dose rate should be 1 mg/kg q12h for the first 1 to 2 days, followed by 1 mg/kg given only in the morning for 5 days, after which 0.5 mg/kg is administered for a further 3 to 5 days. In some cases systemic corticosteroids alone have been sufficient to resolve the condition.
- In the case of granulomas around the urethral process and conjunctivae, excision is the treatment of choice.

Phycomycosis

Phycomycosis, which is more properly called *pythiosis,* is a condition found mainly in the tropics.

KEY POINT ▶ It usually causes a single, large granulomatous lesion with a characteristic pale granulation tissue in the distal limbs.

It arises from prolonged contact with water, where the fungus can infect damaged tissue, particularly wounds.

History and Presenting Signs

- Occurs only in wet tropical areas
- Most lesions are single
- Usually associated with a previous wound

Clinical Findings and Diagnosis

- Phycomycosis should always be on the list of differential diagnoses in any granulomatous condition found in horses kept in moist conditions in tropical climates.

KEY POINT ▶ One of the characteristic features of phycomycosis is the proliferative, large, ulcerative granulomatous reactions. Discharging sinuses are common from the surface of the granulomatous tissue.

- Pruritus is often a feature of the lesions.
- With larger lesions, it is common to find lymphangitis or at least limb edema.

KEY POINT ▶ Positive diagnosis is by biopsy of the granulomatous lesions and histologic demonstration of the fungal hyphae. There is evidence of marked inflammatory response with the additional presence of eosinophils.

Differential Diagnosis

- Sarcoid
- Excessive granulation tissue formation
- Habronemiasis

Treatment

KEY POINT ▶ Because many of the lesions are proliferative and rather large, surgical excision is necessary.

- There should be radical trimming of excess tissue down to below the skin surface. It is common to require repeat surgical excision if new lesions become apparent.
- Topical application of amphotericin B (Treatment No. 7) (50 mg in 10 ml saline and 10 ml dimethylsulfoxide; Treatment No. 34) has been reported to be useful.

- A vaccine prepared from *Phythium* cultures has been reported to be successful in some case of phycomycosis. The recommended regimen is that the vaccine be given weekly for three total vaccinations.

Sarcoid

KEY POINT ▶ Sarcoids are the most common tumor affecting the skin of horses.

They are nonmalignant tumors that have a suspected viral etiology. While sarcoids may arise spontaneously, our experience is that they are more commonly associated with previous skin wounds. While single sarcoids are most common and are relatively easily treated, up to a third of cases will involve multiple sites, and recurrence in these cases is common.

History and Presenting Signs

- History of previous wound
- Progressive granulomatous lesion
- History of recurrence despite excision

Clinical Findings and Diagnosis

KEY POINT ▶ Clinical appearance of sarcoids varies from the common fibroblastic type, which look like chronic granulation tissue, to verrucose lesions that have a more wart-like appearance.

- The fibroblastic type may grow quite large, particularly in areas of the distal limbs.
- Sarcoids are found most commonly around the head, particularly the eyes, followed by the legs and then areas of the trunk.
- In some lesions around the head, sarcoids may not have the classic, or granulomatous, appearance. These lesions can appear slightly scabby and are often intradermal. They may be mistaken for other skin tumors or granulomas. They are sometimes referred to as "occult sarcoids."

KEY POINT ▶ Biopsy and/or excision for diagnosis is important.

- While there is some disagreement among histopathologists about the exact characteristics of certain sarcoids, they are usually typified by fibroblastic proliferation with an abnormal appearance of the fibroblasts.

Differential Diagnosis

- Exuberant granulation tissue
- Viral papillomas
- Habronemiasis
- Phycomycosis
- Bacterial and/or fungal granulomas

Treatment

- Some clinicians favor surgical excision as the primary therapy, but the recurrence rate with surgical excision alone is quite high.

KEY POINT ► For lesions that are not close to the eye, the best clinical results can be obtained by cryosurgery.

- In horses with multiple lesions, we have seen regression of all lesions within 2 to 3 months of cryosurgical treatment of a few of the major lesions. This would seem to indicate that a general immune response is stimulated by excision and cryosurgery.

KEY POINT ► In smaller lesions or in those around the eye, we have found the injection of a mycobacterial cell-wall extract (Equimune, Vetrepharm, Athens, GA) into the base of the lesion has given excellent results.

- The dose that we have used is 1 ml/cm^3 of tissue. The lesion is debulked prior to injection, and the volume of the tissue remaining is estimated so that an appropriate volume of material is injected. Prior to the mycobacterial cell-wall extract preparation, immunotherapy with BCG vaccine was found to be useful, but this is no longer necessary.

Squamous Cell Carcinoma

KEY POINT ► Squamous cell carcinoma is probably the most common of the malignant skin neoplasms. It usually develops in areas around the mucocutaneous junction, such as the eyelids, penis and prepuce, and occasionally, the lips and nose.

While some authors consider that a viral etiology may be involved, most think that this is unlikely. Exposure to the sun may be a predisposing factor. The lesions usually commence without obvious changes to the surrounding tissue. In many cases, lesions may not be noticed in areas that are hidden, such as the penis, prepuce, and vulva. However, the tumor is locally invasive and metastasizes quite readily to the regional lymph nodes. We have seen a few horses presented for swelling of the hindlimbs due to lymphatic obstruction from metastasis of squamous cell carcinoma of the penis.

History and Presenting Signs

- Erosive lesions at a mucocutaneous junction
- Usually affects older horses
- Lesions common around the third eyelid, penis, and prepuce

Clinical Findings and Diagnosis

- The client's attention is usually drawn by the progressive nature of the problem. Lesions often appear ulcerous, and with progression, a granulomatous reaction develops at the site of the tumor.
- While many of the lesions have an erosive appearance, those around the penis and prepuce can sometimes appear cauliflower-shaped.
- Excision and/or biopsy is critical to enable histopathologic diagnosis.

Differential Diagnosis

- Sarcoid
- Exuberant granulation tissue
- Viral papillomas
- Habronemiasis
- Phycomycosis
- Bacterial and/or fungal granulomas

Treatment

- Early diagnosis is important for successful outcome.
- In some cases excision back to normal margins can be satisfactory.
- If the lesion involves the glans of the penis, amputation may be indicated.

KEY POINT ► We have had success with radiation therapy, particularly radon-222 implants. In some cases close to the eye, strontium-90 treatment has been effective.

- Recurrence of the lesion does not seem to be as common as with sarcoids but nevertheless may occur in a small percentage of cases.

NODULAR SKIN DISEASE
Folliculitis

KEY POINT ► Bacterial folliculitis is the most common type of folliculitis found, and the main offending organism is *Staphylococcus aureus*. We have seen it most commonly in young horses in training during the summer.

History and Presenting Signs

- Summer incidence
- Lesions over the saddle area, pastern, and occasionally the tail

Clinical Findings and Diagnosis

- It is thought that the combination of rubbing from the girth and/or the saddle, local sweating, and the ubiquitous nature of staphylococcal organisms leads to the development of the folliculitis.

- While staphylococcal folliculitis is the most common bacterial folliculitis, there is also a form due to *Corynebacterium pseudotuberculosis.*
- Lesions are papular and may be small or progress to larger pustules.
- Horses show signs of pain on palpation of the lesions or when pressure is applied with grooming equipment or tack.

KEY POINT ► Samples of pus from the nondischarging pustules should be collected aseptically for bacterial culture.

- It is important that contamination from skin organisms is avoided, as discussed under Diagnostic Aids. Some of the issues relating to sample collection are further discussed in Chapter 15.

KEY POINT ► Another form of staphylococcal folliculitis is found in horses that traumatize their tails. This form of the disease is difficult to treat successfully.

Differential Diagnosis

- Fly and mosquito bites
- Dermatophilosis
- Dermatophytosis

Treatment

- The initiating local skin moisture and trauma should be avoided by ensuring that the horse is not ridden or driven.

KEY POINT ► Local application of antiseptic solutions, particularly iodophor shampoos (Povidone Shampoo 5%, Butler, Dublin, OH; Iodine Shampoo, Evsco, Buena, NJ), can be helpful in treating the condition.

- If the staphylococci are sensitive to penicillin G, a course of IM procaine penicillin (Treatment No. 83) at a dose rate of 15,000 IU/kg (15 mg/kg) q12h may be useful. The duration of therapy may need to be as long as 2 weeks.

Fly and Mosquito Bites

A number of biting flies and mosquitoes can produce skin weals and papules that may be quite painful and sometimes pruritic. Apart from mosquitoes and sand flies (*Culicoides* spp.), there are a range of stable flies (*Stomoxys* spp.), black flies (*Simulium* spp.), and horse flies (*Tabanid* spp.). Fly and mosquito bites are mainly found in the late summer and fall and cause considerable irritation to horses.

KEY POINT ► Most fly and mosquito bites are located around the limbs and trunks,

although there is a condition associated with *Culicoides* spp. and also horn flies that can cause a ventral midline dermatitis.

History and Presenting Signs

- Papules and weals in a number of body sites
- Seasonal incidence, usually in summer and fall
- Change in horse behavior

Clinical Findings and Diagnosis

- Most fly bites result in small to medium-sized papules with some more extensive skin weals.
- The most common locations for fly bites are the legs and trunk, although the bites of some flies, in particular *Haematobia* spp., have been associated with a ventral midline dermatitis, while the bites of *Simulium* spp. tend to be located around the head, neck, and ears.
- If a skin biopsy is taken, which is seldom necessary, nonspecific changes are found, including perivascular dermatitis and a number of eosinophils.

Differential Diagnosis

- Necrobiosis
- Papilloma
- Insect hypersensitivity (e.g., tick bites)

Treatment

KEY POINT ► Control of insect bites is difficult and is best achieved by management practices.

- Because many of the flies are active during the early morning and later evening, light rugs and hoods may be helpful in decreasing the bites at these times of the day.
- A closed system for disposal of horse manure and bedding can be helpful in reducing the fly population.
- In areas where there are particular problems, confining horses in screened box stalls with the use of timed-misting insecticidal devices can be helpful.
- During competition or for procedures such as radiography and electrocardiography, where the horse should stand still, various fly repellent sprays are helpful for temporary control. These usually contain pyrethrins, citronella, and/or piperonyl butoxide. Commercial products include Flysect Citronella Spray and Flysect Repellent Shampoo (Equicare, Dallas, TX) and Equine Fly Repellent Mist (Vetmate, Suwanee, GA).
- In cases where there are severe reactions to the bites, the use of corticosteroids may be indicated. In many cases a single injection of intravenous dexamethasone (Treatment Nos. 29 and

30) at a dose rate of 0.05 to 0.1 mg/kg is sufficient to control the reaction.

Melanoma

KEY POINT ▶ Melanomas are generally a problem in gray horses, and while melanomas may be located anywhere in the body, the most common site is around the perineum.

Melanomas may occur in single or multiple sites and are usually slow to metastasize. The tumors are firm and nodular in appearance. In chronic cases there may be ulceration. The biologic behavior of melanomas in the horse varies, with the majority being malignant. However, spread appears to be slow, and many horses with metastases to regional lymph nodes can live for many years without adverse clinical signs.

History and Presenting Signs

- Usually found in gray horses
- Small, firm nodules

Clinical Findings and Diagnosis

KEY POINT ▶ Firm nodules located around the perineum, head, and occasionally the distal limbs with characteristic hyperpigmentation are almost always diagnostic for equine melanoma.

- In long-standing cases with multiple nodules at a particular site, ulceration of the skin over the melanomas may be found.
- Some cases have presented as a subcutaneous lump with no apparent changes in the skin. Melanomas have been confirmed in these cases by biopsy or excision.

Differential Diagnosis

- Nodular necrobiosis
- Fly and mosquito bites

Treatment

- In cases where there is a single, isolated nodule, excision may be possible. However, the majority of cases are multiple, and therefore, excision can be difficult. This is particularly the case around the perineum, where wound breakdown is common following excision and there may be non-healing wounds.
- Cimetidine (Treatment No. 26) given orally at a dose rate of 2.5 mg/kg q8h, with a reduction to a once-daily maintenance dose after a clinical response is seen, has been reported to be successful in causing regression of some melanomas. However, our experience is that treatment is expensive and results are not good. Further studies involving large case numbers are needed before the efficacy of cimetidine can be evaluated.

Nodular Necrobiosis (Nodular Granuloma)

KEY POINT ▶ This type of nodular skin reaction, which is quite common, appears to be a reaction to insect bites.

There are usually several firm nodules ranging up to 3 to 4 cm (1.5 in) in diameter, most commonly in the skin over the back, particularly where the saddle is located. In some cases, the typical firm, nodular skin reaction is found in the neck.

History and Presenting Signs

- Firm, localized skin nodules
- No history of pruritus
- Horses usually presented in summer

Clinical Findings and Diagnosis

- The location of the nodules (usually on the back, particularly where the saddle sits) and the lack of pain associated with them indicate the likelihood of nodular necrobiosis.
- The problem is intradermal, and in most cases there is normal hair growth over the site of the nodules.

KEY POINT ▶ Skin biopsy reveals typical histopathologic changes characteristic of collagenolysis, granuloma formation, and eosinophil infiltration.

Differential Diagnosis

- Neoplasia
- Amyloidosis
- Foreign-body granuloma
- Fly and/or mosquito bites
- Viral papular dermatitis

Treatment

KEY POINT ▶ Early in the course of the problem, before calcification occurs, local injection of long-acting corticosteroids such as methylprednisolone acetate (Treatment No. 74) or triamcinolone acetate (Treatment No. 106), up to 0.25 ml per lesion, may be effective in decreasing the size of the lump.

- This treatment is of most use when there are single or only a few nodules. If the reaction is more extensive, prednisolone (Treatment No. 92) may be given orally at a dose rate of 1 mg/kg q12h for 2 to 3 days, followed by 1 mg/kg daily for 7 to 10 days, after which the dose is reduced to 1 mg/kg every second day for a further 10 to 14 days.
- Larger calcified lesions that cause cosmetic problems or where the saddle irritates the local area require surgical excision. However, some care is required, particularly where there are lesions in

the dorsal midline, because nonhealing of the skin wound may result.

Ulcerative Lymphangitis

While a number of microorganisms have been associated with ulcerative lymphangitis, *Corynebacterium pseudotuberculosis* is the most common cause. It is an uncommon disease and is probably associated with poor hygiene and attention to bedding in horses kept in box stalls.

History and Presenting Signs

- Swelling of one or more limbs
- Painful nodules

Clinical Findings and Diagnosis

KEY POINT ▶ Early in the course of the infection there is hindlimb edema followed by development of painful nodules that tend to ulcerate and have a purulent discharge.

- The purulent material is often creamy to green in color.
- The majority of cases seem to involve a hindlimb, and there is localized swelling, often involving the whole of the hindlimb.
- The major difficulty in establishing a diagnosis is obtaining appropriate material for bacteriologic culture. As noted in Chapter 15, inappropriate bacteriologic samples are useless. Swabs from discharging skin lesions are of no diagnostic value.

Differential Diagnosis

- Nonspecific lymphangitis
- Sporotrichosis
- Histoplasmosis
- Phycomycosis

Treatment

- If the disease is associated with poor local environmental conditions, these should be attended to. Ensuring that the horse has clean bedding and that the feet are cleaned daily are important parts of therapy.

KEY POINT ▶ Antibiotics are useful in the early stages of the disease but may be of little use in well established cases.

- Antibiotics that we have found useful include IM procaine penicillin (Treatment No. 83) at a dose rate of 15,000 IU/kg (or 15 mg/kg) q12h and trimethoprim–sulfur combinations (Treatment No. 107) at a combined drug dose rate of 20 mg/kg (PO) or 15 mg/kg (IV) twice daily are the drugs of choice. In some cases that have not been responsive to these antibiotics, we have had response to oxytetracycline given IV at a dose rate of 5 mg/

kg q12h. However, many cases are unresponsive to antibiotic treatment.

Warts (Viral Papilloma)

Papovaviruses are known to cause warts in a variety of species, including horses.

KEY POINT ▶ The term *papillomatosis* has become more common because, while warts are the most common presenting signs in horses with papillomatosis, aural plaques also have been reported.

History and Presenting Signs

- Yearling and 2-year-old horses affected
- Typical warts are found around the lips and nose

Clinical Findings and Diagnosis

- Warts are very characteristic and cannot be mistaken for many other skin disorders.

KEY POINT ▶ There are usually multiple lesions, the most common sites being around the nose and lips, genitalia, and occasionally the distal limbs.

- Aural plaques also may be a feature of papillomatosis in horses. These plaques occur usually bilaterally and affect the inner surface of the ear. Lesions usually progress to form hyperkeratotic plaques.
- Horses with either warts or aural plaques do not show any signs of irritation or pruritus in the majority of cases.
- The typical appearance of the lesions enables a diagnosis to be made without resort to biopsy or other techniques.

Differential Diagnosis

- The wart-type lesions are typical and not confused with other skin conditions.
- The aural plaque lesions may be confused with insect bites, but these are usually on the outer part of the ear.

Treatment

- Papillomatosis is a self-limiting disease, where spontaneous regression of the lesion occurs with time.
- Because the lesions occur in young animals that may be for sale, there is some pressure on the clinician to try some type of treatment.
- A number of topical agents, including podophyllin, have been used but generally are ineffective.

KEY POINT ▶ While lesions are best left untreated, it is important to isolate infected horses so transmission is less likely.

PRURITIC AND ALOPECIC SKIN DISEASE

Contact Dermatitis

Contact dermatitis is quite common in horses, arising occasionally from some plants but more commonly by the application of or access to various irritating chemicals. The most frequently observed contact dermatitis is associated with the use of various iodine-based "blisters." These are commonly used by horse owners and trainers to treat a variety of musculoskeletal problems.

History and Presenting Signs

- Localized inflammatory reaction
- Rapid onset of signs

Clinical Findings and Diagnosis

- The area of involvement is localized, and the most common regions affected are the lips and mouth and distal limbs.
- There is initial edema and erythema at the site progressing to vesicle formation or ulceration.
- In the early stages there is severe irritation at the contact site, with horses showing pain and sometimes pruritus.
- In cases where the reaction has been severe, there may be permanent deformation of the skin with scarring and alopecia.
- A specific diagnosis cannot be made from the findings, and skin biopsy is of little use. Diagnosis is by exclusion of other conditions and the history.

Differential Diagnosis

- Sunburn
- Photodermatitis

Treatment

- Removing the offending agent is obviously critical to effective treatment.
- Topical antibiotic/corticosteroid ointments (Treatment No. 8) are helpful in reducing the extent of local inflammation.

Culicoides Hypersensitivity ("Queensland Itch," "Sweet Itch," "Summer Itch")

KEY POINT ► Hypersensitivity associated with Culicoides (sandfly or midge) bites is one of the most common causes of pruritic and alopecic skin disease throughout the world.

There are a variety of Culicoides spp. that tend to be more of a problem in the summer months, except in the tropics, where they are active through-

out the year. Type I and type IV hypersensitivity reactions are involved, the dorsum of the horse being most frequently afflicted.

History and Presenting Signs

- Most common during summer months
- Mature horses (>3 years old) more commonly affected
- Pruritus and alopecia

Clinical Findings and Diagnosis

- The various Culicoides spp. are most active in the early morning and late afternoon.
- The likely affected areas are the dorsal midline, and the ears, mane, and tail are most commonly involved.
- If the affected horse is part of a herd, it is unlikely that more than one or two horses will show clinical signs of the disease.
- Pruritus is a characteristic feature of Culoides hypersensitivity. Horses will often rub their manes and bases of their tails with the result that the hair becomes quite sparse in these areas.
- In the early stages of this condition, there may be small papules, and with progression of the hypersensitivity, alopecia may be quite widespread, particularly over the dorsum.

KEY POINT ► The classic distribution of lesions, pruritus, and seasonal incidence are diagnostic for Culicoides hypersensitivity.

- If skin biopsies are taken, nonspecific findings such as the presence of perivascular eosinophils are found.

Differential Diagnosis

- Fly and mosquito bites
- Onchocerciasis
- Ectoparasites
- Dermatophilosis
- Dermatophytosis

Treatment

KEY POINT ► Insect control is an important part of management but is often difficult to achieve.

- The gnats are most active in the early evening and early morning, and therefore, stabling horses in insect-proof environments can help to reduce the extent of pruritus. If this is not possible, then rugging the horses with light rugs and hoods may be helpful.

KEY POINT ► The oral use of prednisolone is helpful in controlling the clinical signs.

- Prednisolone (Treatment No. 92) is administered at a dose rate of 1 mg/kg bid for 2 to 3 days, followed by 1 mg/kg given in the morning for a further period (usually 5–10 days) until signs are controlled. After this, dosage can be tapered to 1 mg/kg given in the morning every second day, followed by 0.5 mg/kg every second day.

Drug Eruption

Drug eruptions are uncommon hypersensitivity reactions that can occur after drug administration by any of the routes.

KEY POINT ► Most commonly, these eruptions are seen after antibiotic administration, but they also have been seen after anti-inflammatories, vaccines, and tranquilizers.

History and Presenting Signs

- Variable reaction in the skin
- History of recent or current drug administration

Clinical Findings and Diagnosis

- The extent and type of reaction in the skin are variable, ranging from urticaria to a papular-type dermatitis.
- Because of the variability of the skin reactions, it is difficult to differentiate a drug eruption from a number of other dermatoses.
- Pruritus may or may not be present.

Differential Diagnosis

- Insect hypersensitivity
- Onchocerciasis
- Urticaria
- Pemphigus foliaceus
- Erythema multiforme

Treatment

- Corticosteroids (0.1 mg/kg of dexamethasone IV; Treatment Nos. 29 and 30) can be used, but most drug eruptions are not responsive to this therapy.
- The reaction abates after withdrawal of the drug, but this may take several weeks.

Ectoparasites

KEY POINT ► A number of ectoparasites can cause pruritus and alopecia in horses.

Lice infestation is relatively common, particularly in herds of horses, during the winter months. Two types of lice are found, biting lice (*Damalinia equi*) and sucking lice (*Haematopinus asini*). Mange is less common than lice and consists of three types: sarcoptic mange (caused by *Sarcoptes scabei* var. *equi*), psoroptic mange (caused by *Psoroptes equi*), and chorioptic mange (caused by *Chorioptes equi*). Tick infestation also can occur in horses but seldom causes signs of pruritus.

History and Presenting Signs

- Pruritus
- Alopecia
- Papules
- Crusting and alopecia of skin
- Horses usually not intensively supervised or groomed

Clinical Findings and Diagnosis

► Lice

KEY POINT ► Lice are commonly located around the mane and tail, and horses will often show intense pruritus and rub their manes, bite at their flanks, and rub their tails.

Examination of the coarse mane hairs usually demonstrates eggs, and sometimes the lice can be seen.

► Chorioptic Mange

KEY POINT ► This is usually called *leg mange* and causes irritation to the distal limbs.

- Because the mites live on the surface of the skin, the clinical findings are usually minimal, there being small, crusty lesions and alopecia involving the distal limbs.
- On occasion, horses will stamp their feet because of the irritation.
- Skin scrapings usually show the mites and should be taken from the edge of the skin lesions.

► Psoroptic Mange

- As with chorioptic mange, the mites do not burrow.

KEY POINT ► The common sites for the mites are the mane and tail.

- Extreme pruritus is found, with lesions ranging from papules to scaling and crust formation. There is variable alopecia.
- Skin scrapings usually show the mites and should be taken from the edge of the skin lesions.

► Sarcoptic Mange

KEY POINT ► These mites tend to burrow into the skin, unlike the other types of mange mites.

- Pruritus is characteristic, and lesions may progress from the front of the horse to involve the whole body.
- There may be severe excoriation of affected skin with severe alopecia.
- Deep skin scrapings are needed to identify the mites, which are generally more difficult to find than those causing chorioptic and psoroptic mange.

Differential Diagnosis

- Insect hypersensitivities
- Chorioptic mange
- Lice
- Psoroptic mange
- Sarcoptic mange
- Tick infestation

Treatment

KEY POINT ▶ Most of the ectoparasites respond to treatment with topical organophosphates or pyrethrins (Treatment No. 105).

- Because the eggs of the various ectoparasites hatch after 10 to 14 days, treatment must be repeated about 14 days after the initial spraying.
- It is important to spray all the gear associated with the horse, including rugs, cloths, etc., as well as the box stall or other accommodation.
- Some of the mites and the sucking lice can be treated with ivermectin (Treatment No. 62) administered at a dose rate of 0.2 mg/kg and repeated at 14-day intervals for a total of three treatments.

Onchocerciasis

Onchocerca cervicalis is the main species of *Onchocerca* causing skin lesions in horses in most regions of the world.

KEY POINT ▶ Infection with *Onchocerca* is very widespread in most horse populations, but the majority of horses are asymptomatic.

It is most likely that the clinical signs of disease are related to a hypersensitivity reaction. While the adult worms are located in the ligamentum nuchae, microfilariae are located in the skin, most frequently in the region of the ventral abdomen. Various of the *Culicoides* spp. serve as intermediate hosts for the microfilariae.

History and Presenting Signs

- Mature horses (>3 years old) affected
- Most common in warm to hot weather
- Lesions most common on the ventral abdomen and chest

Clinical Findings and Diagnosis

KEY POINT ▶ Skin lesions are variable and range from thinning of hair and edematous plaques in the early stages to scaly or crusty alopecia in later stages. There may be chronic induration of the affected skin.

- Most lesions are localized to skin over the ventral abdomen but also can be found around the head, neck, and chest.

- The degree of pruritus is variable but in some cases is quite intense. However, in contrast to *Culicoides* hypersensitivity, horses seldom rub around their tails.
- A circular lesion in the center of the forehead is thought to be indicative of cutaneous onchocerciasis but is found only occasionally.
- Microfilariae can be demonstrated by taking a skin biopsy, chopping the sample into fine pieces, and incubating it in 0.9% saline at 37°C (98.6°F) for 10 to 15 minutes. The microfilariae can be seen in the solution. However, because the microfilariae of *Onchocerca* are commonly found in asymptomatic horses, the presence of microfilariae per se does not indicate a clinical problem.

Differential Diagnosis

- Dermatophilosis
- *Culicoides* hypersensitivity
- Ectoparasites
- Fly and mosquito bites

Treatment

- Ivermectin (Treatment No. 62) administered orally at a dose rate of 0.2 mg/kg is effective in eliminating the microfilariae but does not kill the adult *Onchocerca*. Repeated treatments are necessary at 3-month intervals.
- With the death of the microfilariae, there is quite an intense pruritus in some horses, although there is less reaction with ivermectin than with diethylcarbamazine, which previously was used to treat onchocerciasis. This reaction can be avoided or minimized by the prior administration of a short-acting corticosteroid such as dexamethasone disodium phosphate (Treatment Nos. 29 and 30) at a dose rate of 0.1 mg/kg.

Urticaria

Urticarial reactions are the result of hypersensitivity reactions (type I and III) and are caused by a wide range of diseases, medications, feedstuffs, dust, and pollen. Lesions may be localized or generalized.

History and Presenting Signs

- Extensive skin wheals
- May occur in an acute or recurrent form

Clinical Findings and Diagnosis

KEY POINT ▶ The skin wheals that typify an urticarial reaction can be localized and vary in size from small, localized lesions (1–3 cm) to extensive reactions involving a large area of skin.

- Isolated cases of urticaria resolve spontaneously or with medication, but determining the etiologic agent is difficult in recurrent urticaria.

- Recurrent urticarial reactions may require feed elimination trials if some component of the feed is suspected. Intradermal allergy testing also may be useful.

Differential Diagnosis

- Drug eruption
- Vasculitis
- Erythema multiforme
- Purpura hemorrhagica
- Pemphigus foliaceus
- Onchocerciasis

Treatment

KEY POINT ► Intravenous corticosteroids are the treatment of choice in acute reactions, and many cases are responsive.

- Dexamethasone phosphate (Treatment Nos. 29 and 30) can be given IV in a single dose of 0.1 mg/kg.
- If a specific feed or environmental allergen is involved, it may be necessary to modify the environment appropriately to reduce exposure to the offending agent.
- Antihistamines are of value in some cases and pyrilamine (Histavet-P, Schering-Plough, Kenilworth, NJ) can be used at a dose rate of 1 mg/kg given either intramuscularly or slowly intravenously.

NONPRURITIC AND ALOPECIC SKIN DISEASE

Dermatophilosis ("Rain Scald")

KEY POINT ► Dermatophilosis is a common condition affecting horses at pasture and causes a superficial dermatitis with moist, crusty lesions affecting skin over the dorsum.

The microorganism (*Dermatophilus congolensis*) is a Gram-positive anaerobe that is sensitive to penicillin G. Prolonged exposure to rain is a key component in the development of the disease, hence the common name "rain scald."

History and Presenting Signs

- Exposure to heavy rain
- Skin damage
- Matted tufts of hair on dorsum

Clinical Findings and Diagnosis

- The classical skin appearance in *Dermatophilus* infection is an exudative dermatitis, there being matted tufts of hair along the dorsum.

KEY POINT ► Close inspection of the skin reveals multiple, small scabs at the base of the matted hair. If the scabs are lifted, the skin underneath has a raw, bleeding appearance.

- Unlike the various insect hypersensitivities, there is no pruritus. However, the areas are tender, the horses showing sensitivity by crouching away when the lesions are examined or if the hair is clipped.
- In some cases, *Dermatophilus* can affect the distal limbs, but this is less common than the form affecting the dorsum.
- Diagnosis is made from the clinical findings, particularly the typical slightly raised, raw appearance of the skin underneath the crust. Smears can be made from underneath the crust and a Gram stain performed, which reveals typical branching filaments of Gram-positive cocci.

Differential Diagnosis

- Pemphigus foliaceus
- Dermatophytosis (early stages)
- Staphylococcal folliculitis
- Seborrhea

Treatment

- Attention to skin hygiene and the use of topical disinfectants are the keys to successful resolution. However, many horses will recover spontaneously, particularly if the horse is moved to a protected environment such as a box stall.

KEY POINT ► Loosening the scabs and spraying the affected areas with a disinfectant such as chlorhexidine (Nolvasan Solution, Fort Dodge Labs or Aveco, Fort Dodge, IA) or 1% povidone-iodine solution (Treatment No. 91) is the treatment of choice. Treatment should be continued daily for up to 10 days.

- The organism is sensitive to penicillin G, and therefore, in cases where the lesions are extensive, administration of procaine penicillin (Treatment No. 83) at a dose rate of 15,000 IU/kg (15 mg/kg) IM q12h for 3 to 5 days can aid in more rapid resolution of the infection.

Eosinophilic Dermatitis

This disease is thought to be the result of a hypersensitivity reaction, but the initiating cause is not known. The condition, which is quite rare, is also known as *eosinophilic granulomatosis*.

History and Clinical Signs

- More commonly found in winter
- Systemic signs as well as skin disease

Clinical Findings and Diagnosis

- Crusting-type lesions with presence of some scaling. Evidence of exudation is typical of the condition, and there is generalized alopecia. Skin nodules are often present. Although there have been reports of pruritus, this is an uncommon finding.

■ Lesions also may be found at the coronary band, where fissures develop.

KEY POINT ▶ Weight loss is often found, and affected animals may be depressed.

■ Because the intestinal disease is generalized, diarrhea is often found as a result of colonic involvement.

■ D-Glucose or D-xylose absorption tests are usually flattened, indicating malabsorption. Rectal mucosal biopsy (for details, see Chap. 6) may be useful to aid in diagnosis because the eosinophilic infiltrates are present.

■ Skin biopsies are essential to make a diagnosis and reveal eosinophilic infiltrates as well as nonspecific changes such as hyperkeratosis and collagen degeneration.

Differential Diagnosis

■ Dermatophilosis
■ Pemphigus foliaceus
■ Seborrhea
■ Sarcoidosis

Treatment

KEY POINT ▶ Most horses do not recover from this disorder.

We have had experience of two cases that were initially responsive to treatment with systemic corticosteroid therapy. Dexamethasone disodium phosphate (Treatment Nos. 29 and 30) is given IV for 2 to 3 days, after which therapy is continued using oral prednisolone (Treatment No. 92) at a dose rate of 0.5 mg/kg q12h for 3 to 4 days and then 0.5 mg/kg daily for 7 to 10 days. The administration of prednisolone is gradually tapered off over a further 7 to 10 days. This treatment will not cure the condition, but it may provide short-term relief.

Pemphigus Foliaceus

KEY POINT ▶ Pemphigus foliaceus is an autoimmune skin disorder that seems to be more common in hot, humid climates.

There are reports of Appaloosas being predisposed to the disorder. It causes generalized disease, there being alopecia with exudation and the formation of skin crusts.

History and Presenting Signs

■ Generalized skin disease
■ Depression and lethargy
■ Inappetence

Clinical Findings and Diagnosis

■ The disease may commence with vesicles and pustules, progressing to crusting-type lesions and variable scaling of the skin.

■ Lesions most commonly are located on the head, neck, and forelimbs but eventually become widespread.

KEY POINT ▶ Signs of lethargy and inappetence are common, and affected horses often appear depressed.

■ Pruritus is uncommon, but recently developed lesions may be painful.

■ Anemia (PCV < 0.30 L/L) is common, and there may be hypoalbuminemia.

■ In the early stages of the condition, when there are intact vesicles, a needle aspirate for cytology reveals numerous acanthocytes and neutrophils.

■ Skin biopsy of recently developed lesions is vital to diagnosis, there being acantholysis on histologic examination. Biopsy samples for immunofluorescence should be placed in Michel's medium (pH 7.0) (see p. 339), and the testing shows widespread immunoglobulin deposits. False-positive and false-negative results are found with direct immunofluorescence, so it is important that the clinical picture and skin histopathology are given adequate emphasis in making a diagnosis of pemphigus.

Differential Diagnosis

■ Dermatophytosis
■ Dermatophilosis
■ Bacterial folliculitis
■ Onchocerciasis
■ Insect hypersensitivity

Treatment

KEY POINT ▶ Cases of pemphigus do not improve with time, but many cases respond well to systemic corticosteroid administration.

Oral prednisolone (Treatment No. 92) is the treatment of choice because it is inexpensive and there is generally a good response. Initially, a dose rate of 1 mg/kg q12h should be used for a period of 5 to 7 days, at which time the affected horse should be showing signs of improvement. The dose frequency is then decreased to a morning dosage only for a further 10 to 14 days, after which an every-other-day treatment regimen still at a dose rate of 1 mg/kg is used. Treatment needs to be continued indefinitely, and the aim is to maintain the horse on the minimum possible dose rate. In most cases we have found that a twice-weekly treatment regimen is adequate for maintenance.

Photodermatitis

Photodermatitis is an inflammatory skin disease caused by exposure to ultraviolet radiation.

KEY POINT ► The main form of disease is photosensitization that is either primary (from photodynamic agents in plants) or secondary (due to liver disease resulting in phylloerythrin accumulation).

The hepatic form of photosensitization is more common than the primary form and is usually seen with ingestion of plants containing pyrrolizidine alkaloids (see Liver Disease, Chap. 6). Sunburn is the other form of photodermatitis that can occasionally be found in horses that have fine hair coats with areas of skin that are nonpigmented.

History and Presenting Signs

- Nonpigmented skin affected
- Areas where there is less hair covering affected

Clinical Findings and Diagnosis

KEY POINT ► Areas around the head and unpigmented expanses of skin are the regions most affected by photosensitization.

- Skin lesions are severe and include inflammation with crusting and fissuring. After the early inflammatory reaction, there is peeling and sometimes sloughing of the affected skin.
- Pruritus may be found, particularly in the early stages of the condition.
- Blood samples should be collected for hematology and liver function tests (see Chap. 6). This should allow differentiation of primary from secondary photosensitization.
- Diagnosis is often possible by the localized but severe skin abnormalities.

Differential Diagnosis

- Contact dermatitis
- Sunburn

Treatment

KEY POINT ► Stabling the horse to prevent exposure to the sun is important to prevent worsening of the problem.

- Topical application of antibiotic/corticosteroid ointments (Treatment No. 8) can be helpful in decreasing the local inflammation.
- Because secondary photosensitization is more common than primary, the prognosis is often poor because liver failure may supervene (see Chap. 6). Most cases of primary photosensitization recover uneventfully.

Ringworm (Dermatophytosis)

KEY POINT ► Dermatophytosis is one of the most common skin diseases affecting stabled horses. It is found most often in young horses and is caused by two main fungal species, *Microsporum* and *Trichophyton*.

There seems to be a seasonal pattern of the disease in the northern hemisphere, with the majority of cases occurring in winter and fall. Infection is common in racing stables, particularly in yearling and 2-year-old horses. Dermatophytosis can spread via direct contact but more commonly by contaminated grooming equipment, blankets, and cloths. The incubation period may be quite prolonged, with some cases taking up to 4 weeks to show clinical signs. The condition may be spread to humans, and therefore, advice should be given to personnel handling affected horses to ensure that a zoonotic infection does not occur.

History and Presenting Signs

- Horses less than 3 years of age
- Lesions most common in the girth/saddle region
- Alopecia

Clinical Findings and Diagnosis

- In the early stages, dermatophytosis can mimic a range of other skin diseases because there may be papular lesions and/or urticaria. These areas are usually sensitive to the touch.
- After several days, crusts appear, and scaliness of the skin is typical of the infection.
- Alopecia develops that is circumscribed, the skin and hair in the immediate vicinity of the lesions having a normal appearance.
- Because some degree of skin trauma appears to be involved in dermatophytosis becoming established, lesions are most commonly seen in the saddle/girth regions.
- Pruritus may be found, particularly during the early stages of the infection. However, in the majority of cases, pruritus is not a feature of the disease.
- Diagnosis can be made from the typical appearance of the skin lesions in most cases. Skin scrapings may be made to confirm the diagnosis (see Diagnostic Aids, p. 338), with samples examined directly as well as being submitted for fungal culture. The scrapings should be taken from the periphery of the lesions, where the fungi are more likely to be found.

Differential Diagnosis

- Urticaria
- Dermatophilosis
- Pemphigus
- Staphylococcal folliculitis

Treatment

- Dermatophytosis is self-limiting, and most horses recover spontaneously after several months. The condition is highly contagious, and it is important that action be taken to limit the spread via isolation of the affected horse's grooming equipment, blankets, etc. and applying topical antifungal agents to the infected areas of skin.
- Captan (Treatment No. 17), applied as a 3% solution, is an inexpensive and popular treatment for dermatophytosis. Other topical agents that are effective in limiting the spread of disease include iodine (1% available iodine) and lime sulfur (3%) solutions. We have had a good response to topically applied natamycin in some cases of generalized ringworm.
- Oral griseofulvin has been advocated at dose rates around 10 mg/kg per day for 1 to 2 months. We have not had successful results with this therapy, which is quite expensive. Because of this, we do not recommend its use.

Seborrhea

Seborrhea is usually secondary to some other skin disease, but it also can be a primary disorder. It is rarely found as a generalized disease and is most commonly localized around the mane and tail. It is principally a disease of abnormal keratinization and occurs in two forms, one where there is increased oiliness of the skin and the other where the skin becomes scaly in appearance.

History and Presenting Signs

- Prior skin disease
- Presented with scaling or crusting skin lesions
- Lesions usually localized

Clinical Findings and Diagnosis

- Three main forms of the disease have been described. *Seborrhea sicca* is uncommon and is typified by a scaly, dry skin. *Seborrhea oleosa* is the form that is most easily recognized, there being increased oiliness of the skin and associated matting of the oily material in the hair. *Seborrheic dermatitis* can have the combined appearance of the two other forms, and there is usually some degree of bacterial infection of the skin due to alterations in the normal bacterial flora.
- Because primary seborrhea is rare in the horse, initiating causes should be determined. A wide range of skin disease can result in seborrhea, including ectoparasites, pemphigus foliaceus, folliculitis, dermatophytosis, and dermatophilosis.
- Skin biopsy findings may reveal hyperkeratosis.

Differential Diagnosis

- Most important is to identify whether there is a secondary cause for disease.
- Ectoparasites
- Pemphigus foliaceus
- Dermatophilosis
- Dermatophytosis
- Folliculitis

Treatment

- Keratolytic shampoos are useful for seborrhea oleosa. Shampoos that are available include sulfur-salicylate (Sebalyt, DVM, Miami, FL; Sebolux, Allerderm/Virbac, Hurst, TX) and selenium (Seleen, Sanofi, Overland Park, KS). Tar-based shampoos also have been used (Thiomar, Evsco, Buena, NJ; Equitar Shampoo, DVM, Miami, FL).
- Keratolytic shampoos should be avoided in the case of seborrhea sicca because they may worsen the drying of the skin. For this reason, emollient shampoos such as Allergroom (Allerderm/Virbac, Hurst, TX) are best. An after-shampoo rinse containing emollients (Humilac, Allerderm/Virbac, Hurst, TX) is also useful. This product is added at the rate of 5 capfuls per liter of water.

References

Barbet, J. L., Baxter, G. M., and McMullan, W. C.: Diseases of the Skin. In P. T. Colahan, I. G. Mayhew, A. M. Merritt, and J. N. Moore (Eds.), *Equine Medicine and Surgery,* 4th Ed. Goleta, Calif.: American Veterinary Publications, 1991, p. 1569.

Evans, A. G., and Stannard, A. A.: Diagnostic approach to equine skin disease. *Compend. Contin. Educ. Pract. Vet.* 8(9):652, 1986.

Fadok, V. A., and Mullowney, P. C.: Dermatologic diseases of horses: I. Parasitic dermatoses of the horse. *Compend. Contin. Educ. Pract. Vet.* 5:5615, 1983.

Fadok, V. A., and Greiner, E. C.: Equine insect hypersensitivity: Skin test and biopsy results correlated with clinical data. *Equine Vet. J.* 22(4):236, 1990.

Lees, M. J., Fretz, P. B., Bailey, J. V., and Jacobs, K. A.: Principles of grafting. *Compend. Contin. Educ. Pract. Vet.* 11(8):954, 1989.

Lindsay, W. A.: Step-by-step instructions for equine skin grafting techniques. *Vet. Med.* 83(6):598, 1988.

Manning, T., and Sweeney, C.: Immune-mediated equine skin diseases. *Compend. Contin. Educ. Pract. Vet.* 8(12):979, 1986.

Mullowney, P. C.: Dermatologic diseases of horses: IV. Environmental, congenital, and neoplastic diseases. *Compend. Contin. Educ. Pract. Vet.* 7(1):22, 1985.

Mullowney, P. C.: Dermatologic diseases of horses: V. Allergic, immune-mediated, and miscellaneous skin diseases. *Compend. Contin. Educ. Pract. Vet.* 7(4):217, 1985.

Mullowney, P. C., and Fadok, V. A.: Dermatologic diseases of horses: III. Fungal skin diseases. *Compend. Contin. Educ. Pract. Vet.* 6(6):324, 1984.

Scott, D. W.: *Large Animal Dermatology*. Philadelphia: W.B. Saunders, 1988.

Scott, D. W.: Autoimmune skin diseases in the horse. *Equine Pract.* 11(10):20, 1989.

Scott, D. W.: Unusual immune-mediated skin diseases in the horse. *Equine Pract.* 13(2):10, 1991.

White, S. L.: Bullous autoimmune skin diseases in the horse. *Proc. 28th Annu. Conv. Am. Assoc. Equine Pract.,* 1982, p. 113.

Woollen, N., Debowes, R. M., Leipold, H. W., and Schneider, L. A.: A comparison of four types of therapy for the treatment of full-thickness skin wounds of the horse. *Proc. 33rd Annu. Conv. Am. Assoc. Equine Pract.,* 1987, p. 569.

CHAPTER 13

Neurology

Neurologic disease is common in horses. Although the neuroanatomic and neuroendocrine pathways involved in dysfunction of the nervous system are extremely complex, the clinician need not be overwhelmed when dealing with a horse with suspected neurologic disease. If an ordered approach to the examination is undertaken, a diagnosis of the disorder often can be obtained. A thorough examination can be undertaken in 10 to 15 minutes, less time than required for many lameness examinations. Unfortunately, omission of parts of the examination, an all too frequent occurrence, may lead to a failure to identify abnormalities, with resultant adverse effects on treatment.

NEUROLOGIC EXAMINATION

History

Some important aspects to be addressed when presented with the horse with neurologic disease include:

- How old is the horse?
- How long have the signs been present?
- Are there other neurologic signs?
- Is there a history of trauma?
- Is there a history of intercurrent infectious disease?
- Are other horses affected?
- Has the horse's diet been altered recently?
- Are the signs progressive?
- Were the signs sudden or insidious in onset?
- Has the horse received any medications recently?
- Has the horse's behavior altered?
- Is the horse insured?

Physical Examination

KEY POINT ► We have found that the procedure for neurologic examination is simplified if initial efforts are directed toward defining the site of the lesion (i.e., making an anatomic diagnosis).

Subsequently, attempts to delineate the cause of the neurologic dysfunction are made. The examination begins at the head, examining the function of the brain and cranial nerves, and proceeds caudally, investigating the function of the spinal cord and limbs. The tail and peripheral nerves are the final structures to be examined. If this procedure is utilized, it becomes relatively easy to define a lesion to one of the major parts of the nervous system (i.e., cerebrum, brainstem, cerebellum, spinal cord, or peripheral nerves and muscles).

Examination Procedure

Mayhew (1989) has outlined the detailed evaluation of the horse with suspected neurological disease. His approach, which is logical and sequential, is outlined below.

Investigation for evidence of a lesion in the brain or cranial nerves is the first step. If this cannot be found, it is most likely that the lesion lies at a level below the foramen magnum. If there is evidence of a lesion in the brain, then the question to be asked is, Can all the neurologic abnormalities present be the result of this lesion? If not, there is likely to be more than one lesion, with another site or sites of dysfunction outside the brain. Evaluation of the spinal cord follows, focusing on the neck, forelimbs, back, hindlimbs, tail, and anus. Abnormalities of the gait often indicate spinal cord lesions.

Examination of the Head

Demeanor. Information related to the animal's current and previously observed behavior patterns should be obtained from the owner or handler. If the history is suggestive of seizures, the horse should be examined for evidence of such alterations in behavior. Inappropriate behavior (e.g., head pressing, compulsive yawning or wandering, circling, and licking objects, and aggressiveness) is often obvious and reflects cerebral dysfunction.

Responsiveness. This is undertaken with the aim of assessing the horse's state of consciousness. Responsiveness of the horse is related predominantly to brainstem function and to a lesser extent to the cerebral cortex. Response to visual (menace and bright light), touch of the skin, noise, and painful stimuli should be determined.

Head Position. A cerebral lesion may result in the horse circling, with the neck but not the poll deviated to the affected side. In contrast, vestibular lesions frequently result in a head tilt that is characterized by the poll being deviated to the side of the lesion, a body lean to the same side, and nystagmus. These signs may be worsened by application of a blindfold (Fig. 13-1). Cerebellar disease results in jerky movements of the head, (referred to as *intention tremor*), gait abnormalities, and a reduced or absent menace response. A summary of the major deficits resulting from lesions in different sites of the brain is included in Table 13-1.

Examination of the Cranial Nerves

Abnormalities in the cranial nerve (CN) examination are helpful in localizing a lesion to a specific nerve or to the brainstem. Cranial nerves are examined in an orderly manner. Abnormalities in cranial nerve function can be summarized as follows:

I. Olfactory Nerve. Responsible for the sense of smell. Function of this nerve is difficult to assess.

II. Optic Nerve. Responsible for vision and corneal sensation. Assessment of function is made by the menace response, in which a hand is directed toward the eye in a threatening gesture. A normal menace response depends on a functional cranial nerve VII. At times, depression or excitation results in an altered response to a menace test. Neonatal foals may not respond or may become refractory to repeated menace testing. A further assessment of vision may be made by requiring the horse to walk through an obstacle course (Fig. 13-2) or by watching the horse when placed in a strange environment. This nerve can be damaged by head trauma and pituitary tumors.

III. Oculomotor Nerve. Responsible for control of the pupillary diameter (constriction) via parasympathetic fibers. Dilatation of the pupil is controlled by the dilator muscles innervated by sympathetic fibers from the cranial cervical ganglion.

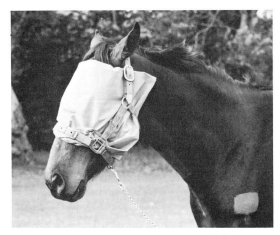

Figure 13–1. Use of a towel as a blindfold for assessment of vestibular function.

When assessing this nerve, the pupils should be checked for size and symmetry and the response to light, both direct and consensual. Dysfunction can be the result of brainstem lesions or ocular trauma. The oculomotor nerve in association with cranial nerves IV and VI are responsible for normal position of the eye due to their innervation of the extraocular muscles. These nerves are tested by observing the position of the eyes within the orbits and eye movement when the head is moved. Strabismus (an abnormal position of the eyes) results when these nerves or muscles are damaged.

IV. Trochlear Nerve. Responsible for normal eye position. Lesions of this nerve are rare, but it may be damaged by fractures to the base of the skull.

V. Trigeminal Nerve. Contains motor fibers to the muscles of mastication and sensory nerve fibers from most of the head. This nerve has three branches: mandibular, maxillary, and ophthalmic. Mandibular nerve palsy results in a dropped jaw and an inability or decreased capacity to chew. The tongue may protrude from the mouth, and drooling of saliva is common. After about 10 days, there is atrophy of the temporal and masseter muscles. Sensory function is tested by assessing sensation to the

TABLE 13–1. Major Findings in Lesions Involving the Brain

Site of the Lesion	Mental Status	Gait Abnormalities	Cranial Nerve Involvement
Cerebrum	Depression, ± coma, ± seizures, ± circling, ± head pressing, ± blindness	Mild ataxia	No
Brain stem	Depression, ± seizures, ± circling, ± head tilt (if caudal lesion)	Variable: none through to ataxia/weakness ± tetraparesis	Yes. Rostral lesion → CNII; midbrain → CNIII–IV; caudal lesion → CNV–XII
Cerebellum	Intention tremor, ± ↓ menace reflex	Dysmetria/spasticity; *no* weakness	No (except ↓ menace response)

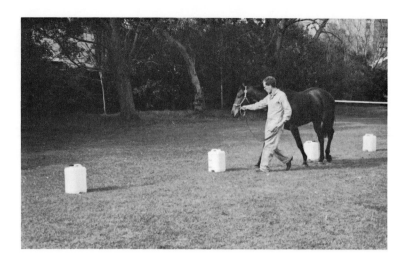

Figure 13–2. Walking through an obstacle course for assessment of vision and proprioceptive function.

head. This is done by tapping or pricking the head and is reflected by movement of the ear, eyelids, and lower lip. These movements also require an intact facial nerve.

VI. Abducens Nerve. Responsible for normal eye position along with cranial nerves III and IV. Lesions of this nerve are rare.

VII. Facial Nerve. Innervates the muscles of facial expression and the lacrimal and salivary glands. This nerve is responsible for the reflexes described when testing the trigeminal nerve. This nerve controls blinking (assessed by the menace, palpebral, and corneal reflexes) and movement of the ears, lips, and nostrils. Facial paralysis results in a drooping of the ear, ptosis of the upper eyelid, decreased tear production, and paralysis of the upper lip, with it being pulled to the unaffected side. Saliva may drool from the mouth.

VIII. Vestibulocochlear Nerve. Responsible for hearing (cochlear division) and balance (vestibular branch). Unilateral hearing loss is difficult to assess. Signs of peripheral vestibular disease may result in the presence of a head tilt toward the side of the lesion. Nystagmus occurs frequently, either with the head in a normal position (spontaneous) or when it is held in various abnormal positions (positional). The direction of nystagmus (fast phase) is *away* from the side of the lesion. Blindfolding will often worsen the signs. Care should be exercised with doing this because some horses may fall down. Signs of vestibular disease will often improve over a period of days as the horse accommodates for the problem. Central vestibular disease will result in similar signs plus abnormalities in proprioception or voluntary limb movement, ataxia, weakness, depression, and possible dysfunction of the other cranial nerves.

IX. Glossopharyngeal Nerve, X. Vagus Nerve. These nerves innervate the pharynx and larynx (sensory and motor). Function of these nerves is tested by observing normal swallowing of food and water and assessing the swallowing reflex by pas-

sage of a nasogastric tube. If required, the larynx and pharynx can be examined endoscopically. Pharyngeal paralysis is characterized by dysphagia, a common manifestation of which is that food and water are dropped from the mouth and discharges are seen from the nostrils.

XI. Accessory Nerve. Provides motor innervation to the trapezius and sternocephalicus muscles. Lesions in this nerve are rare.

XII. Hypoglossal Nerve. Supplies motor innervation to the tongue. Lesions result in weakness of the tongue, as assessed by the withdrawal reflex, changes in symmetry, and atrophy of the muscles of the tongue. Palsy, particularly if bilateral, results in the tongue hanging out and difficulty in prehending food.

Evaluation of Motor Function

Many subtle gait deficits due to neurologic dysfunction can easily be mistaken for musculoskeletal problems.

KEY POINT ► It is important that the examiner assess the gait and determine if there is a musculoskeletal problem.

If such a problem is ruled out, a neurologic deficit is likely, and the gait is assessed to define the deficit. Gait deficits are classified as weakness, ataxia, spasticity, and dysmetria and are graded 0 to 5 depending on severity (Table 13-2). Gait and proprioceptive deficits are assessed with the horse walking, trotting, turning (Fig. 13-3), backing, moving up and down an incline (Fig. 13-4), and after application of a blindfold (see Fig. 13-1). Walking through an obstacle course (see Fig. 13-2) and over a step or curb (Fig. 13-5) is useful for assessing proprioception. Other tests for proprioceptive function involve crossing the forelegs (Fig. 13-6) and forcing the horse to adopt a base-wide stance. This test is most useful for assessing hindlimb proprioception (Fig. 13-7).

TABLE 13–2. Criteria for Grading Ataxia, Weakness, Spasticity, and Dysmetria

Grade	Deficit
0	Normal—no deficit
1	Deficit may be detectable at normal gaits. Exacerbated with manipulative procedures (e.g., turning in tight circles, walking up/down a slope ± elevation of head)
2	Deficit obvious at normal gaits. Signs exacerbated with manipulative procedures (e.g., turning in tight circles, walking up/down a slope ± elevation of head)
3	Signs particularly obvious at normal gaits. Horses give the impression they may fall (but do not) and buckle with manipulative procedures (e.g., circling, backing, walking up/down a slope, tail pull, etc.)
4	Profound deficits at normal gait. Horse frequently stumbles and may fall at normal gaits or when manipulative procedures are utilized (e.g., circling, backing, walking up/down a slope, tail pull, etc.)
5	Recumbent horse

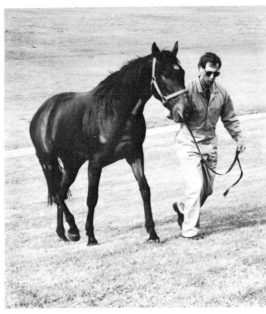

Figure 13–4. Walking up a slope for assessment of the gait. This test is used to worsen abnormalities such as spasticity, dysmetria, weakness, and ataxia.

Ataxia (Incoordination)—Is a proprioceptive deficit that is obvious when the horse moves the limbs.

KEY POINT ► Ataxia causes an unstable (swaying) gait and possibly interference of the affected limbs.

This results in abnormal foot placement, which becomes worse when the horse is walked up and down a slope. Severely affected horses may step on the opposite foot. The limbs are often circumducted, particularly when the horse is required to turn in tight circles. Pivoting on the affected limbs also may occur during this maneuver or when backing the horse.

Weakness (Paresis)—Is demonstrated by dragging the feet, stumbling, and possibly increased wear of the toes. When bearing weight, an affected limb will show increased extension of the fetlocks and possibly shaking of the limb, knuckling, and

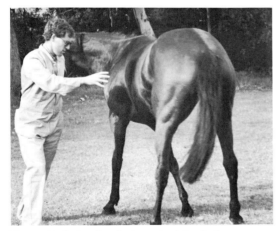

Figure 13–3. Turning the horse in tight circles to assess ataxia and weakness. Particular note should be made of the horse stepping on itself and the degree of circumduction of the outside hindlimb.

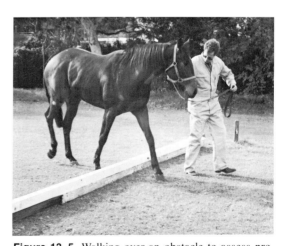

Figure 13–5. Walking over an obstacle to assess proprioceptive function.

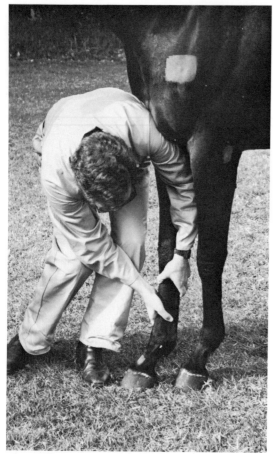

Figure 13–6. Crossing of the forelimbs to evaluate proprioceptive function. A delayed return of the limb to a normal position may indicate neurologic dysfunction. Care should be taken to avoid the legs touching, since skin sensation may provide false results.

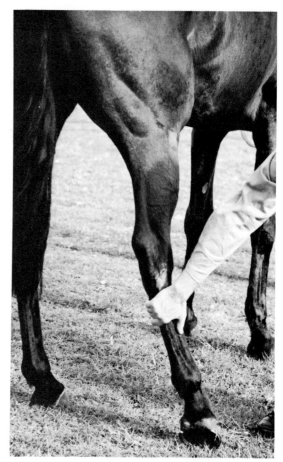

Figure 13–7. Forcing the horse to adopt a base-wide stance in the hindlimbs as an assessment of proprioceptive function. A delayed return of the limb to a normal position may indicate neurologic dysfunction.

dropping of the body as a whole. These changes are worsened when the horse is required to walk in a tight circle or up a slope (particularly with the head elevated) (Fig. 13-8).

Spasticity (Stiffness)—Describes stiff movement of the limbs with reduced flexion of the joints. Affected horses may have a "tin soldier" gait. This sign is often most obvious in the carpus and hock.

KEY POINT ▶ Spasticity can be exaggerated when the horse walks up and down an incline with the head elevated.

Spasticity is common with cervical spinal cord lesions.

Dysmetria—Describes alterations in the range of movement of limbs or joints. It usually occurs as overstepping (hypermetria) with excessive joint movement. This results in an altered stride length. Hypermetria without weakness (plus an intention tremor) is characteristic of cerebellar disease.

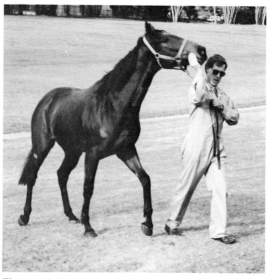

Figure 13–8. Walking the horse up an incline with the head elevated. This test will often exacerbate ataxia, spasticity, and dysmetria.

Ataxia and weakness is more easily recognized than spasticity and dysmetria.

Other Manipulative Procedures for Evaluation of Spinal Cord Function

- Following assessment of the gait, the neck, fore-limbs, trunk/back, and hindlimbs are examined for symmetry, gross skeletal defects, and patchy sweating. Demonstration of abnormalities in any region may assist in localization of the lesion.
- *Skin sensation* should be assessed. This procedure is undertaken to assess spinal reflexes, which are responsible for reaction to skin sensation. A pen or probe is used to assess sensation over the neck. This will result in flinching of the cervical musculature. Prodding caudal to the ear will elicit the cervicofacial reflex, which includes twitching of the ear, closure of the eyelids, and movement of the corner of the mouth on the side being tested. Absence of these reflexes, local muscle wasting, and/or patchy sweating may reveal an abnormality in innervation of the neck. Skin sensation and spinal reflexes of the thorax and body are tested by prodding the skin along the body with a pen and observing for contraction of the cutaneous trunci muscles. If a pen tip is run over the thoracolumbar area (from the wither to the sacrum) near the spine, the normal response is for the horse to extend the thoracolumbar spine. In contrast, running the pen or blunt instrument over the croup should result in flexion of the thoracolumbar spine. Skin sensation on the limbs is then assessed.
- *The neck should be manipulated* dorsoventrally and laterally to assess normal range of movement (Fig. 13-9). Reluctance to flex the neck may reflect cervical pain.
- *The "sway test,"* where the clinician pushes against the horse's shoulders to assess postural reactions (i.e., capacity to resist the force before stepping laterally), should be performed (Fig. 13-10). This test is done with the horse standing and then with it walking. This test often demonstrates weakness and/or ataxia, as reflected by a reduced resistance and stumbling when pressure is applied to the shoulder. Similarly, pushing against the pelvis with the horse standing and walking and assessing the resistance and proprioceptive responses help define weakness and ataxia in the pelvic limbs.
- A *"tail-pull test"* also should be performed. With the horse standing still, a lateral pull is applied to the tail and lead rope simultaneously. This test assesses the strength of each side of the body. A tail pull is also performed to assess the hindlimbs (Fig. 13-11). This is done with the horse standing and walking. Limited resistance to the pull and profound abduction with crossing of the hindlimbs indicate weakness and ataxia, respectively.
- *Perineal response and tail tone* should be tested. The tail is manipulated, and evidence of flaccidity

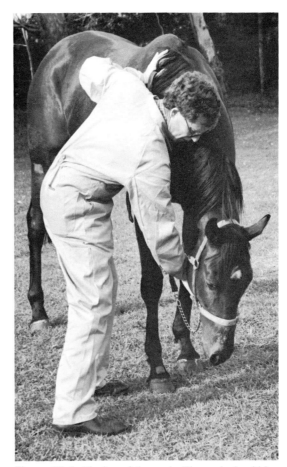

Figure 13–9. Flexion of the neck. The neck should be flexed dorsoventrally and to each side to assess pain.

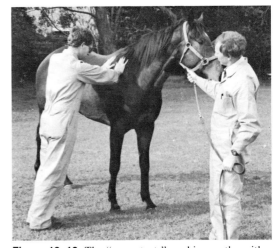

Figure 13–10. The "sway test," pushing on the wither with the horse standing. This test assesses strength and proprioceptive function because the horse should resist the force.

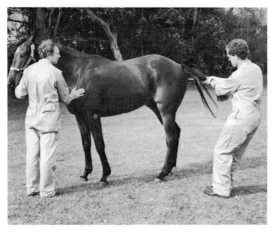

Figure 13–11. The "tail-pull test." With the horse walking, the tail is pulled to the side, and the horse's ability to resist the force and maintain normal foot placement are assessed.

is determined. The perineal reflex is then tested by stimulating the perineum. A normal response occurs with contraction of the anal sphincter and clamping down of the tail.

■ A *rectal examination* should be performed, if required. This will assist in identification of space-occupying lesions and fractures or luxation of the pelvis or lumbar, sacral, and coccygeal vertebrae. The rectum should be assessed for tone and for fecal retention, and the urinary bladder assessed for size and tone. In recumbent adult horses, urination may not occur, and the bladder may become greatly distended. Catheterization to empty the bladder is often required. This will then reduce the volume of the bladder and thereby allow a better examination of the pelvic structures.

Conclusions Following Completion of the Neurologic Examination

Once the neurologic examination is completed, the clinician should be able to determine whether a neurologic deficit is present and, if so, in which major component of the nervous system it is likely to be located. With this information, more logical decisions can be made regarding the likely diagnosis, choice of ancillary diagnostic tests, and treatment strategies.

Neurologic Examination in Foals

Foals have different neurologic responses during the first few weeks of life than those of adult horses. These can be summarized as follows:

■ Restraint of young foals may result in a short-lived catatonic (narcoleptic-like) state.
■ A reduced or absent menace response is common. However, pupillary light reflexes and blinking in response to bright light should be present.

■ Jerky head movements are common.
■ A wide-based stance is often adopted and may not indicate neurologic dysfunction.
■ The gait is characterized by dysmetria and apparent incoordination. Some foals in the first few days of life will pace at slow gaits.
■ Foals should have a normal suck reflex.
■ Responses to the "slap test" of laryngeal adductor and cervical spinal function is quite variable or absent until about 1 month of age.

DIAGNOSTIC AIDS

Laryngeal Adductor ("Slap") Test

KEY POINT ► The "slap test" of laryngeal adductor function can be useful as an aid in assessment of cervical spinal cord disease.

In horses with cervical spinal cord disease, the adductor response of the contralateral arytenoid cartilage to slapping the chest is often absent. This test can be performed without an endoscope by palpating the muscular process of the arytenoid cartilage and feeling the "flick" as the chest wall on the opposite side is slapped.

Cerebrospinal Fluid Collection and Analysis

Analysis of cerebrospinal fluid (CSF) may be useful in some cases where nervous system dysfunction is detected. The common sites for collection of CSF are the atlanto-occipital (A-O) and lumbosacral (L-S) spaces.

Collection from the A-O Space. The horse is placed under general anesthesia, and the poll and rostral neck are clipped and prepared as for surgery. The head is flexed at a right angle to the axis of the neck. The cranial borders of the atlas are palpated and constitute the lateral landmarks for the puncture site. The eminence of the nuchal crest is palpated and used to identify the midline.

KEY POINT ► The site for needle insertion is where the line between the cranial borders of the atlas bisects the midline.

With the clinician wearing sterile surgical gloves, a 9-cm (3.5 in), 18-gauge spinal needle (Becton-Dickinson., Rutherford, NJ) is inserted. The point of the needle is directed toward the lower jaw and is advanced slowly. There is a progressive increase in resistance to penetration as the needle is inserted. However, when the needle penetrates into the subarachnoid space, there is often a noticeable "give" and no further increase in resistance. The subarachnoid space is usually penetrated at a depth of 5 to 7 cm (2 to 3 in) (Fig. 13-12). Care should be exercised not to penetrate the brainstem. Once the needle is in place, CSF is collected aseptically into a sterile syringe.

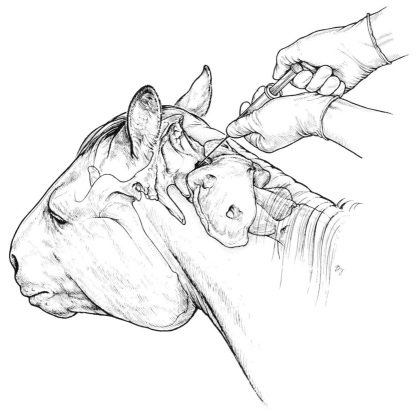

Figure 13–12. Line drawing of the atlanto-occipital space showing the site for insertion of an 18-gauge, 9-cm (3.5 in) spinal needle.

Collection from the L-S Space. This is the most frequently used method for collection of CSF because it can be performed in the conscious standing horse and has fewer inherent risks of complications, since the conus medullaris can be penetrated without damage. In addition, CSF flows caudad, so abnormalities due to spinal cord lesions are more commonly detected in fluid collected from this site. The horse should be restrained in stocks. Sedation usually is unnecessary. The caudal borders of the tuber coxae are identified—a line bisecting these on the midline is often near the site for insertion of the needle. The caudal edge of the sixth lumbar spinous process is palpated, and a depression can commonly be identified just caudal to this. This is the site for insertion of the needle (Fig. 13-13 and 13-14). In some horses, the tuber sacrale can be palpated, and a line between the cranial borders of these also will help identify the site for puncture. In fat horses and geldings and stallions, the tuber sacrale may be very difficult to palpate. A region around this site is clipped and aseptically prepared. Two to 3 ml lidocaine (Treatment No. 67) is injected under the skin, and a stab incision is made with a no. 15 scalpel blade. Small amounts of hemorrhage are controlled prior to insertion of the needle.

KEY POINT ▶ It is most important that the horse stands with weight evenly distributed on both hind feet when the needle is inserted.

With the clinician wearing sterile gloves and standing beside the horse an 18-gauge, 15-cm (6 in) spinal needle (Becton-Dickinson., Rutherford, NJ) is inserted (see Fig. 13-13). It is helpful for an assistant to stand behind the horse to ensure that the

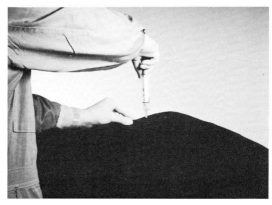

Figure 13–13. Position of an 18-gauge, 15-cm (6 in) spinal needle just anterior to an imaginary line drawn through the tuber coxae to enable collection of cerebrospinal fluid from the lumbosacral space.

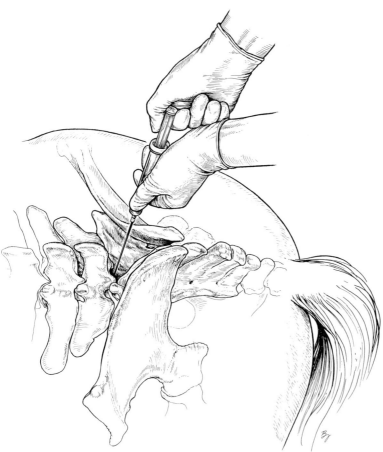

Figure 13–14. Line drawing showing the needle position in the lumbosacral space to enable cerebrospinal fluid collection.

needle is inserted down the plane of the midline, since small errors in direction at the site of insertion will be greatly magnified at the L-S space. In some cases, the clinician may be better able to visualize the plane of insertion if he or she stands on a small platform beside the horse. The needle is inserted to about 11 to 13 cm (4.5 to 5 in) in adult horses before penetration of the subarachnoid space occurs. The sensations for the operator are similar to those described for the A-O procedure. When the subarachnoid space is penetrated, the horse will often flinch. With correct needle placement, aspiration with a 10-ml syringe will yield CSF. Occlusion of the jugular veins may increase the yield of CSF.

CSF Analysis. Following collection, CSF can be subjected to bacteriologic and cytologic examination. In the former case, a sample of the fluid should be placed in a sterile container and forwarded to a bacteriology laboratory. The remainder of the sample should be examined for color, clarity, total and differential nucleated cell counts, red cell count, and total protein. The constituents of normal CSF are provided in Table 13-3.

Radiology

KEY POINT ► Radiology constitutes an extremely valuable tool for defining nervous

system disorders, particularly those due to trauma, malformations, or bony infections.

Diagnostically useful radiographs of the head and cervical spine can often be obtained with small portable x-ray machines and modern high-speed screens. Often, survey films can be taken with the animal standing. If greater definition is required or patient compliance is a problem, general anesthesia should be considered prior to taking radiographs. However, general anesthesia may worsen some neurological problems. Positive contrast radiography (myelography) is now much more widely practiced in larger hospitals and referral centers. The advent of less irritant contrast agents such as iohexol has made this technique much safer in recent years. Radiology remains one of the most commonly employed methods for diagnosis of cervical spinal cord compression ("wobbler" syndrome).

Hematology and Serum Biochemistry

Routine hematology may provide some indication of diseases with an inflammatory component, as reflected by a leukocytosis and possibly increases in fibrinogen. In long-standing cases, anemia of chronic disease may be present. In cases

TABLE 13–3. Characteristics of Cerebrospinal Fluid

Constituent	Normal Value	Abnormal Findings
Appearance	Clear, colorless	• Some infections may → ↑ turbidity • Hemorrhage → xanthochromia
Total nucleated cell count	<6/μl; all should be mononuclear cells	• Bacterial infections → ↑ total number, including ↑ neutrophils • Viral infections → ↑ total number (mainly mononuclear cells) • Parasitic infections (protozoal, helminth) → ↑ total number (+ eosinophils) • Large hemorrhage → ↑ total number (neutrophils, mononuclears)
Red blood cells	0	• ↑ with blood contamination during collection • ↑ with CNS trauma (+ xanthochromia)
Total protein	0.5–1.0 g/L (50–100 mg/dl); predominantly albumin	• ↑ with infectious diseases, trauma, and some toxicoses

where there is suspected trauma and hemorrhage, blood loss may be indicated by a reduction in the packed cell volume and red cell numbers.

Plasma biochemical tests are often useful in assisting the clinician in defining the cause of neurologic dysfunction. Dramatic elevations in liver enzyme activities and bile acid concentrations are indicative of liver disease, a common cause of encephalopathies in horses. Hypocalcemia, hypoglycemia, or hyperkalemia can at times be demonstrated. Each of these disorders may be associated with neurologic dysfunction.

Collection of serum samples for determination of specific antibody titers also may be useful. The potential for diagnosis of myeloencephalopathy due to equine herpesvirus type 1, and the viral encephalitides is strengthened if seroconversion to the offending viral agents can be demonstrated between acute and convalescent samples.

Diseases of the Spinal Cord

Cervical Vertebral Malformation ("Wobbler" Syndrome, Cervical Stenotic Myelopathy)

KEY POINT ► Cervical vertebral malformation predominantly affects young horses, usually before they are 3 years of age.

The disease results from abnormal growth and/or articulation of the cervical vertebral bodies, resulting in focal compression of the spinal cord. This compression can be constant, referred to as *static compression*, or may only occur when there is movement, particularly flexion or extension of the neck, referred to as *dynamic compression*. Osteochondrosis often occurs in the vertebral column (and at other body sites) of affected horses. A large number of causes of cervical vertebral malformation have been proposed, including a genetic predisposition, mineral imbalances, and overnutrition.

History and Presenting Signs

- Young horses less than 3 years of age are usually affected. Younger animals (<18 months) tend to have dynamic compression, whereas those with static compression tend to be older (up to 3 years).
- Predominantly thoroughbreds and quarter horses, although members of most breeds have been affected

- Males more frequently affected than females
- Horses that are well grown for their age
- A history of poor performance, stumbling, falling down, or an obscure lameness

Clinical Findings and Diagnosis

- Ataxia and weakness are the most common clinical findings. Signs usually occur acutely and are usually most severe in the hindlimbs, generally being at least one grade worse than in the forelimbs. Signs are most commonly symmetrical but can be more severe on one side if compression is greater on that side.
- Manipulative procedures (e.g., circling, walking up and down a slope, with and without the head being elevated, backing, and the "sway" and "tail-pull" reactions) will often worsen the clinical signs.
- Progression of signs is often variable, with some horses appearing to improve followed by signs recurring.
- In general, there are no obvious abnormalities detectable in the cervical vertebral column on physical examination.
- Localized alterations in pain perception, muscle atrophy, and sweating may occur in some cases but are rare.
- Diagnosis is based on the clinical signs and radiographic findings.

KEY POINT ▶ Plain radiographs will often demonstrate some bony abnormalities in the cervical vertebral column, including flaring of the caudal metaphyses and alterations in the dorsal articular facets of the vertebrae.

- Signs of osteochondrosis and degenerative joint disease also may be seen. Measurement of the vertebral canal diameter on plain radiographs has been reported to be a valuable means of assisting with the diagnosis of cervical vertebral malformation. Horses with cervical vertebral malformation have been shown to have narrowing of the vertebral spaces of cervical vertebrae two to six.

KEY POINT ▶ Confirmation of the diagnosis is made by the demonstration of a reduction in vertebral column dimensions by positive contrast myelography.

- This procedure is relatively complex, requiring general anesthesia, and it provides some risk to the patient. In our experience, these cases are best handled by experienced individuals in well-equipped referral facilities.
- The most common site for compression is C3–C4, with C4–C5 and C5–C6 also affected. Compression at other multiple sites also occurs.

Differential Diagnosis

- Trauma
- Equine degenerative myeloencephalopathy
- Equine herpesvirus myeloencephalopathy
- Equine protozoal myeloencephalopathy
- Neuritis of the cauda equina
- Vertebral osteomyelitis
- Verminous myelitis
- Rabies
- Congenital abnormalities

Treatment

- Conservative medical management of cervical vertebral malformation is designed to decrease pain and inflammation if the onset is acute. Corticosteroids such as dexamethasone (0.5–2.0 mg/kg IV q24h for 1–2 days; Treatment Nos. 29 and 30) or prednisolone (1–2 mg/kg PO q12h for several days; Treatment No. 92) are commonly prescribed to reduce inflammation. *Note:* High dose rates of dexamethasone have been associated with induction of laminitis. Phenylbutazone (Treatment No. 88) or flunixin meglumine (Treatment No. 52) also may be used for their anti-inflammatory effects. Intravenous administration of dimethylsulfoxide (0.5–0.9 g/kg of a 10%–20% solution q12–24h for 1–2 days; Treatment No. 34) also appears to be of value in cases with a recent acute onset of signs.
- Some horses respond to prolonged rest (2–12 months); however, most horses affected with cervical vertebral malformation will not return to neurologic normality with rest alone.

KEY POINT ▶ Surgery to stabilize the vertebral column by fusion of two or more cervical vertebrae and/or decompression of the spinal cord is performed in a number of surgical referral facilities.

- Interpretation of the results of this procedure tend to be controversial depending on who is analyzing the data. Prognosis for life is improved in many cases following surgery, whereas prognosis for resumption or commencement of an athletic career must be more guarded.
- Euthanasia should be considered in horses that are severely affected and whose clinical signs make them a danger to themselves or to their handlers.

Equine Degenerative Myeloencephalopathy

KEY POINT ▶ Equine degenerative myeloencephalopathy is one of the most common causes of ataxia in young horses.

In several surveys, more than 20% of horses examined at necropsy following a history of ataxia had equine degenerative myeloencephalopathy.

There are characteristic diffuse degenerative changes in the spinal cord and brain in some cases. The specific etiology of equine degenerative myeloencephalopathy is unknown. However, confinement to dirt paddocks, exposure to insecticides and wood preservatives, and consumption of processed or pelleted feeds are thought to be risk factors for the disease.

KEY POINT ▶ Foals born to dams that have previously had a foal with equine degenerative myeloencephalopathy appear much more likely to develop the disease.

Hypovitaminosis E has been implicated as a cause in some outbreaks.

History and Presenting Signs

- Young horses less than 3 years of age
- Insidious onset of incoordination and stumbling is usual, although abrupt onset of signs may occur.
- Horses in dirt yards fed pelleted or processed rations
- Can occur in outbreaks
- Application of insecticides or exposure to wood preservatives
- Familial predisposition reported

Clinical Findings and Diagnosis

KEY POINT ▶ Variable degrees of symmetrical ataxia and paresis that usually are noticeable before the horse is 12 months old.

- All limbs are commonly affected. Signs may be worse in the hindlimbs or similar in all limbs.
- Despite progression of signs early in the disease, tetraplegia rarely develops.
- There may be evidence of thoracic hyporeflexia, as demonstrated by reduced skin sensation over the trunk. This will assist in identification of a thoracic lesion and decrease the likelihood of the ataxia being due to cervical vertebral malformation.
- Some horses with the disease will have low plasma α-tocopherol concentrations (<1.5 mg/L; normal > 2.0 mg/L). However, given the potential daily variation in α-tocopherol values in individual animals and the delay that may exist between the presence of hypovitaminosis E and occurrence of the disease, measurement of plasma α-tocopherol values is more likely to be of use as a herd screening test in outbreaks.
- Diagnosis is based on clinical signs and by ruling out other possible causes of ataxia. Evidence of hypovitaminosis E may be helpful. Definitive diagnosis depends on histopathologic examination of the brain and spinal cord and demonstration of neuraxonal dystrophy, neuronal fiber degeneration, and other changes.

Differential Diagnosis

- Trauma
- Equine cervical vertebral malformation
- Equine herpesvirus myeloencephalopathy
- Equine protozoal myeloencephalopathy
- Neuritis of the cauda equina
- Vertebral osteomyelitis
- Verminous myelitis
- Rabies
- Congenital abnormalities

Treatment

KEY POINT ▶ Once signs have developed, treatment is difficult. Provision of a balanced diet with fresh green feed and administration of vitamin E (100–150 IU/kg q24h) may be effective in reducing clinical signs in some affected horses.

Prevention of equine degenerative myeloencephalopathy may be related to ensuring that foals are not kept in dirt paddocks, are not exposed to insecticides and wood preservatives, and receive a balanced diet, preferably at pasture, that is rich in green feed. Supplementation with vitamin E (50–100 IU/kg q24h), particularly in animals with marginal to low plasma concentrations of α-tocopherol, is thought to be helpful in preventing the disease.

Equine Herpesvirus Myeloencephalopathy

KEY POINT ▶ Equine herpesvirus type 4 (EHV-4) is a major cause of respiratory tract disease in horses, whereas EHV-1 is responsible for abortions, birth of dead or weak foals, mild respiratory infections, and a myeloencephalopathy.

The latter disorder is due to a vasculitis in the central nervous system and frequently results in signs of spinal cord disease, especially ataxia and weakness.

History and Presenting Signs

- Occurs in horses of all ages
- Exposure to horses with signs of respiratory tract disease, abortion, or neurologic deficits may be reported.
- May affect a single horse or occur in outbreaks
- Respiratory tract infection 10 to 14 days prior to acute onset of ataxia

Clinical Findings and Diagnosis

- There may be fever and evidence of mild respiratory tract disease or abortion.

KEY POINT ▶ Neurologic deficits can be highly variable.

- Common findings include symmetrical ataxia and weakness, predominantly in the hindlimbs; thoracic limb involvement is frequently present, albeit to a lesser extent. Urinary incontinence and retention, penile prolapse, fecal retention, and hypalgesia in the tail and perineal regions also will occur. Vestibular signs with or without facial nerve palsy may occur.

KEY POINT ► There is little progression of signs after approximately 24 to 48 hours.

- Analysis of CSF reveals xanthochromia and an increase in protein (albumin), with values increasing to 1.0 to 3.0 g/L (100 to 300 mg/dl). The total nucleated cell count is normally not increased to a level that might be expected from the protein concentration.
- A three- to fourfold increase over 2 to 3 weeks (from the onset of signs) in serum neutralizing or complement-fixing antibody titer to EHV-1 is also strong evidence of a recent infection with the virus. A positive titer for EHV-1 in the CSF also can assist in diagnosis, particularly if the titer is higher than in the serum.

KEY POINT ► Diagnosis is often presumptive based on the history and clinical signs, in particular stabilization of manifestations after 24 to 48 hours, together with characteristic changes in the CSF and seroconversion. Definitive diagnosis is based on histologic demonstration of vasculitis and white and gray matter malacia.

Differential Diagnosis

- Equine cervical vertebral malformation
- Equine protozoal myeloencephalopathy
- Neuritis of the cauda equina
- Viral encephalitides
- Meningitis
- Trauma
- Vertebral osteomyelitis
- Verminous myelitis
- Brain abscess
- Rabies
- Congenital abnormalities

Treatment

- Supportive therapy is critical. In mildly affected horses that can walk, eat, and drink, little or no therapy may be required. Horses with severe ataxia require restriction of movement and ready access to water and palatable feed. Recumbent patients provide a significant therapeutic challenge and usually have the worst prognosis for recovery.
- Horses with urinary retention require bladder catheterization and evacuation. In cases where urinary incontinence persists, placement of an in-

dwelling Foley catheter is indicated. In stallions and geldings, this may need to be performed via a perineal urethrostomy. Once the catheter is inserted, the balloon is inflated, and the free end of the catheter is attached (with Supaglue or Crazyglu) to a urine collection bag or old 5-L fluid bag. This bag is then taped to the horse's leg to allow accumulation of urine by gravity flow. Provision of the bag prevents the occurrence of urine scald. Cystitis is common secondary to urine stasis and bladder catheterization. As a result, antibiotic coverage is indicated, and trimethoprim-sulfadiazine (15–20 mg/kg of the combination PO q12h; Treatment No. 107) is a good choice.
- We have found anti-inflammatory therapy using intravenous dimethylsulfoxide (0.5–0.9 g/kg IV as a 10%–20% solution in normal saline q12h; Treatment No. 34) and dexamethasone (0.05–0.1 mg/kg IV q12h for several days; Treatment Nos. 29 and 30) to be beneficial.

KEY POINT ► Recovery may require weeks in some cases, whereas it is slower or nonexistent in others. Residual deficits may be seen in some horses following convalescence.

- If a horse is severely affected, is not responding to therapy, or the clinician is unable to provide appropriate nursing care, euthanasia should be considered.
- Prevention of disease may be possible using the herpesvirus vaccines (Treatment No. 110).

Equine Protozoal Myeloencephalitis

Equine protozoal myeloencephalitis is a debilitating and potentially fatal disease caused by the protozoan *Sarcocytis neurona*. This organism commonly produces multifocal, asymmetrical lesions in the brain and particularly the spinal cord. Although equine protozoal myeloencephalitis is an infectious disease, it does not appear to be contagious from horse to horse. This is probably so because the organism is in the noninfective merozoite form when found in the central nervous system of horses. It is the most common form of multifocal neurologic disease.

History and Presenting Signs

- All ages affected but most common in horses less than 4 years of age
- Standardbreds and thoroughbreds are overrepresented.
- Onset of signs is usually acute and progressive.
- Reported signs are variable—frequent stumbling and falling are the most commonly reported signs.
- History of an obscure lameness
- This disorder is most common in the Midwest, Northeast and South.

Clinical Findings and Diagnosis

KEY POINT ► Gait abnormalities are usually asymmetrical owing to the multifocal nature of the disease.

■ All limbs are commonly affected. Both upper and lower motor neuron signs can occur, producing severe weakness, ataxia, spasticity, and muscle wasting in some cases. Signs are often progressive and in severe cases result in recumbency.
■ Areas of hypalgesia or complete loss of cutaneous sensation on the head, neck, or body may be demonstrated.
■ If there are lesions in the brain, acute onset of head tilt, depression and facial paralysis, dysphagia, and loss of the menace response are the most common effects.
■ Cerebrospinal fluid may have evidence of xanthochromia and an increase in total nucleated cell count (10–100 × 10⁶/L or 10–100/μl), predominantly lymphocytes and mononuclear cells. Eosinophils may be seen on occasion. Moderate elevations in total protein (1.0–2.0 g/L or 100–200 mg/dl) also occur at times. Identification of sporzoon zooites in CSF is rare.
■ Diagnosis of equine protozoal myeloencephalitis is difficult because there is no specific antemortem method for diagnosis. Therefore, diagnosis is usually made by exclusion and/or response to therapy.

KEY POINT ► Equine protozoal myeloencephalitis should be suspected in any horse with acute onset of progressive, asymmetrical, multifocal neurologic disease characterized by ataxia, weakness, and muscle wasting.

■ If there are changes in CSF similar to those described above, then the likelihood of equine protozoal myeloencephalitis being the cause is increased. Definitive diagnosis can only be made at postmortem examination with demonstration of characteristic histopathologic changes and possible identification of the causative organism.

Differential Diagnosis

■ Equine cervical vertebral malformation
■ Equine herpesvirus myeloencephalopathy
■ Neuritis of the cauda equina
■ Viral encephalitides
■ Meningitis
■ Trauma
■ Vertebral osteomyelitis
■ Verminous myelitis
■ Rabies
■ Brain abscess
■ Congenital abnormalities

Treatment

KEY POINT ► Horses suspected of having equine protozoal myeloencephalitis should be treated with trimethoprim-sulfadiazine (15–20 mg/kg of the combination PO q12h for 4 to 8 weeks; Treatment No. 107) and pyrimethamine (Daraprim, Burroughs Wellcome Co., Research Triangle Park, NC) (0.3–0.7 mg/kg q12h PO for 3 days and then q24h PO for 4–8 weeks).

■ A full blood count should be performed every 2 weeks during therapy because these antifolate drugs may produce folate deficiency, manifested by cytopenia (leukopenia, thrombocytopenia, anemia). This side effect is rare, but if it occurs, pyrimethamine should be discontinued, and folinic acid (0.006–0.010 mg/kg IM q3d) should be administered for several weeks. Anti-inflammatory therapy using intravenous dimethylsulfoxide (Treatment No. 34) at a dose rate of 0.5 to 0.9 g/kg, given as a 10% to 20% solution, and/or nonsteroidal anti-inflammatory drugs such as phenylbutazone (Treatment No. 88) may provide some symptomatic relief early in the disease.
■ Most horses with equine protozoal myeloencephalitis will show clinical improvement within several weeks of starting therapy. Some require several months to achieve the maximum benefit. Residual neurologic deficits may still exist at the conclusion of therapy. Euthanasia should be considered in horses in which the signs progress or who are severely affected initially and show a poor response to treatment.

Neuritis of the Cauda Equina (Polyneuritis Equi)

This is a severe, chronic, granulomatous perineuritis involving the cauda equina and often less severe lesions of spinal nerve roots and cranial nerves (especially V, VII, and VIII) roots. The disorder is thought to be immune-mediated, possibly the result of viral infection.

History and Presenting Signs

■ Usually adult horses
■ There is no sex or breed predisposition
■ Tail rubbing, paralysis of the tail, and hindlimb ataxia are common.

Clinical Findings and Diagnosis

KEY POINT ► Signs may occur acutely, with cranial nerve and/or perineal hyperesthesia being most prominent.

■ This phase of the disease may pass without being identified. Subsequently, the signs tend to become chronic and are characterized by symmetrical hindlimb ataxia (normally mild) and progressive paralysis of the tail, rectum, and bladder. Perineal hyporeflexia and retention of urine and feces are common. The penis often protrudes from the prepuce. Muscle atrophy in the hindlimb area may be apparent.

■ Although sacrococcygeal lesions predominate, head signs also can occur. The latter are often characterized by asymmetrical lesions of cranial nerves V, VII, and VIII, resulting in a head tilt, unilateral facial paralysis, and difficulty in chewing.

■ Cerebrospinal fluid is abnormal in some cases, with increases in protein (1.0–3.0 g/L or 100–300 mg/dl) and total nucleated cell count (predominantly lymphocytes) being demonstrated most frequently.

■ Hematology can reveal evidence of generalized inflammation, as reflected by leukocytosis, hyperfibrinogenemia, and possibly anemia of chronic disease.

KEY POINT ▶ Diagnosis is based on the history, clinical signs, CSF findings, and evidence of progression of the disease.

■ Recently, assays demonstrating antibodies to myelin protein P2 have been developed. Increases in the concentration of anti-P2 antibodies in the CSF of some affected horses have been demonstrated. Unfortunately, these assays are not specific for diagnosis of the disease. Definitive diagnosis is by postmortem examination.

Differential Diagnosis

■ Equine protozoal myeloencephalopathy
■ Equine cervical vertebral malformation
■ Equine herpesvirus myeloencephalopathy
■ Trauma
■ Vertebral osteomyelitis
■ Verminous myelitis
■ Rabies
■ Congenital abnormalities

Treatment

■ There is no effective specific therapy for neuritis of the cauda equina. As a result, supportive therapy is sometimes prescribed. This involves manual evacuation of the rectum, catheterization of the bladder (see Equine Herpesvirus Myeloencephalopathy), and antibiotic and anti-inflammatory therapy, such as dexamethasone (0.05–0.1 mg/kg IV q12h; Treatment Nos. 29 and 30). Unfortunately, the disease progresses insidiously in most cases, and therapy is unrewarding.

■ Euthanasia should be recommended in severely affected horses.

Occipitoatlantoaxial Malformations

Congenital malformations involving the occipital bones, atlas, and axis in horses are relatively rare, but when they occur, may result in signs of brainstem or spinal cord compression. Because of this, clinical signs have varied from none to a foal being dead at birth. The most common neurologic deficits involve ataxia and weakness affecting all limbs.

History and Presenting Signs

■ Young horses (<6 months old)
■ Most common signs relate to progressive spinal cord ataxia and tetraparesis.
■ Occurs in all breeds occasionally
■ Familial predisposition for occipitoatlantoaxial malformation in Arabian horses

Clinical Findings and Diagnosis

KEY POINT ▶ Ataxia and weakness usually affecting all limbs are the most common manifestations of occipitoatlantoaxial malformation.

■ In some cases, spinal cord compression is sufficiently severe that foals are found dead or recumbent and unable to rise.

■ Palpation of the atlanto-occipital articulation in affected foals may reveal swelling, malarticulation, and a reduction in the amount of movement of that joint. In Arab foals with occipitoatlantoaxial malformation, the transverse processes are often small and abnormally shaped. Crepitus or a "clicking" sound may be demonstrable when the head and neck are manipulated.

■ Diagnosis is based on presenting signs and clinical findings. Radiographs are often helpful in establishing the diagnosis. In Arab foals with occipitoatlantoaxial malformation, there is atlanto-occipital fusion, hypoplasia of the atlas and dens, malformation of the axis, and modification of the atlantoaxial joint.

Differential Diagnosis

■ Trauma
■ Equine cervical vertebral malformation
■ Equine herpesvirus myeloencephalopathy
■ Bacterial meningitis
■ Viral encephalitides
■ Rabies
■ Other congenital abnormalities

Treatment

■ Mild cases may require no therapy, although progression of the signs is likely as the foal grows.

■ Surgical stabilization and/or decompression of the affected site has been reported in some cases, particularly those occurring in non-Arabian breeds. However, under most circumstances, treatment is conservative, and if the signs are severe, euthanasia should be recommended.

KEY POINT ► Since the disease has a genetic basis in Arabian horses, parents of known affected animals should not be bred to each other or to related animals.

Spinal Cord Trauma

KEY POINT ► Trauma to the spinal cord is common in the horse.

There are several ways that traumatic injury to the cord occurs. In adult horses, a common site for vertebral fractures and resulting cord damage is the caudal cervical region. In contrast, foals tend to suffer fractures of epiphyseal separations in the caudal thoracic to cranial lumbar regions. Subluxations and luxations of the occipitoatlantoaxial joints and fracture of the dens also can occur. These are common in young horses that are tied up and pull back on the lead rope against a fixed object, particularly when first being handled.

History and Presenting Signs

- All ages affected
- Acute onset of incoordination, weakness, and stumbling
- There may be a history of a fall or incident during times when the horse is being handled.

Clinical Findings and Diagnosis

KEY POINT ► Variable signs of ataxia, weakness, and spasticity are common.

- If the lesion is in the cervical region, all limbs will be affected, whereas there may only be hindlimb signs if the lesion is between T2 and S2. In some cases deficits are quite symmetrical, whereas in others they are asymmetrical.
- Neurologic deficits are usually exacerbated in response to manipulative tests, including circling, walking up and down a slope, backing, etc. If the lesion is severe, local gray matter and sympathetic trunks can be damaged, leading to patchy sweating and localized loss of pain sensation. If the signs persist, muscle atrophy may result and be evident by 10 to 14 days post-injury.
- The recumbent horse provides a particular challenge requiring careful attention to detail when performing the neurologic examination if the site of the lesion is to be correctly identified.

KEY POINT ► Horses that are recumbent and have been so for more than 24 hours have a grave prognosis for survival.

- Analysis of CSF may reveal few abnormalities, even in cases where there is a severe traumatic myelopathy. There may be evidence of hemorrhage into the subarachnoid space, reflected by xanthochromia and an increase in red blood cells in the CSF. Hemorrhage is followed by an increase in the number of nucleated cells (neutrophils and macrophages).

KEY POINT ► Diagnosis is often surprisingly difficult.

- In addition to the history, neurologic deficits localized to the spinal cord, and results of CSF analyses, radiography may be useful in assisting the clinician in ascertaining injuries to the bony spine. However, it must be remembered that radiographs only provide images of tissues in two dimensions and fractures without displacement may show no abnormalities. To optimize the likelihood of demonstrating lesions, lateral and dorsoventral or ventrodorsal views should be taken whenever possible.

Differential Diagnosis

- Equine cervical vertebral malformation
- Equine protozoal myeloencephalopathy
- Equine herpesvirus myeloencephalopathy
- Viral encephalitides
- Hepatoencephalopathy
- Vertebral osteomyelitis
- Bacterial meningitis
- Rabies
- Brain abscess
- Congenital abnormalities

Treatment

KEY POINT ► In mild cases, stall rest and restriction of movement may be all that is necessary.

- In addition to inactivity, medical therapy involves administration of agents to reduce cerebral edema and provide anti-inflammatory effects. Corticosteroid therapy such as dexamethasone (0.1–0.2 mg/kg IV q6–8h for several days; Treatment Nos. 29 and 30) is useful.
- If there is no response to this therapy or a deterioration in signs occurs over the first 4 to 6 hours, more aggressive therapy using the osmotic diuretic agent mannitol (0.25 g/kg IV as a 20% solution; Treatment No. 68) is valuable to reduce swelling in the central nervous system. If there is improvement in the signs, therapy with mannitol can be continued every 6 to 12 hours for up to 48 hours. Care should be exercised to ensure that the patient does not become clinically dehydrated. An alternate and additional treatment to mannitol involves intravenous infusion of dimethylsulfoxide (0.5–0.9 g/kg IV as a 10%–20% solution q12–24h for several days; Treatment No. 34).
- In cases where there is surgically correctable instability of the vertebral column or a failure of response to medical therapy, consideration should be given to referring the horse to a specialist facility for appropriate surgical decompression and stabilization.

Verminous Myelitis/Encephalitis

A number of species of internal parasites have been reported to occasionally undergo aberrant migration through the central nervous system. Parasites reported within the central nervous system include *Strongylus vulgaris, Draschia megastoma, Hypoderma* spp., *Setaria* spp. and *Halicephalobus deletrix.*

History and Presenting Signs

- Usually an acute onset of signs that generally are progressive
- No breed or age predilection
- Dramatic alterations in neurologic function are commonly reported.

Clinical Findings and Diagnosis

KEY POINT ▶ Signs are variable and include blindness, head tilt, depression, circling or aimless walking, seizures, ataxia, weakness, recumbency, and death.

- In most circumstances, verminous myelitis results in asymmetrical neurologic signs.
- Cerebrospinal fluid analysis often provides useful information. Xanthochromia, increased total protein, and elevations in the total number of cells (including neutrophils and eosinophils) occur. These changes are more commonly identified early in the course of the disease.
- Diagnosis is difficult antemortem. History of acute onset of neurologic signs, clinical signs revealing asymmetrical deficits, and the CSF findings can assist the clinician in compiling a list of differential diagnoses, of which verminous myelitis may be under strong consideration. Definitive diagnosis usually only occurs following necropsy and histopathologic examination of central nervous system tissues.

Differential Diagnosis

- Equine protozoal myeloencephalopathy
- Equine herpesvirus myeloencephalopathy
- Trauma
- Viral encephalitides
- Equine cervical vertebral malformation
- Vertebral osteomyelitis
- Mycotoxic encephalomalacia
- Brain abscess
- Rabies
- Congenital abnormalities

Treatment

- Since a definitive diagnosis is rare, treatment tends to be empirical and supportive.

KEY POINT ▶ Administration of ivermectin (0.2 mg/kg PO once; Treatment No. 62) will assist in destruction of parasites within the central nervous system.

- Response to this therapy may be slow because it often takes weeks for the parasites to be killed. Repeating the treatment after 10 to 14 days may be useful.
- Anti-inflammatory therapy is advised. Good choices include flunixin meglumine (1.1 mg/kg IV q24h; Treatment No. 52) or phenylbutazone (4.4 mg/kg PO q24h; Treatment No. 88). Dexamethasone (0.1–0.2 mg/kg IV q24h for 3–4 days; Treatment Nos. 29 and 30) can be beneficial. However, if equine protozoal myeloencephalitis is strongly suspected, glucocorticosteroids *should not* be administered. We have found intravenous administration of dimethylsulfoxide (0.5–0.9 g/kg IV as a 10%–20% solution q24h for several days; Treatment No. 34) to be valuable in diseases where inflammation of central nervous system tissues is present.
- Good supportive care, including provision of shelter, water and palatable, nutritious feeds, is important.
- The prognosis for verminous myelitis must always be guarded. Cases with mild deficits may survive or even return to almost normal function. However, in our experience, many cases have been progressive or resulted in significant residual deficits. In these cases, euthanasia should be considered.

Vertebral Osteomyelitis

KEY POINT ▶ Bacterial osteomyelitis is most common in foals and young horses due to hematogenous spread of organisms to the vertebral bodies secondary to septicemia.

In these cases, *Salmonella* spp., *Streptococcus* spp., *Staphylococcus* spp., *E. coli,* and *Actinobacillus* spp. are the most common causative agents. The condition is relatively rare in adult horses, and when it occurs, it is usually the result of infections with *Mycobacterium* spp. or *Brucella* spp.

History and Presenting Signs

- Normally young horses (<6 months old)
- Possible evidence or history of septicemia (e.g., fever, lethargy, and depression)
- Relatively rapid onset of progressively worsening incoordination
- Localized neck pain or reluctance to move the neck or flex the back

Clinical Findings and Diagnosis

KEY POINT ▶ Evidence of spinal cord compression is demonstrated by ataxia, tetraparesis, spasticity, and dysmetria.

- Manipulative procedures such as circling will often result in worsening of the signs. There may be a reluctance to move the neck or flex the back due to pain.
- Identification of an inflammatory response on routine hematologic examination (leukocytosis, hyperfibrinogenemia, anemia of chronic disease) also can reflect osteomyelitis.
- Radiology may reveal abnormal vertebrae.
- Results from analysis of the CSF can be variable. At times, findings are unremarkable; at other times, there is evidence of spinal cord compression (xanthochromia, increased total nucleated cell count, particularly macrophages and increased total protein). On rare occasions there is evidence of meningitis, reflected by marked increases in CSF nucleated cell counts, especially neutrophils and total protein.
- Diagnosis is based on a combination of the history, clinical signs, and results of ancillary diagnostic tests (e.g., clinical pathology, radiology, and CSF analysis).

Differential Diagnosis

- Trauma
- Septicemia

- Equine cervical malformation
- Equine herpesvirus myeloencephalopathy
- Occipitoatlantoaxial malformations
- Bacterial meningitis
- Viral encephalitides
- Rabies
- Other congenital abnormalities

Treatment

- If an accurate, early diagnosis of vertebral osteomyelitis is made, the disorder may be treatable. Surgical curettage of affected tissue and long-term administration of appropriate antimicrobial agents can be successful in some cases.
- Anti-inflammatory therapy to reduce spinal cord compression may be valuable early in the disease. Nonsteroidal anti-inflammatory drugs such as flunixin meglumine (1.1 mg/kg IV q24h; Treatment No. 52) or phenylbutazone (4.4 mg/kg PO q24h; Treatment No. 88) will provide some pain relief. Intravenous administration of dimethylsulfoxide (0.5–0.9 g/kg IV as a 10%–20% solution q24h for several days; Treatment No. 34) is also useful as an agent with anti-inflammatory properties.

Diseases of the Brain and Cranial Nerves

Bacterial Meningitis

KEY POINT ► Bacterial meningitis is a rare but devastating disease that may be found in young foals as a sequela to septicemia.

In addition, the blood–brain barrier may be more permeable to organisms during the neonatal period.

History and Presenting Signs

- Neonates
- Failure of passive transfer of immunity, signs of infection in other body sites, or septicemia
- Acute onset of signs consistent with diffuse central nervous system dysfunction

Clinical Findings and Diagnosis

- There are specific signs of bacterial meningitis. However, any young horse with an acute onset of signs associated with diffuse central nervous system disease may have meningitis.

KEY POINT ► Concurrent omphalophlebitis, polyarticular septic arthritis, diarrhea, or pneumonia may increase the likelihood of bacterial meningitis.

- Abnormal behaviors including ataxia, wandering, "star gazing," failure to drink, recumbency, seizures, hyperesthesia, and opisthotonus are signs that may occur in association with bacterial meningitis. Unfortunately, fever is not a consistent finding of meningitis in neonates.

■ Hematologic examination may reveal changes consistent with those occurring in septicemia, including leukopenia with the presence of band and toxic neutrophils. Failure of passive transfer of immunoglobulins is common, as reflected by low serum IgG concentrations [<4 g/L (<400 mg/dl)].

KEY POINT ▶ Increases in the number of nucleated cells (neutrophils and mononuclear cells), the concentration of protein, and possibly the presence of bacteria in the CSF are features of the disease.

■ The glucose concentration of the CSF is often low, but this should be compared with blood glucose concentrations, which may be lower than normal in septicemia. Note that normally, CSF glucose concentrations are 60% to 80% of plasma values. Cerebrospinal fluid and blood should be submitted for culture. Common offending bacteria include *Salmonella* spp., *Actinobacillus equuli,* and *Streptococcus* spp.

■ Regardless of treatment, death due to meningitis in foals is common.

Differential Diagnosis

■ Trauma
■ Hypoglycemia
■ Septicemia
■ Neonatal maladjustment syndrome
■ Congenital malformations, hydrocephalus
■ Hepatoencephalopathy
■ Idiopathic seizure syndrome

Treatment

■ Treatment is similar to that described for septicemia and is directed toward controlling the infectious agent. Antibiotic therapy is guided by the results of culture and sensitivity. While awaiting results, initial therapy may involve Na or K penicillin G (20 mg/kg IV or IM q6–12h; Treatment Nos. 84 and 85) and gentamicin (2–3 mg/kg IV q8–12h; Treatment No. 56), trimethoprim-sulfadiazine (30 mg/kg IV or PO q12h; Treatment No. 107), or cefotaxime sodium (80 mg/kg IV q6–8h; Treatment No. 16), which is often effective but expensive. Ceftiofur sodium (2 mg/kg IV q12h; Treatment No. 18) also may be useful. Although the healthy blood–brain barrier is often impermeable to drugs, infection of the meninges makes it permeable to most of these agents. Antibiotic selection is subsequently tailored on the basis of culture and sensitivity results. Therapy for 4 to 6 weeks may be required.

■ If seizures are a problem, treatment with diazepam (0.05–0.1 mg/kg IV as required; Treatment No. 32) is often effective. Longer-term control can be achieved with phenobarbital (20 mg/kg IV over 30 minutes as a loading dose followed by 5–9 mg/kg IV slowly q8h; Treatment No. 87).

■ Therapy may be required to decrease central nervous system edema, such as mannitol (0.25 mg/kg IV as a 20% solution q4–6h; Treatment No. 68) or dimethylsulfoxide (0.5–0.9 g/kg slowly IV as a 10%–20% solution q12–24h; Treatment No. 34).

■ It is imperative to ensure that the foal receives adequate fluids and nutrition during the treatment period and maintains a normal blood glucose concentration (see Chap. 16).

Botulism ("Shaker Foal" Syndrome, "Forage Poisoning")

KEY POINT ▶ Botulism, a disease characterized by progressive flaccid paralysis, is caused by the potent exotoxin liberated from the anaerobic bacterium *Clostridium botulinum.*

There are eight serotypes of *C. botulinum* identified, with types A, B, and C being the most common cause of disease in horses in North America. Type C occurs mainly in the western states, type B in Kentucky and the Northeast, and type C in the Southeast and southern California. In general, the toxin grows in decaying vegetable or animal matter. As a result, silage or hay are common sources for the toxin. Three types of botulism occur. Ingestion of preformed toxin ("forage poisoning") is most common in adult horses and is normally caused by *C. botulinum* type B or C. Production of toxin in the gastrointestinal tract (toxoinfectious botulism) occurs in foals ("shaker foal" syndrome) and is thought to be caused by type B toxin. The last form is referred to as "wound botulism" and results from growth of the organism and liberation of the toxin from a wound. This is an extremely rare form of the disease and will not be discussed. However, signs are similar to those described for "forage poisoning."

History and Presenting Signs
▶ Toxoinfectious Botulism

■ Foals 2 weeks to 8 months old
■ Progressive paralysis
■ Dysphagia
■ Recumbency

▶ Ingestion of Preformed Toxin

■ Adult horses
■ History of eating silage 1 to 7 days previously
■ Paresis
■ Dysphagia
■ Recumbency

Clinical Findings and Diagnosis

▶ Toxoinfectious Botulism

KEY POINT ▶ Affected foals have progressive onset of paresis resulting in a staggering gait and muscle tremors ("shaker foal" disease).

- These signs progress to recumbency, an inability to rise, and eventually death. Dysphagia is common, with milk often seen dribbling from the mouth and/or nose. Secondary aspiration pneumonia is common. Dilated pupils and paralyzed eyelids are also notable features.
- Diagnosis is usually presumptive and based on the history and clinical findings. Most reported cases of toxoinfectious botulism have occurred in Kentucky and the mid-Atlantic states. Definitive diagnosis requires identification of the toxin in serum and/or gastrointestinal contents from dead foals. Such attempts are often unrewarding.

KEY POINT ▶ Identification of *C. botulinum* spores in the feces is also useful, since more than 75% of foals suffering from toxoinfectious botulism shed spores in the feces. There is almost no shedding of spores in normal, uninfected foals in the same region.

▶ Ingestion of Preformed Toxin

KEY POINT ▶ Typical signs are progressive weakness resulting in a hesitant, stumbling gait, progression to recumbency, respiratory compromise, and death within days of eating contaminated feedstuffs.

- Muscle tremor is often a common feature. Dysphagia with the horse unable to raise its head is regarded as a classical early sign of the disorder. If the disease progresses slowly, dependent edema of the head ensues. The tongue will often hang out, and saliva will dribble from the mouth. The pupils may be dilated, and there is a poor response to light. Urinary and fecal retention is common.
- The diagnostic principles are similar to those described for toxoinfectious botulism. Diagnosis is presumptive and often not confirmed. Attempts to identify the toxin in feed samples, blood, or gut contents are almost always disappointing. Approximately 20% of horses with botulism will shed spores in the feces.

Differential Diagnosis

▶ Toxoinfectious Botulism

- Septicemia
- Trauma
- Nutritional myonecrosis

- Esophageal obstruction
- Hypoglycemia

▶ Ingestion of Preformed Toxin

- Equine protozoal encephalomyelitis
- Esophageal obstruction
- Trauma
- Nigropallidal encephalomalacia ("yellow star thistle poisoning")
- Nutritional myonecrosis (masseter myopathy)
- Guttural pouch diseases
- Hypocalcemia
- Hyperkalemic periodic paralysis

Treatment

- The principles of therapy are similar for all forms of the disease and will be covered together.

KEY POINT ▶ Use of polyvalent botulinum antitoxin (100–200 IU/kg IV or IM, obtained from the University of Pennsylvania) is useful, although often extremely expensive.

- Antitoxin will adsorb free toxin but not that which is already bound to receptors. Therefore, antitoxin administration is most useful in horses who are still standing and who are experiencing a slow progression of signs.
- Restriction of movement together with nursing care is important to ensure adequate fluid and nutritional intake. Administration of mare's milk to foals or feed gruels and electrolyte–carbohydrate mixtures via nasogastric tube is beneficial. We have found a commercially available liquid diet (Osmolite HN, Ross Laboratories, Columbus, OH) to be a valuable calorie source for horses with dysphagia. From recent research work at the University of Pennsylvania (Sweeney and Hansen, 1990), it is advised to feed 8 ml/kg then 16, 24 and finally 32 ml/kg total daily dose on successive days. The dose is divided and given every 8 hours. The high dose constitutes maintenance calorie requirements for an adult horse. *Note:* Additional water is required for maintenance (total daily fluid intake of 50–75 ml/kg). Administration of mineral oil may help relieve constipation. Catheterization of the bladder is indicated in horses with urinary retention.
- Parenteral nutrition for foals with botulism has been described but is expensive and time-consuming and is normally only reserved for valuable animals.
- Treatment of complications (e.g., aspiration pneumonia) is important.
- Recovery may take several weeks.
- Prevention of toxoinfectious botulism in endemic areas has been undertaken using a *C. botulinum* type B toxoid (Bot Tox-B, Neogen Biologics Corp., Lansing, MI). Mares are vaccinated at 8, 9, and 10 months of gestation. An annual booster

for pregnant mares in the last month of gestation is indicated.
- Silage contaminated with botulinum toxin should be removed from the diet of other susceptible horses.

Brain Abscess

Abscesses in the cerebral hemispheres usually occur in horses less than 5 years old as a sequela to "strangles" (infection with *Streptococcus equi* var. *equi*).

History and Presenting Signs

- Young horses less than 5 years old
- Previous "strangles" infection or a history of "strangles" in the herd
- Behavioral changes and blindness

Clinical Findings and Diagnosis

- There may be fever, inappetence, and evidence of "strangles" abscesses elsewhere.
- Circling, head pressing, blindness, deviation of the head to the side, and ataxia are common features of brain abscesses.
- Antemortem diagnosis is difficult and is based on the history, clinical signs of cerebral disease, and results of ancillary tests. There may be a leukocytosis (with neutrophilia), hyperfibrinogenemia, and hyperglobulinemia. Cerebrospinal fluid often has increased protein and total nucleated cell count (neutrophilia and monocytosis). On rare occasions, bacteria may be identified. Postmortem examination reveals a pyogenic abscess in the cerebrum or elsewhere in the brain.

Differential Diagnosis

- Viral encephalitides
- Hepatoencephalopathy
- Trauma
- Equine herpesvirus myeloencephalopathy
- Equine protozoal myeloencephalopathy
- Bacterial meningitis
- Mycotoxic encephalomalacia
- Verminous encephalitis
- Parasitic thromboembolism
- Neuritis of the cauda equina

Treatment

KEY POINT ► Treatment is very difficult and often unrewarding.

Long-term therapy with procaine penicillin [15,000 IU (15 mg/kg) IM q12h; Treatment No. 83] or trimethoprim-sulfadiazine (20 mg/kg PO of combined drugs q12h; Treatment No. 107) for 4 to 6 weeks has been used but is mostly unsuccessful.

Cerebellar Abiotrophy

KEY POINT ► Cerebellar abiotrophy is a heritable disorder in Arabian (pure and crossbred), and Oldenberg horses and Götland ponies.

History and Presenting Signs

- Foals less than 6 months of age—Arabian, Arabian cross, Oldenberg horses, and Götland ponies.
- Abnormal gait
- Signs are progressive.

Clinical Findings and Diagnosis

KEY POINT ► Affected foals have a base-wide stance and gait abnormalities characterized by ataxia, dysmetria, and a tendency to pace.

- There is no evidence of weakness. An intention tremor and absence of the menace response occur. Signs progress over weeks to months.
- Cerebrospinal fluid protein concentration may be elevated (>2.0 g/L or 200 mg/dl). Other clinical pathology findings are unremarkable.
- Presumptive diagnosis is based on the history, breed, and clinical manifestations. Definitive diagnosis is made on histologic postmortem examination of the cerebellum.

Differential Diagnosis

- Trauma
- Acquired cerebellar diseases (e.g., herpesvirus myeloencephalopathy)
- Septicemia
- Congenital malformations
- Spinal cord diseases

Treatment

- There is no successful therapy for cerebellar abiotrophy.
- Parents of affected foals should not be bred.

Cranial Nerve Palsies

These are common in horses and usually result from trauma to the particular nerve or an inflammatory process secondary to a primary infectious process. In this section, only the most commonly affected cranial nerves will be discussed.

History and Presenting Signs

► **Trigeminal Nerve**

- Trauma
- Dropped jaw and dropping of food and water from the mouth

► Facial Nerve

- Trauma
- General anesthesia
- Halter that is too tight with the horse pulling back
- Altered facial expression

► Vestibular Nerve

- Acute onset of vestibular signs (e.g., head tilt, circling, ataxia)
- Trauma

Clinical Findings and Diagnosis

► Trigeminal Nerve

KEY POINT ► Dropped jaw and food falling from the mouth may be observed.

- After 10 to 14 days, masseter, digastricus, and temporalis muscle atrophy can be marked. Enophthalmus and drooping of the eyelids may be seen. Lesions can be unilateral or bilateral.
- Diagnosis is based on the physical findings. Trigeminal nerve palsy can occur as a result of trauma (e.g., fractures of the mandible and/or stylohyoid bones) or as a result of equine protozoal myeloencephalitis or neuritis of the cauda equina. Diagnosis of fractures is aided by radiography. The findings associated with equine protozoal myeloencephalitis (p. 368) and neuritis of the cauda equina (p. 369) are described elsewhere in this section.

► Facial Nerve

KEY POINT ► There is drooping of the lips and paralysis of the muscles of facial expression, with the muzzle being pulled away from the affected side.

- Ptosis is common, and the ear droops. If there is only damage to the buccal branches of the nerve, as frequently occurs following damage during general anesthesia or as a result of application of a halter that is too tight, ptosis and ear droop may not be present.
- Exposure keratitis is a common sequela to facial nerve palsy, resulting from ptosis and reduced tear production.
- With persistence of the palsy (>6 months), there is fibrosis of affected muscles, making return to normal function less likely.
- With bilateral lesions, dysphagia is common.

► Vestibular Nerve

KEY POINT ► Head tilt, leaning, and circling—all toward the side of the lesion— staggering, and nystagmus (with the fast phase away from the lesion) are the predominant signs.

- With peripheral lesions, the nystagmus is usually horizontal. Application of a blindfold frequently exacerbates the signs.
- Facial nerve paralysis may occur in association with vestibular disease.
- Central lesions resulting in vestibular dysfunction may have other signs, including vertical or rotary nystagmus, weakness, and depression, and possibly involvement of other cranial nerves.
- The most common causes of vestibular syndrome are trauma, osteoarthritis of the temperohyoid region, and idiopathic vestibular syndrome. Osteoarthritis of the temperohyoid region may result from chronic otitis/interna. There is no identified cause for idiopathic vestibular disease, which occurs spontaneously in adult horses.
- Diagnosis of trauma is difficult, but it may be aided by the history, physical signs, and clinico-pathologic and radiographic findings. Osteoarthritis of the temperohyoid region is diagnosed on the basis of radiographic changes (e.g., proliferation, sclerosis, joint fusion, fractures) and possibly hemorrhage into the guttural pouches.
- Idiopathic vestibular syndrome is diagnosed by ruling out other possible causes of vestibular dysfunction.

Differential Diagnosis

► Trigeminal Nerve

- Equine protozoal myeloencephalitis
- Botulism
- Nigropallidal encephalomalacia
- Neuritis of the cauda equina
- Masseter muscle myopathy (nutritional myodegeneration)

► Facial Nerve

- Equine protozoal myeloencephalitis
- Otitis media/interna
- Verminous myelitis
- Neuritis of the cauda equina
- Brain abscess
- Viral encephalitides
- Neoplasia

► Vestibular Nerve

- Equine protozoal myeloencephalitis
- Otitis media/interna
- Verminous myelitis
- Neuritis of the corda equina
- Lightning strike
- Neoplasia

Treatment

► Trigeminal Nerve

There is no specific therapy for trigeminal palsy. Anti-inflammatory therapy using flunixin meglumine (1.1 mg/kg IV q12–24h; Treatment No. 52) and dimethylsulfoxide (0.5–0.9 g/kg IV as a 10%–20% solution q12–24h; Treatment No. 34) may be beneficial.

▶ Facial Nerve

- If the nerve has been severed, there is some potential therapeutic benefit obtained from rejoining the severed ends of the nerve. However, in most cases the injury results from contusion and stretching without breakage in the skin or severance of the nerve. As a result, anti-inflammatory therapy such as flunixin meglumine (0.6–1.1 mg/kg IV q12–24h for up to 5 days) and/or dimethylsulfoxide (0.5–0.9 g/kg IV as a 10%–20% solution q24h) may provide benefit.
- The prognosis for return of normal function, particularly if there is a peripheral lesion due to pressure on the nerve, is generally good if the insult is short-lived. Palsy due to central lesions (e.g., equine protozoal myeloencephalitis) has a less favorable prognosis.

▶ Vestibular Nerve

- Therapy for trauma involves anti-inflammatory medications such as flunixin meglumine (0.6–1.1 mg/kg IV q12–24h for up to 5 days; Treatment No. 52) and/or dimethylsulfoxide (0.5–0.9 g/kg IV as a 10%–20% solution q24h; Treatment No. 34).
- Osteoarthritis of the temperohyoid region may respond to anti-inflammatory therapy (see above) and chronic administration of antibiotics such as trimethoprim-sulfadiazine (20 mg/kg of the combination PO q12h; Treatment No. 107) for at least 2 weeks.
- Idiopathic vestibular syndrome tends to resolve spontaneously irrespective of treatment.

Cranial Trauma (Head Trauma)

Cranial trauma is common in horses as a consequence of kicks, collisions, penetrating wounds, or rearing over backwards. Any traumatic episode can result in injury to the brain and/or spinal cord. Spinal cord trauma is discussed elsewhere in this section (p. 371). When horses are tied to a fixed object and attempt to pull away, they tend to rear over backwards. These incidents can result in basisphenoid or basioccipital fractures and injury to the brainstem.

KEY POINT ▶ In many cases, cranial trauma is complicated by ongoing hemorrhage within the calvarium that induces significant increases in intracranial pressure and necrosis of nervous tissue, resulting in a progression of signs.

History and Presenting Signs

- All ages affected
- History of trauma (e.g., rearing over backwards, being kicked, hit by a car, fall in a race)
- Neurologic signs will depend on the site and severity of the lesion.
- Evidence of skin contusions
- Stupor, head tilt, recumbency, blindness, etc.

Clinical Findings and Diagnosis

- Clinical signs depend on the site of the injury. Penetrating wounds, fracture fragments, or indications of blunt trauma may be evident. Evidence of blood (fresh or dried) discharging from the ear canals or nostrils should be noted. In some cases, CSF may discharge from an ear canal.

KEY POINT ▶ With cerebral injuries, changes in behavior (e.g., depression, stupor, seizures and coma) and gait (e.g., ataxia, weakness, and possibly recumbency) are common.

- Circling to the side of the lesion may be a feature, and blindness is frequently noted. The pupils may be asymmetrical and variably responsive to light. Progression to coma and unresponsive bilateral mydriasis indicates midbrain involvement and a grave prognosis.
- Lesions of the brainstem often result in motor dysfunction (e.g., ataxia, paresis), cranial nerve deficits, and effects on heart and respiratory rates.
- Injury and hemorrhage near the inner ear may result in vestibular signs (e.g., head tilt, circling to the side of the lesion, nystagmus—with the fast phase away from the side of the lesion). Facial nerve palsy may occur in association with these lesions.
- Diagnosis is usually based on history, circumstantial evidence, and clinical signs, as well as by ruling out other possible causes of the signs. Radiographs are helpful, particularly when there is obvious evidence of trauma.

KEY POINT ▶ However, it should be noted that nondistracted fractures (e.g., those of the basisphenoid or basioccipital bones) may be extremely difficult to detect on radiographs.

Differential Diagnosis

- Viral encephalitides
- Hepatoencephalopathy
- Verminous encephalitis
- Equine herpesvirus myeloencephalopathy
- Bacterial meningitis/brain abscess
- Hypocalcemia
- Tetanus
- Botulism

- Septicemia (foals)
- Benign idiopathic seizure syndrome (Arabian foals)
- Congenital malformations (foals)

Treatment

- In mild cases, stall rest and restriction of movement may result in full recovery.

KEY POINT ► Mostly, aggressive medical therapy is necessary.

- This involves administration of anti-inflammatory drugs and agents to reduce cerebral edema. Dexamethasone (0.1–0.2 mg/kg IV q6–8h for several days; Treatment Nos. 29 and 30) is useful to decrease intracranial pressure and central nervous system edema.
- If there is no response to this therapy or a deterioration in signs over the first 4 to 6 hours, more aggressive therapy using the osmotic diuretic agent mannitol (0.25 g/kg IV as a 20% solution; Treatment No. 68) is indicated. This should assist in reducing swelling in the central nervous system. If there is improvement in the signs, therapy with mannitol can be continued every 6 to 12 hours for up to 48 hours. *Note:* Care should be exercised to ensure that the patient does not become clinically dehydrated. Intravenous infusion of dimethylsulfoxide (0.5–0.9 g/kg IV as a 10%–20% solution q12–24h for several days; Treatment No. 34) may also be valuable.
- Administration of nonsteroidal anti-inflammatory drugs such as flunixin meglumine (1.1 mg/kg IV q24h; Treatment No. 52) will assist in decreasing tissue swelling and pain.
- Complications of the injuries include progression of signs leading to death or the necessity for euthanasia. Other factors that may impede successful treatment include infections (e.g., aspiration pneumonia, decubital sores in recumbent patients), bladder paralysis, and cystitis.
- Nursing care and maintenance of fluid and electrolyte balance are important.
- In some cases, a craniotomy to allow decompression and removal of bone fragments may be possible. In these cases, referral of the horse to a specialist facility for appropriate surgical decompression should be considered.
- Some horses recover uneventfully despite profound clinical manifestations soon after the trauma. In others, signs progress or significant complications arise, resulting in death or the necessity for euthanasia. Some horses improve initially, but residual deficits remain. For example, permanent blindness can occur as a result of damage to the optic nerve roots.

Equine Togaviral Encephalomyelitides

Infection with alphaviruses is responsible for induction of eastern (EEE), western (WEE) and Venezuelan (VEE) equine encephalomyelitis. These viruses have birds as their reservoir host, with mosquitoes being responsible for spread of the virus to horses. Spread of the disease is therefore dependent on the presence of the reservoir hosts and insect vectors. As a result, viral encephalitides can occur year round in the Southeast. They are more common in the North during the summer and fall. The viral encephalitides have a reasonably predictable geographic distribution, with EEE and WEE being most common in the United States. As the names of the diseases imply, WEE occurs in the West, Midwest and South, whereas EEE is found in the East. There is a large area, approximately 1600 km (1000 miles) wide, down the center of the United States where both diseases occur. In contrast, VEE only occurs in the most southern regions of the United States. All three viral encephalitides occur in Mexico and South America.

History and Presenting Signs

- All ages of horses affected, but rare in young foals
- Acute onset of lethargy, depression, and colic
- Signs progress to include alterations in behavior and other neurologic abnormalities

Clinical Findings and Diagnosis

- Fever, depression, head pressing, circling, blindness, seizures, and coma are common. These signs are the result of cerebral invasion, necrosis, and inflammation in response to the virus. Infection with EEE and VEE is often fatal, whereas death following WEE is less frequent.

KEY POINT ► Diagnosis is based on the history, with emphasis being focused on the time of the year and geographic location, the clinical signs, and the results of diagnostic tests.

- Analysis of the CSF reveals xanthochromia, increased total protein (>1.5 g/L or 150 mg/dl), and leukocytosis (50–400 $\times$ 10^6/L or 50–400/μl). With EEE, the leukocytosis is often the result of a neutrophilia, whereas a monocytic pleocytosis tends to occur with WEE. Serology is useful in assisting with diagnosis. In general, seroconversion has occurred by the time encephalitic signs occur. As a result, a fourfold increase in titer between samples collected in the acute phase of the disease and those collected 10 to 14 days later may not occur. However, a high titer in an unvaccinated horse with clinical signs of cerebral disease will increase the likelihood of viral encephalitis. Postmortem analysis of tissues reveals relatively characteristic changes. The offending virus often can be cultured from central nervous system tissues.

Differential Diagnosis

- Other togaviral encephalitides
- Hepatoencephalopathy
- Trauma
- Equine protozoal myeloencephalopathy
- Bacterial meningitis
- Rabies
- Mycotoxic encephalomalacia
- Verminous encephalitis

Treatment

- There is no specific therapy for the viral encephalitides. As a result, treatment is supportive and mainly involves nursing care. Anti-inflammatory therapy with nonsteroidal anti-inflammatory drugs such as flunixin meglumine (1.1 mg/kg q24h; Treatment No. 52) or phenylbutazone (4.4 mg/kg q24h; Treatment No. 88) is indicated. In addition, intravenous administration of dimethylsulfoxide (0.5 to 0.9 g/kg IV as a 10% to 20% solution q12–24h for several days; Treatment No. 34) appears to provide some palliative effects. Use of corticosteroids for short periods early in the disease, such as dexamethasone (0.1–0.2 mg/kg IV q6–8h for 1–2 days; Treatment Nos. 29 and 30), may be of benefit. If seizures are occurring, administration of diazepam (0.05–0.5 mg/kg IV as required; Treatment No. 32) or phenobarbital (4–10 mg/kg IV slowly; Treatment No. 87) is often useful.
- Attention to maintenance of hydration and nutritional status is important. Administration of mineral oil (Treatment No. 77) may be indicated to assist in prevention of gastrointestinal impaction. Horses who remain anorexic can be fed gruels via stomach tube (see Chap. 16) or dietary supplements (Osmolite HN, Ross Laboratories, Columbus, OH).
- Full recovery from the viral encephalitides is rare. If neurologic signs are present, mortality is common, being greater than 80% for horses with EEE, up to 50% for WEE, and up to 75% for VEE.
- Prevention of the disease has been afforded by insect-control programs and vaccination.

KEY POINT ▶ Administration of formalin-inactivated vaccines to horses at risk affords good protection (Treatment No. 109).

- If vaccinating for protection against VEE, a trivalent vaccine containing inactivated EEE, WEE, and VEE should be given. Vaccination should always be conducted in the spring before the insect numbers increase. In endemic areas, or if there is a prolonged presence of vectors, vaccination should be repeated every 4 to 6 months. Mares should be vaccinated in the month prior to foaling. Vaccination in the face of an outbreak is indicated.

Hepatoencephalopathy

Hepatoencephalopathy is a disorder of cerebral function resulting in dementia, head pressing, and altered behavior in horses as a consequence of hepatic dysfunction. The signs, causes, and management of hepatoencephalopathy are discussed in the section dealing with liver diseases in Chapter 6.

Mycotoxic encephalomalacia (Leukoencephalomalacia, "Moldy Corn" Poisoning, "Blind Staggers")

Mycotoxic encephalomalacia is a disorder resulting from liberation of the toxin fumonisin B_1 from the mold *Fusarium moniliforme,* which grows readily on cereal grains, in particular corn. In high doses this toxin produces a hepatopathy, whereas in lower doses an encephalopathy results.

History and Presenting Signs

- History of eating corn for at least 2 weeks
- Occurs mostly from late fall to spring
- Often occurs in outbreaks
- Sudden death is common.
- Inappetence followed by behavioral changes

Clinical Findings and Diagnosis

- In addition to signs noted above, the disease is often characterized by asymmetrical cranial nerve deficits, depression, mania, blindness, and circling. Ataxia and weakness followed by recumbency, coma, or seizures also can occur.

KEY POINT ▶ The activity of liver-specific enzymes in the plasma is normally elevated due to the hepatotoxic effects of fumonisin B_1.

- Analysis of the CSF provides variable results depending on the extent and site of the lesion. In most cases, increases in the number of neutrophils and total protein are found.
- Antemortem diagnosis is difficult. The history, clinical signs, and laboratory data (altered CSF in particular) should increase the clinician's suspicion of mycotoxic encephalomalacia. Large numbers of spores of *F. monoliforme* in feed samples also will increase the likelihood of mycotoxicosis. Definitive diagnosis is made at postmortem examination by the demonstration of a characteristic liquefactive cerebral necrosis.

Differential Diagnosis

- Trauma
- Hepatoencephalopathy
- Viral encephalitides
- Bacterial meningitis/brain abscess
- Verminous encephalitis
- Botulism

- Equine herpesvirus myeloencephalopathy
- Equine protozoal myeloencephalopathy
- Neuritis of the cauda equina

Treatment

- There is no specific treatment for mycotoxic encephalitis. Supportive therapy may be helpful. Flunixin meglumine (1.1 mg/kg IV q24h; Treatment No. 52) or phenylbutazone (4.4 mg/kg PO q24h; Treatment No. 88) may have anti-inflammatory effects. Empirically dexamethasone (0.1–0.2 mg/kg IV q24h for 3–4 days; Treatment Nos. 29 and 30) is also of value. Mannitol (0.25 mg/kg IV as a 20% solution q4–6h for 1 day; Treatment No. 68) may help decrease brain edema. Dimethylsulfoxide (0.5–0.9 g/kg IV as a 10%–20% solution q12–24h for several days; Treatment No. 34) also may be useful in decreasing clinical signs.
- Good supportive care, including provision of shelter, water, and palatable, nutritious feeds, is important.

KEY POINT ► The prognosis is always poor. Some cases may make a partial recovery, but in most circumstances the disease can be considered fatal.

Narcolepsy (Fainting Disease)

Narcolepsy is a rare disorder in horses characterized by repeated episodes of sudden onset of muscle weakness and abnormal sleep-like activity.

History and Presenting Signs

- Onset of signs usually before 1 year of age
- History of muscle weakness or collapse
- Signs may be initiated when the horse is stimulated (e.g., feeding, return to herd mates, and various treatment procedures).
- Familial in some Suffolk and Shetland foals

Clinical Findings and Diagnosis

KEY POINT ► Clinical manifestations can be variable, with episodes being infrequent (weeks apart) or relatively constant.

- We saw one horse that had an episode every 5 to 10 minutes. During episodes, there can be mild muscle weakness through to collapse. Horses often buckle at the knees and stumble. Some horses may be extremely difficult to arouse and to make walk during episodes; others are more easily stimulated. Ataxia is common during episodes. Signs last from seconds to minutes.
- Between episodes, affected horses are normal.
- Diagnosis is based on the history, clinical manifestations, and possibly response to physostigmine salicylate (0.06–0.08 mg/kg slowly IV; An-

tilirium, Forest, Maryland Heights, MO). In many horses with narcolepsy, this agent induces signs in under 15 minutes. In severely affected horses, atropine (0.06 mg/kg IV; Treatment No. 11) will decrease the severity of signs for a number of hours.

Differential Diagnosis

- Trauma
- Hyperkalemic periodic paralysis
- Exertional rhabdomyolysis
- Syncope
- Hypocalcemia
- Restraint of neonates leading to a narcoleptic-like state
- Botulism (foals)
- Hypoglycemia (foals)
- Septicemia (foals)

Treatment

Treatment of narcolepsy is often unrewarding. Imipramine (Tofranil, Geigy Pharmaceuticals, Summit, NJ) at a dose rate of 0.5 mg/kg IV or 1.5 mg/kg PO q8h is of value in some narcoleptic horses, although in our experience the results of therapy are quite variable.

KEY POINT ► The prognosis for this disorder varies enormously among individual cases. Some foals have several episodes and then appear to recover spontaneously. In others, signs persist for life.

Nigropallidal Encephalomalacia ("Yellow Star Thistle Poisoning")

Nigropallidal encephalomalacia is a fatal disease of horses caused by toxins in yellow star thistle or Russian knapweed. There is a highly specific lesion in the substantia nigra and globus pallidus resulting in dysphagia.

History and Presenting Signs

- All ages
- Western states
- History of eating Centaurea solstitialis (yellow star thistle) or Centaurea repens (Russian knapweed) for at least several weeks. Dried plants in hay are also toxic. Horses tend to develop a desire to selectively eat these plants.
- Dysphagia and weight loss are the most common presenting signs.

Clinical Findings and Diagnosis

- Affected horses have a sudden onset of dysfunction of the muscles of mastication characterized by rigidity and fasciculation. Horses cannot move their mouths normally or chew food. Some horses also show behavioral abnormalities.

- We have seen several cases with pronounced facial and lip edema.
- Clinical pathology tests are unremarkable. There may be evidence of dehydration.
- The diagnosis is based on the history and clinical findings.

Differential Diagnosis

- Botulism
- Guttural pouch mycosis
- Viral encephalitides
- Hepatoencephalopathy
- Bacterial meningitis/brain abscess
- Verminous encephalitis
- Equine protozoal myeloencephalopathy
- Masseter myopathy (nutritional myodegeneration)
- Neuritis of the cauda equina
- Trigeminal nerve palsy

Treatment

There is no successful treatment for this disorder. Affected horses usually die from starvation.

Parasitic Thromboembolism

Parasitic thromboembolism is an acute disorder occurring as a result of thromboemoli formed following the migration of *Strongylus vulgaris* larvae through the vasculature of the central nervous system.

History and Presenting Signs

- Usually horses less than 3 years old
- Acute onset of behavioral changes, depression, recumbency, and possibly seizures

Clinical Findings and Diagnosis

- Signs are often asymmetrical. In horses that are standing, blindness, aimless wandering, pacing, and circling to the affected side can occur. Beligerent behavior or depression also may be features. Mild ataxia is common. Death can ensue.
- In many cases, signs do not progress and may improve over time.
- Diagnosis is difficult and often speculative. Clinical signs may help, and CSF usually has nonspecific manifestations such as xanthochromia and mildly increased protein and total nucleated cell counts.

Differential Diagnosis

- Trauma
- Hepatoencephalopathy
- Viral encephalitides
- Bacterial meningitis/brain abscess

- Verminous encephalitis
- Botulism
- Mycotoxic encephalomalacia
- Equine herpesvirus myeloencephalopathy
- Equine protozoal myeloencephalopathy
- Neuritis of the cauda equina

Treatment

- Since a definitive diagnosis is rarely made, treatment is empirical and supportive. If it is assumed that migrating parasites are still present, administration of ivermectin (0.2 mg/kg PO once; Treatment No. 62) is indicated. Repeating the therapy after 10 to 14 days is often useful.
- Anti-inflammatory therapy is advised. Good choices include flunixin meglumine (1.1 mg/kg IV q24h; Treatment No. 52) or phenylbutazone (4.4 mg/kg PO q24h; Treatment No. 88). Dexamethasone (0.1–0.2 mg/kg IV q24h for 3–4 days; Treatment Nos. 29 and 30) also can provide benefit. However, if equine protozoal myeloencephalitis is strongly suspected, glucocorticosteroids *should not* be administered. Intravenous administration of mannitol (0.25 mg/kg IV as a 20% solution q4–6h for 1 day; Treatment No. 68) and/or dimethylsulfoxide (0.5–0.9 g/kg IV as a 10%–20% solution q12–24h for several days; Treatment No. 34) may be valuable because increased intracranial pressure is likely.
- Good supportive care is important, including provision of shelter, water, and palatable, nutritious feeds.
- The prognosis must always be guarded. Cases with mild deficits may survive or even return to normal function. In more severely affected or recumbent patients, euthanasia should be considered.

Rabies

Rabies is a disease associated with profound public health implications because it can occur in all warm-blooded domestic species and humans. Mandatory vaccination of dogs has made the disease rare in North America. Rabies is normally spread by bites from infected wildlife, particularly racoons, skunks, and possibly foxes. The virus ascends tracts within the nervous system. Initial infection of a tract produces local hyperactivity, reflected by hyperesthesia and tremors. Affected neurons subsequently die, resulting in flaccidity and failure of neuronal activation. Death of the horse is inevitable. There are three main forms of the disease. When there are manifestations of cerebral disease, the disorder is sometimes referred to as the *furious form* of rabies. Signs reflecting predominantly brainstem disease are referred to as the *dumb form*. A third manifestation of the disease relates to the spinal cord and is referred to as the *paralytic form* of rabies.

History and Presenting Signs

- All ages and breeds affected
- There may be a history of a bite by a raccoon or skunk, although the bite may occur months before the onset of signs
- Behavioral changes may include aggression, self-mutilation, and signs of colic and depression
- Obscure lameness, ataxia, paresis, and paralysis
- Death occurs within 5 to 14 days after the onset of signs

Clinical Findings and Diagnosis

- Because there are no specific signs of rabies, diagnosis is difficult.
- In all cases, progression of the disease is rapid, with death normally occurring within 2 weeks of the onset of signs.
- In the furious form, signs consistent with cerebral dysfunction are common. These may include aggression, hyperesthesia, photophobia and extraocular muscle spasms, blindness, straining, inappetence, and in the terminal stages chewing and seizures.
- With the brainstem, or dumb form, ataxia, depression, and dysphagia with increased drooling of saliva often occur.
- In the spinal cord form of rabies, the most predominant signs are of progressive ataxia, paresis, and paralysis. In some cases there may be regional hyperesthesia, or the horse may have a tendency for self-mutilation. In the spinal cord form of the disease, signs will progress to involve the brainstem. Once brainstem signs are present, the disease is usually rapidly fatal. However, in some cases, death may not occur until there is involvement of the cerebrum.

KEY POINT ► Rabies should always be considered in any rapidly progressive neurologic disorder in a horse.

- If rabies is suspected, the clinician must be cautious regarding further handling of the animal because the disease can spread to humans.
- Antemortem diagnosis is difficult. Full-thickness skin biopsies containing tactile hairs may be used for demonstration of fluorescent antibodies. Biopsies should be collected, chilled, and sent to a laboratory capable of performing the test. Many horses with rabies do not show a positive response to this test until late in the disease.
- Corneal impression smears may be used for the same purpose.
- Seroconversion of the CSF is slow and does not occur until clinical signs have been present for at least a week.

KEY POINT ► In a dead horse, the head (and possibly the spinal cord if only spinal cord signs are present) should be shipped to a diagnostic laboratory equipped to handle tissues from rabies suspects.

- The laboratory should be contacted regarding the most appropriate tissues and methods of handling, storage, and transportation. Diagnosis is based on the presence of fluorescent antibodies and histopathologic demonstration of Negri bodies.

Differential Diagnosis

- Viral encephalitides
- Hepatoencephalopathy
- Trauma
- Botulism
- Bacterial meningitis
- Mycotoxic encephalomalacia
- Verminous encephalitis
- Parasitic thromboembolism
- Equine cervical vertebral malformation
- Equine herpesvirus myeloencephalopathy
- Equine protozoal myeloencephalopathy

Treatment

- There is no successful treatment for rabies. Antiinflammatory therapy may prolong the course.
- Prevention is based on vaccination with killed-virus vaccines (Treatment No. 113). These vaccines are registered for use in horses older than 3 months. Annual boosters are recommended.

Seizures (Fits, Convulsions)

Seizures are due to abnormal electrical activity in the cerebrum and are more common in foals than in adults. In most cases the onset of seizures is usually abrupt, with the convulsion running a finite course and then concluding relatively quickly. There is normally a phase of altered behavior prior to the onset of the seizure that may last from seconds to hours. After the seizure, temporary blindness and depression are common. A variety of causes of seizures exist and include the following:

Benign Epilepsy of Arabian Foals. A seizure disorder in foals, particularly Arabians, that is present in the first year of life. The clinical manifestations normally abate by the time the foal reaches adulthood.

Hypocalcemia. Low serum calcium concentrations may result in seizure activity in horses. This disorder is discussed elsewhere in this chapter (p. 388).

Inadvertent Intracarotid Injection. Inadvertent administration of substances into the carotid artery when attempting intravenous injection is a common cause of a single convulsive episode.

Organophosphate Toxicity. Exposure of horses to toxic doses of these anticholinesterase preparations commonly results in seizure activity. Toxicity is quite common because these agents are used widely for medicinal purposes in horses and have a low therapeutic index. Anticholinesterase compounds are also used commonly for agricultural purposes, posing the risk of unintended exposure of horses to toxic amounts of the preparations.

History and Presenting Signs

► Benign Epilepsy of Arabian Foals

- Foals less than 12 months old
- Intermittent violent convulsions
- Unexplained head injuries

► Inadvertent Intracarotid Injection

- Attempt to administer drugs into the jugular vein
- The horse moved or jumped during injection
- Behavior change followed by blindness, recumbency, and convulsions

► Organophosphate Toxicity

- All ages
- Recent exposure to these agents—topical, via the gastrointestinal tract, or possibly from agricultural sources
- Evidence of weakness, tremors, colic, increased salivation

Clinical Findings and Diagnosis

► Benign Epilepsy of Arabian Foals

- When seizure activity is not present, foals are normal on neurologic examination. Some foals will have evidence of trauma as a result of the seizures, including head and eye injuries and contusions of the gums and skin.
- During convulsions, the foals become unaware of their environment, recumbent, and convulse, quite violently at times. Subsequent to the episode, affected foals are depressed and may show signs of cerebral dysfunction similar to those occurring with the neonatal maladjustment syndrome. Signs include wandering aimlessly, failure to drink, inability to recognize the dam, depression, head pressing, and blindness.
- There are no specific clinicopathologic findings associated with this disease.
- Diagnosis is based on the age and breed of the foal and history or evidence of signs, and by ruling out other causes of seizure activity.

► Inadvertent Intracarotid Injection

- Following the injection of material into the carotid artery, there may be a range of effects depending on the volume and type of agent administered.
- On many occasions, no change in behavior or a short period of apparent agitation may ensue.
- In more severe cases, there is a brief period of apparent anxiety, possibly some muscle twitch-ing, particularly on the face, followed by recumbency and convulsive activity. Horses often paddle and appear quite violent. After a variable period (seconds to minutes), signs become less intent. Many horses regain their feet but remain blind, depressed, and apparently disoriented, signs that may last for days. In some cases, permanent, irreversible effects including death occur.
- In most circumstances, water-based sedatives (e.g., xylazine) are inadvertently administered into the carotid artery. These agents tend to be associated with the fewest residual effects. In some cases, damage to the recurrent laryngeal nerve may result in subsequent laryngeal hemiplegia.
- Diagnosis is based on the knowledge of an injection into the carotid artery or on the dramatic results following an injection into what was thought to be the jugular vein.

► Organophosphate Toxicity

- Clinical manifestations include nystagmus, tremor, salivation, patchy sweating, dyspnea, colic, diarrhea, muscle weakness, ataxia, and occasionally seizures.
- Diagnosis is based on a history of exposure to one of the chemicals in this group, the clinical signs, and laboratory analysis. Determination of acetylcholinesterase activity in red blood cells or plasma helps support the diagnosis.

Differential Diagnosis

► Benign Epilepsy of Arabian Foals

- Trauma
- Neonatal maladjustment syndrome
- Septicemia
- Bacterial meningitis/brain abscess
- Viral encephalitides
- Hepatoencephalopathy
- Verminous encephalitis
- Equine herpesvirus myeloencephalopathy
- Severe hyponatremia (neonates)
- Hyperkalemic periodic paralysis (older foals)
- Heat stroke

► Inadvertent Intracarotid Injection

- Trauma
- Anaphylaxis
- Hyperkalemic periodic paralysis

► Organophosphate Toxicity

- Trauma
- Viral encephalitides
- Hepatoencephalopathy
- Verminous encephalitis
- Equine herpesvirus myeloencephalopathy
- Hyperkalemic periodic paralysis

- Bacterial meningitis/brain abscess
- Colic
- Respiratory disease

Treatment

Doses of drugs commonly used for the treatment of seizures are provided in Table 13-4.

KEY POINT ▶ The phenothiazine-derivative tranquilizers (e.g., acepromazine) are contraindicated because they may worsen seizures.

▶ Benign Epilepsy of Arabian Foals

- Many foals with mild signs and infrequent convulsive episodes probably do not require specific therapy. In those which are more severely affected, maintenance anticonvulsant therapy is indicated.

KEY POINT ▶ We have found phenobarbitone to be useful for this purpose (20 mg/kg IV as a loading dose followed by maintenance doses of 4–10 mg/kg PO q12h; Treatment No. 87).

- Therapy is continued for 4 to 12 weeks, and then the foal is weaned from the drug over 10 to 14 days. If signs recur, reinstitution of therapy is indicated.
- Symptomatic therapy for head injuries and corneal ulcers is indicated.
- In the majority of foals, convulsive activity abates by the time they are 12 months old.

▶ Inadvertent Intracarotid Injection

- In general, no treatment is necessary. If the seizure activity is prolonged, administration of diazepam (0.05–0.2 mg/kg IV as required; Treatment No. 32) is useful.
- In horses with residual effects, treatment with flunixin meglumine (1.1 mg/kg IV q24h; Treatment No. 52) and dimethylsulfoxide (0.5–0.9 g/kg IV as a 10%–20% solution q12–24h for 1–3 days; Treatment No. 34) may be of benefit.

▶ Organophosphate Toxicity

- If seizures are present, treatment with diazepam (0.05–0.2 mg/kg IV as required; Treatment No. 32) is indicated. Atropine (0.2 mg/kg IV or SC every 60 minutes until salivation is decreased and mydriasis occurs; Treatment No. 11) is helpful in controlling symptoms. *Note:* Large doses of atropine will cause ileus. Administration of 2-PAM (20 mg/kg initial dose IV followed by similar or lesser doses q4–6h as required; Protopam Chloride, Wyeth-Ayerst, Philadelphia, PA) is useful.
- Intravenous fluids to assist in promoting diuresis and removal of free drug from the circulation can be of value (see Chap. 17). Other supportive therapy may be necessary.
- If the drug has been absorbed from the skin, washing the horse with shampoo and water is necessary. Similarly, if the route of absorption is the gastrointestinal tract, administration of dioctyl sodium sulfosuccinate (10–20 mg/kg PO as a 5% solution; Treatment No. 35) helps promote expulsion of the toxic agent from the tract.

Tetanus ("Lockjaw")

Tetanus is caused by toxins liberated from the bacterium *Clostridium tetani*. Spores from this organism are capable of persisting in the soil for many years. As a result, horses may be frequently exposed to the infective form of the bacteria. Tetanus usually occurs as a consequence of deposition of infective spores in a deep, penetrating wound. The depth and devitalized tissue in these types of wounds provide a suitable (anaerobic) environment for growth of the organism. Exotoxins are released by the organisms and enter the nervous system by passing up peripheral nerve roots. Clinical signs occur because the toxin causes central potentiation of normal sensory stimuli, resulting in a state of constant muscular spasticity leading to exaggerated responses to relatively innocuous stimuli.

History and Presenting Signs

- All ages, particularly those with *no* history of vaccination
- History of puncture wounds (e.g., subsolar abscess of the foot)
- The incubation period is usually 1 to 3 weeks
- Stiff gait initially

TABLE 13–4. Doses and Routes of Administration of Drugs for the Control of Seizures in Horses and Foals

Drug	Dose for Acute Control of Seizure Activity	Maintenance Dose
Diazepam	0.05–0.2 mg/kg IV as required	Not indicated
Xylazine	0.5–2.0 mg/kg IV as required	Not indicated
Pentobarbital	5–20 mg/kg calculated dose; administer to effect	Not indicated
Chloral hydrate	25–100 mg/kg IV (*Note:* Irritant perivascularly)	Not indicated
Phenobarbital	5–20 mg/kg in 25 ml saline slowly IV as a loading dose	4–10 mg/kg PO q8–12h
Phenytoin	1–5 mg/kg IV or PO q4h for up to 24 h	1–5 mg/kg PO q12h

Clinical Findings and Diagnosis

KEY POINT ► Initially, there is a general increase in muscle stiffness accompanied by muscle tremor.

- This is followed by restriction of jaw movements, prolapse of the third eyelid, and an unsteady, straddling gait.
- The tail is often held out stiffly, particularly when the horse is required to back or turn.
- There may be an anxious, alert expression, erect carriage of ears, and dilation of the nostrils.
- The horse is reluctant to eat from the ground, and saliva may drool from the mouth. Dysphagia is common.
- Many of the clinical signs are exaggerated by external stimuli. As the disease progresses, mastication is prevented by tetany, hence the name "lockjaw."
- Colic, constipation, and urine retention are common because horses cannot posture to void feces or urine. Eventually, the tetany becomes sufficiently severe that the horse assumes a "sawhorse" posture and has great difficulty walking. Some horses may fall and their limbs remain in tetany.
- Terminally, opisthotonus is marked, and there may be convulsions. Death occurs due to asphyxiation as a result of tetany of the respiratory muscles.
- The course of clinical disease is usually 5 to 10 days, although signs may persist for weeks in some horses.
- Diagnosis is based on the history and clinical signs. Horses that have not been vaccinated and have characteristic clinical signs can be assumed to have tetanus. Unfortunately, location of the site of infection is extremely difficult and isolation of the organism almost impossible.

Differential Diagnosis

- Laminitis
- Exertional rhabdomyolysis
- Pleuropneumonia
- Hypocalcemia
- Heat stroke

Treatment

KEY POINT ► The aims of therapy include (1) elimination of causative organisms, (2) neutralization of residual toxin, and (3) control of neuromuscular derangements.

- Elimination of causative bacteria involves local wound treatment (e.g., debridement, drainage, and exposure to the atmosphere) and administration of antibiotics. Na or K penicillin [20,000 IU IV q6h; Treatment Nos. 84 and 85; or 15,000–20,000 IU/kg, 15–20 mg/kg IM q12h (procaine); Treatment No. 83] for at least 7 days is indicated.
- Methods for neutralization of residual toxin include vaccination with tetanus toxoid and administration of tetanus antitoxin. In the latter case, antitoxin (100 U/kg IV, IM, or SC q72h; Treatment No. 115) will help neutralize any free toxin. However, it will have no effect on toxin already bound within the central nervous system because parenterally administered antisera does not cross the blood–brain barrier.

KEY POINT ► Intrathecal administration of antitoxin may be of value.

- The horse should be placed under general anesthesia. Ketamine should not be used as the induction agent. A spinal needle is inserted into the atlanto-occipital space (see Fig. 13-12), and 50 ml of CSF is withdrawn with an equal amount of antitoxin being replaced. We have had quite variable response with this form of therapy. Some horses have shown rapid response to treatment, whereas others have not responded or have developed laminitis following injection.
- Control of neuromuscular derangements is accomplished by administration of tranquilizers. We find acepromazine (0.05 mg/kg IV or IM q12h; Treatment No. 1) to be moderately effective.
- It is imperative to keep the horse in a dark stall and as free from external stimuli as possible.
- Attention to hydration and electrolyte status is important. Administration of fluids via a small nasogastric tube is possible in many cases, although those horses with pharyngeal dysfunction will require intravenous fluids. Manual evacuation of feces and urinary catheterization may be required.
- The prognosis for horses with tetanus must always be considered guarded and grave if treatment is not offered. Complications of tetanus include laminitis, aspiration pneumonia, and pleuropneumonia.
- Prevention of tetanus is readily achieved by the administration of tetanus toxoid (Treatment No. 116). A primary dose is given, a second dose 1 month later, and annual boosters thereafter. This vaccine is one of the most effective equine vaccines available, and its use in all domestic horses should be strongly encouraged. Recovery from tetanus *does not* result in effective immunity.

Diseases of the Peripheral Nerves and Muscles

Hyperkalemic Periodic Paralysis

KEY POINT ► Hyperkalemic periodic paralysis is a familial disorder affecting pure and crossbred quarter horses in North America.

Affected horses undergo episodes of muscular weakness similar to those reported in humans with hyperkalemic periodic paralysis.

History and Presenting Signs

- Young (<4 years old), pure or crossbred quarter horses
- Most common in colts
- Intermittent episodes of muscular weakness and recumbency
- Normal between episodes
- Sudden death may be the only finding in some horses

Clinical Findings and Diagnosis

- Affected horses have good muscular development and are usually normal when examined between episodes.
- Stimuli, such as exercise or transport, may precipitate clinical manifestations of the disorder, but this association is by no means direct, and the onset of signs is often unpredictable.

KEY POINT ► Clinical episodes begin with a brief period of stiffness.

- In some horses, prolapse of the third eyelid occurs at the onset of signs. Sweating is common, and muscular fasciculations may be observed. Some horses may "dog sit," whereas severely affected animals become recumbent with muscle flaccidity developing within minutes. In less severely affected horses, stimulation and attempts to move may worsen muscular fasciculations.
- Muscular weakness is characteristic of this disease, but affected horses remain bright and alert during episodes. Responses to noise and painful stimuli remain intact during episodes.

- Clinical episodes last for variable periods, usually 15 to 60 minutes. Some horses die during fulminant episodes.

KEY POINT ► Provisional diagnosis is based on historical and/or direct evidence consistent with episodic weakness in a relatively young quarter horse.

- A possible familial predisposition also should be considered; a history of similar signs in other family members may support the diagnosis.
- The classical finding of normal serum or plasma potassium concentrations between episodes (3-5 mmol/L or mEq/L) that rises to 7 to 12 mmol/L (mEq/L) during episodic weakness also supports the diagnosis. Serum or plasma potassium concentration returns to normal following abatement of clinical signs. Reduction in clinical signs parallels diminution of serum or plasma potassium concentration. Reduced serum or plasma sodium and calcium concentrations and increases in total plasma protein concentration and the hematocrit also occur during clinical episodes in many horses. Indicators of myonecrosis, such as serum or plasma creatine kinase activity, are unaltered in response to these periods of episodic weakness.

KEY POINT ► Further support for the diagnosis can be provided by the administration of a potassium chloride provocation test to horses suspected of having the disease.

- Potassium chloride (90–150 mg/kg dissolved in 1–2 L of water, via nasogastric tube, *following an overnight fast*) will often provoke clinical manifestations of the disorder and high serum potassium concentrations in affected animals. Begin with the low dose rate and increase the dose by 25% daily. Some affected horses do not show clinical signs at the low dose rates, making the progressive increase necessary. This dose of potassium chloride will have no detrimental effect in a normal horse. This test should not be administered to horses with cardiac or renal disease. *Note:* Caution should be exercised in using the provocation test, particularly at the high dose rates, because it may produce life-threatening hyperkalemia in a small percentage of affected horses. However, clinical signs can be rapidly reversed by administration of treatment (see below).

Differential Diagnosis

- Colic
- Exertional rhabdomyolysis
- Seizures
- Narcolepsy

Treatment

- During severe acute episodes, administration of calcium gluconate (40–90 mg/kg IV; dilute the calculated dose in 1–2 L of 5% dextrose usually results in rapid remission of signs. Alternative treatments include dextrose (4–6 ml/kg IV of a 5% solution) or sodium bicarbonate (1 mmol/kg or mEq/kg IV as a 5% solution).
- Maintenance therapy should be directed at decreasing potassium intake in the diet. Removal of alfalfa (lucerne) hay (high in potassium) from the diet and replacing it with oats or grass hay may be useful. Feeding oats two or three times daily and allowing the horse free access to salt is also helpful in many cases. If possible, the horse should be kept at pasture and allowed to exercise. Rapid changes in diet should be avoided.
- Treatment with acetazolamide (2–4 mg/kg PO q8–12h; Diamox, Lederle, Pearl River, NY) has been utilized with some success in horses that do not respond to dietary management.
- Given the genetic basis of the disease, affected horses should not be allowed to breed.

Hypocalcemia (Lactation Tetany, Transit Tetany, Idiopathic Hypocalcemia, Eclampsia, Hypocalcemic Tetany)

KEY POINT ► Hypocalcemia is rare in horses and occurs most frequently in lactating mares or following prolonged transport with food deprivation.

The severity of clinical signs is related to the serum (ionized) calcium concentration.

History and Presenting Signs

- Lactating mares
- Following transport
- Stiff gait, muscle fasciculations, sweating, recumbency
- In severe cases, convulsions may be noted.

Clinical Findings and Diagnosis

- Clinical manifestations are variable, depending on the degree of hypocalcemia. Increased muscle tone, a stiff, stilted gait, hindlimb ataxia, muscle fasciculations (especially temporal, masseter, and triceps muscles), trismus, dysphagia, salivation, anxiety, profuse sweating, tachycardia, fever, cardiac arrhythmias, synchronous diaphragmatic flutter, convulsions, coma, and death all can occur. Signs may progress over 24 to 48 hours, especially in lactating mares.
- Excitability or anxiousness are the most common signs when serum total calcium concentrations exceed 2 to 2.5 mmol/L (8 to 10 mg/dl), whereas concentrations of 1.2 to 2 mmol/L (5–8 mg/dl) usually produce tetanic spasms and incoordination, and concentrations less than 1 mmol/L (4 mg/dl) usually result in recumbency and stupor.
- A diagnosis of hypocalcemia should be suspected on the basis of the history and clinical signs, which are often quite characteristic. Definitive diagnosis depends on laboratory demonstration of hypocalcemia, with serum or plasma calcium values as low as 1 mmol/L (4 mg/dl) found in some cases. In addition, hypo- or hypermagnesemia and hyper- or hypophosphatemia have been associated with hypocalcemia in horses.

Differential Diagnosis

- Trauma
- Tetanus
- Viral encephalitides
- Hepatoencephalopathy
- Equine herpesvirus myeloencephalopathy
- Equine protozoal myeloencephalopathy
- Hyperkalemic periodic paralysis
- Neuritis of the cauda equina
- Bacterial meningitis/brain abscess
- Verminous encephalitis

Treatment

- Mildly affected horses may recover without specific treatment.

KEY POINT ► Since hypocalcemia can be life-threatening, therapy should be undertaken when significant hypocalcemia (<2 mmol/L or 8 mg/dl) is recognized in affected horses.

- Treatment involves intravenous administration of calcium solutions, such as 20% calcium borogluconate or those recommended for treatment of parturient paresis ("downer cow syndrome") in cattle. Administration of these solutions IV at 250 to 500 ml/500 kg diluted 1 : 4 with isotonic saline or dextrose and given over 15 to 30 minutes often results in full recovery, although in some cases this may take several days.

- Relapses can occur, and the clinician should be mindful of this possibility.
- Calcium preparations should be infused slowly, with close monitoring of the cardiovascular response. Dilution of the calcium solutions in saline or dextrose allows for more rapid administration and decreases the chance of cardiotoxicity. Normally, there is a positive inotropic effect. However, alterations in heart rate or rhythm indicate the need to suspend the infusion. If there is no response to an initial infusion, a second dose may be given 15 to 30 minutes later. Most horses respond to this form of therapy, although some require repeated treatments.

Myotonia

Myotonia is a sustained contraction of muscle following stimulation. Some forms of myotonia in horses have a genetic basis, particularly in certain families of quarter horses. The cause of the disorder is not known, but alterations in ion conductance across muscle membranes is implicated.

History and Presenting Signs

- Young horses
- Quarter horses more commonly affected
- Affected animals may appear to be "double muscled."
- Reports or evidence of a stiff, stilted gait

Clinical Findings and Diagnosis

- Affected animals commonly display mild hindlimb stiffness. Gait abnormalities are most pronounced when exercise begins and often diminish as exercise continues.

KEY POINT ▶ Bilateral bulging of the thigh and rump muscles may give the impression that the horse is overdeveloped or "double muscled." This finding may be an initial diagnostic clue.

- Stimulation of affected muscles, especially by percussion, induces a prolonged, localized muscle contraction evident as a firm, raised lump referred to as "dimpling." Affected muscles may remain contracted for up to a minute or more, with subsequent slow relaxation.
- Most horses with myotonia have involvement of skeletal muscle and do not demonstrate progression of clinical signs beyond 6 to 12 months of age. However, in some cases, signs may be severe, progressive, and possibly involve a variety of organ systems, similar to myotonia dystrophica in humans.
- A tentative diagnosis of myotonia can often be made on the basis of age and breed, a stiff gait (particularly at the onset of exercise), muscle bulging, and prolonged, localized contraction after muscle percussion. Definitive diagnosis is based on electromyographic examination. Usually this is performed only in university or specialist referral clinics. Affected muscle manifests pathognomonic crescendo–decrescendo, high-frequency repetitive electrical bursts with a characteristic "dive bomber" or, more correctly, "revving motorcycle" type of sound.

Treatment

- Considering the uncertainties regarding the pathophysiologic basis of myotonia, recommendations for effective therapy are not possible.
- The prognosis for horses with myotonia is often variable, depending on the severity of clinical signs. Mildly affected animals may have some amelioration of clinical signs with age. Other more severely affected horses may have a progression of signs associated with fibrosis and pseudohypertrophy, to the point where the animal is no longer able to move without great pain and apparent difficulty. Euthanasia of such animals is warranted.

KEY POINT ▶ Although conclusive evidence regarding the genetic basis of this disorder is still not available, owners of affected horses should be cautioned as to the possible heritability of this disease.

Peripheral Neuropathies

Peripheral nerve palsies are common in horses and can result from direct trauma to the nerve or as a result of local inflammatory changes involving the nerve.

History and Presenting Signs
▶ Suprascapular Nerve ("Sweeny")

- Trauma to the front of the shoulder
- Forelimb lameness
- Atrophy of the shoulder muscles ("sweeny")

▶ Radial Nerve

- Most common following general anesthesia or in combination with injury to the brachial plexus
- In association with fractures of the humerus

▶ Avulsion of the Brachial Plexus

- Trauma to the shoulder

▶ Sciatic Nerve

- Mostly foals
- Inappropriate placement of intramuscular injections

▶ Peroneal Nerve

- Common following general anesthesia in adults
- Trauma to the lateral stifle

Clinical Findings and Diagnosis

▶ Suprascapular Nerve

- Initially after the injury there is a lateral deviation or subluxation of the shoulder when the horse bears weight on the limb. This is thought to be due to damage to other supporting structures in addition to the suprascapular nerve. Over the next 2 to 4 weeks, atrophy of the supraspinatus and infraspinatus muscles occurs.
- Diagnosis is based on the history and clinical signs. Some referral clinics perform electromyographic studies, which assist in diagnosis.

▶ Radial Nerve

- Affected horses are unable to extend the elbow, making weight bearing almost impossible. The dorsum of the foot may face the ground. Horses have a characteristic gait when attempting to walk, since they use their body to propel the leg forward.
- Diagnosis is based on history and physical signs.

▶ Avulsion of the Brachial Plexus

- This injury usually results from compression of the brachial plexus resulting in an inability to bear weight, dropping of the elbow, and great difficulty in advancing the limb when walking. Sensory loss up to the elbow is usual.

▶ Sciatic Nerve

- Affected foals cannot flex and advance the hindlimb. If the lower limb is manually extended, affected foals can bear weight. However, under most circumstances, foals have the dorsum of the foot on the ground. They can bear some weight when in this posture.

▶ Peroneal Nerve

- There is an inability to flex the hock and extend the foot. The fetlock is flexed and may touch and be dragged along the ground when attempting to walk. Even if the foot is manually extended, weight bearing is compromised.

Differential Diagnosis

▶ Suprascapular Nerve

- Other causes of forelimb lameness
- Avulsion of the brachial plexus
- Radial nerve paralysis

▶ Radial Nerve

- Other causes of forelimb lameness
- Avulsion of the brachial plexus
- Suprascapular nerve palsy

▶ Avulsion of the Brachial Plexus

- Other causes of forelimb lameness
- Radial nerve palsy
- Suprascapular nerve palsy

▶ Sciatic Nerve

- Fractures of the limb or pelvis
- Other causes of hindlimb lameness
- Peroneal or tibial nerve palsy

▶ Peroneal Nerve

- Fractures of the limb or pelvis
- Other causes of hindlimb lameness
- Sciatic or tibial nerve palsy

Treatment

▶ Suprascapular Nerve

Initially, conservative treatment involving rest and anti-inflammatory therapy is indicated. In cases where signs persist, surgical exploration and removal of any tissue entrapping the nerve are possible. Further details of treatment are given in Chapter 3 in the section on sweeney.

▶ Radial Nerve

Treatment is normally symptomatic, involving anti-inflammatory therapy such as flunixin meglumine (1.1 mg/kg IV q12–24h; Treatment No. 52) and possibly dimethyl sulfoxide (0.5–0.9 g/kg IV as a 20% solution in dextrose q24h; Treatment No. 34). In most cases where radial nerve palsy occurs as a result of pressure during general anesthesia, remission of signs often occurs within hours to days.

▶ Avulsion of the Brachial Plexus

Treatment is as described for radial nerve palsy. Improvement in signs occurs in some cases in about 1 month. In those cases which do not improve in this time, the prognosis is guarded.

▶ Sciatic Nerve

Principles of therapy are similar to those described for radial nerve palsy. The prognosis must always be guarded.

▶ Peroneal Nerve

Principles of therapy are similar to those described for radial nerve palsy. Return to normal function in cases following general anesthesia is relatively common. Direct trauma to the nerve in the form of a kick or cut has a more variable prognosis.

Stringhalt

Stringhalt refers to intermittent or continuous exaggerated flexion of the hindlimbs (one or both) when the horse moves. This disease occurs as an isolated event in adult light horses and in an outbreak form as described elsewhere in the text (see Chap. 3).

References

Adams, R.: Evaluation of the neurologic status of the newborn foal. *Proc. 29th Annu. Conv. Am. Assoc. Equine Pract.,* 1983, p. 153.

Andrews, F. M., and Matthews, H. K.: Localizing the source of neurologic problems in horses. *Vet. Med.* 85:1107, 1990.

Andrews, F. M., Matthews, H. K., and Reed, S. M.: Medical, surgical, and physical therapy for horses with neurologic disease. *Vet. Med.* 85:1331, 1990.

Beech, J.: Differential diagnosis of neurologic disease in the horse. *Proc. 31st Annu. Conv. Am. Assoc. Equine Pract.,* 1985, p. 27.

Beech, J.: Neurologic Diseases. In N. E. Robinson (Ed.): *Current Therapy in Equine Medicine,* Vol. 2. Philadelphia: W. B. Saunders, 1987.

Blythe, L. L., Hultgren, B. D., Craig, A. M., et al.: Clinical, viral, and genetic evaluation of equine degenerative myeloencephalopathy in a family of Appaloosas. *J. Am. Vet. Med. Assoc.* 198:1005, 1991.

Bolon, B., and Buergelt, C. D.: A simple field necropsy technique for examination of the equine cervical spinal cord. *Equine Pract.* 12:26, 1990.

Collatos, C.: Neurology: Seizures in foals. Pathophysiology, evaluation and treatment. *Compend. Contin. Educ. Pract. Vet.* 12:393, 1990.

Cox, J., and Debowes, R.: Neurology: Episodic weakness caused by hyperkalemic periodic paralysis in horses. *Compend. Contin. Educ. Pract. Vet.* 12:83, 1990.

Dill, S. G., Correa, M. T., Erb, H. N., et al.: Factors associated with the development of equine degenerative myeloencephalopathy. *Am. J. Vet. Res.* 51:1300, 1990.

Fayer, R., Mayhew, I., Baird, J., et al.: Epidemiology of equine protozoal myeloencephalitis in North America based on histologically confirmed cases: A report. *J. Vet. Intern. Med.* 4:54, 1990.

Foreman, J. H., and Santschi, E. M.: Equine bacterial meningitis, part II. *Compend. Contin. Educ. Pract. Vet.* 11:640, 1989.

George, L. W.: Localization and differentiation of neurologic diseases, In B. P. Smith (Ed.), *Large Animal Internal Medicine.* St. Louis, MO: Mosby, 1990, p. 145.

Huntington, P. J., Jeffcott, L. B., Friend, S. C. E., et al.: Australian stringhalt-epidemiological, clinical and neurological investigations. *Equine Vet. J.* 21:266, 1989.

Matthews, H. K., and Andrews, F.: Performing a neurologic examination in a standing or recumbent horse. *Vet. Med.* 85:1229, 1990.

Mayhew, I. G.: *Large Animal Neurology: A Handbook for Veterinary Clinicians.* Philadelphia: Lea and Febiger, 1989.

McCue, P. M.: Equine leukoencephalomalacia. *Compend. Contin. Educ. Pract. Vet.* 11:646, 1989.

McKerrell, R. E.: Myotonia in man and animals: Confusing comparisons. *Equine Vet. J.* 19:266, 1987.

Ostlund, E. H., Powell, D., and Bryans, J. T.: Equine herpesvirus 1: A review. *Proc. 36th Annu. Conv. Am. Assoc. Equine Pract.,* 1990, p. 387.

Reed, S. M., and Fenner, W. R.: The approach to spinal cord disease in horses. *Proc. 31st Annu. Conv. Am. Assoc. Equine Pract.,* 1985, p. 19.

Santschi, E. M., and Foreman, J. H.: Equine bacterial meningitis, part I. *Compend. Contin. Educ. Pract. Vet.* 11:479, 1989.

Smith, J. M., Debowes, R. M., and Cox, J. H.: Central nervous system disease in adult horses: III. Differential diagnosis and comparison of common disorders. *Compend. Contin. Educ. Pract. Vet.* 9:1042, 1987.

Sojka, J. E., Brisson Kimmick, S., Carlson, G. P., and Coppoc, G. L.: Dimethyl sulfoxide update: New applications and dosing methods. *Proc. 36th Annu. Conv. Am. Assoc. Equine Pract.,* 1990, p. 683.

Sommardahl, C. S., Henton, J. E., and Peterson, M. G.: Rabies in a horse. *Equine Pract.* 12:11, 1990.

Spier, S. J., Carlson, G. P., Holliday, T. A., et al.: Hyperkalemic periodic paralysis in horses. *J. Am. Vet. Med. Assoc.* 197:1009, 1990.

Sweeney, R. W., and Hansen, T. O.: Use of a liquid diet as the sole source of nutrition in six dysphagic horses and as a dietary supplement in seven hypophagic horses. *J. Am. Vet. Med. Assoc.* 197:1030, 1990.

Endocrinology

Endocrine disorders are rare in horses and are mostly found in older animals. Disorders of the endocrine system seldom manifest themselves with any clarity, and often presenting signs may be nonspecific, such as weight loss, lethargy, and change in appetite. When such signs occur, endocrine diseases should be on a list of differential diagnoses. This brief section will focus on only the most common endocrine problems.

EXAMINATION OF THE ENDOCRINE SYSTEM

The endocrine system is not accessible for examination in most cases, with the thyroid gland being one of the few structures that can be palpated in some horses.

History

Important questions when considering the possibility of endocrine alterations include:

- Is the problem acute or chronic?
- Have there been increases or decreases in appetite?
- Has there been a change in water consumption or urine output?
- Is there an alteration in the horse's behavior?
- Is there a change in the appearance of the skin or hair coat?

Physical Examination

A routine examination should be performed, and given the nonspecific nature of the history, all body systems should be examined carefully. Since some pituitary disorders result in abnormal characteristics of the hair coat, note should be taken in cases where the age range and history could indicate a pituitary adenoma. Changes in appetite and water consumption are important considerations in endocrine disorders, and these should be carefully quantitated.

DIAGNOSTIC AIDS

The *hemogram* is an essential part of examination for a potential endocrine disorder. The neutrophil-to-lymphocyte ratio is useful as a rough screening for alterations in plasma or serum cortisol values. Lowered cortisol values are associated with a low neutrophil-to-lymphocyte ratio, whereas normal values are around 1.5:1. High values for plasma cortisol are reflected by neutrophil-to-lymphocyte ratios above 2:1 with disappearance of eosinophils from the peripheral circulation.

Serum or plasma biochemistry profiles may be useful to rule out specific organ diseases, particularly renal and hepatic disease, which may present with similar features to some endocrine diseases. Normal values for various measurements are presented in Appendix 2.

Hormonal measurements in both serum and plasma that can be determined by most laboratories include ACTH, cortisol, and T_3 and T_4. Normal values for these are given in Table 14-1, together with various suppression or stimulation tests to enable assessment of endocrine function.

Endocrine Diseases

Hypoadrenocorticism

Hypoadrenocorticism is a rare disorder, which has been reported in some cases of "poor performance" in racehorses. Hyperadrenocorticism as a primary disorder has not been recognized in the horse.

History and Presenting Signs

- History of corticosteroid administration
- Depression
- Reduced exercise tolerance
- Loss of weight
- Change in hair coat

Clinical Findings and Diagnosis

- Some cases are horses that have been administered doses of oral prednisolone or have had repeated IM doses of long-acting corticosteroids. For this reason, a careful history should be taken in horses that may have received corticosteroid therapy. Lower than normal plasma cortisol values may be present for up to 4 to 6 weeks after a single IM dose of long-acting corticosteroids.

- A useful screening test for low plasma cortisol values is a white cell count and differential. Horses with hypoadrenocorticism often have a decreased total white cell count and a neutrophil-to-lymphocyte ratio of less than 1.
- Baseline cortisol should be measured, followed by an ACTH stimulation test, as outlined in Table 14-1. The ACTH stimulation test results in a blunted cortisol response.

Differential Diagnosis

- Pituitary adenoma
- Hypothyroidism
- Pancreatic disorders

Treatment

- Reduction of environmental stress is important, and if horses are in training, the training should be discontinued.
- Some clinicians have used mineralocorticoids in an attempt to ameliorate the signs of the disorder, but such therapy is seldom necessary.

TABLE 14–1. Normal Hormonal Values and Endocrine Function Tests in Horses

Test	Reference Value or Response
Serum or plasma cortisol	<13 μg/dl
ACTH stimulation test, 1 U/kg ACTH gel IM	Doubling or trebling of cortisol values at 8 hours
Dexamethasone suppression, 0.04 mg/kg given IM	66% decrease in serum cortisol by 12 hours
Insulin tolerance 0.05 U/kg crystalline insulin IV	30% to 50% decrease in plasma glucose at 15 minutes, 60% decrease at 30 minutes, with normal values at 2 hours
Glucose tolerance, 0.5 g/kg of 50% dextrose solution IV	Four- to sevenfold increase in serum insulin level at 15 to 30 minutes, followed by rapid decrease
Serum or plasma ACTH	Early A.M.: <60 pg/ml, with values in the late P.M. being lower
Serum or plasma T_3	90 ± 20 ng/dl (foals 100–300 ng/dl)
Serum or plasma T_4	1.8 ± 0.8 μg/dl (3–5 μg/dl)
TSH response test, 5 IU TSH IV	Twofold increase over baseline in serum or plasma T_4 at 4 to 6 hours
Thyroid-releasing hormone response test, plasma cortisol before, 15, 30, 60, 120, and 180 minutes after 1 mg TRH IV	No change in baseline cortisol levels

Source: From J. Beech: Tumors of the Pituitary Gland (Pars Intermedia). In N.E. Robinson (Ed.), *Current Therapy in Equine Medicine 2*. Philadelphia: W.B. Saunders, 1987, with permission.

Hypothyroidism

Thyroid disease is rare in the horse, and while some cases of hypothyroidism have been reported, there have been no reported cases of hyperthyroidism. Suspected horses may present with depression and lethargy, but in foals, an array of clinical signs has been reported. There have been some reports of hypothyroid-related myopathies.

History and Presenting Signs

- Depression
- Edema of distal limbs
- Changes in skin and hair coat

Clinical Findings and Diagnosis

- In foals, a number of signs, including contraction of the flexor tendons, reduced sucking, tarsal and carpal bone malformations, incoordination, and hypothermia, have been reported. However, the incidence of hypothyroidism in foals appears to be very low.
- Findings in adult horses, apart from the presenting signs indicated above, include hypothermia, sensitivity to the cold, and, in some cases, nonspecific distal limb edema involving the hindlimbs.
- Measurements of T_3 and T_4 are useful for diagnosis, but it should be remembered that considerable variation may be found in normal values for T_3, which are affected by sex (higher in stallions) and show some diurnal variation. For this reason, a diagnosis of hypothyroidism can only be reached by conducting a thyroid-stimulating hormone (TSH) test, as indicated in Table 14-1. In normal horses, a doubling of T_4 values is usually found 4 to 5 hours after 5 IU of TSH is given IV.

KEY POINT ▶ Note that when samples for T_3 and T_4 are submitted to a laboratory dealing with human samples, values are about 25% of human values, and therefore, the assay must be modified. Normal T_3 and T_4 values for foals are higher than adults (see Table 14-1).

Differential Diagnosis

- Pituitary adenoma
- Pancreatic disorders
- Hypoadrenocorticism
- Hyperlipemia

Treatment

- Treatment with sodium levothyroxine (Synthroid, Flint) at a dose rate of 20 µg/kg PO q24h (10 mg for a 500-kg horse) has been reported to be effective. After 2 weeks, check the T_3 and T_4 levels and adjust the dose rate accordingly.

- Iodinated casein also has been described as effective at a dose rate of 5 g PO q24h.

Pancreatic Disorders

There have been some reports of diabetes mellitus and rare cases of neoplasia of the pancreas resulting in hypoglycemia. It is extremely unlikely that a case of pancreatic dysfunction would be encountered during the average year in a busy equine practice. However, acute pancreatitis may result in signs of colic. These cases result in a mild peritonitis, and abdominal fluid examination reveals increases in lipase and amylase activity.

History and Presenting Signs

- Usually an older horse
- Weight loss
- Depression
- Polydipsia
- Polyuria
- Polyphagia

Clinical Findings and Diagnosis

- It is extremely unlikely that functional pancreatic disorders will be found in practice, but screening horses for changes in plasma glucose is usually part of the workup of cases presenting for weight loss, polydipsia, polyuria, or disorders of the hair coat.
- Increased or decreased plasma glucose values provide an indication of the possibility of pancreatic dysfunction. Insulin-secreting tumors will result in hypoglycemia, with resulting central nervous system signs. In one case reported, the hypoglycemia was isolated to the time of feeding, and glucose concentrations were normal at other times of the day.
- If blood samples cannot be processed soon after collection, the blood should be taken into tubes containing fluoride oxalate to inhibit glycolysis.

Differential Diagnosis

- Pituitary adenoma
- Hypoadrenocorticism
- Hypothyroidism
- Colic

Treatment

- There is little experience with the use of insulin in the treatment of functional diabetes mellitus. In such cases, the horse should be referred to a university clinic or specialist practice should the client elect to try therapy.
- Acute pancreatitis should be treated by supportive therapy (see Medical Treatment of Colic, Chap. 6)

Pituitary Adenoma (Adenoma of the Pars Intermedia)

This condition occurs in older horses, the usual presenting complaint being polyuria and polydipsia and the hair coat having a shaggy appearance. The condition can produce an array of signs, and once the diagnosis is made, there is little in the way of effective therapy.

History and Presenting Signs

- Coarse and wavy hair coat
- Polyuria and polydipsia
- Weight loss
- Lethargy
- Vision disturbances
- Laminitis

Clinical Findings and Diagnosis

- There are a variety of clinical findings, the most common presenting complaints being listed above.
- The most obvious change in long-standing cases is the appearance of the hair coat, which becomes coarse and has a curly appearance.
- Other findings may include *Dermatophilus* infections, pot-bellied appearance, and, in some cases, laminitis.
- Specific diagnostic tests are not available, but a thyroid-releasing hormone response test can be helpful. Details are provided in Table 14-1. An abnormal response is an increase in baseline plasma cortisol values.
- Variations in plasma glucose concentrations have been reported in tumors of the pars intermedia with no consistent findings.

Differential Diagnosis

- Hyperlipemia
- Diabetes mellitus
- Hypothyroidism
- Laminitis
- Hypoadrenocorticism

Treatment

Although treatment of pituitary adenomas is likely to be unrewarding, the use of cyproheptadine hydrochloride (Periactin, Merck Sharpe and Dohme, West Point, PA) at a dosage schedule of 60 mg/450 kg PO q24h in the morning for 1 to 2 weeks with the dosage slowly increased to 120 mg/450 kg PO q12–24h has been found helpful. Response, if it occurs, should be present in 6 to 8 weeks. After 3 months of therapy, reduction to alternate-day treatment can be considered.

References

Beech, J.: Tumors of the Pituitary Gland (Pars Intermedia). In N. E. Robinson (Ed.), *Current Therapy in Equine Medicine 2*. Philadelphia: W.B. Saunders, 1987.

Beech, J., and Garcia, M. C.: Diseases of the Endocrine System. In P. T. Colahan, I. G. Mayhew, A. M. Merritt, and J. N. Moore (Eds.), *Equine Medicine and Surgery*, 4th Ed. Goleta, Calif.: American Veterinary Publications, 1991, p. 1737.

Duckett, W. M., Manning, J. P., and Weston, P. G.: Thyroid hormone periodicity in healthy adult geldings. *Equine Vet. J.* 21:123, 1989.

Freestone, J. F., Wolfscheimer, K. J., Ford, R. B., et al.: Triglyceride, insulin, and cortisol responses of ponies to fasting and dexamethasone administration. *J. Vet. Intern. Med.* 5:15, 1991.

Freestone, J. F., Wolfsheimer, K. J., Kamerling, S. G., et al.: Exercise-induced hormonal and metabolic changes in thoroughbred horses: Effects of conditioning and acepromazine. *Equine Vet. J.* 23:219, 1991.

Lothrop, C. D., and Nolan, H. L.: Equine thyroid function assessment with the thyrotropin-releasing hormone response test. *Am. J. Vet. Res.* 47:942, 1986.

Shaftoe, S.: Thyroid-stimulating hormone response tests in one-day-old foals. *J. Equine Vet. Sci.* 8:310, 1988.

CHAPTER 15

Clinical Bacteriology

![black bar]

Daria N. Love

Clinical bacteriology is a very useful adjunct to other services offered within an equine practice. If samples for bacteriology are collected and handled appropriately and results of culture and sensitivity interpreted correctly, the information obtained can be of great value. However, if samples are collected or handled inappropriately or the results of culture and sensitivity testing are misinterpreted, the outcome may be detrimental to the care of cases.

This chapter outlines many of the procedures involved in clinical bacteriology. Most of these procedures are simple and can be performed within the confines of most practices. Some samples, however, may require more sophisticated culture and sensitivity testing, and I recommend that these be sent to a referral laboratory that is appropriately equipped to perform these procedures.

SAMPLE COLLECTION

General Principles of Sample Collection

- Collection of appropriate samples is essential for accurate interpretation of bacteriologic results and proper selection of antimicrobial therapy.
- Specimen collection and subsequent processing of the sample will vary depending on (1) the type of bacteria expected within the sample and (2) the site to be sampled.

If Aerobic and Facultatively Anaerobic Bacteria Are Suspected

Normally Sterile Sites

- These sites include blood, CSF, joint fluid, urine from the bladder, and tissues beneath the skin.

KEY POINT ► Since these sites are normally sterile, sampling technique must be aseptic so that organisms are not introduced or surface bacteria do not contaminate the sample.

- An appropriate technique for the collection of blood, CSF, joint fluid, subcutaneous tissue is as follows:

    1. Clip hair.
    2. Wash thoroughly with soap and water or use a povidone-iodine scrub.
    3. Swab with 70% alcohol, and then swab with tincture of iodine (2% iodine in 70% alcohol) or povidone-iodine (Treatment No. 91), and allow to dry before sampling.

KEY POINT ► It is also preferable to wear a surgical mask when sampling CSF and joint fluid and to wear sterile gloves if the area is to be palpated to facilitate collection. This is to prevent introduction of the collector's pharyngeal bacteria (such as

Staphylococcus spp.) into the sterile site during sample collection.

Sites with Normal Flora

KEY POINT ▶ Normal flora will be present in the sample, and culture results have to be interpreted in the light of knowledge of the normal flora at the site. The presence of inflammation is an important indicator of disease at these sites.

■ When collecting samples from these sites, try to eliminate the normal flora if possible. For example, if sampling skin lesions, select an intact pustule rather than ulcers or erosions. The surface of the pustule should be swabbed with alcohol, and then the pustule can be incised with a sterile scalpel blade and underlying tissues sampled using moistened swabs.
■ Alternatively, if the lesion is large enough, a fine-needle aspiration of infected tissue may be obtained.
■ For sites where avoidance of normal flora is impossible (e.g., lesions within mucous membranes of the mouth or vagina), use a dry swab to remove as much of the secretions and surface flora as possible before sampling with a moistened swab.

If Strictly Anaerobic Bacteria Are Suspected

KEY POINT ▶ Anaerobic bacteria may be the sole etiologic agent in an infectious process or they may be a part of mixed infections (e.g., abscesses, osteomyelitis, postoperative infection of the gastrointestinal and female genital tracts, pleuritis, pneumonia, and peritonitis).

Routine isolation and identification of anaerobes are often unwarranted. Such work is time-consuming and expensive, and anaerobes are part of the normal flora in many sites. It is important, therefore, to decide when it is necessary to attempt isolation of the anaerobes.

Criteria for Suspecting Anaerobic Infection

■ Location of infection—sites associated with or close to areas where anaerobes are a component of the normal flora (e.g., submandibular abscess, osteomyelitis after a compound fracture, pleuritis, injection abscess)
■ Presence of gas at site of infection
■ Black discoloration of a site of infection
■ Foul odor
■ Morphology of bacteria seen in the initial Gram stain [e.g., gram-negative rods and filaments (*Bacteroides* spp., *Fusobacterium* spp.), branch-ing gram-positive filaments (possibly *Actinomyces* spp.), or large gram-positive, gram-variable, or gram-negative rods which may or may not be sporing (*Clostridium* spp.)]
■ Infections secondary to an animal bite
■ Prior therapy with aminoglycoside antibiotics (e.g., kanamycin, neomycin, gentamicin, amikacin)

KEY POINT ▶ Anaerobes are resistant to aminoglycosides (as are facultative bacteria multiplying anaerobically) because these antibiotics require oxygen for transport into cells; the aminoglycosides often kill off the other normal bacterial flora at the site and thus allow unchecked multiplication of anaerobes.

Collection Techniques

KEY POINT ▶ A thin smear *must* be made at the time of collection regardless of the method of collection.

Place one drop of the sample onto a clean microscope slide, smear the material as you would a blood smear, and submit the smear to the laboratory for a Gram stain. If the sample is a piece of solid tissue, the sample can be prepared and placed onto a slide as for an impression smear.

Swabs

If Aerobes and Facultatively Anaerobic Bacteria Are Suspected

■ Dry swabs should be moistened prior to collection (e.g., BBL Transport Systems, BBL Division of Becton Dickinson and Co., Cockeysville, MD).
■ Alternatively, swabs may be placed onto appropriate transport media immediately after collection (e.g., Stuart's medium for most specimens collected onto swabs). This medium is used in the Marion Scientific Culturette specimen transport system (Marion Scientific, Kansas City, MO).
■ If the contagious equine metritis organism (*Taylorella equigenitalis*) is suspected, Amies medium should be used to moisten and transport swabs after collection.
■ Swabs should be processed as soon as possible after collection.

KEY POINT ▶ It can be difficult to interpret the significance of bacteria isolated from a sample collected and transported on a dry swab. Dry swabs may only yield the more hardy organism(s), and the more delicate organism may have been the etiologic agent.

If Strictly Anaerobic Bacteria Are Suspected

- Swabs are *definitely inferior* for collection of specimens with suspected anaerobic bacteria. They should only be used when the sample cannot be obtained by another means.
- If swabs have to be used, the swab should be placed immediately into a commercial transport system that is suitable for anaerobic bacteria (e.g., Port-A-Cul Tube, BBL Division of Becton-Dickinson and Co., Cockeysville, MD; BD Vacutainer Anaerobic Specimen Collector, BD Division of Becton-Dickinson and Co., Rutherford, NJ; or the Scott Two-Tube System, Scott Laboratories, Inc., Fiskeville, RI).

Fluids (Pus, Synovial Fluid, CSF, Peritoneal Fluid)

If Aerobic or Facultatively Anaerobic Bacteria Are Suspected

- These samples are best transported in a syringe with all the air expelled.
- Remove the needle from the syringe, and cap it effectively to prevent leakage.
- If bottles are used, use one that leaves minimal airspace, and tape lid to prevent leakage.
- If a delay is anticipated between collection and processing, the sample should be inoculated into a commercially available culture medium that will sustain growth of aerobic and facultatively anaerobic bacteria (e.g., Culture Collection and Transport System, Curtin Matheson Scientific, Inc., Precision Dynamic Corporation, Burbank, CA).

If Strictly Anaerobic Bacteria Are Suspected

- Draw the sample into syringe through a wide-bore needle. Expel any air, and insert the needle into a rubber stopper to exclude air, or replace plastic cap.
- Alternatively, commercially available media may be used, especially if a delay is anticipated. This may be either a medium that supports both aerobic and anaerobic bacteria (e.g., Port-A-Cul Vials, BBL Microbiology Systems, P.O. Box 243, Cockeysville, MD) or a transport system that has been strictly adapted for anaerobic bacteria (e.g., BD Vacutainer Anaerobic Specimen Collector, Becton-Dickinson and Co., Rutherford, NJ).

Solid Tissues

If Aerobic and Facultatively Anaerobic Bacteria Are Suspected

- Place the tissue collected into a sterile screw-capped container with minimal airspace.

KEY POINT ► If a delay is anticipated between collection and processing, place the tissue into a syringe by removing the hub and inserting the material, replace the hub, and expel the air. If necessary, draw up a small amount of sterile saline or broth to prevent drying out.

- A commercial transport medium (e.g., BBL Port-A-Cul Transport System Vial, BBL Division of Becton-Dickinson and Co., Cockeysville, MD) also can be useful for the transport of solid material.

If Strictly Anaerobic Bacteria Are Suspected

- Place tissue into a sterile container with minimal airspace, or alternatively, place into a commercially available medium that is capable of supporting the growth of strictly anaerobic bacteria (e.g., Port-A-Cul Vial, BBL Division of Becton-Dickinson and Co., Cockeysville, MD).
- Do not refrigerate the sample, but place in a cool place and submit to the laboratory within 6 to 12 hours. If the delay in submission is longer, the sample should be refrigerated.
- It is imperative to have as short a delay as possible between collection and processing because it can be very difficult to maintain viability of anaerobic bacteria.

Urine

- Collect samples in sterile screw-capped containers.
- Keep samples upright, and make sure that they do not leak during transportation.
- Transport to the laboratory as quickly as possible, and keep the temperature less than 15°C. If a delay of greater than 20 minutes occurs, place at 5°C.
- Anaerobes rarely cause cystitis, and samples are not routinely cultured anaerobically.

Blood

Blood samples require special consideration when culturing. Several factors should be kept in mind prior to collection and transportation of these samples.

Selection of Patient

- To obtain the most reliable results, a blood culture should be performed when *no* prior antibiotic therapy has been given in the previous 24 hours.
- If it is not practical, at least a previously unused vein should be prepared to ensure maximal sterility.

Selection of Sampling Time

KEY POINT ► Often, blood is free from significant numbers of organisms at the time of peak fever.

■ Fever clears the blood of organisms, so if the blood sample is cultured at this time, the yield will be low. Therefore, if the patient has a history of fever spikes or some predictable pattern of fever peaks, it is best to try to take the sample approximately 1 hour prior to the next fever peak.

KEY POINT ► If it is not possible to select the sampling time in this way, a number of samples should be taken to try to obtain a sample during a peak of bacteremia.

■ In a truly septicemic animal, multiple cultures are seldom required because numbers of bacteria are usually quite high. However, in some septicemic states (e.g., *R. equi* infections), where it may be difficult to sample alternate sites, the numbers of organisms in the blood may be disappointingly low, and multiple samples may be required.

KEY POINT ► It is important to remember that small bacterial numbers can occur even when the bacteremia is significant. This fact will play a role when interpreting smears and when judging time for incubation before a negative result is reported.

Collection and Submission of Sample

■ The area over the selected vein should be prepared as described above, using a surgical preparation.
■ Then 10 to 20 ml of blood should be obtained from the patient using a new needle and syringe. Use only minimum negative pressure to collect the sample. Vacutainer tubes (Becton-Dickinson and Co., Rutherford, NJ) should not be used to collect blood for culture because the excessive vacuum will often contaminate the sample.
■ Send the samples to the laboratory immediately if the laboratory is adjacent to the practice.
■ If the sample has been collected in the field, it may be necessary to inoculate samples immediately to prevent clotting. In these cases, the sample should be inoculated either into a commercially available blood culture medium (e.g., Signal Blood Culturing System, Oxoid USA, Columbia, MD) or medium that has been preprepared in your laboratory [e.g., Brain Heart Infusion Broth (BHIB), Oxoid USA, Columbia, MD].
■ Smears *must* also be made at the time of sampling (see below for details), and these should be submitted to the laboratory with the samples.

KEY POINT ► All procedures must be done rapidly, before the blood clots (up to 2 minutes).

■ Owing to the possibility of contamination at the time of sampling with normal flora of the skin, it may be advisable to inoculate several vials of BHIB or two separate commercial blood culture bottles after the sample is taken. In this way, if

bacteria grow in one culture bottle but not another, the bacteria that is growing is *probably* a contaminant.
■ There are occasions when anaerobes may be involved in bacteremia/septicemia (e.g., neonatal infections associated with umbilical trauma).
■ If anaerobes are suspected, the procedures for collection and transportation of blood cultures should be followed, except that the media to be inoculated should be boiled to drive off dissolved oxygen and cooled before inoculation, and anaerobic culture methods should be used.
■ Alternatively, commercial media that support the growth of anaerobic bacteria are also available (e.g., Signal Blood Culture Bottles, Oxoid USA, Columbia, MD).

GENERAL PRINCIPLES FOR HANDLING SAMPLES AFTER COLLECTION

■ All specimens *must* be collected in an appropriate manner (see above). They must be handled so that specimen viability is maintained and they do not spill or discharge into the environment.
■ There are basically two aims when handling samples after collection:

1. Preserve viability of organisms.
2. Preserve original numbers and proportion of species.

■ These aims are best achieved by processing the sample as soon as possible.

KEY POINT ► The sample must *not* be allowed to dry out. Swabs are particularly vulnerable.

■ Transport media are available to help prevent the sample from drying out [e.g., Stuart's medium, Amies' charcoal, BBL Port-A-Cul Transport System (Becton-Dickinson, Cockeysville, MD)].

KEY POINT ► Body fluids such as blood, CSF, joint fluid, urine, and conjunctival secretions contain factors that inhibit or kill microorganisms.

■ It is therefore imperative to process without delay. Inflammatory cells also deteriorate/disintegrate if left in fluid for more than a few hours, which is especially relevant to urine.
■ The second aim is more difficult to achieve because different genera of bacteria can multiply at different rates, whereas others may die out completely during the processing of the sample.
■ Furthermore, although transport media prevent drying of the sample, they do not inhibit multiplication of bacteria. Thus the number and proportion of bacteria present within the sample at the time of collection may be greatly altered after transportation.

- One way to try to prevent unchecked multiplication of bacteria is to keep the sample cool but preferably not frozen.

KEY POINT ▶ Uncontrolled freezing kills a large percentage of bacteria. Cooling keeps the organisms alive but retards their multiplication.

KEY POINT ▶ A smear should be made at the time of sampling so that visual examination will give some idea of the numbers and proportion of species present at the time of sample collection.

- Smears are mandatory when sampling blood, for samples placed in transport medium, and for samples with suspected anaerobic organisms.
- Furthermore, smears performed at the time of sampling will help interpretation of culture results (i.e., is the bacteria cultured consistent with that observed in the original smear).
- Otherwise, it can be difficult to determine the significance of bacteria isolated when there is no knowledge of original proportions of bacteria, whether inflammatory cells were present, whether there was evidence of phagocytosis, etc.

INITIAL PROCESSING AND EXAMINATION OF SAMPLES

Criteria for Sample Rejection

- Dried swabs should not be processed (see above).
- Samples with gross external contamination should be rejected if an *appropriate* representative sample cannot be taken from a central portion of the lesion.
- Samples from autopsy when the organ/tissue has been subjected to room temperature for greater than 4 hours, or where samples arrive at room temperature, should not be processed without noting and using guarded interpretation.
- Urine samples should be rejected if not refrigerated.

Initial Processing

KEY POINT ▶ A Gram stain must be performed on all material and examined before culturing.

- Special stains or wet preparations [KOH, india ink (see Appendix 15A) or wet film using sterile saline] also may be required depending on the sample received.

KEY POINT ▶ A blood film should be made immediately upon receipt of blood

cultures but should be examined after processing of samples because this may require a protracted time for examination.

- Selection of the appropriate medium is done on the basis of the sample obtained and the presence or otherwise of possible swarming bacteria (e.g., *Proteus* spp.).

Microscopy
Gram Stains

- Make a smear by rolling the swab onto the surface of a slide, or prepare a thin film from pus or macerated material.
- Allow smears to dry thoroughly *in air*.
- Stain with Burke's Gram stain.
- Record relative numbers of each morphologic type of bacteria (it may be helpful to draw, using colored pens, the morphology and Gram reaction of all organisms). Note numbers and types of inflammatory and other cells.

Special Stains

Acid-Fast Stain. If it is suspected that *Mycobacterium* spp. (e.g., *M. tuberculosis*) may be involved, an acid-fast stain should be performed on the sample submitted. If tuberculoid mycobacteria are suspected (e.g., *M. smegmatis, M. kansasii,* or *M. xenopi*), 15% sulfuric acid for 5 minutes should be used as the decolorizer rather than the acid/alcohol decolorizer.

KEY POINT ▶ Only tubercle bacilli are acid/alcohol-fast.

Modified Acid-Fast Stain. If it is suspected that *Brucella, Campylobacter, Nocardia,* or *Rickettsia* may be involved, a modified acid-fast stain should be performed on the sample submitted (see Appendix 15A).

Wet Films

Indian Ink Preparations (see Appendix 15A)

- If it is suspected that *Cryptococcus neoformans* is involved
- This procedure also can be used with CSF samples

10% KOH (see Appendix 15A)

- If filamentous fungi are suspected

Saline Wet Films

- If yeasts are suspected
- This technique also may be used to determine motility and morphology of bacteria

PROCESSING OF SAMPLES

General Processing for All Samples

Tissues

- If the sample is a piece of tissue, place the specimen into a sterile Petri dish, or dissect the sample directly in the delivery container.
- Dissect out an appropriate piece of tissue, place it into a sterile plastic bag along with a small amount of sterile medium (e.g., BHIB, Oxoid USA, Columbia, MD), and process in a Stomacher 80 lab blender (Tekmar Co., Cincinnati, OH). This machine gently extracts the bacteria or fungi from tissues and so enhances culture of bacteria.
- With a flamed platinum loop, obtain a loopful of the processed tissue and inoculate onto appropriate agar plates.

Fluids

Fluids (e.g., pus, peritoneal fluid, joint fluid) should be inoculated into a liquid culture medium (see below) and also may be inoculated directly onto solid medium.

Media

- For optimal recovery of microorganisms, it is essential to inoculate appropriate primary isolation media with the specimen as soon as possible.
- Most (if not all) of the media listed below are available as prepoured plates or broths from bacteriologic suppliers and are a relatively inexpensive alternative to pouring your own plates. It is necessary, however, to ensure the quality of the basal medium. To get growth of streptococci and delicate gram-negative organisms, there is a need to ensure that yeast or other extract is incorporated into the medium. Many blood agar bases and nutrient broths and agar do not contain extract, and thus severely limit the range of bacteria grown.
- The media listed below are some of the basic requirements that would be useful in a practice. More specialized media are also available, if required, for biochemical tests or for isolation of more fastidious bacteria (e.g., *Mycoplasma*).

Solid Media

2% and 4% Agar Blood Plates

- These plates should be used for most samples because this medium will support the growth of most fastidious bacteria (e.g., *Streptococcus* spp.) as well as less fastidious bacteria (e.g., *Staphylococcus* spp., Enterobacteriaceae, *Pseudomonas aeruginosa*).

- If swarming bacteria (e.g., *Proteus* spp.) are suspected, the sample should be placed onto a 4% agar blood plate as well. The increased agar concentration retards swarming of *Proteus* spp. It is worth remembering that on this medium the typical colonial morphology of bacteria may not be seen because of the surface-restricting properties of the medium.

MacConkey's Agar Plates. If the sample collected is thought to contain Enterobacteriaceae, it is also desirable to place the sample onto a MacConkey's agar plate.

Sabouraud's and Mycosel Agar Plates

- If the sample is thought to contain *yeasts* and/or filamentous *fungi* (other than dermatophytes), inoculate the sample onto a Sabouraud's agar plate with or without added chloramphenicol and gentamicin.
- If dermatophytes are suspected, Mycosel (BBL Division of Becton-Dickinson and Co., Cockeysville, MD), which has chloramphenicol and cycloheximide added, should be inoculated with your sample.
- Incubate plates at room temperature (25–30°C).

Chocolate Agar

- This medium is used for specimens that may contain *Taylorella equigenitalis* (the causative agent of contagious equine metritis).
- Inoculate samples onto a Columbia base (Oxoid USA, Columbia, MD) chocolate horse agar and incubate in 5% to 10% CO_2 in humidified air for 48 to 72 hours at 37°C.
- Some authors also recommend addition of L-cysteine HCl (100 mg/L).

Liquid Media

Brain Heart Infusion Broth

KEY POINT ► Blood or inflammatory cells contain substances that are inhibitory for bacterial growth. Hence, if large amounts of these fluids or cells are present in the preparation, place the sample into liquid medium (e.g., Brain Heart Infusion Broth, Oxoid USA, Columbia, MD) so that these substances are diluted out, as well as onto a suitable solid medium.

The volume may vary from 2 to 10 ml depending on the numbers of organisms seen and the amount of blood (generally a dilution of 1:5 to 1:10 is required).

Cooked Meat Medium or Prereduced Medium (e.g., Thioglycolate Broth). This may be used if it is suspected that strictly anaerobic bacteria may be involved in the disease process. These media have reducing agents that support the growth of anaerobes.

Commercially Available Media. Special media are available for cultivation of blood (see below) and also may be used for other fluids (e.g., joint fluid, CSF, etc) if you are concerned about the presence of inhibitory substances. Care must be taken in the use of commercial media for joint fluid and CSF so that you do not dilute organisms so much that growth does not occur.

Atmospheric Conditions and Temperature for Incubation

All specimens should be placed into the appropriate atmospheric conditions depending on the clinical history and appearance of the Gram stain. It is usually possible to determine if microaerophilic and/or anaerobic bacteria are present from these two criteria.

Aerobic Conditions

Aerobic conditions can be achieved by incubation under normal atmospheric conditions, usually at 37°C or room temperature if molds are suspected.

Microaerophilic Conditions

- Microaerophilic conditions should be used *only* if required for primary isolation of organisms, and this is determined by the history and clinical signs.
- Microaerophilic conditions can be achieved either by the addition of a commercially available gas-generating system similar to that used for anaerobic bacteria [CO_2-generating kits (Oxoid USA, Columbia, MD) or a candle jar].

Anaerobic Conditions

- Anaerobic conditions should be used only if required for primary isolation of organisms. Remember that it is not recommended to perform anaerobic culture on specimens that have a significant population of normal floral anaerobes.
- The simplest method for achieving anaerobic conditions in a clinical setting is with the use of Gas Pak Jar (BBL, Division of Becton Dickinson and Co., Cockeysville, MD) or Oxoid Anaerobic Jars (Oxoid USA, Columbia, MD).
- Both these systems use disposable gas-generating envelopes. These liberate H_2 and CO_2 and remove oxygen from the chambers by reaction of hydrogen with a palladium catalyst.
- The use of a catalyst in each system is important, and we recommend the "cold" catalysts available from Oxoid (Oxoid USA, Columbia, MD). All catalysts should be rejuvenated after each use by heating to 160°C for 1½ hours to drive off moisture and H_2S. While still hot, they should be placed into a desiccator.
- A disposable resazurin indicator strip (which also can be bought from the above companies) is also required as an indicator that anaerobic conditions have been reached. Anaerobic conditions should occur approximately 3 hours after incubation, and the jars should be checked at that time to ensure that the indicator strip is white (indicating anaerobic conditions).

Storage of Samples

- Store the remainder of samples in a sterile bijou bottle or in a syringe from which air has been excluded.
- Specimens should be stored at 5°C for up to 3 days after primary setup.
- Plates should be kept at room temperature for up to 3 days before discarding.

Special Laboratory Procedures for Selected Tissues

Laboratory Procedures for Blood Cultures

Initial Processing and Blood Smears

- Blood samples must be submitted immediately to the laboratory (or must be inoculated directly into the culture medium at the site of collection, after making a smear, as described below) so that processing can commence before clotting of the sample.
- On receipt of the blood, slides for the blood smears should be prepared by swabbing the slide with 70% alcohol and allowing to dry. These slides should then be handled such that fingerprints and squames and dust cannot contaminate the slide.
- The sample should arrive in a new sterile syringe which has been used to collect the specimen, and after sampling, a fresh sterile needle should be used to cover the end of the syringe.
- On receipt of the blood sample in the laboratory, the syringe should be rotated to mix blood, the cap and needle should be removed, and 4 drops of blood should be expelled aseptically into an appropriate disinfectant (e.g., Lysol).
- A small drop of blood should be placed onto a slide, and the edge of another prepared slide should be dipped into the drop of blood so that approximately ¼ drop adheres to edge of slide. This slide is then used to smear a third slide so that a thin blood film is achieved. It is best to prepare several thin slides for Gram staining.
- Stain the blood films with a Burke's Gram stain (see Appendix 15A), but cut down the staining cycles to 10 seconds each.

KEY POINT ► Remember to blot the slide dry after decolorization and before application of safranin. This procedure is necessary for accurate staining of blood-containing smears of any origin.

If this step is not performed, the red blood cells will appear refractile and often out of the focal plane.

- Examination of blood smears may be immediately rewarding because bacteria may be observed directly. Alternatively, examination may require a search of up to 20 to 30 minutes. If examination is immediately rewarding, the samples should be cultured appropriately depending on the results of the Gram stain. If a search is required, you will have to guess the best culture conditions and proceed before the blood clots in the syringe.

KEY POINT ► It is obvious that accurate observation and interpretation of the Gram-stained original smear are of major diagnostic significance.

Blood Culture Media

- Blood contains bacteriostatic agents (e.g., acidic polypeptides released from neutrophils) that will inhibit growth of significant numbers of bacteria if these substances are present in high concentrations (e.g., if cultured on blood plates). Blood also clots, preventing the growth of bacteria.
- Therefore, all blood should be inoculated into a broth medium at a dilution of 5:1 (i.e., 5 parts broth to 1 part blood). This dilution will overcome the inhibitory phenomena and allow bacteria to grow within the culture medium.
- Brain Heart Infusion Broth (BHIB, Oxoid USA, Columbia, MD) dispensed in aliquots of 10 ml will sustain the growth of most bacteria causing septicemia in the horse and can be used routinely to culture blood samples.

KEY POINT ► Commercial blood culture bottles are available that contain a substance that "neutralizes" the neutrophils and antimicrobial agents in the sample and which prevents clotting. The substance is sodium polyanetholesulfonate (SPS).

- SPS is a polyanionic anticoagulant that is supplemented at the rate of 0.025% to 0.05%. It acts to inhibit complement and lysozyme activity, interferes with phagocytosis, and inactivates residual clinically achievable concentrations of aminoglycosides not neutralized by dilution.
- An example of this type of medium is the Signal Blood Culture System (Oxoid USA, Columbia, MD). This system utilizes a single blood culture bottle for isolation of bacteria from blood samples.
- A further advantage of the Signal Blood Culture System is that strictly anaerobic and microaerophilic bacteria also will grow in this medium, so it can be used when these organisms are suspected as the cause of the septicemia.
- Alternatively, prereduced anaerobically sterilized Brain Heart Infusion Broth (Oxoid USA, Columbia, MD) may be used for blood cultures.

Inoculation of Media and Assessment of Positive Cultures

- Ten ml of blood should be inoculated into a blood culture bottle as per manufacturer's instructions or 2 ml of blood can be added to each of four to five BHIB bottles. Cultures should be incubated for 24 hours at 37°C.
- If commercially available media bottles are used, it is recommended to use at least two bottles per animal (10 ml of blood per bottle). This is to check for contamination, which can occur at the time of sampling or when sampling broth cultures for bacterial growth.
- After 24 hours, the blood cultures should be observed for evidence of bacterial growth (either turbidity within the medium or by small white colonies on top of the settled red blood cells).
- If growth is evident, the blood cultures can be sampled for Gram stains and for subculturing onto a blood agar plate.
- It may take 4 to 7 days for a positive sample to show growth; therefore, do not discard your cultures before this length of time. Incubation time will depend on the number of organisms present and the species of organism growing.

KEY POINT ► It is important to use aseptic procedure when sampling broths to ensure that false-positive results do not occur. Always leave at least one broth undisturbed to try to check the relevance of any isolate.

- Once organisms have been subcultured to a blood agar plate, identification and sensitivity testing can proceed as with any organism.

Laboratory Procedures for Cerebrospinal Fluid (CSF), Joint Fluid, Pleural Fluid, Abdominal Fluid, and Transtracheal Aspirates

- Samples from CSF, synovial fluid, transtracheal aspirates, and pleural and abdominal fluid also contain inhibitory substances and possibly neutrophils if an inflammatory process is in progress.

KEY POINT ► Usually samples from these sites will not yield bacteria even if centrifuged deposit samples are placed onto blood plates. Positive results will occur usually only after inoculation of deposit samples into liquid medium.

- Centrifuge the fluid sample to deposit inflammatory cells and bacteria. Supernatant fluid is discarded, and the deposit is resuspended in a small amount of nutrient broth (e.g., BHIB, Oxoid USA, Columbia, MD).
- A Gram-stained smear is made for visualization of bacteria and cells, and a record of these should be made.

- Samples are inoculated into a nutrient broth (e.g., BHIB, Oxoid USA, Columbia, MD). Alternatively, liquid culture medium used for blood cultures may be used (e.g., Signal Blood Culture System, Oxoid USA, Columbia, MD).
- If, on inspection of the smear, the number of bacteria is greater than the number of neutrophils, it may be worthwhile inoculating a blood agar with the sample as well in case viable colonies result. Moreover, in acute disease, when time is vital, it may be wise to commit one drop of the pellet of the centrifuged sample, which has been resuspended in nutrient broth, to a blood agar plate for incubation.
- If the organisms outnumber the inhibitory substances in the preparation, the organisms may grow on the agar plate and allow the saving of at least 12 hours of time for the sample.
- Samples are treated subsequently in a similar manner to blood cultures (i.e., the broth is subcultured onto blood agar plates, etc.).

Laboratory Procedures for Urine

KEY POINT ▶ Urine samples are handled and interpreted differently from most other samples.

- There are a strict set of criteria drawn up for cultivation and interpretation of human urine samples. Similar work has not been done in veterinary medicine, but there are some guidelines (based on these studies) that are generally followed.
- Urine should be collected to avoid contamination with normal urethral/vaginal flora (e.g., a midstream voided sample is useful only if the vulva/prepuce/penis has been cleaned and dried thoroughly before voiding).
- Catheterized samples are preferable to decrease the contamination from normal flora of the lower urinary tract.

KEY POINT ▶ All urine samples should be refrigerated immediately after collection. Even 20 minutes at room temperature can change results significantly.

- A full urinalysis should be carried out on each sample submitted for bacteriology. This is necessary to allow interpretation of the findings.

Initial Processing

- If urine is turbid (unfortunately normal for horse urine), make a smear, Gram stain, and examine for bacteria and inflammatory cells. It is usual to consider a possible urinary tract infection if greater than 10 white blood cells and greater than 20 bacteria are seen per oil-immersion field ($\times$ 1000).
- When using a direct cell count of the urine sample with a disposable chamber (e.g., Kova Glass-

tic Slide 10 with grids, Hycor Biomedical, Inc., USA), if greater than 10^4 white blood cells per milliliter of urine are present, then the possibility of a urinary tract infection should be considered.
- The Gram reaction and morphology of bacteria present should be noted, as well as the relative proportions of each type of bacteria. The number and type of inflammatory and other cells seen in the smear also *must* be noted, since these will help in the interpretation of culture results.

Culture of Urine Samples

- For valid interpretation of urine cultures, quantitative urine cultures should be performed.
- Since cystitis is relatively uncommon in the horse, most practices will have little or no experience with urine cultures. Therefore, if there is evidence of a urinary tract infection, after urinalysis and evaluation of a Gram-stained smear of the urine, the samples can be submitted to a referral laboratory for quantitation and identification of the bacteria.
- A sensitivity test also should be requested because the bacteria that commonly cause cystitis in the horse do not have predictable sensitivities (e.g., *E. coli, P. mirabilis, Klebsiella* spp., *Enterobacter* spp.).
- It is important to remember when submitting urine samples for culture that the urine must be kept cold (4°C) until processed because bacteria can multiply rapidly in urine at room temperature and so will invalidate quantitative tests performed on the urine sample.
- Urine may be stored at 4°C for 24 hours without any significant change in the numbers of bacteria. However, leukocytes will disintegrate after several hours, and the viability of bacteria will decrease on extended storage. Both these factors adversely affect interpretation of results.
- After results of the culture and sensitivity are received and the animal is placed on the appropriate antimicrobial agent, the urine should be reexamined after 5 to 7 days of therapy to check that the therapy is effective. It may be sufficient to obtain a *fresh* midstream urine sample for this examination.
- Examination will consist of a check of pH, presence of inflammatory cells, and presence of bacteria.
- It may be necessary to centrifuge the sample and examine the deposit. If bacteria are seen, reculture should be attempted.

Laboratory Procedures for Feces

KEY POINT ▶ Feces should only be cultured for specific organisms.

Since feces can contain a multitude of organisms, many of which are not pathogenic, the search should be directed to the question, "Does this fecal sample contain such-and-such?"

Salmonella

KEY POINT ► Since *Salmonella* may be shed in very low numbers in feces of horses with salmonellosis, a total of three to six fecal samples (approximately 5 g of feces) should be collected at 12-hour intervals to increase the possibility of diagnosis.

- Owing to the presence of large numbers of normal flora of the gastrointestinal tract in fecal samples, the feces have to be inoculated into enrichment media that retard the growth of many of the normal flora and selectively enrich the growth of *Salmonella*.
- Hence feces should be inoculated into tetrathionate or selenite broth cultures (Oxoid USA, Columbia, MD; Difco, BBL Division of Becton Dickinson and Co., Cockeysville, MD).
- Direct plating onto MacConkey's or XLD agar (Oxoid USA, Columbia, MD) also may be useful at this stage on the off chance that *Salmonella* are present in high numbers.
- The tetrathionate or selenite broth cultures should be subcultured to MacConkey's or XLD agar at 12 and 24 hours before incubated a further 12 to 24 hours at 37°C.
- Suspect colonies (non-lactose-fermenting colonies if MacConkey's agar is used or black colonies if XLD is used) should be subcultured and tested to determine if *Salmonella* is present (see below under Biochemical Tests).
- Colonies from a nutrient agar plate also should be tested to see whether they are smooth using fresh acriflavine solution. Smooth colonies should be tested against poly-O and poly-H *Salmonella* typing sera (e.g., BBL Division of Becton-Dickinson and Co., Cockeysville, MD).

HANDLING OF BACTERIA FOR SUBCULTURE AND BIOCHEMICAL TESTS

Biochemical tests are used to determine the genus or species to which a bacterial isolate belongs. These tests should only be performed in a clinical situation if this information influences treatment, prognosis, or control of the case in question.

KEY POINT ► The subculture of bacteria for biochemical tests is aimed at keeping organisms in log phase of growth. This is imperative to ensure optimal enzymatic activity for biochemical testing and also optimal growth for antibiotic sensitivity testing.

Time for Subculture

This will depend on the growth cycle of the organism.

Rapidly Growing Organisms

- These bacteria grow to maximum colonial size in 16 to 18 hours. Colony size will be 2 to 4 mm.
- Examples include Enterobacteriaceae, *Staphylococcus* spp., *Pseudomonas aeruginosa*, *Bacteroides fragilis* types, *Fusobacterium necrophorum*, some *Clostridium* spp., and *Bacillus* spp.
- These organisms can be handled rapidly (i.e., after overnight growth).
- Subculture a portion of one colony to another blood agar plate or one colony into 4 ml of broth.
- For antibiotic sensitivity testing, subculture one colony into 2 ml of broth and incubate 2 to 3 hours until optimal density is obtained as compared with a barium sulfate standard.
- The rapidly growing organisms can usually be mishandled and still allow all their biochemical tests to be performed correctly because they have great biochemical reserves.

Organisms that Grow Well

- These bacteria grow to maximum colonial size in 24 to 36 hours. Colony size is 2 to 4 mm.
- Examples include *Pasteurella multocida*, *Actinobacillus* spp., *Streptococcus equi* ss. *equi*, and *Rhodococcus equi*.
- These organisms require specific media and may have limited viability on the surfaces of agar plates.
- Organisms in the "good grower" category require frequent 24-hour subculturing, say three times, before committing them to broth media for biochemical testing. They should be subcultured to a level where the broth shows turbidity. It may then be possible to subculture those to biochemical tests some 8 hours later.

Organisms That Grow Poorly

- These bacteria take 48 hours to reach maximum size. Colonies reach 1 to 2 mm.
- Examples include some capsulated *Streptococcus equi*, *Brucella* spp., *Actinomyces* spp., *Corynebacterium* spp. (*Cryptococcus neoformans* may require 4 to 5 days).
- The "poor growers" will require subculturing at 48-hour intervals before placing into appropriate broth media and incubation for 18 hours before biochemical testing.
- Some anaerobes will need 24 to 48 hours of incubation in broth inoculated to 10% (i.e., 1 ml well-grown broth per 10 ml nutrient broth).

Media for Biochemical Testing

- The introduction of packaged microbial identification systems by several microbiologic supply laboratories has made the biochemical testing of bacteria easier to perform for the person in clinical practice.

- Packaged bacterial identification kits were initially designed for differentiating members of the family Enterobacteriaceae, primarily because of the frequency of isolation from human clinical specimens (also true in veterinary medicine) and their relatively rapid growth and generally distinct, readily visible biochemical reactions.
- In more recent years, the number of packaged systems available has expanded to include the identification of additional groups of microorganisms such as the nonfermentative gram-negative bacteria, some fastidious species of bacteria, anaerobic bacteria, and yeasts.
- Semiautomated or fully automated instruments are also available, but these would rarely be cost-effective within the confines of most equine practices.
- The range of packaged identification systems that would be useful within a practice situation will depend on (1) the types of samples commonly seen in the practice and (2) the reliability of the system involved.
- For example, in most practices, systems that differentiate the oxidase-negative, gram-negative rods (for the most part these are members of the family Enterobacteriaceae) would be useful, and these systems are very reliable.
- On the other hand, oxidase-positive, gram-negative rods are not nearly so commonly involved in infectious diseases in horses, and furthermore, the systems that differentiate this group of bacteria are not particularly reliable. More traditional means of differentiating among the bacteria in this group are recommended.
- Considerable care must be taken in the use of these media. Only a single colony should be used to inoculate media (to overcome use of mixed culture results from different organisms with the same Gram reaction and morphology being used). Extensive bacteriologic experience is also required to enable accurate and reliable use of

these tests and especially to ensure that aberrant and inconsistent reactions can be detected. Commercial media can give incorrect naming of organisms, which may go undetected by inexperienced personnel.
- Examples of the systems that are available, their manufacturers, and their applications are given in Table 15-1.

Interpretation of Laboratory Results

KEY POINT ► Unless the specimen has been taken thoughtfully and carefully, obeying the principles set out earlier, meaningful interpretations of laboratory results are often impossible.

Even with a well-taken specimen, interpretations can be difficult. This task will be easier if you have the following attributes:

1. A knowledge of the normal flora (species and approximate distribution) in various sites.
2. A knowledge of the likely pathogens in various sites (see Table 15-2).
3. The realization that the pathogenic organism(s) can originate from (a) outside the horse (e.g., wound contamination), (b) the horse's own normal flora (e.g., fecal contamination of a wound, abscess communicating with the oral cavity), or (c) overgrowth of one species in the gastrointestinal tract due to unwise antibiotic usage.
4. The realization that laboratory results must be correlated with the clinical signs in the horse.
5. The use of other laboratory data that may be available to help you with interpretation of the significance of your isolate.
Hematology. Infections are *usually* accompanied by a neutrophilia.
Urinalysis. A high white cell count and alkaline urine may indicate urinary tract infections.

TABLE 15–1. Packaged Systems That Identify Bacteria by Biochemical Testing

System Manufacturer	Name	Organisms Identified
Abbott Laboratories	MS-2	Enterobacteriaceae MIC susceptibility testing
American Scientific	Microscan	Gram-negative rods
Analytab Products	API 20E	Enterobacteriaceae and nonfermentative gram-negative rods
	API 20	Anaerobic bacteria
	API 20C	Yeast
	API 3600S	MIC susceptibility testing
Bioquest (BBL)	Minitek	Enterobacteriaceae, anaerobic bacteria, and yeasts
Flow Laboratories	Uni-N/F Tek	Nonfermentative and other gram-negative bacteria
	Uni-Yeast Tek	Yeast
	Enteric-Tek	Enterobacteriaceae
	Anaerobe-Tek	Anaerobic bacteria
Gibco	Sensititre	MIC susceptibility testing
Johnston Laboratories	Bactec	Early detection of bacteria in blood
Roche Diagnostics	EnteroTube-II	Enterobacteriaceae
	Oxi/Ferm Tube	Nonfermentative gram-negative rods

Cytology. Were there neutrophils present in your original smear of your sample? If so, how many, and what percentage of cells present (usually PMNs are the predominant cell type in acute bacterial infections). Can you observe phagocytosis?

Histopathology. To diagnose systemic fungal infection, invasion of tissue must be demonstrated.

Serology. Was there a high antibody titer to the organism that you isolated? Was there a rising titer to the organism you isolated? Serology for the preceding diagnostic purposes is seldom attempted nowadays.

Interpretation of a Pure Culture

KEY POINT ▶ If the primary blood agar plate yields a pure culture, do not immediately assume that it is the organism responsible for the infection.

- You may be justified if the bacteria has been isolated from a normally sterile site and if the bacteria is known to have pathogenic potential at that site.
- However, the possibility still exists that the real causative organism has not grown, and your organism is simply multiplying in a favorable environment.
- Gram stains of the original material will aid the interpretation in this case.

Interpretation of Isolation of Bacteria from Sites with Normal Flora

If you have cultured bacteria from samples obtained from a site with normal flora, three investigations are possible:

- Full investigation with identification of all organisms found. This is time-consuming and only appropriate for a research laboratory.
- Exclusion of known pathogens (i.e., has one of the bacteria that you have cultured previously been shown to cause disease in this site?). This should be done thoroughly.
- Exclusion of known pathogens plus a partial investigation of the normal flora. This is the preferred approach.

KEY POINT ▶ In many cases, the pathogenic organism(s) belongs to the normal flora, and it may only be present in excess in clinical cases.

On the other hand, the predominance of one species of the normal flora does not necessarily mean it is causing disease. It may simply reflect an imbalance in the flora due to another factor(s). The real pathogen may be suppressed for some reason (e.g., antibiotics, host responses, inappropriate laboratory media, or inappropriate sampling and transport). It is important in these cases to try to determine what is going on. The other laboratory data

that you have collected may be of some value in these cases.

The knowledge that the bacteria that you have isolated can cause disease in the site from where it was isolated also may help in the interpretation of these cases. Some of the common disease-causing organisms isolated from various sites are outlined in Table 15-2.

ANTIBIOTIC SENSITIVITY TESTING

A number of different types of antimicrobial sensitivity testing are available to the veterinary practitioner. However, a few basic principles exist that are true for all bacterial isolates and all the types of sensitivity testing:

1. Only perform antibiotic sensitivity tests on an organism that you have isolated and consider to be pathogenic in the given situation.
2. If you believe that more than one organism is significant, then test each one separately.
3. Antibiotic susceptibility testing should be used only for those organisms which do not have a predictable sensitivity.

KEY POINT ▶ In life-threatening situations, where therapy must be initiated immediately, use clinical judgment based on experience in treating such infections.

Two things may be of value in assisting your choice of antimicrobials in these situations:

1. A Gram stain, which shows the morphology and gram reaction of the bacteria involved
2. Previously published reports or previously accumulated data from your own practice of the sensitivity patterns of the bacteria frequently involved in the same clinical situation as your current sample

KEY POINT ▶ Try to take a sample for isolation of the causative organism before treatment begins.

KEY POINT ▶ Some bacteria which may be recognizable (a) in a Gram stain, (b) by culture, or (c) by subsequent identification have predictable sensitivity patterns, and susceptibility testing is not therefore necessary. Other bacteria do not have a predictable sensitivity pattern and require sensitivity testing before therapy is instituted.

Bacteria with predictable and unpredictable antibiotic sensitivities are given in Table 15-3.

KEY POINT ▶ All the bacteria with predictable sensitivities are sensitive to benzylpenicillin, except *Rickettsia*, which are sensitive to tetracyclines.

TABLE 15–2. Organisms That May Cause Disease at Various Sites in the Horse

Site	Common Isolates	Uncommon Isolates
Lower respiratory tract	*Streptococcus equi ss. zooepidemicus* Obligate anaerobes, e.g., *Bacteroides* spp., *Fusobacterium* spp. Enterobacteriaceae, e.g., *Escherichia coli, Klebsiella pneumoniae* *Pasteurella* spp. *Bordetella bronchiseptica* *R. equi* (foals)	*Streptococcus pneumoniae* (foals) *Streptococcus equi ss. equi* (foals) *Salmonella* (foals) *Mycoplasma* *Pseudomonas aeruginosa*
Uterus	*Streptococcus equi ss. zooepidemicus* *Streptococcus dysgalactiae* (equisimilis) Enterobacteriaceae, e.g., *Escherichia coli, Klebsiella pneumoniae* *Pseudomonas aeruginosa*	*Actinobacillus equuli* *Salmonella abortus-equi* *Taylorella equigenitalis* *Staphylococcus aureus*
Thoracic/peritoneal cavities	Obligate anaerobes, e.g., *Bacteroides* spp. Enterobacteriaceae, e.g., *Escherichia coli* *Streptococcus equi ss. zooepidemicus*	*Actinobacillus equuli* *Corynebacterium* spp. *Actinomyces pyogenes*
Abscesses	*Streptococcus equi ss. zooepidemicus* *Corynebacterium pseudotuberculosis* Obligate anaerobes *Escherichia coli* *Staphylococcus aureus*	*Pseudomonas aeruginosa* *Actinomyces pyogenes*
Bone/joints	*Staphylococcus aureus* *Escherichia coli* *Streptococcus equi ss. zooepidemicus* *Actinobacillus equuli* (foals) *Salmonella* (foals)	*Fusobacterium necrophorum* *Rhodococcus equi* (foals) Other coliforms
Gastrointestinal tract	*Salmonella* *Clostridium perfringens* *Ehrlichia risticii* *Rhodococcus equi* (foals)	*Clostridium difficile* (foals) *Clostridium cadaveris*
Skin	*Staphylococcus aureus* *Dermatophilus congolensis*	*Corynebacterium pseudotuberculosis* *Rhodococcus equi* *Streptococcus* spp.
Septicemia	*Actinobacillus equuli* (foals) *Escherichia coli* *Salmonella* (foals)	*Enterobacter* spp. (foals) *Serratia* spp. (foals)
Eye	*Streptococcus equi ss. zooepidemicus* *Staphylococcus aureus* *Corynebacterium* spp. *Pseudomonas aeruginosa*	*Bacillus cereus* *Klebsiella* spp.
Nervous system	—	*Listeria monocytogenes* *Streptococcus equi ss. zooepidemicus*
Bladder (urine)	*Escherichia coli* *Proteus mirabalis* *Klebsiella* spp. *Staphylococcus* spp.	*Corynebacterium* spp. *Enterobacter* spp.

TABLE 15–3. Indications of Bacteria with Predictable and Nonpredictable Antibiotic Sensitivity Patterns

Predictable	Not Predictable
Beta-hemolytic *Streptococcus* spp.	*Staphylococcus* spp.
Clostridium spp.	Alpha-hemolytic *Streptococcus* spp.
Corynebacterium spp.	*Nocardia asteroides*
Most *Bacteroides* spp.	*Bacteroides fragilis*
Erysipelothrix rhusopathiae	Most gram-negative facultatively anaerobic bacteria e.g., *Escherichia coli*,
Bacillus anthracis	*Klebsiella pneumoniae, Salmonella* spp., *Actinobacillus equuli*,
Pasteurella multocida (in horses)	*Bordetella bronchiseptica, Enterobacter* spp.
Listeria monocytogenes	
Actinomyces spp.	
Dermatophilus congolensis	
Fusobacterium spp.	
All gram-positive strict anaerobes	
All *Rickettsia* (e.g., *Ehrlichia*)	

Antimicrobial Sensitivity Tests

The range of sensitivity tests available include the following:

Direct Antibiotic Sensitivity Testing

■ Direct antibiotic sensitivity testing is the placement of antibiotic disks onto the surface of a plate, seeded over its surface with an original clinical sample.

KEY POINT ► *Direct* antibiotic sensitivity testing of the original sample is rarely, *if ever*, warranted.

■ The original sample may yield insufficient growth on the plate or a mixture of organisms. In either case, a meaningful result is impossible.
■ If there is a mixture of organisms, how do you know which one is important, which is producing antibiotics, bacteriocins of their own, etc.?
■ It is argued that direct sensitivity testing gives a quick result. However, a quick, wrong result is worse than useless. Often it is possible to achieve an equally quick result with proper techniques.

Modified Kirby-Bauer Disk Diffusion Method

KEY POINT ► Testing should be done with the standardized technique as outlined in microbiological manuals. Without a standardized test, it is not possible to determine zone size for "zone size interpretation."

■ The Kirby-Bauer technique is simple, quick, and gives a much more reliable indication of the best antibiotic to use than uncontrolled sensitivity testing.
■ However, this test is only valid for (a) organisms in log phase at the time of disk application and (b) organisms that grow rapidly (i.e., 16 hours to full size).

■ One criticism of this test in veterinary medicine is that interpretation of the zone sizes (and hence whether a bacterial isolate is sensitive or resistant) is determined by achievable levels of antibiotics within the blood of *humans* (and not domestic species) after a standard dose of antibiotic. However, with most of the antibiotics used commonly in equine practice, if the test is performed in a meticulous and standard manner, and if the antibiotics used are bactericidal agents (e.g., penicillins, aminoglycosides), the interpretation of this test appears to be valid.
■ If this test is performed in your practice, strict adherence to the guidelines set out for conducting this assay should be practiced. These guidelines are available from standard bacteriologic texts or the National Council of Laboratory Testing.

Broth Dilution Tests (MICs)

KEY POINT ► This method is used in more accurate work when the pharmacokinetics of an antibiotic are to be determined. It is not usual to employ this method for more routine work.

■ In broth dilution tests, doubling dilutions of antibiotic in broth are inoculated with small numbers of the bacterium being tested, incubated usually for 18 hours, and examined to find the smallest concentration that has completely inhibited macroscopic growth of the test organisms (i.e., turbidity). This concentration of antibiotic is called the *minimum inhibitory concentration (MIC)*.

KEY POINT ► A variation of this theme is presented in the form of commercially available microtiter plates containing particular antibiotics at concentrations that should cover the range of sensitivities of most of the organisms encountered in veterinary practice.

■ The organisms are grown on plates, picked off, and emulsified in broth to a specific concentration. Drops of the organism are placed into the wells and incubated along with the appropriate controls.
■ With this assay, it is possible to determine the minimum inhibitory concentration (MIC) of the organism under test overnight.
■ This test may be of value if the MIC can be interpreted in light of the dose schedules given to animals, but this is a major limitation of the current disk test system.

Agar Dilution Tests

KEY POINT ► Agar dilution tests are the most practical form of test for moderate to large volumes of work.

■ They are used more commonly in larger laboratories to obtain the same accurate information as the broth dilution tests, yet without the consumption of large amounts of time and materials.
■ Agar dilution tests also may be used when it is desired to determine the minimum inhibitory concentrations of a number of strains of bacteria, using doubling dilution over a range, as in broth dilution tests.

Appendix 15A

STAINS

Gram Stain

■ Label slide with a diamond pen to determine which side of the slide has been stained and to mark the center of the smear area.
■ Make a thin smear of your sample by either:

1. Rolling a swab onto the surface of the slide if the sample is presented on a swab.
2. Placing a small loopful of pus/fluid onto the slide and spreading with the wire loop into a thin smear.
3. Solid material may be emulsified in saline or broth and smeared as in 2.
4. Impression smear may be made from solid tissue.

■ Allow to dry thoroughly in air
■ Stain with Burke's Gram stain:

1. Cover the slide with Burke's crystal violet, add 3 drops of Burke's solution B (sodium bicarbonate buffer), and wait 3 minutes.
2. Wash off the crystal violet with tap water, cover the slide with Burke's iodine, and wait 3 minutes.

3. Wash off the iodine with tap water.
4. Hold the slide between the thumb and forefinger, and flood the surface with a few drops of acetone-alcohol decolorizer until no violet color washes off. This usually requires about 10 seconds or less.
5. Cover the slide with safranin counterstain, and wait for 1 minute. Wash the slide with tap water.

KEY POINT ► Thin smears stained by experienced personnel may be performed by staining steps 1, 2, and 5 for 10 to 15 seconds only.

6. Place the smear in an upright position, allow the excess water to drain off, and let the smear dry or, preferably, blot dry.
7. Examine the stained smear under 100× (oil) immersion objective of the microscope. *Gram-positive bacteria stain dark blue/purple; gram-negative bacteria appear pink/red.*

■ Record the relative numbers and morphology of each bacterial type observed. Note numbers and types of inflammatory and other cells (e.g., squames).

Modified Acid-Fast Stain

1. Freshly dilute to 10% v/v stock carbol fuchsin.
2. Flood slide, and stain for 3 to 5 minutes.
3. Remove stain with water, drain.
4. Add 0.3% v/v acetic acid, leave for up to 30 seconds to decolorize (time depends on species suspected).
5. Wash off with water.
6. Counterstain 1 minute with 1% aqueous methylene blue, wash off with water, and blot dry.

Indian Ink Stain

This stain is used for direct microscopic examination of the capsules of microorganisms. This technique is particularly useful in visualizing the large capsules of *Cryptococcus neoformans* from clinical samples.

1. Rub a small amount of sample with a loopful of india ink.
2. Add a very clean coverslip, and examine after removing excess india ink thus: Fold blotting paper over surface of coverslip, and using handle of loopholder, roll it gently but firmly over the coverslip, pressing it into a thin film.
3. Dispose of blotting paper immediately to autoclave bucket.
4. Flame loophandle before returning it to bench.
5. Examine for budding and thick capsules.

KEY POINT ► Ensure you do not mistake neutrophils or other phagocytes for the yeast forms.

KOH for Filamentous Fungi

The KOH mount is used to aid in detecting fungal elements in thick mucoid material or in specimens containing keratinous material, such as skin scales, nails or hair. The KOH dissolves the background keratin, unmasking the fungal elements to make them more apparent.

1. Add 1 drop of 40% KOH to slide.
2. Add sample and mix with loop, glass rod, or straight wire. Add coverslip.
3. Heat gently over bunsen flame (do not boil). Seal edges of coverslip with wax to prevent evaporation. Allow to incubate at room temperature for approximately 15 to 30 minutes.
4. Examine with reduced light and 10× and 40× objectives.

Tissue samples may require overnight incubation at 30°C in a humidified atmosphere to allow sufficient digestion of tissue to enable visualization of fungal elements.

Saline Wet Film for Yeasts or for Motility and Morphology

This technique is used to determine the biologic activity of microorganisms, including crude motility.

1. Add 1 drop of saline to slide.
2. Add sample and mix with a glass rod or straight wire.
3. Add coverslip and examine with reduced light and 40× objective.

To prevent streaming if motility is being assessed, seal the edge of the coverslip with petrolatum.

Hanging-Drop Preparation for Motility Tests

This is needed especially for judging motility of *Listeria* spp.

1. Place a loopful of specimen onto the center of a clean coverslip.
2. Heat gently a flat metal washer, 1.5 cm diameter, with approximately 0.5-cm-diameter central hole.
3. Place washer into petrolatum and rotate gently to cover in a thin film of petrolatum.
4. Place this washer onto the center of a slide. Press lightly, and leave petrolatum to cool on slide.
5. When the petrolatum is set, invert the slide and gently push the covered washer onto the coverslip in such a way that the drop of fluid is in the center of the hole in the washer.
6. Lift the slide and return it into position so that the coverslip is uppermost.
7. Examine the slide under the microscope and reduced light. Focus on the edge of the drop on the coverslip to optimize visualization of organisms and their motility.

This method eliminates streaming (since there is no evaporation of fluid or presence of air bubbles under the coverslip). The suspended drop allows easy visualization of tumbling motility.

Dark-Field Examination

Dark-field examinations are used to visualize certain microorganisms that are not visible by bright-field optics or stain only with great difficulty. This technique is particularly useful in demonstrating spirochetes in biologic materials, particularly in urine or placental tissues suspected of containing *Leptospira* spp. that are too thin to see in bright field and which do not stain with Gram or polychrome stains. It is also excellent to enable differentiation of cocci and coccobacilli, which may not be possible in Gram stains.

1. Place a small quantity of the secretions to be examined on a microscope slide. Gently lower scrupulously clean slide on top, avoiding

air bubbles. (Press down to make very thin, since dark field will not be possible if the film is too thick.)

2. Ring a coverslip with petrolatum to prevent evaporation and streaming.

3. Examine the mount directly under a microscope fitted with a dark-field condenser with a 40× or 100× objective.

4. Spirochetes will appear as motile, bright "corkscrews" against a black background.

Reference

Dow, W., Jones, R. L., and Rosychuk, R. A. W.: Bacteriologic specimens: Selection, collection, and transport for optimum results. *Compend. Cont. Educ. Pract. Vet.* 11:686, 1989.

CHAPTER 16

Clinical Nutrition

John R. Kohnke

Horses are able to use a wide variety of different feedstuffs, and the cost and availabilities of feeds are important factors that can influence the final composition of any ration. Not all horse owners are able to purchase or select the best-quality feed for their horses, particularly when seasonal conditions influence availability, quality, and cost.

Many horses are overfed in their relation to growth and exercise demand. The National Research Council (NRC) and other specialist groups provide scientific guidelines for all types of horses related to body weight, age, exercise, and production demand. However, the busy practitioner requires some practical guidelines for giving sound advice on feeding horses. The dietary guidelines outlined in this summary of practical feeding are formulated to meet the growth, exercise, and clinical needs of the average horse maturing to, or maintaining, 450 kg (1000 lb) of body weight according to NRC (1989) recommendations. To avoid variations in nutrient supply caused by differing quality of feedstuffs, feeds should be measured by weight rather than volume. However, since most horse owners relate intake to volume, calculations based on weights and volumes of average-quality feeds have been included as advice to clients.

PRACTICAL FEEDING HINTS

A degree of common sense applies to the art of feeding horses. However, clients new to horses should adopt certain basic "rules" to avoid ailments related to feeding. Proper feeding management will ensure that a horse maintains good health and receives maximum benefit from the ration. As a veterinarian, you can give qualified advice on the "do's" and "don'ts" of feeding.

The Do's

- The ration should be balanced between roughages (hay, chopped hay or cubes, pasture) and concentrates (grains, wheat bran, protein meals, etc.)

KEY POINT ► Ideally, the grain-to-roughage ratio should be 70:30 maximum by volume and roughly 50:50 by weight. Stabled horses should be provided with roughage as hay or cubes to 1% of their body weight.

- Excessive amounts of poor-quality roughage may lead to "hay belly" due to too much fibrous food, and too much concentrate can lead to digestive upsets, such as colic and laminitis. Horses can safely eat quantities of fiber up to 1% of their total body weight. However, once horses start losing condition or fail to grow adequately, then supplementary feeding is required. In most cases, good-quality hay is a suitable supplement. Concentrate feeds are generally required only for horses in training, for pregnant and lactating mares, and for young, growing horses.

■ The ration should match the animal's requirements. The majority of cared for horses are idle, and therefore, adult horses require only a maintenance diet. Horses at pasture need little supplementary feeding except under conditions of nutritional stress or when growing, for mares in foal or nursing a foal, or for performance horses in training. Nutritional stress most commonly occurs under conditions of high stocking rate or when the pasture has little nutritional value. Short, green winter pasture or lush spring pasture often has low nutritional content, and horses may not be able to consume sufficient nutrients to meet their needs. Dry summer grass also has lowered feed value, and supplementary feeding may need to be carried out. Once a horse is stabled, the formulation of the ration becomes more important.

KEY POINT ► Horses in light work only require a diet consisting of good-quality hay, chopped hay, and minimal grain. If the horse is required to perform strenuous exercise, the grain portion can be increased accordingly.

■ The ration should be modified to suit individual horses. Horses differ in appetite, "likes and dislikes," so the ration should be modified to suit the individual horse and to ensure adequate nutritional intake and benefit.

KEY POINT ► If a horse is not eating well, the ration can be made more attractive by adding boiled barley or molasses or supplementing with B-complex vitamins. Also check the teeth for sharp edges.

■ It is useful to condition young horses to accept a variety of feeds (e.g., oats, corn, barley, lupins, soya bean, linseed, etc.) because they are less likely to develop distinct "likes" and "dislikes" and reject unavoidable changes in feed.
■ The ration should be fed at regular times. The horse is a creature of habit and comes to expect to be fed at the same time every day. Its digestion patterns will coincide accordingly. Regular feeding is especially important in stabled horses in training.
■ The ration should be fed at least two or three times daily. The horse has a small stomach and

no gallbladder, and it chews its food slowly. Therefore, an almost continuous supply of food should be available, especially with hand-fed, stabled horses. Racing horses in training should be fed at least three to four times a day. Slow eaters should be fed little and often.

KEY POINT ► Space the feed times equally throughout the day, with the last feed consisting of quality hay as roughage to occupy the horse overnight.

■ The feed should be good quality. It is useful to monitor the quality of feed available by checking the weight-to-volume ratio of each new batch of feed, since requirements are based on weight of feed. This avoids changes in energy as well as unnecessary cost. New sources of grain should be weighed to allow for differences in quality due to foreign matter and seasonal and district variations.
■ The ration also should be complemented by good husbandry. Careful attention to general health, teeth care, parasite control, and regular exercise will ensure good utilization of feed and maximum work capacity. Internal parasites and poor teeth are the most common cause of poor condition or ill-thrift even when a suitable ration is fed.

The Don'ts

There are certain precautions that should be observed when feeding horses, especially when horses are being fed concentrates.

■ Do not make sudden changes in ration proportion or ingredients. Sudden food changes can lead to digestive upsets or loss of appetite. A slow replacement over 10 days or more is necessary for changes such as old to new season's hay or grain.
■ Avoid sudden changes in grain content or sudden introduction to highly concentrated rations. To increase the grain content of the ration of a horse brought in from pasture, initially add about 5 to 10 percent of the planned level and gradually increase it over a week or so.
■ Do not feed dusty, moldy, or contaminated ingredients. Dusty foods can cause respiratory problems. Either sieve the grain or dampen the ration with warm water or a 50 percent molasses–water mixture.
■ Do not feed full grain ration on idle days. Reduce grain content to about one-third of the normal amount on idle days to decrease incidence of "tying up" and digestive upsets when the horse is exercised again.

KEY POINT ► In performance horses, it is also best to reduce the grain level of the feed ration the night before the idle day.

- Rapid ingestion of concentrates can lead to digestive upsets. Carefully mix the grain, etc. with the roughage component, or place a stone or brick (e.g., a salt brick) in the base of the feeder so the horse has to search to pick up the concentrates.
- Do not feed from dirty feeders or waterers. Regularly clean out feed bins to prevent molds and other toxic products from building up. Water troughs should be checked daily and cleaned regularly to prevent buildup of algae and sludges of chewed food. Some horse owners separate the feeding area and watering point to reduce the buildup of grains and food in water troughs where horses that have a habit of eating and drinking alternatively.

- Do not feed concentrates on the ground. Feed on the ground is quickly scattered, pawed, and wasted. Parasite and sand intake can be increased when horses are encouraged to fossick on the ground for tasty concentrate feeds. Provide an adequate container with no sharp edges and enough weight to prevent the horse tipping it over.

References

Cunha, J. T.: *Horse Feeding and Nutrition*, 2d Ed. New York: Academic Press, 1991.
Hintz, H. F.: *Horse Nutrition: A Practical Guide*. New York: Agro, 1983.

Growing Horses

Orphan Foals

Orphan foals need careful feeding and management, particularly if they are orphaned at or soon after birth. It is most important that all newborn foals receive sufficient colostrum to provide immunoglobin defence against environmental pathogens (see Failure of Passive Transfer, Chap. 8). The recommendations given below are for foals of 45 to 50 kg (90–110 lb) birth weight maturing to 450 kg (1000 lb) body weight.

For orphan foals, extra colostrum can be collected within 12 hours of foaling, preferably from mares that have a dead foal, have lost their foals soon after birth, or are overproductive milkers.

KEY POINT ▶ Foals orphaned at birth should receive approximately 1200 ml (2 pints) of good-quality colostrum by bottle if they will suck, over the tongue by syringe, or by nasogastric tube within 12 hours of birth to meet immunologic competence. A foal's gut is unable to absorb antibodies past 24 hours after birth.

Note: In foals less than 24 hours of age, *do not* feed milk or water until colostrum is given, since the gastrointestinal tract will cease immunoglobulin uptake.

Feeding the Orphan Foal

In newly born foals, foster mothering is usually successful, provided a suitable nurse mare, or even a goat on a raised platform, is available. Where a foster mother or nurse mare is not available, the foal will need to be hand reared.

Dietary Guidelines: First Week of Age

Bottle feeds can be given for the first 5 to 7 days with a commercial milk replacer formulated for foals. However, most foals from 2 to 3 days of age can be taught to drink from a bucket. If commercial fed milk replacer is unavailable, whole fresh milk, full cream powdered milk, or calf milk replacers can be used. Cow's milk contains more fat and less sugar than mare's milk. Cow's milk should be fortified with 6% to 7% additional sugar to give the approximate composition of mare's milk. Where possible, it is best to house orphan foals in a loose box, preferably with a companion, for the first 1 to 2 weeks, particularly during cold or wet weather.

Preparation of Milk

Specialized commercial foal milk replacers are available, and these are convenient and provide good results when fed as directed. However, where these are not available, milk for young foals can be made up by dissolving approximately 60 to 70 g (2–2.5 oz or 4 tablespoons) lactose (preferably), dextrose, or brown sugar in each 1000 ml (approximately 2 pints) of cow's milk or accurately reconstituted milk powder mixture.

KEY POINT ► In each liter (2 pints), mix in two level teaspoons (10 g) of dicalcium phosphate powder and, if available, 5 mg iron in a commercial supplement, since cow's milk is low in these essential bone and blood building nutrients.

Make up freshly as required. A commercial baby's bottle (e.g., a plastic bottle with screw-down teat, with hole large enough for a drip to collect when full bottle is held teat downward) or a soda drink bottle fitted with a small lamb's teat is recommended. Feed at blood temperature (37°C) (drip some on inside of wrist; it feels just warm), and shake the bottle occasionally during feeding. Milk temperature can be gradually lowered to room temperature (20–25°C) by 1 week of age as bucket feeding is introduced.

Feeding Volumes: First 5 to 7 Days

Note: Guidelines on the volume of milk are based on thoroughbred-sized foals of 40 to 50 kg (88–110 lb) birth weight—adjust to foal's demands (see Table 16–1):

KEY POINT ► If the foal is hungry and seeks more milk, give an extra half volume in between the 2-hour feeds to decrease the risk of diarrhea.

Dietary Guidelines: 7 Days and Older

Most foals at 2 to 3 days of age can be taught to drink from a bucket. Bucket feeding should certainly be commenced after the first week.

Bottle to Bucket Change. Studies have shown that most foals will accept bucket feeding after a day or so.

KEY POINT ► In foals less than 1 week of age or those that will not drink, stimulate the sucking reflex by letting the foal suck on a finger (dip the finger in milk; moving it against the palate and tongue often helps). Once the foal starts to suck, lift the dish of milk until the foal drinks the milk; then remove the finger. Forcing the foal's head down into the milk is

counterproductive. Repeat the process until the foal learns to drink.

Generally, young foals will nurse on a finger and will readily learn to drink once the milk has been tasted after one or two attempts. Foals that have been bottle fed for the first week are usually accustomed to drinking milk mixture. Put the milk in a wide, shallow container in a small enclosure with the foal. Show the foal where the milk is, and splash milk on its nose. A foal will usually start drinking once it becomes hungry.

KEY POINT ► Once the foal learns to drink from the dish, a shallow plastic bucket 300 mm (12 in) in diameter, 200 to 250 mm (8–10 in) deep, secured 600 mm (24 in) above the ground is ideal to prevent the foal from standing in it, tipping it over, or fouling it.

Preparation of Milk. Although the milk mixture for young foals (see above) can be used for bucket feeds, recent research has shown that powdered milk replacers diluted 1:10 with water and supplemented with good-quality concentrate feed will ensure adequate growth and development in foals over 2 weeks of age. The volume of milk is allowed as *ad lib* drinks between replenishments. Discard any leftovers, but ensure that the foal is drinking at least 75% of the milk allocation between feeds. A feeding guideline for a foal 7 to 14 days of age is given in Table 16-1.

Concentrate Feeds. Most young foals will nibble supplementary feeds and milk-based pellets from 7 to 10 days of age. Many commercial supplementary feeds containing 12% to 14% crude protein are available as creep or supplementary feeds for young foals. Alternatively, a palatable, high-quality protein, low-fiber ration suitable for foals can be mixed as shown in Table 16-2.

The dry feed base can be mixed and stored for a few days. Add the molasses and water and mix freshly each day. If a commercial feed is used, additional vitamin E and molasses sweetener may be mixed into the feed.

After 2 to 3 weeks, most orphans and nursing foals will begin to graze to supplement their milk intake if green pasture is available. Alternatively, leafy, good-quality alfalfa hay or grass hay, dampened and sweetened with a 50:50 molasses and water mix, can be provided in a shallow, safe trough. Dampening the hay or cubes will soften them for chewing and will be better accepted.

Foals 6 to 16 Weeks

After about 6 weeks of age, reduce milk powder by 100 g (3 oz) per week, and substitute with 100 g (3 oz) soybean meal. Milk powder in the ration may give slightly higher growth rates (because of its better digestibility in young foals) than comparable amounts of soybean meal. Soybean meal is gener-

TABLE 16–1. Feeding Guidelines: Thoroughbred Foal, 45 kg (100 lb)

Age	Volume/Day	Suggested Feeding Times
0–7 days (bottle feeding)	3 liters (5 pints) daily, 300 ml (10 oz) per feed (about 1–1.5 cups at each of 10 feeds)	Every 2 hours, 6:00 A.M. to 10:00 P.M., once at 2:00 A.M.
7 to 14 days (bucket feeding): Provide 1 kg (2 lb) of concentrate "sweet" feed in a shallow dish near feeding bucket for foal to nibble between meals (see formulation below).	Increase to 5 to 6 L (9–11 pints) daily, 1000 to 1250 ml (2–2.5 pints) per feed.	4 hourly, 6:00 A.M. to 10:00 P.M., (5 feeds)
14 to 21 days: Provide 1.5 kg (3.5 lb) of concentrate "sweet" feed 12% protein *ad lib* daily.	Increase to 6 to 8 L (11–14 pints) daily, 1.5 to 2 L (3–4 pints) per feed.	6 hourly, 6:00 A.M. to 10:00 P.M., 4 feeds
21 days to 8 weeks: Provide concentrate feed.	Start on 8 L (15 pints) daily; increase by 2 L (3.5 pints) weekly.	8 hourly, 6:00 A.M. (*ad lib* to appetite) increasing to 4 L (7 pints) at 2:00 P.M. feed
After 8 weeks: (Feed *ad lib* to appetite). Start to wean off milk onto concentrate feed and good pasture.	Provide 6 L (11 pints) twice daily.	Morning and evening provide *ad lib* concentrate feed, 12% protein; reduce milk by 1 L (1.5 pints) per feed each week until milk is no longer taken.

ally less expensive and is a well-balanced protein source for older foals. Where molasses is used as an appetizer, feeds should be made fresh each day.

KEY POINT ▶ As a "rule of thumb," foals can be provided with concentrate feed at the rate of 2.0% of body weight (1 kg/ 50 kg; 2 lb/100 lb) daily, with additional access to good-quality pasture or alfalfa hay.

TABLE 16–2. Dietary Guidelines: Foals 1 to 6 Weeks of Age

Ingredient	Weight	Approx. Volume
Crimped or crushed oats	2.0 kg (4.5 lb)	4 L (7 pints)
Cracked corn	1.0 kg (2 lb)	1.5 L (3 pints)
Full cream milk powder	300 g (10 oz)	2 cups
Soybean meal	200 g (7 oz)	2 cups
Alfalfa cubes, crushed	500 g (1 lb)	1 L (2 pints)
Dicalcium phosphate	30 g (1 oz)	1.5 tablespoons
Vitamin E	250 IU	—
Salt	15 g (0.5 oz)	3 teaspoons
Molasses	1 cup in 1 cup warm water mixed into feed	
Commercial vitamin/mineral supplement	Foal dosage	

GUIDE TO HAND REARING

▶ Feeding Rules

Certain rules of feeding should be observed to prevent gastric upsets, diarrhea, or food refusal:

- Changes in diet must be made gradually.
- The earliest feeds should be offered at blood heat (37°C). After a week, this can be gradually lowered to room temperature.
- Change formulas over 2 or 3 days.
- Do not overfeed—it is best to feed small feeds more frequently to demand rather than large milk feeds during the first 1 to 2 weeks of age.
- Gradually wean the foal off milk at 2 to 2.5 months of age, depending on its rate of development and appetite for concentrate food and available grazing.

▶ Prevent Diarrhea

Increased intake of fibrous feeds, such as green grass, can cause mild diarrhea from 7 to 10 days of age. Milk overload can cause diarrhea in foals during the first week. This can be avoided by reducing the volume and increase the frequency of feeding. Control of intestinal threadworms (*Strongyloides westeri*) may be necessary if the foal develops a persistent "brown bubbly" type of diarrhea despite careful feeding and a normal body temperature. A sample of fresh feces may be examined for the characteristic embryonated strongyle-type eggs within 2 hours of collection. *Note:* Infections are not patent for 8 to 14 days.

▶ Exercise and Sunlight

Ensure that the foal has sufficient area to exercise and receives at least 2 to 3 hours of sunlight per day, preferably more. The foal should be taught to lead as soon as possible.

▶ Parasite Control

The foal can be treated for internal parasites routinely at 4 to 6 weeks of age with an anthelmintic paste formulation (see Anthelmintics, Chap. 17). Repeat deworming every 4 to 6 weeks, shifting to a new pasture after each worming, if possible.

▶ General Observation

Instruct your clients to observe for signs of ill-health, colic, and poor appetite.

KEY POINT ▶ It is also good practice to give the newborn foal tetanus antitoxin. In weaker foals, consider an additional immunoglobulin boost during the first week and at 1 month of age with commercial immunoglobulin preparations.

▶ Discipline

An orphan foal can become rather cheeky and difficult to manage because it does not receive its mother's discipline and has no herd position. Care and strictness in handling the foal are therefore important. It is best not to allow a foal to play games with its handlers.

Nursing Foals

The most rapid period of growth and development of the young foal occurs during the first 3 months of age. The peak of lactation occurs from 6 to 10 weeks after foaling. In most cases, the nutritional needs of the growing foal will be provided by milk intake and access to good-quality pasture or nibbling at supplementary concentrates provided for the mare.

However, where the contribution from grazing falls short of requirements due to seasonal availability or heavy stocking rates, then supplementary concentrate feeds may be necessary to maintain optimal, but not excessive, growth rates.

KEY POINT ▶ Foals that are supplemented with a good-quality, palatable ration from 2 to 3 months of age will suffer less nutritional setback at weaning.

Where a mare's milk supply dries up due to mastitis, injury, sickness, or malnutrition, or in aged mares with poor milk supply, it is best to wean the foal at less than 4 weeks of age and rear it as an orphan.

Generally, concentrate feeds in a separate "creep" feed area are of no advantage to foals growing at an average rate. Studies indicate that average thoroughbred-sized foals (450 to 500 kg mature weight) gain approximately 1 to 1.4 kg (2–3 lb) daily for the first 90 days after birth. Weight gain drops to 700 g (1.5 lb) daily at 6 months of age and to 500 g (1 lb) daily after weaning.

In poor seasons, creep feeding may be beneficial, but uncontrolled feeding can result in excess energy intake, with risk of developmental orthopedic disease (DOD). Studies have shown that excess energy intake relative to exercise and growth results in a higher incidence of DOD. Most younger foals prefer to cofeed with their mothers, sharing a good-quality lactating mare concentrate ration, since this provides security and develops eating habits. Paddock exercise is important to ensure adequate development. If the opportunity for the foal to exercise is restricted, then the mare and foal ideally should be walked together for 15 to 20 minutes daily.

KEY POINT ▶ In practice, young foals can be supplemented until weaning with a 10% to 12% CP, 1.5% calcium, 3.0 Mcal/kg ration at the rate of 1% to 1.5% of body weight [1–1.5 kg (2–3 lb) per 100 kg (220 lb) of body weight] with *ad lib* paddock exercise without risk of overfeeding and DOD problems (Table 16-3).

Foals that develop evidence of DOD, with epiphysitis or contracted tendons, can be restricted in growth by reducing supplementary feed intake for

TABLE 16–3. Dietary Guidelines: Young Foal

Age: 8 weeks to weaning
Frequency: Ad lib in creep area

Ingredient	Weight	Approx. Volume
Rolled barley	1.0 kg (2 lb)	2 L (3.5 pints)
Cracked corn	500 g (1 lb)	1 L (1.5 pints)
Skim milk powder	100 g (3 oz)	0.7 cup
Soybean meal	200 g (7 oz)	1.3 cups
Alfalfa cubes, crushed	300 g (10 oz)	700 ml (1.5 pints)
Dicalcium phosphate	20 g (0.6 oz)	1 tablespoon
Salt	15 g (0.5 oz)	3 teaspoons
Molasses	Half cup in half cup of warm water mixed into feed	
Commercial vitamin/mineral supplement at foal dosage		

3 to 4 weeks and ensuring regular exercise. This is most easily done by teaching affected foals to lead, walking them for 10 to 15 minutes daily, or leading the mare with the foal at foot.

Many good-quality commercial creep feeds are now available, and these are convenient and can be provided on an *ad lib* basis from a self-feeder in a creep area. However, for owners wishing to mix their own feeds, a suitable palatable creep feed ration can be made up as shown in Table 16-3.

The ration can be offered at the rate of 1 to 1.5 kg (2–3 lb) per 100 kg (220 lb) of body weight, adjusted to body weight as foal develops, increasing by approximately 200 g (7 oz) weekly or to appetite. However, body development should be monitored weekly, and the creep should be withdrawn or limited in foals that are developing too quickly due to excessive energy intake. Where pasture is limited, good-quality grass hay can be provided to appetite.

Weanlings

A well-managed weaning process minimizes any psychological, nutritional, or health stress on the young horse. Nutritional or disease-related setbacks at weaning can affect the subsequent age of maturity of the horse. Most foals, by 5 to 6 months of age, have little nutritional reliance on nursing, and if they are provided with good pasture or are accustomed to consuming concentrate feed, they will suffer no significant setback at weaning.

KEY POINT ▶ Foals should be weaned before 7 months of age. Early weaning at less than 4 months of age has no significant benefit, except where a mare has inadequate milk to feed her foal.

Fretting is common in younger weanlings for the first 5 to 7 days, and they may lose their appetite. It is important that a palatable concentrate feed and good, clean pasture be available.

Weanlings should gain about 500 g (1 lb) daily until 12 months of age. Provision of concentrate (12%–14% CP, 3 Mcal/kg) at a rate of 1.25 to 1.5 kg (2.5–3 lb) per 100 kg (220 lb) of body weight daily, supplemented *ad lib* by good-quality alfalfa–grass hay mix or plentiful paddock grazing, and free exercise will maintain an adequate rate of growth and development. Placement of feeders well apart from water troughs also will encourage exercise.

KEY POINT ▶ As the foal gets older, the ration should be increased by more roughage in the form of good-quality mixed hay, leaving the grain intake relatively constant.

The ration must be adjusted in proportion to body weight. The quality and availability of the pasture should be monitored regularly, particularly during autumn and winter periods. If the grazing pasture becomes dominant in either grass or legume, additional sources of phosphorus (to bal-

ance calcium intake from legumes and alfalfa hay) and calcium (to balance low calcium intake from grasses) may be necessary to maintain an optimal calcium-to-phosphorus ratio of 1.2 to 2.0:1.0 in growing horses. Under most conditions, addition of 1.5% calcium powder (15 g/kg calcium carbonate) to cereal-based rations and 1.0% phosphorus (100 g wheat bran per kilogram) to alfalfa-based rations is a useful guideline to balance the calcium/phosphorus intake.

Weanlings grazing topical grass species containing high oxalate content, which interferes with calcium absorption, may develop symptoms of DOD over 2 to 3 months after weaning. Concentrate feeds should contain 2% calcium powder (20 g/kg calcium carbonate or commercial supplement). It is best to feed the weanlings in a small yard or fenced corner area to ensure that the concentrate is consumed.

Ration Guidelines

Commercial rations such as sweet feed mixes or pelleted feeds are popular because of convenience; uniformity of energy, protein, and calcium/phosphorus levels; and savings in time of mixing. Home-mixed rations must be palatable to tempt young weanlings to feed (Table 16-4). If the ration is offered *ad lib* from automatic feeders, then care should be taken to avoid overeating under cold conditions.

TABLE 16–4. Dietary Guidelines: Weanlings

Body weight: 200 to 250 kg (450–550-lb) weanling
Age: 6 months of age, maturing to 450 to 500 kg (1000–1100 lb), medium growth rate
Frequency of feeding: Access to good-quality mixed pasture, one feed per day

Ingredient	Weight	Approx. Volume
Rolled barley or oats	2.0 kg (4 lb)	4 L (7 pints)
Cracked corn	1.0 kg (2 lb)	1.5 L (3 pints)
Soybean meal	350 g (12 oz)	2 cups
Alfalfa cubes, broken for mixing, or chopped hay	1.5 kg (3 lb)	3 L (5.5 pints)
Dicalcium phosphate	60 g (2 oz)	3 tablespoons
Calcium carbonate	30 g (1 oz)	1.5 tablespoons
Salt	20 g (0.7 oz)	1 tablespoon
Molasses	1 cup in 1 cup of warm water mixed into feed	
Commercial vitamin/mineral supplement containing vitamin A and vitamin D in the winter months, when grazing green, cereal-based pastures		

Increase the amount fed and the hay or roughage in the ration by approximately 250 g (9 oz) per fortnight in proportion to growth rate. Regular weekly assessments of growth and development and feed adjustments relative to weight gain, quality of pasture, weather conditions, and individual foal appetite and development should be carried out.

Yearlings

KEY POINT ▶ Most well-grown young horses should have achieved 90% of their mature height and 70% of their adult body weight at 12 to 15 months of age.

The yearling age is ideal to assess the growth and development of the young horse, and nutritional management can be modified to achieve the standards desired.

Preparation of a yearling for sale requires careful attention to nutrition and exercise, particularly in the final 3 to 4 months prior to sale (Table 16-5). Each sale yearling must be assessed individually, so adjustment to feeding and overall preparation can be targeted to achieve the standards required.

TABLE 16–5. Dietary Guidelines: Yearling

Body weight: 325 kg (700-lb) yearling maturing to 450 kg (1000 lb)
Frequency of feeding: Access to pasture, one feed daily
Provision: 75% NRC (1989) plus grazing to maintain growth and condition

Ingredient	Weight	Approx. Volume
Rolled barley/ whole oats	3.0 kg (6.5 lb)	5.5 L (10 pints)
Soybean meal	350 g (12 oz)	2.5 cups
Alfalfa cubes	2.0 kg (4.5 lb)	4 L (7 pints)
Dicalcium phosphate	60 g (2 oz)	3 tablespoons
Calcium carbonate	30 g (1 oz)	1.5 tablespoons
Salt	20 g (0.6 oz)	1 tablespoon
Molasses	1 cup in 1 cup warm water mixed into feed	

Good-quality grass hay [1.5–1.8 kg (3–4 lb)] may be provided with the meal for semiconfined horses on poor grazing. A commercial vitamin/mineral supplement containing zinc and copper (40 ppm) and 750 to 1000 IU vitamin E may be mixed into the concentrate ration for performance horses or potential sale animals.

An approximate daily rate of commercial concentrate feeding of 1.25 kg (2.5 lb) per 100 kg (220 lb) of body weight with up to 1.5 kg (3 lb) where pasture is limited with regular increases to body weight gain will allow adequate growth and development. However, since individual animals differ in metabolic efficiency, the animal should be assessed weekly and fed to maintain an even growth rate, being careful to avoid higher energy intake than required and the risk of DOD problems.

Where predominately cereal-based pastures are available that contain phosphorus in excess of calcium intake, provision of *ad lib* alfalfa hay as well as the preceding concentrate is recommended to help maintain a positive calcium-to-phosphorus ratio. Young horses grazing topical grass pasture with high oxalate content should be provided with *ad lib* alfalfa hay and brought into a yard to consume the concentrate feed with added calcium if there is a history of DOD.

If pastures are legume-based, containing alfalfa or clover species, then total phosphorus intake relative to calcium may not meet the requirements of the growing horse. In this case, the concentrate feed should contain only half the amount of dicalcium phosphate, and extra phosphorus should be provided by mixing in 360 g (12 oz) or 2 L (3 pints) of wheat bran.

References

Cunha, J. T.: *Horse Feeding and Nutrition,* 2d Ed. New York: Academic Press, 1991.

Frape, D. L.: *Equine Nutrition and Feeding.* Essex, England: Longmans, 1986.

Kronfeld, D. S., Meacham, J. N., and Donoghue, S.: Dietary Aspects of Developmental Orthopedic Disease in Young Horses. In *Veterinary Clinics of North America: Equine Practice (Clinical Nutrition).* Philadelphia: W.B. Saunders, 1990, p. 451.

National Research Council: *Nutrient Requirements of Horses,* 5th Ed. Washington: National Academy of Sciences, 1989.

Performance Horses

The ration of racing, showjumping, eventing, polo, and endurance horses must be tailored to meet the needs of the individual horse, related to its age and build, duration, type, distance and intensity of exercise, stage of training, temperament, and climatic conditions, as well as appetite and eating habits.

KEY POINT ▶ A performance horse will consume from 2.0% to 2.5% of its body weight per day in dry feeds as fed, with a minimum content of 25% of the feed as good-quality roughage.

Smaller-framed horses may eat less, whereas hard-working horses may consume feed at up to 3.0% of their body weight per day.

The feeding routine must be regular, designed to mirror the natural feeding pattern, with three to four meals per day in stabled horses, providing a nutritionally balanced, palatable diet. Rations need not be complicated mixtures. A balanced diet can be formulated using one or two sources of energy, a protein source if required, and adequate roughage consisting of either hay, chopped hay, or cubed hay. Supplementary calcium, phosphorus, electrolytes, or trace mineral/vitamin additives may be required to balance the ration or meet elevated needs relative to exercise intensity. It is essential that horses in training have free access to potable water at all times.

KEY POINT ▶ Feeding must be in proportion to daily exercise demand.

High-energy feeds, such as grains, must be reduced by about one-third on light days, or preferably the night before a rest day, to avoid overactive behavior and the risk of metabolic problems such as myopathies on resumption of regular exercise. The feeding routine must be designed to limit boredom in horses on concentrate rations confined to stables, particularly overnight, to avoid such vices as wood chewing, stall walking, and windsucking. Provision of good-quality alfalfa or grass hay with the evening feed is recommended.

KEY POINT ▶ A horse's appetite reflects its well-being and acceptance of the ration.

The most common causes of reduced appetite are overwork or excessively fast work for the stage of training. The use of molasses and B-complex sup-

plements in sweet feeds helps to maintain the appetite and acceptance of the ration.

Racing Horses

A number of breeds of horses are used in competitive racing, and the ration must be tailored to the stage and intensity of training, body weight, build, and eating habits of the individual animal.

Energy

KEY POINT ▶ The energy content of the ration must be in proportion to the exercise duration and intensity so as to maintain a desired body weight, temperament, and level of performance.

Horses less than 4 years old require adequate energy for growth, development, and performance. Horses housed under cold conditions or nervous horses will require higher energy intake to maintain body condition.

Cereal grains such as corn, barley, oats, and milo are common sources of energy depending on availability, cost, and individual palatability. Smaller-framed horses, such as standardbreds and Arabians, or horses that have consistently poor appetites are best fed rations based on higher-energy-density feeds such as corn and fats to help reduce the overall volume of the ration to a bulk that can be comfortably consumed.

In hotter climates, or in horses exercising over longer distances, corn and polyunsaturated fats such as corn oil or other vegetable oils, or even tallow, can be substituted for more fibrous grains such as barley and oats to increase the energy density of the ration and reduce heat increment from fermentation. Where fat is used as an energy source, at least 1 cup or 230 ml (8 oz) is the minimum amount that is worthwhile adding to replace cereal grains in the feed.

KEY POINT ▶ One cup of corn oil will replace 6 cups of whole oats, 4.5 cups of rolled barley, and 3 cups of cracked corn in the ration.

Protein

KEY POINT ▶ In working horses, protein intake is related to energy need. Generally, as the energy content of the ration is increased by the addition of grain, the corresponding increase in protein supplied by the additional grain will meet normal everyday needs in racing horses, particularly where alfalfa hay or cubes form the roughage base of the concentrate ration.

Excess protein intake requires additional energy and higher water requirement for excretion. However, during early training or in 2- to 3-year-old horses, additional protein provided by 1 to 2 cups of protein meal (e.g., soybean meal) may assist body and skeletal development. Where fats are used as an energy source and the protein contribution from grains is reduced accordingly, 1 cup of protein meal per cup of fat added will maintain adequate protein intake. Provision of an additional 1 to 2 cups protein meal (e.g., soybean meal) in the two evening feeds following hard exercise, competition, or racing may assist recovery.

Fiber

KEY POINT ▶ All rations should be based on hay, chopped hay, or roughage cubes. Adequate good-quality fiber to a minimum 0.5% to 1.0% of body weight, or 25% to 50% by weight of the ration, must be provided, although a reduction in large bowel volume may be desirable in racing horses.

Provision of hay overnight and, where possible, access to field exercise and grazing are helpful to reduce boredom.

Excessively dusty hay can increase the incidence of lower respiratory tract disease in confined horses. Dry, brittle, or dusty hay should be dampened by soaking in clean water for 10 to 15 minutes and draining prior to feeding. In stabled or confined horses, supplementary hay should be provided in a trough located below chest height, preferably on the stable floor. Bedding should be as dust-free as practically possible.

Minerals

KEY POINT ▶ The minerals of major concern in horses on high-energy, grain-based diets are the macrominerals calcium, phosphorus, and sodium and the microminerals iron, copper, zinc, and selenium. Heavily sweating horses require higher amounts of calcium, sodium, potassium, and iron to replace sweat loss.

Provision of calcium to balance the relatively higher intake of phosphorus on grain- and grass hay–based rations is essential to maintain skeletal integrity and reduce bone and joint disease in young horses in training. About 60 to 90 g (2–3 oz) of calcium carbonate (ground limestone) added to cereal grass–based rations or 60 to 90 g (2–3 oz) of dicalcium phosphate to alfalfa/legume-based feeds will satisfy basic needs for 450- to 500-kg (1000–1100-lb) working horses. Many commercial supplements are also available.

Where alfalfa hay, chopped hay, or cubes are used as a primary roughage source, additional phosphorus may be required to meet the needs and maintain the calcium-to-phosphorus ratio to within 1:1 to 2:1. Addition of 60 to 90 g (2–3 oz) or 3 to 4.5 tablespoons of dicalcium phosphate to the concentrate feed or 270 to 360 g (9–12 oz) of wheat bran will help provide additional phosphorus.

Trace minerals are best provided by a commercial supplement containing 50% NRC (1989) requirements of iron, copper, zinc, selenium, and iodine. Supplementation with 60 ml polyunsaturated oil (e.g., corn oil) daily to a 500-kg (1100-lb) equestrian horse will help promote and maintain haircoat condition.

Electrolytes

The addition of 60 g (2 oz) or 3 tablespoons of salt daily will assist in meeting sodium needs, maintaining fluid intake, and increasing acceptance of concentrate rations in horses with little or no regular access to pasture. In heavily sweating horses, supplementation with additional potassium chloride contained in Lite salt and magnesium contained in epsom salts will assist in replacing electrolytes lost in sweat outputs of 15 to 30 L daily in hot weather or extended exercise periods. Horses must have access to water at all times when supplemented with electrolyte mixtures.

Vitamins

KEY POINT ▶ Rations based on cereal grains and grass hays with little access to pasture may be relatively deficient in vitamins A, D, and E and some B-complex vitamins.

Sun-cured alfalfa hay will provide vitamin D to meet needs in racing horses. Provision of up to 1000 IU vitamin E daily is considered beneficial in performance horses.

Where polyunsaturated oils are used to increase the energy density in small-framed horses or horses with a poor appetite, an additional 250 IU of vitamin E per cup of oil is recommended above the basal 1000 IU vitamin E daily. Because of the inherent instability of vitamin E in vitamin–mineral mixes, it is best to provide additional vitamin E as an individual supplement.

In horses in hard work with restricted access to pasture or green feed, a commercial supplement containing A, D, and B-complex vitamins is useful to maintain appetite.

Water

Racing and performance horses should have access to clean, cool water at all times, particularly during hot weather and when electrolytes are being added to the diet.

Weight of Rider

Tables 16-6 and 16-7 present dietary guidelines calculated to allow for a rider weight range of 50 to 75 kg in ridden horses.

Early Training Notes

1. If the horse is not eating all its feed, reduce the bulk of the hay to ensure that the full concentrate intake is maintained. If the horse consumes all the ration and appears hungry, increase the overnight portion of hay.
2. Concentrate feeds may be dampened with molasses and water if desired to reduce dust and increase acceptance.
3. Wheat bran [240 g (8 oz)] can be added to the evening meal to provide additional phosphorus and encourage acceptance. For young horses in early training, 1 cup of soybean meal may be mixed into the morning and evening feeds.
4. During hot weather or in apprehensive fillies or small-framed horses unable to consume the bulk of concentrate ration, polyunsaturated oil (e.g., corn oil) can be substituted for some of the rolled barley or whole oats on a volume basis of 1 cup corn oil replacing 6 cups (2.5 pints) whole oats or 4.5 cups (2 pints) rolled barley. During the conditioning exercise period, 1 cup corn oil can be fed morning and evening, introduced in a step-wise manner over 5 to 7 days, reducing the grain accordingly. Where more than 1 cup of corn oil is added, add 1 cup soybean meal per additional cup of corn oil to replace protein previously contributed by the grain.
5. A commercial electrolyte replacer may replace the salt and Lite salt.
6. On light work days, delete corn from the ration, and on rest days, reduce barley or oats to half (including the evening meal prior to the rest day) and increase the bulk of the ration with alfalfa or grass hay.

Advanced Training Notes

1. The value of fat as an energy source for fast exercise and racing has not been fully established.
2. Adjust grain intake to maintain body weight relative to the individual horse's exercise program.
3. An additional protein meal is not required in this ration where alfalfa is used as the concentrate base. If alfalfa is replaced by grass hay, 1 cup of soybean meal and 40 g (1.3 oz) or 2 tablespoons of calcium carbonate should be added to the morning and evening meals.

4. Supplementary B-complex vitamins may be given to help improve the appetite if green grass or grazing is not available.

Eventing/Horse Trialing

Competition in the cross-country or steeplechase phase of 3-day eventing or horse trialing is one of the most demanding types of equine athletic activity. The horse must be well conditioned and physically fit, yet calm and obedient to compete successfully and score well in all three phases.

▶ Early Training

Initial training regimens include trotting and cantering exercise for 30 to 40 minutes daily, with dressage and jumping training for up to 60 minutes on alternate days. The dietary requirements for a 500-kg (1100-lb) eventing horse for these regimens are similar to those for a racing horse in early training, as outlined in Table 16-6.

If the horse has access to pasture during the day and is stabled overnight, then the midday feed of hay can be deleted. If the horse is confined for most of the time, then the three feeds as outlined in Table 16-6 should be offered. The dietary composition and intake should be adjusted to suit the individual training regimen and the horse's appetite limit.

If the animal is small-framed or has a nervous temperament, up to 2 cups of corn oil can be substituted for cereal grains to increase energy density and provide an alternative noncarbohydrate slow-release form of energy.

▶ Advanced Training

Once the horse begins cantering and galloping exercise for 20 minutes daily in preparation for steeplechase and cross-country phases, the energy density of the ration must be increased accordingly. The ration guideline for a racing horse outlined in Table 16-7 may be adopted, deleting the midday concentrate feed.

On showjumping, dressage practice, or competition days, the amount of barley or oats should be reduced to 1 kg morning and evening, with corn deleted from the morning feed on that day. Reduce grain on light work days and rest days as recommended in Table 16-6.

Polo/Polocross Horses

Polo and polocross competition encompass a variety of exercise speeds, with energy and protein needs similar to a racehorse in training. However, many polo horses are smaller-framed than thoroughbred racehorses, and often the bulk of the ration has to be reduced to increase the energy density in proportion to the horse's appetite and body weight.

TABLE 16–6. Dietary Guidelines: Racehorse, Early Training

Body weight: Racing horse, 450 to 500 kg (1000–1100 lb)
Stage of training: First 6 weeks, moderate work up to 30 to 40 minutes daily
Frequency of feeding: Three feeds daily, stabled; evening feed home-mixed sweet feed
Provision: 100% daily requirement (NRC, 1989)

Ingredient	Weight	Approx. Volume
Morning Feed		
Rolled barley or whole oats	1.5 kg (3 lb)	3 L (5.5 pints)
Corn	450 g (1 lb)	600 ml (1 pint)
Alfalfa cubes	1.0 kg (2 lb)	2 L (3.5 pints)
Vitamin E	1000 IU	—
Salt	30 g (1 oz)	1.5 tablespoons
Midday–Early Afternoon Feed		

1.0 kg (2 lb) dampened, dust-free grass hay, adjust to appetite. If available, 1 to 2 hours of grazing late morning after concentrate feed has been consumed. Alternatively, graze on lead midafternoon or 2.0 kg (4.5 lb) green grass in stable and afternoon walking exercise.

Ingredient	Weight	Approx. Volume
Evening Feed		
Rolled barley or whole oats	1.5 kg (3 lb)	3 L (5.5 pints)
Corn	450 g (1 lb)	600 ml (1 pint)
Alfalfa cubes	1.5 kg (3 lb)	3 L (5.5 pints)
Molasses	1 cup in 1 cup warm water mixed into feed	
Dicalcium phosphate	30 g (1 oz)	1.5 tablespoons
Lightly Sweating Horses—Cool Weather		
Salt	30 g (1 oz)	1.5 tablespoons
Heavily Sweating Horses—Hot Weather		
Salt	30 g (1 oz)	1.5 tablespoons
Lite salt	30 g (1 oz)	1.5 tablespoons
Magnesium sulfate	30 g (1 oz)	1.5 tablespoons
Dicalcium phosphate	30 g (1 oz)	1.5 tablespoons
Dextrose glucose	60 g (2 oz)	3 tablespoons (optional)

Commercial vitamin/mineral supplement containing vitamins A, D, and B-complex and trace minerals

Overnight	1.0 kg dampened grass hay	

TABLE 16–7. Dietary Guidelines: Racehorse, Advanced Training

Body weight: Racing horse, 450 to 500 kg (1000–1100 lb)
Stage of training: Advanced training, breezed 3 times weekly, intense work 10 to 15 minutes daily
Frequency of feeding: Three to four feeds daily, stabled; evening feed home-mixed sweet feed
Provision: 100% daily requirement (NRC, 1989)

Ingredient	Weight	Approx. Volume
Morning Feed		
Rolled barley or whole oats	1.5 kg (3 lb)	3 L (5.5 pints)
Corn	1.0 kg (2 lb)	1.5 L (3 pints)
Alfalfa cubes	1.0 kg (2 lb)	2 L (3.5 pints)
Vitamin E	1000 IU	—
Salt	30 g (1 oz)	1.5 tablespoons
Midday–Early Afternoon Feed		
Rolled barley	1.0 kg (2 lb)	2 L (3.5 pints)
Corn	450 g (1 lb)	600 ml (1 pint)

This feed may be dampened with water: 1.0 kg (2 lb) dampened, dust-free grass hay to appetite. If available, 1 to 2 hours of grazing later after concentrate feed has been consumed. Alternatively, graze on lead midafternoon or 2.0 kg (4.5 lb) green grass in stable and afternoon walking exercise.

Ingredient	Weight	Approx. Volume
Evening Feed		
Rolled barley or whole oats	1.5 kg (3 lb)	3 L (5.5 pints)
Corn	750 g (1.5 lb)	1 L (2 pints)
Alfalfa cubes	1.5 kg (3 lb)	3 L (5.5 pints)
Wheat bran (optional)	240 g (8 oz)	1.5 cups
Molasses	1 cup in 2 cups warm water mixed into feed	
Dicalcium phosphate	90 g (3 oz)	5 tablespoons
Lightly Sweating Horses—Cool Weather		
Salt	30 g (1 oz)	1.5 tablespoons
Heavily Sweating Horses—Hot Weather		
Salt mix consisting of:		
Salt	30 g (1 oz)	1.5 tablespoons
Lite Salt	30 g (1 oz)	1.5 tablespoons
Magnesium sulfate	30 g (1 oz)	1.5 tablespoons
Calcium carbonate	30 g (1 oz)	1.5 tablespoons
Glucose/dextrose	60 g (2 oz)	3 tablespoons (optional)

Commercial vitamin/mineral supplement containing vitamins A, D, and B-complex and trace minerals

Overnight	2.0 kg dampened grass hay	

During routine training at varied exercise intensity for 30 to 40 minutes daily, the requirements of a 400- to 450-kg (900–1000-lb) polo horse would be satisfied on a diet as recommended in Table 16-6, with a decrease in bulk of the ration by providing the total grain intake as 50% barley or oats and 50% corn. Polyunsaturated oils, such as corn oil, are also useful to increase energy density, with grain intake and protein supplementation manipulated as outlined in the notes for early training (p. 423).

Showjumpers/Hunters/Western Pleasure Horses

Showjumpers, hunters, and roping/cutting horses train and compete at medium intensities, with a ration requirement for a 500- to 550-kg (1100–1200-lb) horse similar to the diet outlined in Table 16-6 in energy and protein requirements. The substitution of barley for corn and corn oil as a slow-release energy source and reducing the bulk of the ration in horses to meet appetite limits are practical ways of ensuring adequate performance and manageable temperament.

Hack/Dressage Horses

While performance demand in terms of speed is not required for these horses, adequate energy must be provided to meet 40 to 60 minutes of daily training, while maintaining a controllable temperament and optimal coat and body condition.

Grain intake is normally limited to 2 to 2.5 kg (4.5–5.5 lb) daily for a 500- to 550-kg (1100–1200-lb) equestrian horse, with roughage intake increased by 50% on levels outlined in Table 16-6. The use of corn oil as an alternative energy source is recommended for horses with nervous temperaments. Since good coat condition is essential, addition of 60 ml (2 oz) corn oil daily to the basic ration promotes a glossy hair coat, which is aided by a vitamin/mineral supplement containing vitamins A and D, iron, copper, and zinc. Supplementation with vitamin E may be reduced to alternate days, particularly where natural-source vitamin E is used.

Endurance/Trail Riding Horses

The sports of endurance riding and, to a lesser extent, trail riding have grown in popularity. Endurance horses undergo long-term conditioning over a period of many months leading up to a competitive ride. Most top endurance horses are trained for up to 2 to 3 years to prepare them for regular competition. Many have access to daily grazing, with concentrate feeds being provided in the morning and evening.

Studies have indicated that endurance horses expend up to ten times more energy in a 100-km (60-mi) ride than a racing horse in a distance race. However, many successful Arabian-bred endurance horses receive only half the amounts of cereal grain of racing horses. Endurance horses seem to be more sensitive to carbohydrate intake than other performance horses. Fats, such as corn and vegetable oils, can boost the energy density of the ration, and metabolism of fats at medium-intensity exercise may have a glycogen-sparing effect in endurance horses.

Where horses are regularly trained over 10 to 15 km (6 to 8 mi) daily, use of corn and fat in the ration will increase energy density to enable the horse to consume adequate energy to its appetite limit (Table 16-8). Corn oil ranging in volumes from 500 ml (1 pint or 2 cups) to 1 L (2 pints or 4 cups), divided between morning and evening feeds, has been used with success in endurance horses on minimal grain diets. Oils and fats should be introduced in a stepwise manner until the desired dose is reached in 7 to 10 days. Additional vitamin E (250 IU vitamin E per cup of oil in addition to 1000 IU vitamin E, the standard daily supplementation) is recommended, as well as 1 cup protein meal (e.g., soybean) per cup of fat added in excess of the first cup of oil.

Adequate fiber from grazing or hay is essential to maintain efficient digestive function on grain and fat-concentrate diets. Fiber traps water in the large bowel and may provide a fluid reservoir to replace sweat loss and combat dehydration during a long-distance ride. However, excessive fiber intake increases digestive bulk and body weight and may reduce competitiveness.

Supplements of calcium to maintain skeletal integrity and replace sweat loss during prolonged training periods must be provided in concentrate feeds. Daily provision of trace elements such as copper, iron, zinc, manganese, and selenium to 50% NRC (1989) levels in a commercial supplement is also recommended.

Supplements of 25,000 IU vitamin A, 1000 IU vitamin E, and a range of B-complex vitamins are beneficial to maintain appetite, general vitality, and stamina in endurance horses. Doses of 3000 to 4000 IU vitamin E daily for 7 to 10 days prior to competition are often provided. Electrolyte depletion from sweat losses of up to 10 to 20 L daily during training in hot weather must be replaced by daily supplementation of salt mixes containing sodium, potassium, chloride, magnesium, and calcium to help prevent dehydration, exercise myopathies, and synchronous diaphragmatic flutter (the "thumps").

The first requirement after exercise is water, followed by electrolytes and feed.

Endurance Training Notes

Refer to general feeding notes for early training (p. 423). Feeding for competition involves the following:

1. *Preride Feeding:* Many riders reduce roughage levels to reduce digestive mass and body weight during the 4 to 5 days prior to a competitive ride. This can be achieved by increasing corn by 25%

TABLE 16–8. Dietary Guidelines: Endurance Horse

Body weight: Endurance horse, 400 to 450 kg (900–1000 lb)
Stage of training: 15 to 20 km daily ride at walk, trot, and canter
Frequency of feeding: Daily grazing, stabled overnight, two concentrate feeds daily
Provision: 80% NRC (1989) requirements from concentrates, 20% pasture contribution

Ingredient	Weight	Approx. Volume
Morning Feed		
Rolled barley or whole oats	1.5 kg (3 lb)	3 L (5.5 pints)
Corn	450 kg (1 lb)	600 ml (1 pint)
Alfalfa cubes	1.0 kg (2 lb)	2 L (3.5 pints)
Polyunsaturated oil	250 ml (8 oz)	1 cup
Vitamin E	1250–1500 IU	—
Salt	30 g (1 oz)	1.5 tablespoons
Midday–Early Afternoon Feed		
Depending on grazing intake, provide up to 1.0 kg (2 lb) dampened, dust-free grass or alfalfa hay to appetite.		
Evening Feed		
Rolled barley or whole oats	1.0 kg (2 lb)	2 L (3.5 pints)
Corn	450 g (1.5 lb)	600 ml (1 pint)
Alfalfa cubes	1.5 kg (3 lb)	3 L (5.5 pints)
Soybean meal	150 g (5 oz)	1 cup
Polyunsaturated oil	250 ml (8 oz)	1 cup
Molasses	1 cup in 1 cup warm water mixed into feed	
Dicalcium phosphate	60 g (2 oz)	3 tablespoons
Medium Sweating Horses (45 Minutes Exercise)		
Salt	30 g (1 oz)	1.5 tablespoons
Lite salt	30 g (1 oz)	1.5 tablespoons
Heavily Sweating Horses (Long Rides/Hot Weather) (45 to 60 Minutes Exercise)		
Salt mix consisting of		
Salt	30 g (1 oz)	1.5 tablespoons
Lite salt	30 g (1 oz)	1.5 tablespoons
Magnesium sulfate	30 g (1 oz)	1.5 tablespoons
Calcium carbonate	30 g (1 oz)	1.5 tablespoons
Dextrose/ glucose	60 g (2 oz)	3 tablespoons
Commercial vitamin/mineral supplement containing vitamins A, D, and B-complex and trace minerals		
Overnight	1.0 kg dampened grass hay	

and replacing overnight grass hay with 1 kg (2 lb) alfalfa hay to maintain calcium and protein intake.

2. *Ride day:* On the day of the ride, offer a dampened mixture of 2.0 kg (4.5 lb) crushed corn and 2.0 kg (4.5 lb) broken-up alfalfa cubes dampened with 1 cup 50:50 molasses–water mix. Mix in half the evening allowance of salt mix for a heavily sweating horse. Allow free access to water until the start of the ride.

3. *During the ride:* If available, allow the horse to drink small quantities of fresh water from streams, etc. This is particularly important during a ride under hot, humid conditions. Often horses will not drink sufficiently at checkpoints because of fatigue or excitement.

4. *At the checkpoints:* Place a bucket of cool (not cold) water in reach of the horse to allow it to drink as it requires. During humid weather, where a horse has sweated heavily during a ride, it may be useful to give 40 g (1.3 oz) or 2 tablespoons of heavy sweat salt mix (see Table 16–8), made into a paste with 1 tablespoon of honey, deposited over the tongue by syringe, with access to water at all times. About 4 to 6 L (1–1.5 gal) of 50:50 corn/alfalfa sweet feed as recommended prior to the start or a commercial sweet feed may be offered at checkpoints, although many horses prefer to nibble at dampened alfalfa or sweet grass hay provided in a hay net. A similar feed with electrolytes and water can be given at completion of a ride.

Refererences

Cunha, J. T.: *Horse Feeding and Nutrition,* 2d Ed. New York: Academic Press, 1991.
Frape, D. L.: *Equine Nutrition and Feeding.* Essex, England: Longmans, 1986.
Lewis, L. D.: *Feeding and Care of the Horse.* Philadelphia: Lea & Febiger, 1982.
National Research Council: *Nutrient Requirements of Horses,* 5th Ed. Washington: National Academy of Sciences, 1989.
Snow, D. H., and Vogel, C. J.: *Equine Fitness: The Care and Training of the Athletic Horse.* London: David and Charles, 1987.

Breeding Horses

Mares

Brood mares may be classified into three groups: nonpregnant, pregnant, and lactating. Nonpregnant mares can be divided into maiden mares (fillies) and older nonpregnant mares that have bred previously.

Nonpregnant Mares

Mares in Poor Condition

In practical terms, thin or poorly conditioned mares should be fed to give a rising plane of nutrition in the 4 to 6 weeks until mating, and heavier mares should be maintained at a constant body weight without obesity. There is no advantage to a "flushing" feeding regimen, but poorly conditioned mares should be fed to increase body weight to a fleshy condition for breeding (Table 16-9).

Maiden Mares

Young maiden mares are often chased away from feed bins by older mares, and extra feed bins positioned away from the main feeding area should be provided to ensure that they feed without stress and disturbance. It is best to segregate maiden mares on larger breeding farms.

Mares in Training

Mares sent for breeding direct from training stables often lose condition once the high-energy ration is discontinued, and they may fail to cycle and conceive. It is best to maintain these mares on their normal ration and exercise regimens and breed the mare while in work. Once pregnancy is confirmed, the ration can be slowly reduced over a 4- to 6-week period to the level recommended for pregnancy.

Older Mares

Many older thoroughbred mares may lose condition during the winter months or as a result of teeth problems, advanced age, or heavy parasite burdens. Loss of body weight can cause inward sloping of the perineal area and increase fecal contamination of the vulva and risk of pneumovagina and breeding-tract infection. It is best to place older underweight mares into a separate group, check their teeth, treat for parasites, and feed a higher-energy ration to build up body condition and ensure a more upright perineal conformation.

Pregnant Mares

First 8 Months after Breeding

Many owners tend to overfeed pregnant mares and underfeed the lactating mares. The dietary guidelines outlined in Table 16-9 are recommended, with individual adjustments to maintain body weight. In many cases, spring pastures will maintain pregnant mares in good condition, with supplementary hay to appetite provided overnight.

TABLE 16–9. Dietary Guidelines: Mares Prior to Breeding

Body weight: 450 to 500-kg (1000–1100-lb) mare
Condition: Non-pregnant, 4 weeks before breeding, poor general condition
Frequency of feeding: Grazing, one concentrate feed daily in evening, hay overnight in sheltered area
Provision: Maintenance and 10%.

Ingredient	Weight	Approx. Volume
Rolled barley or whole oats	2.5 kg (5.5 lb)	5 L (9 pints)
Alfalfa cubes or chopped hay	2.5 kg (5.5 lb)	5 L (9 pints)
Vitamin E	500 IU	—
Salt	20 g (0.6 oz)	1 tablespoon
Molasses	1 cup in 1 cup warm water mixed into feed	
Dicalcium phosphate	30 g (1 oz)	1.5 tablespoons
Commercial vitamin/mineral supplement containing vitamin A		
Overnight	2.0 kg dampened grass or alfalfa hay or *ad lib* in hay rack; adjust the amount of feed to achieve and maintain a fleshy body weight to time of breeding.	

However, in winter grazing, availability should be monitored daily and supplementary concentrates or hay provided to pony mares, particularly if grazing is restricted due to adverse weather, to avoid hyperlipemia.

Last 90 Days Prior to Foaling

The energy, protein, and calcium intake should increase during the last 90 days of gestation as the unborn foal makes half its growth during this period. The increase in energy, protein, and calcium can be achieved by substituting 3 kg (6.6 lb) alfalfa hay for grass hay as a supplementary feed. Alternatively, each month until foaling, add an extra 500 g (1 lb) barley or oats, 100 g (3 oz) soybean meal, and 20 g (0.6 oz) or 1 tablespoon dicalcium phosphate to the ration outlined in Table 16-9.

Pastured mares will usually exercise sufficiently to maintain a good body condition without excessive weight gain. Exercise can be encouraged by locating feeding and watering facilities well apart. Where a heavily pregnant mare is confined to a small yard, regular walking on the lead for 15 to 20 minutes at least every second day will provide beneficial exercise.

Lactating Mares

The dietary intake of the lactating mare must be monitored carefully because the mare must produce adequate milk to feed her foal as well as maintain fertility and body weight to breed back in the current season. A good-quality ration also will serve as a cofeed for the foal to encourage it to develop individual eating habits, which can help reduce nutritional stress at weaning (Table 9-10).

In overly fat mares, it is important to avoid weight loss during the first 2 to 3 months of lactation; otherwise, milk production and subsequent fertility may be reduced. The peak of lactation occurs 6 to 8 weeks after foaling, with mares producing up to 3% of their body weight in milk each day. The failure of many lactating mares to breed successfully within the first 3 months after foaling may be related to deficiencies of energy, protein, and phosphorus content of the diet below those required for breeding. In cold weather, the concentrate ration of a lactating mare should be increased by 10% to 15% to meet elevated demands for maintenance.

Lactation: 3 Months to Weaning

Once a mare has passed her lactation peak, then the demand for energy, protein, calcium, and phosphorus is reduced. Using the ration outlined in Table 16-10 for a 500-kg (1100-lb) mare, the amount of grain can be reduced by 500 g (1 lb) per month, the soybean and bran omitted, and the dicalcium phosphate reduced to 60 g (2 oz) daily, with hay fed to appetite to maintain a good body condition. If the mare failed to conceive during the first 3 months of

TABLE 16–10. Dietary Guidelines: Mares–Lactation

Body weight: 500-kg (1100-lb) mare
Condition: First 3 months of lactation
Frequency of feeding: Grazing, one concentrate feed daily in evening, hay overnight in sheltered area
Provision: 80% NRC (1989) supplemented by grazing on spring pastures; the processed grain in the ration enables it to be used as a cofeed for a foal.

Ingredient	Weight	Approx. Volume
Rolled barley or crushed oats	3.0 kg (6.6 lb)	6 L (11 pints)
Cracked corn	1.5 kg (3 lb)	2.5 L (5 pints)
Alfalfa cubes or chopped hay	4.0 kg (9 lb)	8 L (14.5 pints)
Soybean meal	300 g (10 oz)	2 cups
Wheat bran	450 g (1 lb)	2.5 L (5 pints)
Salt	30 g (1 oz)	1.5 tablespoons
Molasses	1 cup in 2 cups warm water mixed into feed	
Vitamin E	500 IU	—
Dicalcium phosphate	120 g (4 oz)	6 tablespoons

Commercial vitamin/mineral supplement containing vitamin A, vitamin D, zinc, copper, and other trace minerals
1.0 kg (2.2 lb) supplementary alfalfa or grass hay can be provided to appetite, depending on pasture availability.

lactation, then the energy level of the ration should be maintained to avoid body-weight loss until the mare is bred successfully.

STALLIONS
Breeding Season

In practice, the nutritional need during the breeding season is related to the condition of the stallion and the number of times he is bred each week. Some stud owners prefer stallions in "show condition" to exhibit to visiting owners of mares, but breeding stallions should not be allowed to become excessively fat. A diet containing 12% to 13% protein is adequate for breeding purposes, since higher-protein diets are unlikely to increase fertility and libido. Only good-quality feeds and hays should be used. Stallions should be kept fit by regular exercise by lunging for 5 to 10 minutes every 1 to 2 days, but excessive exercise may lead to fatigue and reduced breeding libido.

A diet as outlined in Table 16-6 for a horse in training, omitting the corn, would be adequate to maintain a 500-kg (1100-lb) working stallion during the breeding season. A daily supplement of 60 ml polyunsaturated oil will help promote coat condition.

References

Cunha, J. T.: *Horse Feeding and Nutrition,* 2d Ed. New York: Academic Press, 1991.

Donaghue, S., Meacham, T. N., and Kronfeld, D. S.: A Conceptual Approach to Optimal Nutrition of Brood Mares. In *Veterinary Clinics of North America: Equine Practice (Clinical Nutrition).* Philadelphia: W.B. Saunders, 1990, p. 373.

Frape, D. L.: *Equine Nutrition and Feeding.* Essex, England: Longmans, 1986.

Lawrence, L. M.: Nutrition and Fuel Utilization in the Athletic Horse. In *Veterinary Clinics of North America: Equine Practice (Clinical Nutrition).* Philadelphia: W.B. Saunders, 1990, p. 393.

Lewis, L. D.: *Feeding and Care of the Horse.* Philadelphia: Lea & Febiger, 1982.

National Research Council: *Nutrient Requirements of Horses.* Washington: National Academy of Sciences, 1989.

Clinical Nutrition of Sick Horses

Horses often become inappetent following minor disease, injury, or excessively hard work. The provision of a more palatable diet, along with oral or parenteral supplementation with B-complex vitamins, may improve the horse's interest in feed and allow it to regain its appetite.

The recovery and health of horses suffering from trauma, sepsis, or specific organ disease will be enhanced by especially formulated diets. The diet formulated for sick horses must be palatable, meet the specific needs of the animal, and in the case of recovery from organ disease, avoid overloads that could delay recovery. Diets can be formulated either for complete nutritional support or partial supplementation, depending on the horse's appetite and ability to eat and digest feeds.

The dietary guidelines are based on a 450-kg (1000-lb) adult horse and can be apportioned to individual patient body weight. Since these specialized diets are meant only for short-term nutrition of sick horses, no special recommendations for young horses, working horses, or lactating mares are given. Adjustments to meet their specific needs may be necessary if the diets are fed for extended periods.

Infection and Sepsis

Septic conditions commonly encountered in horses include peritonitis, pleural effusion, and severe cellulitis following trauma. Prompt nutritional intervention may improve a horse's clinical state and retard the rate of catabolism and amino acid drain that occurs in severely traumatized horses and horses with septic conditions.

KEY POINT ► Horses recovering from sepsis require a digestible, highly palatable diet that is rich in available nutrients.

Since the infection itself may be partitioning nutrients from general metabolism, higher amounts of protein, energy, B-complex vitamins, and vitamins E and C are required to supplement normal gut synthesis of vitamins and maximize the immune response to infection during the recovery phase (Table 16-11).

Chopped apples and carrots may be useful to rekindle interest in feeding. Good-quality alfalfa hay (dampened) or Timothy hay can be provided to appetite. In stabled horses, fresh green grass [1.5 kg (3 lb)] may stimulate interest in feed. For growing horses, add an extra 1 cup of soybean meal and 60 g (2 oz) dicalcium phosphate to total ration daily, and feed *ad lib.*

Wheat bran [225 g (8 oz)] may be soaked in boiling water and added to the mix when warm. Boiled linseed meal (15 minutes boiling, then cool) is often more palatable for sick horses than soybean meal initially, with 350 g (12 oz) soybean meal being substituted with 450 g (1 lb) boiled linseed meal to maintain protein intake, gradually phasing in soy-

TABLE 16–11. Dietary Guidelines: Severe Trauma or Infection

Body weight: Adult, 450 kg (1000 lb)
Frequency of feeding: Divide into two or three feeds daily, hay *ad lib*
Provision: Maintenance plus 20%

Ingredient	Weight	Approx. Volume
Cracked corn	2.0 kg (4.5 lb)	3 L (5.5 pints)
Boiled barley (wet)	2.0 kg (4.5 lb)	3 L (5.5 pints)
Soybean meal	350 g (12 oz)	2.5 cups
Alfalfa cubes	2.0 kg (4.5 lb)	4 L (7.5 pints)
Polyunsaturated oil	250 ml (8 oz)	1 cup
Brewers yeast	60 g (2 oz)	4 tablespoons
Vitamin E	1000 IU	—
Dicalcium phosphate	60 g (2 oz)	3 tablespoons
Salt	20 g (0.6 oz)	1 tablespoon
Molasses	1 cup with 1 cup hot water mixed into feed	

bean meal over 5 to 7 days as the appetite is regained.

KEY POINT ► Overloading with energy and amino acids must be avoided, since excessive nutrient intake can lead to other complications such as laminitis and diarrhea during the recovery phase.

Good-quality commercial sweet feeds containing 12% to 14% protein, fortified with 1 cup of soybean meal per 2.5 kg (5.5 lb) good-quality sweet feed with added molasses, often helps to improve the appetite and provide additional nutrients. Brewers yeast [60 g (2 oz)] added to this mix or, alternatively, an oral vitamin B-complex supplement may help stimulate the appetite.

A parenteral dose of vitamin B complex daily, or on alternate days, may help to improve general well-being and appetite. Theoretically, provision of up to 10 g vitamin C, 1000 IU vitamin E, and a supplement containing 25,000 IU vitamin A and 200 g zinc may be beneficial to aid healing in the case of burns and large areas of traumatized skin and tissue. In the case of peritonitis, it is best to offer small amounts of feed up to 2.0 kg (4.5 lb) every 4 to 6 hours to avoid digestive overload from large, infrequent feeds and minimize insulin responses to large intakes of carbohydrate in less frequent feeds.

Often sick or inappetent horses can be tempted with chopped apples or carrots, and many prefer to nibble fresh grass or dampened hay from the floor of the stable. In severe cases where the horse is totally inappetent, force feeding of a slurry by nasogastric tube is required (Table 16-12).

The alfalfa cubes should be soaked in warm water until swollen and then should be broken up to mix into a slurry. The amount of feed can be adjusted, increasing as the animal's clinical condition improves over 7 to 10 days. Provide *ad lib* good-quality dampened grass hay or fresh green feed, if available, to reduce boredom between meals and encourage interest in food.

Esophageal Disease

In horses with esophageal complications, semiliquid or slurry diets may be passed through an indwelling nasogastric tube or through an esophagostomy entrance placed in the middle to lower third of the neck. Dietary guidelines for a slurry diet are suggested under trauma and infection (Table 16-12) and may be administered every 8 hours. The animal should be observed regularly for signs of metabolic complications such as laminitis and medical problems such as diarrhea.

Enterolithiasis

Manipulation of the diet to reduce cecal pH has been reported to be effective in decreasing the recurrence of enteroliths in susceptible horses. Provision of a diet as suggested for a 450-kg (1000-lb) geriatric horse is suitable, with the addition of 120 ml (4 oz) or ½ cup apple cider vinegar to each of two feeds daily or 250 ml (8 oz) or 1 cup to a single feed and may decrease the incidence of enteroliths.

TABLE 16–12. Dietary Guidelines: Severe Burns, Trauma, and Inappetence

Body weight: Adult, 450 kg (1000 lb)
Frequency of feeding: Every 8 hours (3 times daily)
Provision: Maintenance plus 25%
Slurry composition feed every 8 hours

Ingredient (Each 8 Hourly Mix Contains)	Weight	Approx. Volume
Dehydrated cottage cheese	225 g (8 oz)	300 ml (0.75 pints)
Dextrose/glucose powder	120 g (4 oz)	8 tablespoons
Alfalfa cubes	1.0 kg (2 lb)	1.5 L (3 pints)
Polyunsaturated oil	125 ml (4 oz)	0.5 cup
Salt	15 g (0.5 oz)	1 tablespoon
Dicalcium phosphate	20 g (0.6 oz)	1 tablespoon
Brewers yeast	20 g (0.6 oz)	1 tablespoon
Vitamin E	500 IU	—
Vitamin C	2.5 g	1/2 teaspoon
Water	qs to a liquid slurry suitable for flow through a large-bore nasogastric tube [approx. 4 L (7 pints)]	

Where these diets are found to encourage wood chewing as triggered by reduced cecal pH, 2.0 kg (4.5 lb) grass hay dampened with 50:50 molasses–water solution in a trough and offered overnight to stabled horses may reduce the risk of this chewing habit.

Chronic Diarrhea

In most cases, diarrhea in adult horses results from large bowel dysfunction. Common primary causes include an abnormal or disrupted fermentation process, chemical- or plant-induced hypermotility of the bowel, altered fluid absorption, and physical irritation of the bowel wall in heavily parasitized horses. Release of large numbers of hypobiotic cyathostomes from gut reservoirs 4 to 7 days following anthelmintic treatment or seasonal pasture flushes also should be considered.

Resting the Large Bowel

It is unwise to fast horses to reduce large bowel activity for more than 18 to 24 hours, because hypoproteinemia may exacerbate the diarrhea. There is also an increased risk of anaerobic bacterial colonization of the divitalized, starved bowel and blood-borne septicemia.

Reduced-Residue Diets

A maintenance ration with a lower fiber residue, containing high protein with available amino acids (Table 16-13), will maintain normal small intestinal function and protein and energy uptake while reducing large bowel activity. Where available, specialized high-protein commercial liquid diets administered by nasogastric tube will minimize residues and rest the large bowel.

Reestablishing Normal Fermentation

If abnormal fermentation is suspected following a history of chronic diarrhea or high-dose antibiotic therapy, as evidenced by passage of poorly fermented food or sour, pasty-type feces following grain overload, large bowel flora can be reestablished in otherwise clinically normal horses (Table 16-14). A diet higher in chopped fiber should be fed to encourage fermentation. Diets with a high alfalfa content can prolong recovery, so it may be beneficial to use a fiber base of chopped grass hay dampened to reduce dust.

Specialized commercial *acidophilus* cultures are available from health food shops for human use and may be used at 5 to 7 times human dose for a 450-kg (1000-lb) horse. These cultures may be given for 2 to 3 days initially, divided between two feeds, and continued for 4 to 5 days if response is slow.

Diarrhea in Working Horses

Occasionally, horses in training will develop a low-grade chronic form of diarrhea on higher-energy rations, and this may respond to a dry bland diet (Table 16-15) while enabling the horse to stay in training. Once the consistency of the feces has returned to normal, gradually change back to the normal racing diet.

Provide good-quality grass hay *ad lib* overnight. Avoid feeding alfalfa hay or cubes initially, but these may be gradually reintroduced over 4 to 5 days for half the grass hay overnight as a choice, reducing the calcium carbonate to 30 g (1 oz). Nat-

TABLE 16–13. Dietary Guidelines: Persistent Diarrhea

Body weight: Adult, 450 kg (1000 lb)
Frequency of feeding: Divide into four feeds daily [approx. 2 L (3.5 pints) per feed]
Provision: Maintenance

Ingredient	Weight	Approx. Volume
Cracked corn	2 kg (4.4 lb)	3.5 L (6.5 pints)
Soybean meal	450 g (1 lb)	3 cups
Boiled linseed meal	300 g (10 oz)	2 cups
Polyunsaturated oil	375 ml (13 oz)	1.5 cups
Alfalfa cubes	1.0 kg (2 lb)	2 L (4 pints)
Brewers yeast	60 g (2 oz)	3 tablespoons
Salt	60 g (2 oz)	3 tablespoons
Vitamin E	1000 IU	—
Molasses	Half cup in half cup hot water mixed into feed	
If acidotic, add 60 g (3 tablespoons) sodium bicarbonate to morning and evening feeds		

TABLE 16–14. Dietary Guidelines: Reestablishment of Large Bowel Fermentation

Body weight: Adult, 450 kg (1000 lb)
Frequency of feeding: Divide into three feeds daily
Provision: Maintenance

Ingredient	Weight	Approx. Volume
Rolled barley/oats	2.0 kg (4.5 lb)	3.5 L (6 pints)
Alfalfa cubes	3.0 kg (6.5 lb)	6 L (11 pints)
Wheat bran	400 g (1 lb)	2 L (4.0 pints)
Brewers yeast	60 g (2 oz)	3 tablespoons
Dicalcium phosphate	30 g (1 oz)	1.5 tablespoons
Salt	20 g (0.6 oz)	1 tablespoon
Molasses	1 cup in 1 cup hot water mixed into feed	
Mixed into each feed prior to feeding:		
Yogurt (natural)	100 ml (3 oz)	5 tablespoons
Alternatively, the yogurt can be given over the tongue prior to feeding.		
Good-quality grass hay can be offered *ad lib* to increase roughage mass for fermentation.		

TABLE 16–15. Dietary Guidelines: Low-Grade Diarrhea in Working Horses

Body weight: 450 kg (1000 lb)
Frequency of feeding: Divide into three equal feeds
Provision: 30 minutes medium-intensity exercise daily

Ingredient	Weight	Approx. Volume
Rolled barley	3.5 kg (7.5 lb)	6.5 L (12 pints)
Cracked corn	2.0 kg (4.5 lb)	3 L (5.5 pints)
Soybean meal	450 g (1 lb)	3 cups
Wheat, fine middling or flour	225 g (8 oz)	2 cups
Grated apples, red	6	(Let stand for 1–3 hours after grating before mixing into feed)
Grass hay, chopped	900 g (2 lb)	6 L (11 pints)
Glucose powder (sweetener)	100 g (3 oz)	6 tablespoons
Salt	60 g (2 oz)	3 tablespoons
Lite salt	30 g (1 oz)	1.5 tablespoons
Calcium carbonate	60 g (2 oz)	3 tablespoons
Dicalcium phosphate	60 g (2 oz)	3 tablespoons
Vitamin E	1000 IU	

Commercial vitamin/mineral supplement
The ration may be slightly dampened with warm water.

ural-flavored yogurt [60 ml (3 oz)] may be given by syringe over the tongue prior to the morning and evening feeds for 2 to 3 days if reduced fermentation is suspected.

Renal Disease

A short-term maintenance diet to restrict protein, calcium, and phosphorus intake should be considered for horses with renal disease.

KEY POINT ▶ Limitation of calcium intake is necessary in equine patients to prevent hypercalcemia.

The diet should be based on grass hay or chopped hay with a low protein energy source such as corn, oats, or brown rice (Table 16-16). Legume hays or chopped alfalfa hay or pellets should be avoided to limit protein and calcium intake, and wheat bran should be eliminated because of its high phosphorus content.

In inappetent horses, divide the ration into four equal parts, add sufficient water to make a slurry, and administer by nasogastric tube every 6 hours until the horse regains its appetite. A parenteral dose once daily of B-complex vitamins also may help to stimulate the appetite.

TABLE 16–16. Dietary Guidelines: Renal Disease

Body weight: Adult, 450 kg (1000 lb)
Frequency of feeding: Divide into three feeds daily
Provision: Maintenance

Ingredient	Weight	Approx. Volume
Crushed oats	1.4 kg (3 lb)	3 L (5.5 pints)
Boiled barley (wet weight)	1.4 kg (3 lb)	2.5 L (4.5 pints)
Cracked corn	1.0 kg (2 lb)	1.5 L (3 pints)
Cereal chopped hay	2.0 kg (4.5 lb)	11 L (21 pints)
Brewers yeast	30 g (1 oz)	1.5 tablespoons
Molasses	1 cup in 1 cup water, mixed into feed	
Salt	20 g (0.6 oz)	1 tablespoon

Good-quality grass hay should be provided, approximately 2 kg, to appetite.

Hepatic Disease

The liver is the first organ to receive nutrients after absorption from the bowel lumen. Where reduced hepatic function is present, diets must provide energy and protein in addition to maintenance requirements to allow normal regenerative processes. There is no need to restrict protein below maintenance, but good-quality protein sources must be provided, based mainly on cereal grains and hays, to reduce hepatic overload with aromatic amino acids. Small amounts of soybean meal may be provided to ensure adequate protein intake. Although polyunsaturated oils are useful to boost energy intake, they should be avoided because hepatic accumulation may occur as a result of reduced metabolic function.

Supplementary B-complex vitamins, either orally or parenterally, and oral vitamin E are recommended. Small, frequent feeds, preferably six times daily, are useful to avoid peak loading of the liver (Table 16-17).

Since many horses with liver disease have reduced appetite, provision of 1.0 kg (2 lb) fresh grass, morning and evening, may improve interest in food and provide additional roughage without risking excessive energy intake. Avoid legume greenfeed.

Geriatric Horses

Aged horses in retirement at pasture often lose condition during winter or summer when the pasture is sparse or dry, despite adequate supplementary hay. Health problems related to poor dentition, thyroid-pituitary adenomas, and reduced ability to digest fiber and protein and absorb phosphorus, as compared with young horses, also may result in weight loss and reduced appetite. Old mares have been shown to have lower plasma vitamin C levels as compared with younger horses.

TABLE 16–17. Dietary Guidelines: Hepatic Disease

Body weight: Adult, 450 kg (1000 lb)
Frequency of feeding: Divided into six feeds daily
Provision: Maintenance

Ingredient	Weight	Approx. Volume
Cracked corn	1.4 g (3 lb)	1 L (3.5 pints)
Rolled barley	2.0 kg (4.5 lb)	3.5 L (6.5 pints)
Cereal chopped hay	2.0 kg (4.5 lb)	11 L (21 pints)
Soybean meal	250 g (8 oz)	2 cups
Molasses	1 cup in 1 cup warm water mixed into feed	
Dicalcium phosphate	30 g (1 oz)	1.5 tablespoons
Calcium carbonate	60 g (2 oz)	3 tablespoons
Salt	20 g (0.6 oz)	1 tablespoon
Vitamin C	10 g	2 teaspoons
Vitamin E	1000 IU	—
Commercial B-complex supplement (use in preference to brewers yeast), 60 g (2 oz)		

In old horses with poor dentition, dampened commercial pelleted feeds are convenient with added vitamins and will avoid problems such as "choke" in old horses unable to chew normal feeds effectively. A suggested diet for geriatric horses is given in Table 16-18.

Boiled barley [3.0 kg (6.5 lb) wet weight] can be added during cold weather or as a twice-weekly

TABLE 16–18. Dietary Guidelines: Geriatric Horse

Body weight: Adult, 450 kg (1000 lb)
Frequency of feeding: Divide into two feeds daily, one where good pasture is available
Provision: Maintenance plus 10%

Ingredient	Weight	Approx. Volume
Rolled barley	2.0 kg (4.5 lb)	4 L (7 pints)
Crushed corn	2.0 kg (4.5 lb)	3 L (5 pints)
Soybean meal	250 g (8 oz)	2 cups
Alfalfa cubes	1.0 kg (2 lb)	2 L (4 pints)
Dicalcium phosphate	30 g (1 oz)	1.5 tablespoons
Calcium carbonate	30 g (1 oz)	1.5 tablespoons
Salt	20 g (0.6 oz)	1 tablespoon
Molasses	1 cup in 2 cups warm water to soften feed soaked for 30–60 minutes before feeding; add only-half volume of water if boiled barley used	
A commercial mineral/vitamin supplement may be added for horses in poor condition.		

treat. Additional calcium should be added to the ration of horses over 16 years of age owing to less efficient uptake, increasing dicalcium phosphate to 90 g (3 oz) or 5 tablespoons daily. However, in old horses with renal disease, the calcium supplement, soybean, and alfalfa should be restricted to half the recommended amount. An equivalent amount of grass or chopped hay should be added to replace the roughage contributed by the alfalfa cubes in this case.

In old mares, 5 g (1.5 teaspoons) daily of vitamin C (ascorbic acid) may be included in the ration. If extra roughage is provided, dampened chopped alfalfa or grass hays are preferable in old horses with poor dentition where hay cannot be fully utilized. The ration can be divided into two feeds where grazing is restricted or given as a night feed where pasture is palatable and the horse is able to graze during the day. Alternatively, for a 450-kg (1000-lb) aged horse, a pelleted ration [3 Mcal (12.6 MJ)/kg 10%–12% crude protein] can be offered at the rate of 4 kg (9 lb) mixed into 2.0 kg (4.5 lb) alfalfa cubes dampened with 1 cup molasses in 2 cups warm water to soften the meal as an evening feed or divided into two feeds.

During cold weather or when the aged horse needs to gain body weight, the ration volume can be increased by 15% to 20% and adjusted to appetite and condition.

KEY POINT ▶ Where appetite is reduced or other internal disease limits the bulk or volume that can be consumed, grain content can be decreased and vegetable oils added to increase energy density.

The general substitution rate is 1 cup [250 ml (8 oz)] vegetable oil replaces 4 cups pellets or 6 cups crushed oats or 3 cups crushed corn. Normally, up to 2 cups of vegetable oil can be mixed into the ration, with a corresponding reduction in grain content. When the grain content is reduced by the inclusion of oil, introduce oil on a step-wise increment over 5 to 7 days, and add an extra cup of soybean meal per cup of oil added, to meet protein needs. Ensure adequate roughage by providing additional alfalfa cubes to make up the volume of the ration.

Fattening an Underweight Horse

The three most common causes of poor condition in horses are heavy parasite burdens, teeth problems, and inadequate quantities or poor quality of feeds. Feeding times interrupted by vices, such as aerophagia or "windsucking," can result in ill-thrift despite an adequate ration. An individual horse's likes and dislikes may affect appetite and feed acceptance. Position in the group pecking order in a herd of grazing horses can affect feed intake in those intimidated by aggression. Sudden withdrawal of high-energy rations when a horse is turned out from training can lead to significant weight loss in 7 to 10 days.

Once the underlying cause of weight loss is recognized and remedied, a step-wise increase in the quality and quantity of the ration, complemented by appropriate exercise, will assist recovery (Table 16-19).

KEY POINT ► The improvement in health and condition should be incremental over a 6- to 8-week period to avoid metabolic and digestive problems.

A repeat deworming 3 weeks after the initial treatment will remove developing cyathostomes released from hypobiotic gut reservoirs within 4 to 7 days of the initial worming in horses where high *Strongyloides* spp. fecal egg counts were part of the underlying cause of ill-thrift.

Reducing the Weight of a Fat Horse

Dietary restriction and controlled exercise can be used to reduce body weight in an obese horse. Obesity is a common problem in horses on rations that exceed their energy and exercise needs. It is best to provide low-energy feeds and water with adequate protein, vitamins, minerals, and electrolytes combined with controlled exercise.

Horses should not be denied feed, since this may lead to hypoproteinemia and perhaps reduced immune competence. Ponies and some thoroughbreds are particularly susceptible to hyperlipidemia by fasting. Overweight ponies with laminitis should not be starved.

In horses with access to good-quality pasture, restricting grazing to 30 minutes each morning and evening, with provision of 250 g (8 oz) low-energy cereal hay per 100 kg (220 lb) of body weight overnight to prevent boredom, is effective when complemented by 10 to 20 minutes of daily aerobic exercise at the trot and loping canter under saddle or on the lunge. Horses should be confined to a bare yard or stable in cold weather with unpalatable bedding of rice hulls or saw dust.

A ration to provide half the maintenance energy, plus adequate protein, minerals, and vitamins (Table 16-20), will assist in weight loss.

Horses at Rest

Mature horses that have retired or rested at grass will maintain body condition on good-quality pasture. Supplementary feed of good-quality alfalfa or cereal-mixed hay may be offered when pasture is sparse, short, or of poor feed value. A commercial ration or pelleted concentrate feed may be necessary when a horse is kept indoors for the winter period. Some guidelines for maintenance of a horse at rest are given in Table 16-21.

TABLE 16–19. Dietary Guidelines: Increasing Body Weight

Body weight: Adult, 400 kg (900 lb)
Condition: Thin, 50 to 100 kg (100–220 lb) underweight
Frequency of feeding: Divide into three feeds for stabled horses, with supplementary hay; one feed daily in pastured horses, with supplementary hay if required
Provision: Maintenance plus 30% with light exercise

Ingredient	Weight	Approx. Volume
Rolled barley or whole oats	1.5 kg (3 lb)	3 L (5.5 pints)
Cracked corn	1.0 kg (2 lb)	1.5 L (3 pints)
Alfalfa, crushed or cubes	2.0 kg (4.5 lb)	6 L (11 pints)
Molasses	1 cup in 1 cup warm water mixed into feed if appetite poor and *ad lib* to appetite overnight.	
Brewers yeast or equivalent commercial vitamin/ mineral supplement	60 g (2 oz)	3 tablespoons
Grass hay	3.0 kg (6.5 lb) or 1.0 kg (2 lb) at each feed, *ad lib* overnight to appetite	
Salt	20 g (0.6 oz)	1 tablespoon
Ad lib alfalfa or cereal grain hay to appetite		

TABLE 16–20. Dietary Guidelines: Weight Reduction

Body weight: Adult, 600 kg (1300 lb)
Condition: 50 to 150 kg (110–330 lb) too heavy
Frequency of feeding: Divide into three feeds daily in stabled horses to prevent boredom
Provision: Low energy, encourage fat cabolism

Ingredient	Weight	Approx. Volume
Alfalfa cubes, crushed	3.0 kg (6.5 lb)	6 L (11 pints)
Oat hulls or clean chopped straw	2.0 kg (4.5 lb)	11 L (21 pints)
Soybean meal	450 g (1 lb)	3 cups
Wheat bran	180 g (6 oz)	1 L (2 pints)
Brewers yeast (or commercial B-complex supplement)	60 g (2 oz)	3 tablespoons
Salt	25 g (1 oz)	1.5 tablespoons
Dicalcium phosphate	75 g (2.5 oz)	3.5 tablespoons
Molasses	1 cup in 1 cup warm water mixed into feed to reduce dust	
Overnight in stabled horses	500 g (1 lb) grass hay or 2.0 kg (4.5 lb) green feed	

TABLE 16–21. Dietary Guidelines: Maintenance

Body weight: Adult, 450 kg (1000 lb)
Condition: Horse at rest on little pasture or confined
Frequency of feeding: One feed, hay other feed
Provision: Maintenance

Ingredient	Weight	Approx. Volume
Rolled barley	2.0 kg (4.5 lb)	4 L (7 pints)
Alfalfa cubes	2.0 kg (4.5 lb)	4 L (7 pints)
Dicalcium phosphate	30 g (1 oz)	1.5 tablespoons
Molasses	1 cup in 1 cup warm water mixed into feed	
Salt	20 g (0.6 oz)	1 tablespoons
Confined Horses		
Grass hay (usually overnight)	3.0 kg (6.5 lb)	—

Ad lib good-quality grass hay can be provided to appetite, rather than specific portions, particularly overnight in confined horses. Body weight and condition should be monitored, and the ration adjusted accordingly. Confined horses should be given some light exercise by lunging for up to 5 minutes or 30 minutes of walking daily to maintain vitality and appetite and reduce boredom.

Behavioral Disorders Associated with Feeding

Horses can show a variety of behavioral disorders such as wood chewing, eating dirt, and aggressive behavior related to feeding. Some of the common behavioral disorders, the predisposing causes, and their prevention are outlined in Table 16-22.

References

Clarke, L. L., Roberts, M. C., and Argenzio, R. A.: Feeding and Digestive Problems in Horses: Physiologic Responses to a Concentrated Meal. In *Veterinary Clinics of North America: Equine Practice (Clinical Nutrition)*. Philadelphia: W.B. Saunders, 1990, p. 433.

National Research Council: *Nutrient Requirements of Horses,* 5th Ed. Washington: National Academy of Sciences, 1989.

Ralston, S. L.: Clinical Nutrition of the Adult Horse. In *Veterinary Clinics of North America: Equine Practice (Clinical Nutrition)*. Philadelphia: W.B. Saunders, 1990, p. 339.

TABLE 16–22. Behavioral Disorders Associated with Feeding

Problem	Clinical Signs	Predisposing Causes	Dietary/Management Prevention
Behavioral eating habits	Scattering feed	Greediness Sudden feed changes Boredom	Change feed over 7–10 days Provide deep feed bins Relieve boredom in stables: hay overnight, exercise during day
	Aggressive feeding	Aggressive nature Food withdrawal Confinement and set feeding times	Feed away from other horses Firm discipline
	Impatience when feeding: kicking walls and bins, pawing floor	Unknown Impatient nature Irregular feed times	Feed horse first Ensure regularly spaced feed times in stabled horses
	Dropping of feed: quidding	Sharp-edged cheek teeth Dark feed area: feeder located in dark, solid-walled corner.	Check molar teeth for sharp edges Relocate feed bin to open area near window, aisle, doorway Ensure visual contact with other horses
	Rapid feed intake: gorging	Irregular feed times Aggressive nature Sharp-edged teeth	Check molar teeth for sharp edges Smooth stone or salt block in feeder to slow consumption Feed chopped hay 30 minutes before concentrates

TABLE 16–22. Continued

Problem	Clinical Signs	Predisposing Causes	Dietary/Management Prevention
	Slow feed intake: selective eater, poor appetite	Teeth problems Distraction at feed times Nervous, pain Unpalatable feeds Respiratory conditions Bulky feeds Early fast work	Check molar teeth for sharp edges Provide palatable feeds, reduce bulk of feeds to minimum safe levels of 0.5% roughage by body weight Treat underlying medical conditions Avoid fast exercise too early in training: introduce fast work in increments over 2–3 weeks After 1 minute rest to regain breathing and oxygenation, cooldown exercise at medium trot to reduce muscle lactic acid accumulation
Pica/abnormal eating habits	Coprophagy: eating manure	Boredom/confinement Low-fiber diets Imbalanced diets	Provide chopped hay overnight Vitamin B_{12} therapy: 5000 μg IV once weekly for 3 weeks, 1000 μg fed daily for 10–14 days Mineral/vitamin supplement Drench with 500 ml cooking oil as a single dose
	Pica, crib biting, wood chewing	Boredom/confinement Lack of phosphorus Pelleted rations Low-fiber rations	Ensure correct Ca:P ratio Cap rails, gates, etc. Deterrent preparations Dilute pellets with chopped hay or moistened cubes
	Aerophagia/windsucking, poor condition	Boredom/confinement Pleasurable sensation	Windsucking neck straps: 3-inch-wide leather strap Deterrent preparations on target surfaces
	Tail and mane chewing	Young horses in cold weather Mineral deficiencies	Deterrent preparations smeared into tail hairs Provide adequate roughage overnight, feed on time, three feeds daily
	Dirt or sand eating	Boredom/confinement Mineral deficiencies	Shift to new pastures Bimonthly drenching with mucilloids or paraffin oil [400 g (30 oz)] to remove sand Mix 60 g clay (bentonite) into feed daily for 10–14 days
	Obesity/overeating	Too much feed in relation to exercise	Reduce ration Increase exercise Do not starve ponies

TABLE 16–22. Continued

Problem	Clinical Signs	Predisposing Causes	Dietary/Management Prevention
	Nervous temperaments	Excess soluble carbohydrates in relation to exercise Heavy sweat loss	Alternate feeds: barley, sunflower seeds, rice-based feeds to limit CHO availability Tranquilizers, e.g., acepromazine orally 60 mg in feed/450 kg (1000 lb); detectable in competition horses Vitamin B_1, high dose, 3 g orally/450 kg (100 lb) daily for 3 weeks

CHAPTER 17

Therapy

Sedation and Anesthesia

The use of sedation and anesthesia is part of the daily routine of equine practice. In the past only one or two agents were available to the general practitioner, whereas now there are a wide array of sedatives and anesthetics that can be used. In this section we will not attempt to cover all agents that are available or to discuss some of the complex areas of anesthesia, which are best left to specialist textbooks. However, we will attempt to give an overview of the agents and techniques that we feel can be undertaken by the general equine practitioner.

MAKING THE DECISION FOR SEDATION OR GENERAL ANESTHESIA

- In most cases, the decision to use tranquilization or anesthesia is clear-cut. To assist in restraint for radiography and suturing of minor lacerations, short-term sedation is required, and the major decision is the extent of sedation needed.
- In other situations, such as major lacerations, cast application, cast removal, and various procedures that will result in a degree of pain, it may be necessary to choose between profound sedation and general anesthesia.

KEY POINT ▶ If a horse is not being treated in an equine hospital, the surroundings and areas for recovery from anesthesia

play important roles in making a decision for or against general anesthesia.

- If a safe induction and recovery cannot be ensured, there may be no choice other than to use sedation for the procedure or transport the horse to a hospital facility.

KEY POINT ▶ While many sedatives cause profound tranquilization and some analgesia, horses may still kick and cause injury to the operator.

- It is important to consider the position of the operator, the likely duration of the procedure, and the possibility of pain when deciding on sedation or general anesthesia.

SEDATIVES

Acepromazine (Treatment No. 1)

Background

Acepromazine has been used by equine practitioners for more than 30 years and has proven to be a safe and effective drug for mild sedation. It is one of the phenothiazine-derivative tranquilizers, the other major agent being promazine hydrochloride. It is used for minor sedation and as a preanesthetic agent.

Clinical and Pharmacologic Effects

- Because it is an alpha-2 adrenergic blocker, acepromazine causes peripheral vasodilatation and hypotension. These effects make acepromazine useful in the treatment of some cases of acute laminitis and recurrent rhabdomyolysis.
- The extent of sedation is mild, and the horse is easily roused from the sedated state. In excited horses, the drug appears to be less effective.

KEY POINT ► One of the major disadvantages of the drug for a busy practitioner is that the onset of maximum sedation is not until 20 to 30 minutes after intravenous administration. However, the duration of sedation is several hours.

- While the degree of sedation is usually reasonably consistent, in some horses there is little or no apparent sedation. In these cases, increasing the dose rate will not result in sedation, but the hypotensive effects of acepromazine will be intensified.

Contraindications

- Because acepromazine can lower systolic pressure from normal values of 120 to 80 mmHg, the drug should be avoided in any horse with signs of dehydration or shock.
- If there is any likelihood of painful stimuli during the course of the procedure, acepromazine should not be used.

KEY POINT ► The drug should not be used in stallions if there is an alternative because of the possibility of penile paralysis. This effect is also found with the other phenothiazine-derivative tranquilizers such as promazine and proprionylpromazine.

Recommended Use and Dose Rate

- The drug is useful as a preanesthetic agent and for minor procedures that do not involve any pain.
- To examine the penis and prepuce of geldings, acepromazine is very effective because it causes temporary prolapse of the penis. If the drug is to be given to a stallion, the owner should be warned of the possibility of permanent penile paralysis.
- Some practitioners use acepromazine with one of the narcotic drugs to provide some analgesia and more profound sedation than acepromazine alone.

KEY POINT ► Acepromazine is usually administered intravenously at a dose rate of 0.03 to 0.06 mg/kg (15–30 mg for a 450–500-kg horse).

- The lower dose rate is used for preanesthetic sedation. In some countries, acepromazine is also available as an oral paste.

Xylazine (Treatment No. 108)

Background

Xylazine became available to equine practitioners in the early 1970s and is now the most widely used agent for sedation and preanesthetic tranquilization. Its favor with equine practitioners is because of the rapid onset of sedation and predictable effects.

Clinical and Pharmacologic Effects

- Xylazine produces some degree of analgesia and muscle relaxation as well as profound sedation that is dose-dependent. Ataxia may be quite severe after high dose rates of xylazine.
- After an early increase in mean blood pressure, there is a dose-related decrease in pressure together with a decrease in heart rate and cardiac output and some reduction in myocardial contractility.
- An increase in vagal tone produces transient second-degree atrioventricular block.
- Its central effect is by stimulation of alpha-2 receptors.

KEY POINT ► Onset of action is within 60 seconds of IV administration, and full effect of the dose used is seen within 5 minutes. The duration of sedation is dependent on the dose used but is usually around 30 to 45 minutes.

Contraindications

- Should not be given except at reduced dose rates to horses with signs of dehydration or shock owing to its hypotensive effect and reduction in cardiac output.
- Should not be used if endoscopic examination of the larynx is required. It causes quite profound laryngeal relaxation so that laryngeal asymmetry is difficult to assess.
- In colic cases, if there is a possibility of a vascular compromise of the intestine, xylazine should be used with caution because of adverse effects on intestinal metabolism and blood supply.
- Should be avoided in mares during the last trimester of pregnancy because of the possibility of induction of parturition, although this is unlikely.
- In rare cases, profuse sweating may be seen after xylazine, and sudden death also has been reported after IV administration.

KEY POINT ► While horses can appear as though they are asleep, they may still be sensitive to stimuli. The operator should take care not to stand where he or she can be kicked or struck.

Recommended Use and Dose Rate

- Useful for minor procedures such as radiography and ultrasound examination.
- Often used in combination with a narcotic or narcotic-like drug to produce more profound sedation and/or analgesia than xylazine alone. In these cases, the xylazine should be administered 3 to 5 minutes before the narcotic.

KEY POINT ► Xylazine is given IV, and the minimum dose rate is 0.2 mg/kg (~100 mg for an adult horse), which provides a satisfactory degree of sedation for minor procedures. The maximum dose used is 1.1 mg/kg, which results in profound sedation, lowering of the head, and ataxia.

Detomidine (Treatment No. 28)

Background

Detomidine has been available to equine practitioners for the past few years and has found a place in practice as an agent that causes profound and long-lasting sedation with some analgesia.

KEY POINT ► It is a similar drug to xylazine but is more potent and produces a greater degree of sedation and analgesia.

Clinical and Pharmacologic Effects

- Detomidine produces profound sedation that is dose-dependent. There is some muscle relaxation and ataxia, which at the highest dose rates is severe.
- Detomidine is an alpha-2 agonist, and the cardiovascular effects are similar to those of xylazine.
- Second-degree atrioventricular block is common and results in a severe bradycardia.

KEY POINT ► There is a rapid onset of action after IV administration, and a peak effect is found after 5 minutes. The duration of action is variable but can be as long as 2 hours.

- Useful in performing a standing castration because of the combination of analgesia and sedation.

Contraindications

- Similar contraindications to xylazine.
- The degree of ataxia with detomidine is more severe than with xylazine, and therefore, detomidine should be avoided if ataxia is likely to be a problem.

Recommended Use and Dose Rate

Detomidine is considerably more expensive than xylazine but may be useful in situations where more profound sedation and analgesia are required than with xylazine.

KEY POINT ► Dose rates vary from 10 to 80 μg/kg (0.01–0.08 mg/kg) administered IV.

Combinations of Sedatives with Narcotics or Narcotic-Like Drugs

Background

KEY POINT ► The narcotic and narcotic-like drugs are useful when combined with one of the sedatives (acepromazine, xylazine, or detomidine) to produce more profound sedation than the sedative effect with some analgesias.

Most of the narcotics will result in central nervous system stimulation when used without a sedative. When using the combination of sedatives and narcotics, the sedative should be administered at least 5 minutes prior to the narcotic.

Clinical and Pharmacologic Effects

- Before the advent of the newer sedatives and narcotic-like drugs, most equine practitioners used acepromazine together with meperidine. This combination was extremely useful but sometimes caused profound sweating and, occasionally, excitement.
- Most combinations of sedatives and narcotics do not produce the degree of arterial hypotension that is found when the sedatives are administered alone.
- There is profound sedation and ataxia with most combinations. Horses are reluctant to move, and the head drops close to the ground.
- The extent of analgesia is related to the potency of the narcotic or narcotic-like drug used. However, in all cases, the analgesia is much greater than when the sedatives are used alone.

Contraindications

- Excitement may occur if the narcotic or narcotic-like drug is administered before the sedative effects are apparent.

KEY POINT ► With some narcotics (particularly morphine), excitement may be seen after the effect of the sedative wears off because of the longer duration of action of the narcotic.

- Should not be used in situations where ataxia is likely to be a problem.

Recommended Use and Dose Rate

- The combination of drugs is not used as much in practice since the introduction of detomidine, which causes similar sedation and some analgesia.
- We still find the combination of sedatives and narcotics to be useful to perform standing castrations, standing patellar desmotomy, and suturing some severe lacerations.
- The combination of sedatives and narcotics should not be used in foals.
- The suggested dose rates for the various combinations are presented in Table 17-1. Other drug combinations also have been used, including the combination of acepromazine, xylazine, and a narcotic or narcotic-like drug.

ANESTHETICS

Intravenous Anesthesia

In routine equine practice, most veterinarians use intravenous short-term anesthesia for procedures that require 5 to 30 minutes of general anesthesia. Prior to administration of the induction agent, a sedative is given, which results in smoother induction and recovery from anesthesia. We prefer small doses of xylazine (0.2–0.3 mg/kg) as preanesthetic sedative, which at these dose rates has little effect on cardiovascular function. No other premedicant is necessary in horses.

It is important that food be withheld for a few hours before anesthesia and that the mouth be washed out prior to anesthetic induction.

KEY POINT ▶ In case of obstruction to the airway, an endotracheal tube should

always be available prior to induction of anesthesia, even if maintenance with a gaseous agent is not planned.

▶ Thiobarbiturates

Background

Chloral hydrate combinations (with magnesium sulfate and pentobarbitone) were widely used for intravenous anesthesia before the thiobarbiturates became available in the late 1950s. Since then, the thiobarbiturates have been the most commonly used induction agents prior to gaseous anesthesia. The two most commonly used thiobarbiturates are *thiopental* (Pentothal, Sanofi, Overland Park, KS) and *thiamylal* (Anestatal, Fermenta, Kansas City, MO; Bio-Tal, Bio-Ceutic, St. Joseph, MO).

KEY POINT ▶ These agents may be used as sole induction agents where they result in anesthesia of short duration (5–10 minutes) or in combination with guaifenesin where the duration of anesthesia is longer (10–20 minutes).

Clinical Use

- Both drugs are similar, but some clinical experience indicates that thiamylal may result in a slightly smoother recovery than thiopental.
- The drugs are administered IV rapidly (<5 s) in a 10% solution (add 50 ml of saline or sterile water to 5 g of powder) through a 12- or 14-gauge catheter, after which the horse loses consciousness in 20 to 30 seconds.

KEY POINT ▶ The usual dose rate after a sedative is 7 to 8 mg/kg, and it is important that the required dose be

TABLE 17–1. Dose Rates of Sedative/Narcotic Combinations* for Use in Horses

Drug Combination	Dose Rate	Comments
Acepromazine + meperidine (Demerol, Winthrop)	Acepromazine 0.04–0.05 mg/kg Meperidine 0.5–0.8 mg/kg	May produce excitement and sweating
Acepromazine + buprenorphine (Buprenex, Norwich)	Acepromazine 0.02–0.04 mg/kg Buprenorphine 0.005 mg/kg (5 μg/kg)	Does not produce profound sedation or analgesia
Xylazine† + morphine	Xylazine 0.2–0.5 mg/kg Morphine 0.2–0.5 mg/kg	Produces excellent sedation and analgesia
Xylazine† + buprenorphine (Buprenex, Norwich)	Xylazine 0.2–0.5 mg/kg Buprenorphine 0.005 mg/kg (5 μg/kg)	Good sedation and some analgesia
Xylazine† + butorphanol (Torbugesic, Aveco)	Xylazine 0.2–0.5 mg/kg Butorphanol 0.03–0.08 mg/kg	Excellent sedation and analgesia, particularly for visceral pain
Xylazine† + pentazocine (Talwin-V, Upjohn)	Xylazine 0.2–0.5 mg/kg Pentazocine 0.3 mg/kg	Good sedation and analgesia but short duration of action

*Note that with all drug combinations, the sedative must be given at least 5 to 10 minutes prior to the narcotic or narcotic-like drug.
†Detomidine may be used at dose rates of 0.02–0.04 mg/kg instead of xylazine.
Note also that all drugs are given intravenously.

given as quickly as possible (<5 seconds) or there may be excitement and paddling after induction of anesthesia.

- Because the effect of the calculated dose rate is variable, a further 1 g (10 ml of a 10% solution) should be kept on hand in case a "top up" is needed. In adult horses of 400 to 550 kg, the "top up" dose is usually 0.5 g.

KEY POINT ▶ Note that "top up" doses of the thiobarbiturates may produce greatly prolonged recovery from anesthesia.

Advantages

- A minimum of equipment is necessary to administer these agents.
- Experience with these agents results in reliable induction of anesthesia.

Disadvantages

KEY POINT ▶ The concentrated thiobarbiturates cause severe phlebitis and will result in sloughing of the jugular vein if injected perivascularly.

- It is essential to administer via a catheter and to draw back on the syringe before and after injection to ensure that the solution was given intravascularly. If there is any possibility of perivascular injection, 2 to 3 L of saline or polyionic fluids should be deposited subcutaneously around the jugular vein to dilute the concentrated barbiturate and lessen the likelihood of phlebitis.
- In fit athletic horses, apnea is common after induction, particularly if the horse is connected to oxygen.
- An experienced handler is needed for induction because horses can sometimes crash to the ground or attempt to rear over backwards.
- Poor-quality recovery from anesthesia also may be found.

▶ Guaifenesin plus Thiobarbiturates

Background

Guaifenesin (Guailaxin, Fort Dodge, Aveco, Fort Dodge, IA) is a centrally acting muscle relaxant that also has some sedative effect. It potentiates a variety of intravenous anesthetic agents. The combination of guaifenesin and thiobarbiturates has become a popular induction technique in the past 20 years because of its reliability and relative lack of excitement when compared with the thiobarbiturates alone. The duration of anesthesia is usually around 20 minutes.

Clinical Use

- Guaifenesin is usually used in combination with either thiopental or thiamylal (see preceding sec-

tion). It can be given to effect followed by a calculated dose of thiobarbiturates or administered as an infusion with the thiobarbiturate incorporated in the solution.

KEY POINT ▶ If guaifenesin is administered with the thiobarbiturate incorporated in the solution, some type of pressure pump is required to ensure rapid administration (1–2 min); otherwise, excitement will occur during induction.

KEY POINT ▶ Guaifenesin is made up to a 5% or 10% solution from 50 g powder and administered at an approximate dose rate of 2 ml/kg of the 5% solution or 1 ml/kg of the 10% solution.

- These solutions are not stable and should generally be used within 24 hours or before they become cloudy. In some countries, guaifenesin is available as a 10% solution in a propylene glycol–ethyl alcohol base.
- If guaifenesin is administered prior to the injection of barbiturate, it is given rapidly intravenously, and when signs of sedation and/or slight ataxia are seen, thiopental or thiamylal is given IV in a 10% solution at a dose rate of 4 to 5 mg/kg.
- If a combination of guaifenesin and barbiturate is to be infused, 2.5 g thiopental or thiamylal is added to the guaifenesin prior to administration and the infusion given to effect. For an average 450-kg horse, it usually requires 800 to 900 ml of 5% solution plus thiobarbiturate to result in anesthetic induction.

KEY POINT ▶ The administration of guaifenesin can be combined with other induction agents such as xylazine and ketamine.

- The xylazine is usually given 5 to 10 minutes prior to the guaifenesin, which is administered at a dose rate of 2 ml of 5% solution per kilogram body weight and a bolus of 2 mg/kg ketamine administered IV once there are signs of ataxia from the guaifenesin. The main advantage of this combination over xylazine and ketamine alone is less motor movement and muscle rigidity after induction together with a slightly longer duration of anesthesia.

Advantages

- Both induction and recovery are relatively smooth in comparison with the thiobarbiturates alone.
- Less respiratory depression occurs, and there is less hypotension than with sole administration of the thiobarbiturates.

Disadvantages

- It is difficult to anesthetize a horse by yourself because of the need for someone to hold the bottle, pump in the solution, and remove the drip set or flutter valve at the appropriate time.

■ High concentrations of guaifenesin can cause hemolysis.

▶ Xylazine plus Ketamine

Background

This has become the most popular induction technique with equine practitioners over the past 10 years.

KEY POINT ▶ The great advantage of this drug combination is the simplicity of administration and the reliable induction and recovery from anesthesia.

It has become popular with most equine practitioners because the veterinarian can induce anesthesia single-handed. Duration of anesthesia is from 10 to 20 minutes.

Clinical Use

■ Xylazine is administered at a dose rate of 1.1 mg/kg IV, and a period of at least 5 minutes is allowed for the maximum effect of the sedation.

KEY POINT ▶ It is extremely important to ensure that the horse is profoundly sedated prior to administration of ketamine.

■ After this, 2.2 mg/kg of ketamine which is available as a 100-mg/ml solution (Ketaset, Veco, Fort Dodge, IA, Vetalar, Aveco, Fort Dodge, IA) is injected rapidly intravenously via a 19-gauge needle.

■ After administration of the ketamine, it may take as long as 90 seconds for the horse to become recumbent. However, unlike a thiopentone or guaifenesin–thiopentone induction, the horse does not fall heavily to the ground but rather appears simply to lie down.

■ It is difficult to judge the depth of anesthesia with xylazine and ketamine. Horses will often rouse suddenly and may stand.

KEY POINT ▶ If prolongation of anesthesia is required and gaseous anesthesia is not available, it is best to use a solution of guaifenesin and thiopental (2.5 g thiopental in 1 L of 5% guaifenesin), administered to effect.

Advantages

■ Minimum of equipment and personnel are required. Both agents can be administered using standard needles and syringes.

■ The drugs are not irritant, so there is no possibility of jugular vein sloughing.

■ There is reliable and quiet induction and rapid recovery without ataxia.

■ The combination of xylazine and ketamine is an excellent choice for quick procedures such as castration.

Disadvantages

■ Unless the xylazine produces profound sedation, there will be excitement and muscle rigidity during induction.

■ It is difficult to control anesthetic depth, and there is poor muscle relaxation. Combining the agents with guaifenesin will counter this effect.

▶ "Triple Drip" Anesthesia (Combination of Guaifenesin–Ketamine–Sedative)

Background

KEY POINT ▶ Where anesthesia is likely to be necessary for longer than 15 minutes but less than 1 hour, the combination of guaifenesin with ketamine and some form of sedative (usually xylazine or detomidine) is a reliable and effective form of anesthesia.

The advantages of the technique are that no equipment is necessary for administering gaseous anesthesia and recovery from anesthesia is excellent.

Clinical Use

■ Ketamine (1 g) and xylazine (500 mg) is added to either a 5% solution (1 L) or 10% solution (500 ml) of guaifenesin. After induction of anesthesia with xylazine and ketamine, an infusion rate of approximately 2 ml/kg per hour is used for the 5% solution and 1 ml/kg per hour for the 10% solution.

■ It is possible to replace the xylazine with detomidine at 5 mg/L of the 5% solution and 5 mg/500 ml if a 10% solution is used.

■ Blood pressure is well maintained with less hypotension than with halothane anesthesia, and the recovery from anesthesia is generally smooth.

Advantages

■ Prolonged anesthesia is possible with a minimum of anesthetic equipment.

■ Smooth recovery from general anesthesia is usual.

Disadvantages

■ It is more difficult to control anesthetic depth than with gaseous anesthesia.

■ Recovery from anesthesia can sometimes be prolonged.

Inhalation Anesthesia

Where anesthesia is to be prolonged beyond 30 minutes or for any form of surgery where dorsal recumbency is required, it is best to maintain anesthesia using gaseous or inhalation anesthesia. More skill and experience are needed with gaseous than with intravenous anesthesia.

KEY POINT ▶ There are two main problems for the anesthetist with the use of most inhalation agents: hypoxemia and hypotension.

Hypoxemia

■ Because of ventilation–perfusion mismatch, hypoxemia is found in all anesthetized horses breathing room air.
■ At sea level, the normal arterial oxygen tension (PaO_2) is around 100 mmHg in the standing conscious horse but during anesthesia may decrease to 50 to 60 mmHg. This decrease in PaO_2 provides some of the stimulus to respiration which may be abolished when the horse breathes 100% oxygen during inhalation anesthesia.

KEY POINT ▶ Hypoxemia also may be found during inhalation anesthesia when the horse is breathing 100% oxygen.

■ This is unusual when the horse is in lateral recumbency, but in dorsal recumbency, the ventilation–perfusion mismatch is more severe and the PaO_2 may decrease to be in the range 50 to 100 mmHg. This is particularly the case when dorsal recumbency is combined with hypotension (as is frequently the case during colic surgery). For this reason, it is helpful to have access to a blood gas machine to determine PaO_2 and carbon dioxide tensions where prolonged inhalation anesthesia requiring dorsal recumbency is anticipated.
■ If severe hypoxemia is found, there are few clinical solutions other than placing the horse in lateral recumbency as soon as possible. Preliminary experience with high-frequency ventilation has shown that some improvement in arterial oxygen tensions may occur.

Hypotension

■ Most of the inhalation agents used cause some degree of hypotension. This effect may be exacerbated by the choice of premedicant (e.g., acepromazine causes significant hypotension).

KEY POINT ▶ More important, the extent of hypotension is related to the depth of anesthesia, so if the anesthetic depth is too great, there can be quite profound hypotension (systolic pressure < 60 mmHg).

■ It is important to note pulse pressure during anesthesia and to monitor systolic pressure. This is most easily performed using a pressure cuff around the tail and a Doppler device to detect flow in the coccygeal artery.
■ Because of the possibility of serious hypotension during inhalation anesthesia, IV polyionic fluids (3–6 ml/kg/h) should be given, which also provides an IV line should pressor agents such as dobutamine be required.

KEY POINT ▶ If there is profound hypotension (systolic pressure < 60 mmHg), dobutamine can be given as an infusion at a dose rate of 1-4 μg/kg per minute.

Apparatus for Gaseous Anesthesia

■ A number of machines are commercially available for closed-circuit anesthesia.
■ Most of these are circle absorbers with one-way valves and a canister containing soda lime for absorption of the CO_2. Many machines are satisfactory, but some have a limited capacity for absorption of CO_2 because the amount of soda lime is too small, particularly when anesthesia is prolonged beyond 1 hour. Soda lime canisters with a volume of at least 15 to 20 kg are required for satisfactory CO_2 absorption in adult horses of 400 to 600 kg body weight.
■ Because CO_2 absorption generates an exothermic reaction, the adequacy of CO_2 removal can be partially determined by monitoring the heat in the canister while the horse is under anesthesia.

KEY POINT ▶ Where infrequent inhalational anesthesia is carried out and the expense of a circle absorber cannot be justified, a "to-and-fro" apparatus can be simply built using a 20-L (5-gal) bucket with a tight-fitting lid and plumbing fittings that allow the attachment of a rebreathing bag near the top of the bucket and an endotracheal tube at the bottom of the bucket on the opposite side (Fig. 17-1).

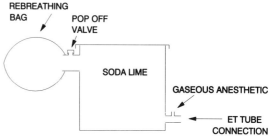

Figure 17–1. Cross-sectional drawing showing a "to-and-fro" anesthetic machine constructed using a plastic bucket with a top that is capable of sealing.

- To prevent soda lime from being inhaled into the endotracheal tube, mesh is inserted near the opening for connection to the endotracheal tube. All that is required is a vaporizer and oxygen to deliver the anesthetic gas to the "to-and-fro" machine, and a standard small animal anesthetic machine can be used for this purpose.
- Vaporizers for delivery of the volatile anesthetics should be temperature, flow, and back-pressure compensated.

Halothane–Oxygen Anesthesia

- Halothane and oxygen have been the most commonly used inhalation anesthetic combination for the last 20 years.
- The advantages of halothane are that anesthetic depth can be well judged using the combination of palpebral reflex, eye position, and appearance together with assessment of anal tone.

KEY POINT ► In the lighter planes of anesthesia there is a very active palpebral reflex with the presence of nystagmus and a brisk anal reflex.

- This plane of anesthesia is adequate for minor procedures. For most surgery, a slightly deeper plane of anesthesia is required where there is no nystagmus, the eye moves slightly ventrally, but there is still some palpebral reflex. Anesthesia is too deep when the eye becomes central and has a dry appearance, there is no palpebral reflex, and the corneal reflex is also lost.
- The main difficulty with halothane anesthesia is hypotension, which is directly related to the depth of anesthesia.
- Following induction with an intravenous agent, around 4% to 5% halothane is required until a surgical plane of anesthesia is established. For most surgery, delivery of 1.5% to 2% halothane is adequate to maintain anesthesia.
- The flow rate of oxygen used depends on the efficiency of the circle absorber for removal of CO_2. If there is a large (20–30 L) canister enabling efficient CO_2 absorption, only low flow rates (2–4 ml/kg/min) are required with the closed system being used. If small-volume (5–10 L) soda lime canisters are used, higher flow rates, around 20 ml/kg per minute, are required so that if there is some CO_2 accumulation, discharge is possible via the pop-off valve.

Isoflurane–Oxygen Anesthesia

- Isoflurane has a number of advantages over halothane because it is less soluble and therefore produces more rapid onset of action and rapid recovery upon termination of anesthesia.
- Isoflurane produces less cardiovascular depression than halothane, resulting in a similar decrease in arterial pressure but less depression of cardiac output for a given plane of anesthesia. However, there appears to be more respiratory depression than with halothane.
- Maintenance concentrations of isoflurane for surgery are usually 1% to 2%, with 3% to 4% being required for establishing surgical anesthesia following induction.

KEY POINT ► The major disadvantages of isoflurane are that it is extremely expensive and more difficult to judge anesthetic depth compared with halothane.

Inhalation Anesthesia Induction in Foals

KEY POINT ► In foals up to 1 month of age, anesthesia can be induced using oxygen and either halothane or isoflurane administered using a standard human circle absorber anesthetic machine. Because of its cost advantage, we prefer the use of halothane.

- The advantage of an inhalation induction is that there is no concern about metabolism of agents such as the barbiturates, recovery is rapid, and most foals tolerate a gaseous induction very well.
- We use either a mask attached to the Y piece of the circle absorber or a nasotracheal tube (Bivona, Inc., Gary, IN).

References

Abrahamsen, E. J., Hubbell, J. A., Bednarski, R. M., et al.: Xylazine and tiletamine–zolazepam for induction of anaesthesia maintained with halothane in 19 horses. *Equine Vet. J.* 23:224, 1991.
Allert, J. A., and Adams, H. R.: Pharmacologic considerations in selection of tranquilizers, sedatives, and muscle relaxant drugs used in inducing animal restraint. *J. Am. Vet. Med. Assoc.* 191:1241, 1987.
Brock, N., and Hildebrand, S. V.: A comparison of xylazine–ketamine and xylazine–guaifenesin–ketamine in equine anesthesia. *Vet. Surg.* 19:468–474.
Clarke, K. W., and Gerring, E. L.: Detomidine as a sedative and premedicant in the horse. *Proc. 36th Annu. Conv. Am. Assoc. Equine Pract.*, 1990, p. 629.
Hamm, D., and Jochle, W.: Sedation and analgesia in horses treated with various doses of domosedan: Blind studies on efficacy and the duration of effects. *Proc. 30th Annu. Conv. Am. Assoc. Equine Pract.*, 1984, p. 235.
Muir, W. W.: Cardiopulmonary resuscitation and the prevention of hypotensive emergencies in horses. *Proc. 30th Annu. Conv. Am. Assoc. Equine Pract.*, 1984, p. 117.

Nilsfors, L., Kvart, C., Kallings, P., and Carlsten, J.: Cardiorespiratory and sedative effects of a combination of acepromazine, xylazine, and methadone in the horse. *Equine Vet. J.* 20:364, 1988.

Riebold, T., and Schmotzer, W.: Anesthesia for the compromised or exhausted patient. *Proc. 34th Annu. Conv. Am. Assoc. Equine Pract.*, 1988, p. 509.

Rose, R., Rose, E., and Peterson, C.: Clinical experience with isoflurane anesthesia in foals and adult horses. *Proc. 34th Annu. Conv. Am. Assoc. Equine Pract.*, 1988, p. 555.

Anthelmintics

A wide range of anthelmintics are available for the treatment of internal parasites. Most of these are now available in paste form, which can be administered by owners and trainers. Unfortunately, these are sometimes administered incorrectly, and because of this, some larger horse farms have returned to the administration of anthelmintics by the veterinarian using nasogastric intubation.

KEY POINT ► Details of the various anthelmintics that are available for oral use or nasogastric administration are presented in Table 17-2.

Many of these drugs are effective against large and small strongyles (cyathastomes), but only a few effective in treatment of *Gastrophilus* spp., *Parascaris equorum*, *Habronema muscae*, *Onchocerca* spp., and tapeworms. Many of the available anthelmintics for horses are part of the benzimidazole group (oxibendazole, oxfendazole, fenbendazole, mebendazole), for which there is variable resistance among the strongyles.

KEY POINT ► The most important clinical problem arising from parasite infestation is verminous arteritis.

This results from the migrating stages of larvae of *Strongylus vulgaris,* which cause variable damage to the arterial intestinal supply, particularly the cranial mesenteric artery (see Chap. 6). Clinical signs vary from mild to severe colic and, occasionally, diarrhea due to intestinal damage during larval migration. Some anthelmintics are larvicidal, the most commonly used being ivermectin. Because of this and the wide range of parasites that are sensitive to ivermectin, it has become the most widely used of the anthelmintics. Some of the benzimidazole agents are also larvicidal at higher dose rates but usually require dosages over several days and may produce diarrhea. These include fenbendazole at 50 mg/kg daily for 3 days and thiabendazole at 440 mg/kg on successive days.

TABLE 17–2. Dose Rates, Formulations, and Indications for Use of Various Anthelmintics Employed in Horses

Drug	Trade Name	Formulation and Dose Rate	Range of Parasites Treated
Oxibendazole	Anthelcide (SmithKline Beecham), Equipar (Coopers)	Paste or suspension, 10–15 mg/kg	*S. equinus, S. edentatus, S. vulgaris,* small strongyles, *Parascaris equorum, Oxyuris equi, Strongyloides westeri*
Oxfendazole	Benzelmin (Syntex)	Powder, paste, suspension, 10 mg/kg	*S. equinus, S. edentatus, S. vulgaris,* small strongyles, *Parascaris equorum, Oxyuris equi*
Oxfendazole + trichlorfon	Benzelmin Plus (Syntex)	Paste, 2.5 mg/kg oxfendazole, 40 mg/kg trichlorfon	Same as oxfendazole plus bots (*Gastrophilus* spp)
Febantel + trichlorfon	Combotel (Haver/Diamond Scientific), Negabot-Plus (Cutter)	Paste, 6 mg/kg febantel, 40 mg/kg trichlorfon	*S. equinus, S. edentatus, S. vulgaris,* small strongyles, *Parascaris equorum, Oxyuris equi, Gastrophilus* spp
Febantel	Cutter Paste Wormer (Cutter), Rintal (Haver/Diamond Scientific)	Paste, liquid, 6 mg/kg febantel	*S. equinus, S. edentatus, S. vulgaris,* small strongyles, *Parascaris equorum, Oxyuris equi*
Ivermectin	Eqvalan (MSD-Agvet)	Paste, liquid, 0.2 mg/kg	*S. equinus, S. edentatus, S. vulgaris,* small strongyles, *Parascaris equorum, Oxyuris equi, Habronema muscae, Onchocerca* spp, *Gastrophilus* spp, *Dictyocaulus arnfeldi, Strongyloides westeri*
Fenbendazole	Panacur (Hoechst-Roussel), Safe-Guard (Hoechst-Roussel)	Paste, granules, liquid, 5 mg/kg	*S. equinus, S. edentatus, S. vulgaris,* small strongyles, *Parascaris equorum, Oxyuris equi*
Pyrantel	Strongid (Pfizer), Imathal Equine (SmithKline Beecham)	Paste, liquid, 6.6 mg/kg of base	*S. equinus, S. edentatus, S. vulgaris,* small strongyles, *Parascaris equorum, Oxyuris equi,* Cestodes (tapeworms)
Mebendazole	Telmin (Pitman-Moore)	Paste, liquid, 9 mg/kg	*S. equinus, S. edentatus, S. vulgaris,* small strongyles, *Oxyuris equi*
Trichlorfon	Combot (Haver/Diamond Scientific)	Liquid, 40 mg/kg	*Gastrophilus* spp, *Oxyuris equi, Parascaris equorum*
Dichlorvos	Cutter Dichlorvos Horse Wormer (Cutter)	Powder, 170 mg/kg	*S. equinus, S. edentatus, S. vulgaris,* small strongyles, *Parascaris equorum, Oxyuris equi, Gastrophilus* spp
Piperazine		Powder, 67 mg/kg	Efficacy 100% against *Parascaris equorum*

Antibiotic Therapy

R. J. Rose and Daria N. Love

Antibiotics are probably the group of drugs most widely misused in equine practice.

KEY POINT ▶ Inappropriate antibiotic selection, incorrect dose rates, prolonged intervals between doses, and incorrect duration of therapy are a few of the common misuses.

Antimicrobial therapy can kill off the normal bacterial flora and may allow some organisms to multiply unchecked by either the antibiotic or by competition from the normal bacteria. Resistance of microorganisms to antibiotics is also becoming an increasing problem. Whatever the ultimate mechanism of such acquired resistance, the prevalence of antibiotic-resistant strains is generally proportional to the extent of use of any particular antibiotic. A particular antibiotic acts as a powerful selection factor in the spread of resistant bacteria, and restriction of its use should reduce the proportion of resistant strains.

A more careful approach to antibiotic use is required by equine practitioners. Therapy should be based on bacteriologic information, which, if not known in the individual case, is based on likely causes and published information. Too often broad-spectrum agents are used without thought for their potential adverse effects. If bacteriologic samples are to be taken, they should not be taken after days or weeks of antibiotics that have been unsuccessful but rather prior to therapy being commenced.

STRATEGY OF ANTIBIOTIC THERAPY

The ideal management of patients with infections in which it is intended to use antibiotics is:

- Establish a clinical diagnosis.
- Confirm the nature of this infection by isolation of the causative organism.
- Prescribe the antibiotic as directed by sensitivity testing.
- Carry out follow-up examinations so that clinical and biologic cures can be checked.

It is usually only possible and practical to follow such a strategic plan in a minority of cases in hospital and even fewer in a practice setting.

Most horses diagnosed as suffering from bacterial infections are treated with antibiotics on an empirical basis. Generally, the results of such treatment are good, in large part because the natural defenses of the body are adequate to overcome the infection. Antibiotics merely assist these mechanisms rather than being the principal reason for recovery. Many infectious diseases do not require antibiotics for a successful outcome, although it is a difficult clinical decision to withhold such therapy, which is anticipated by clients.

In serious infections, horses will require chemotherapy urgently as a life-saving measure. Although every effort should be made to isolate the causal organism and examine its specific antibacterial sensitivities, therapy must be started at the earliest possible moment on the basis of experience in treatment of such infections.

KEY POINT ▶ Wherever possible, a specimen for laboratory examination should be collected from the patient before the start of therapy.

If material cannot be obtained from the animal before therapy is begun, the isolation of microorganisms from tissues and circulating body fluids after antimicrobial therapy has begun is much more difficult. Even when only one dose of antibiotic has been given, it may make it difficult to see and/or culture the causal organism.

KEY POINT ▶ There are many situations in equine practice where examination of simple smear preparations (e.g., from transtracheal aspirate, pleural fluid, abscess aspiration) will allow a presumptive diagnosis and rational antibiotic therapy to be instituted (e.g., streptococcal infections, actinomyces, and corynebacteria are uniformly sensitive to benzylpenicillin).

In other circumstances (unless imminently life-threatening), therapy should be withheld until a correctly performed antibiotic sensitivity assay is available. The result of this will determine therapy to be given—and this should be given for sufficient time to enable resolution of the infection. Changing antibiotic medication after a few days "because it does not appear to be working" is not recommended.

Treatment of Clostridial Infections in Muscle

A common sequela to intramuscular injections administered by clients with unsterile syringes or needles is infection with *Clostridium* spp. This infection is extremely serious, and steps should be taken to begin appropriate therapy immediately. Any horse that shows local swelling, fever, depression, and inappetence 12 to 24 hours after an intramuscular injection should be regarded as being a likely candidate for a clostridial infection. With some clostridial species there will be local gas production, but others may show only swelling and pain. Where possible, samples should be collected from the center of the swelling by aspirating with a needle and syringe. Fluid and/or purulent material in a capped syringe should be submitted for Gram stain and appropriate culture (see Chap. 15), after which antibiotic therapy is begun. Either sodium or potassium benzyl penicillin (Treatment Nos. 84 and 85) should be given intravenously at a dose rate of 20,000 IU/kg q6h until there is clinical improvement. Once the infection has localized, surgical drainage of the area should be carried out and the area exposed to the air, which will inhibit growth of the clostridia.

APPROACH TO ANTIBIOTIC THERAPY

The most important consideration in initiating antibiotic therapy is to decide if the horse has a definite bacterial infection. Antibiotics are often given on the basis of elevated body temperature, where there may be no bacterial infection. In our clinic, we have found that many horses will have a transient increase in temperature that resolves spontaneously in 12 to 24 hours.

KEY POINT ▶ Many clinicians use nonsteroidal anti-inflammatory drugs to decrease the temperature, but in many cases this is poor-quality medicine.

Monitoring a temperature rise is useful in evaluating progress of an infection and response to therapy, and in most cases, antipyretic drugs should not be given. The steps to consider before starting antibiotic therapy are as follows:

1. Make a Diagnosis

Various diagnostic techniques should be considered to establish a bacteriologic cause of the disease. Techniques such as blood culture, transtracheal aspiration, thoracocentesis, abscess aspiration, and joint fluid collection may be useful, de-

pending on the particular problem. Worse than no bacteriology is inappropriate bacteriology.

KEY POINT ▶ For example, collecting bacteriologic samples from discharging wounds is never indicated.

Such samples will invariably result in growth of a mixed bacterial flora and give no indication of the causative organism. It is important that contamination of the sample for bacteriology does not occur during the collection procedure. The most common sources of contamination are from the hair or skin of the horse and occasionally from the person taking the sample. Contamination can be minimized by attention to skin disinfection and protection of the operator using sterile gloves and in certain situations a cap and mask. If possible, it is best to submit an aspirate in a sterile syringe rather than a bacteriologic swab. Unfortunately, a number of laboratories resist receiving samples in sterile syringes, and therefore, arrangements should be made in advance and an explanation given.

Many sites, such as the respiratory and reproductive tracts, have a normal bacterial flora, and thus the mere finding of bacteria on culture does not necessarily indicate an infection. Note should be made of the cytologic findings and the degree of bacterial growth (for details, see Chap. 15).

2. Use a Bactericidal Antibiotic if Possible

Bactericidal antibiotics are preferable to bacteriostatic antibiotics because in many situations (e.g., septic arthritis, pleuritis) there is compromised host phagocytic activity, and therefore, bacteriostatic antibiotics may not eliminate the infection.

KEY POINT ▶ Bactericidal antibiotics include benzylpenicillin, semisynthetic penicillins (amoxycillin, ampicillin), isoxazolyl penicillins (cloxacillin, flucloxacillin), cephalosporins, and the aminoglycosides (streptomycin, neomycin, amikacin, kanamycin, gentamicin).

Bacteriostatic antibiotics include chloramphenicol, erythromycin, tetracyclines, and sulphonamides.

3. Use a Narrow-Spectrum Antibiotic

Although broad-spectrum antibiotics are often favored by clinicians, it is better therapeutic practice to use a narrow-spectrum agent (e.g., penicillin) to avoid complications such as killing off the normal bacterial flora, superinfection, and bacterial resistance. A failure of therapy with a narrow-spectrum agent provides an indication of the likely range of bacteria causing the infection and allows more rational adjustment of the antibiotic regimen.

4. Maintain Effective Blood Levels of Antibiotics

It has been established that maintenance of therapeutic blood concentrations of antibiotics is not necessary to successfully treat an infection. This is so because intermittent antibiotic "peaks" (particularly with bactericidal antibiotics) can successfully eliminate an infection. Nevertheless, most bacterial disease responds best to maintenance of effective antibiotic levels in the bloodstream. Because it is difficult to determine the concentrations of antibiotics at the site of infection, maintenance of effective blood concentrations for a period of treatment is usual. It is generally accepted that the concentration that should be maintained is two to four times the minimum inhibitory concentration (MIC) of antibiotic for the particular bacteria. With most antibiotics, this requires treatment two to four times daily. As a generalization, the so-called long-acting antibiotics only maintain adequate levels against the most sensitive bacteria for the 2 to 3 days claimed by the manufacturer. In most cases these antibiotics do not maintain effective blood levels of antibiotics.

5. Choose an Antibiotic Likely to be Effective Against Equine Bacterial Pathogens

Consider the following points when making a decision to use a certain antibiotic:

Amoxicillin and Ampicillin—Most gram-negative equine pathogens are resistant to the semisynthetic penicillins owing to beta-lactamase production by bacteria. Thus these antibiotics are not cost-effective, given that they are less active but considerably more expensive than penicillin G against gram-positive species.

Chloramphenicol—Whether given intravenously, intramuscularly, or orally, chloramphenicol has such a short half-life that it is not a useful antibiotic for treating horses. Furthermore, with the horse being used as a food-producing animal, there is also a public health risk.

Streptomycin—Streptomycin is still used widely in combination with penicillin for the treatment of infections in horses. However, most gram-negative pathogens are resistant to streptomycin, and therefore, unless sensitivity tests indicate otherwise, it should not be used in horses.

Oral Antibiotics—Oral antibiotics may not provide reliable blood and tissue concentrations in adult horses. Problems include variable absorption and diarrhea, particularly with penicillins. However, trimethoprim–sulfadiazine combinations are often useful in either paste form or powder administered in the feed.

6. Decide on the Duration of Therapy

The length of treatment should be decided by the specific problem and response to therapy.

KEY POINT ► As a general rule, for antibiotics that are bactericidal, the time required for treatment of acute infections should be equivalent to the time that the animal has been clinically ill plus 3 days.

Acute infections usually require therapy for some 5 to 7 days.

KEY POINT ► However, it may be necessary to treat some staphylococcal infections and others that are intracellular survivors for some weeks to ensure that the organisms which have been phagocytosed are killed as they emerge from phagocytes.

It is imperative that organisms that are intracellular survivors and multipliers are treated with bactericidal antibiotics if there is to be quick resolution to the infection. It may be necessary to treat and monitor these infections for many months if they require bacteriostatic antibiotics.

Some guides to the duration of antibiotic therapy are as follows:

- Surgical prophylaxis—12 to 24 hours
- Acute infection—5 to 7 days
- Septic arthritis—10 to 21 days
- Urinary tract infection—14 to 28 days
- Chronic pneumonia (e.g., *R. equi* in foals)—1 to 3 months

7. Decide if Antibiotics Should Be Used Prophylactically

It is important to be sure there is likely to be a bacterial infection before chemoprophylaxis is used. Unless a problem has been identified (e.g., a particular neonatal foal infection on a stud farm), prophylactic antibiotic use is of no value. Routine antibiotic prophylaxis (e.g., before and after surgery) is often used whether or not it is necessary. Important considerations in chemoprophylaxis associated with surgery include the site (i.e., whether contaminated or not), operating time, degree of tissue trauma, and likelihood of contamination.

Antibiotics have been employed as agents in chemoprophylaxis for four purposes:

- To protect healthy animals against invasions by a microorganism to which they have been exposed.
- To prevent secondary bacterial infection in individual animals acutely ill with disease, especially viruses, for which antibiotics are of no direct help.
- To reduce the risk of infection in animals with various types of chronic illness.

■ To inhibit the spread of disease from areas of localized infection or to prevent infection in patients subjected to accidental or surgical trauma.

The following generalizations have been found to apply when antibiotics are administered prophylactically:

KEY POINT ► When a single, effective drug is used when bacterial infection is present but not clinically evident, the results are highly successful.

■ If the aim is to prevent colonization and/or infection by any and all microorganisms that may be present in the internal or external environment, results are often unsatisfactory.
■ The incidence of superinfection is directly related to the time of exposure to broad-spectrum antibiotics. To reduce the likelihood of superinfection, chemoprophylaxis should be used for only a short period.
■ One of the great controversies in chemoprophylaxis is antibiotic use in viral respiratory disease. There have been no clinical trials to support or oppose the use of antibiotics in this situation. However, in principle, it is difficult to advocate the prophylactic administration of antibiotics for treatment of viral respiratory disease.

8. Antibiotic Dose Rates

The dose rates for various commonly used antibiotics, together with some specific considerations in their use, is presented in Table 17-3. Antibiotics used in foals are discussed in Chapter 8.

REASONS FOR FAILURE OF ANTIBIOTIC THERAPY

Failure of antibiotic therapy often leads the clinician to blame the antibiotic rather than looking carefully at likely reasons why the therapy has been unsuccessful. Some of the common reasons for failure of antibiotic therapy are discussed below.

Treatment of Untreatable Infections

One of the most common reasons for antibiotic failure is their use to treat viral infections. Treatment either fails or is deemed to be successful because when given for sufficient period of time, the horse eventually recovers by natural defense mechanisms.

Improper Dosage or Duration of Therapy

Too Much—May be harmful in instances, especially where impaired elimination is present. This is particularly the case with the aminoglycosides, which can cause renal toxicity, especially in cases of shock and dehydration.

Too Little or Too Short a Time—Is probably the most common area of antibiotic misuse. Underestimating the body weight and providing treatment only once daily can result in failure of therapy.

Too Long—It seems general practice to treat horses for too long, especially for acute infections. In most infections, if there has not been clinical improvement after 5 days, you should be looking for an underlying problem that is making the animal refractory to treatment. It may be that you did not have the correct diagnosis and treatment in the first place or that the organism has become resistant to the antibiotic during the course of the treatment. It also may be a problem that will not respond to antibiotic therapy alone (e.g., infected tooth root, discharging sinus, septic arthritis).

Reliance on Chemotherapy with Omission of Surgical Drainage

This often places a demand on antibiotics they cannot always satisfy (e.g., lesions where there are appreciable quantities of purulent exudate or necrotic or avascular infected tissues). Where substantial quantities of pus or necrotic tissue or a foreign body is a problem, the most effective treatment is a combination of antibiotic given in adequate dose plus a properly performed surgical procedure to provide effective drainage.

Certain drugs may be inactivated by microbial or other enzymes. Some drugs will not be as effective at low Eh or at low pH (situations likely to be encountered in abscesses). In some situations, the organisms may not be multiplying fast enough so that antibiotics directed against cell-wall or protein synthesis are effective in inactivating the organism. Likewise, phagocytic cells will not be able to function effectively in such an environment. This will be of particular consequence for antibiotics that depend for ultimate elimination of the organism on phagocytosis.

Lack of Adequate Bacteriologic Information

In human medicine, it has been documented that for hospitalized patients, half the courses of antimicrobial therapy are administered in the absence of support from microbiology. The great bulk of drugs used is based on clinical judgment alone. A high proportion of the use is for chemoprophylaxis of questionable value.

Bacterial samples are often inappropriately taken, and culture reports are therefore inaccurate and/or inappropriate. Bacterial cultures are obtained too infrequently, and results, where available, may be disregarded by the clinician when selecting the antibiotic.

KEY POINT ► Routine use of drug combinations is a cover for diagnostic imprecision.

TABLE 17–3. Dose Rates of Antibiotics for Use in Adult Horses

Antibiotic	Dose Rate (per kg)	Interval	Route	Aspects of Treatment
Na or K benzylpenicillin	20,000 IU	q6h	IM, IV	Blood levels maintained for longer after IM than IV injection. Use to achieve high circulating and tissue levels at start of therapy.
Procaine penicillin	15,000 IU or 15 mg	q12h	IM only	Most useful antibiotic in equine practice for gram-positive pathogens. Excitement reactions may be seen after injection and occasionally anaphylaxis.
Long-acting penicillin (e.g., benzathine)	15,000–25,000	q24–48h	IM	*Do not use except where the organisms concerned have very low MICs as low blood levels of penicillin maintained.*
Na amoxicillin or ampicillin	15–40 mg	q8h	IM, IV	These drugs have a similar spectrum of activity but have less activity than penicillin against susceptible organisms. Little efficacy against gram-negative pathogens in horses.
Na cloxacillin or oxacillin	30 mg	q8h	IM, IV	Used exclusively to treat beta-lactamase–producing *Staphylococcus aureus* infections, particularly in septic arthritis.
Cephalothin or cephalopirin	10–20 mg	q8h	IM, IV	Should not be used unless there is microbiologic evidence for efficacy. Use may result in diarrhea.
Ceftiofur	2–4 mg	q12h	IM, IV	Useful to treat some pneumonias. May cause diarrhea, particularly at higher dose rates.
Kanamycin	5 mg	q8h	IV, IM	Useful to treat some gram-negative infections. However, because only a small range of bacteria are sensitive, there should be culture and sensitivity evidence of potential efficacy.
Gentamicin	2–3 mg	q8h	IV, IM	The most common aminoglycoside used. Effective against a wide range of gram-negative pathogens. Best to use IV because IM administration causes localized myositis.
Amikacin	7 mg	q12h or q8h	IV, IM	Should not be used unless sensitivity tests show no other aminoglycoside that is effective. Gentamicin should be the primary aminoglycoside used.
Oxytetracycline hydrochloride	5 mg	q12h	IV	Because it is a bacteriostatic drug, should only be used if bacteriologic tests indicate sensitivity. May cause diarrhea.
Trimethoprim plus one of the sulfonamides	15–20 mg of combined drugs	q12h	IV, PO	Higher dose with oral use of drug. Useful to treat a wide range of equine bacterial pathogens. At high dose rates may cause diarrhea.
Metronidazole	15-mg loading dose then 7–15 mg	q6h	PO	Useful to treat anaerobic infections, particularly some cases of pleuritis caused by *B. fragilis* infections.

The agents selected are more likely to be those of habit rather than for special indications, and the dosages employed are routine.

References

Adamson, P. J., Wilson, W. D., Hirsch, D. C., et al.: Susceptibility of equine bacterial isolates to antimicrobial agents. *Am. J. Vet. Res.* 46:447, 1985.

Baggot, J. D., and Prescott, J. F.: Antimicrobial selection and dosage in the treatment of equine bacterial infections. *Equine Vet. J.* 19:92, 1987.

Baggot, J. D., Love, D. N., Rose, R. J., and Raus, R.: Selection of an aminoglycoside antibiotic for administration to horses. *Equine Vet. J.* 17:30, 1985.

Hillidge, C. J.: Review of *Corynebacterium (Rhodococcus) equi* lung abscesses in foals: Pathogenesis, diagnosis and treatment. *Vet. Rec.* 119:261, 1986.

Koterba, A., Torchia, J., Silverthorne, C., et al.: Nosocomial infections and bacterial antibiotic resistance in a university equine hospital. *J. Am. Vet. Med. Assoc.* 189:185, 1986.

Love, D. N., Rose, R. J., Martin, I. C. A., and Bailey, M.: Serum concentrations of penicillin in the horse after administration of a variety of penicillin preparations. *Equine Vet. J.* 15:43, 1983.

Prescott, J. F., and Sweeney, C. R.: Treatment of *Corynebacterium equi* pneumonia of foals: A review. *J. Am. Vet. Med. Assoc.* 187:725, 1985.

Anti-Inflammatory Therapy

The anti-inflammatory drugs used in equine practice can be classed in two major groups:

- Nonsteroidal anti-inflammatory drugs (NSAIDs)
- Corticosteroids

NONSTEROIDAL ANTI-INFLAMMATORY DRUGS

There are two major subdivisions of the NSAIDs that can be made:

- Enolic acids—the major drug in this group is phenylbutazone.
- Carboxylic acids—flunixin, meclofenamic acid, ketoprofen, and naproxen are in this group.

A third drug that is gaining more acceptance in equine practice is aspirin, which is also classified with the NSAIDs.

- The NSAIDs block a part of the cyclooxygenase pathway and suppress synthesis of several chemical mediators of inflammation, such as thromboxane, prostacyclin, and prostaglandins.
- The NSAIDs reduce prostaglandin-induced heat, swelling, and pain in inflamed tissues. They are widely used for the treatment of skeletal and soft-tissue injuries and for reducing body temperature.
- While all the NSAIDs have similar modes of action, clinical experience has dictated the use of different drugs for the range of clinical conditions encountered in practice. The two most widely used of the NSAIDs are phenylbutazone and flunixin meglumine. More recently, ketofen (Treatment No. 66) has become available and is efficacious in treating musculoskeletal and abdominal pain. Aspirin, despite its short half-life, is becoming more widely used in equine practice.

Phenylbutazone (Treatment No. 88)

- Phenylbutazone is by far the most commonly used NSAID and has been described as "the equine practitioner's friend."
- Phenylbutazone is the least expensive of the NSAIDs and has been found to be effective in the treatment of a wide range of conditions.
- Most consistent responses have been found in the treatment of soft-tissue injuries and musculoskeletal problems, particularly low-grade lameness.
- Phenylbutazone also has an antipyretic effect and will reduce body temperature when there is a fever, which may be a problem if temperature is being monitored as a guide to possible infection.

However, at low dose rates of phenylbutazone (2.2 mg/kg daily), there appears to be little effect on body temperature.

KEY POINT ► We use phenylbutazone routinely after surgery for 3 to 5 days to reduce the extent of soft-tissue swelling and find that it is also useful after suturing lacerations because the degree of swelling, and therefore tension on sutures, is minimized.

- Because the NSAIDs do not inhibit the cellular inflammatory response, they may be used without delaying wound healing.
- Phenylbutazone is available in oral formulations as tablets, granules, and paste, as well as a solution (200 mg/ml) for intravenous injection (see Treatment No. 88).
- The recommended dose rate for phenylbutazone is a loading dose of 4.4 mg/kg on the first day of administration, followed by 2.2 mg/kg twice daily for up to 4 days, and then 2.2 mg/kg for 7 days. Higher doses than these can be used if necessary to obtain the degree of pain relief required, but the horse should be monitored closely for any adverse effects.

Flunixin Meglumine (Treatment No. 52)

- Flunixin is considerably more expensive than phenylbutazone, but experience by most equine practitioners indicates that it is more effective than phenylbutazone in the treatment of visceral pain (colic) and in the symptomatic control of endotoxemia.
- Oral formulations include granules and paste, and flunixin is also available as a solution for intramuscular or intravenous (preferred route) injection.
- A dose rate of 1 mg/kg has been recommended for treatment of visceral pain, but the dose for control of endotoxic manifestations is as little as 0.2 mg/kg.

Ketoprofen (Treatment No. 66)

- Ketoprofen is a NSAID in the propionic acid group (similar to naproxen) that has been available for a few years and appears to be valuable in the treatment of musculoskeletal disorders. Some clinical experience has shown that it is also useful for the treatment of colic and uveitis. Ketoprofen has some effect on signs of endotoxemia but is not as effective as flunixin in relieving abdominal pain. One of the advantages of ketoprofen is that no adverse effects on gastrointestinal function have been reported even at five times the normal dose rate. It has a relatively long half-life, so treatment is only required every 24 hours.
- Ketoprofen is only available in a solution for intravenous injection. The concentration of the solution is 100 mg/ml.

- The recommended dose rate is 1 to 2 mg/kg given IV every 24 hours.

Aspirin (Treatment No. 9)

- Aspirin recently has become a popular drug with equine practitioners because it appears to have a more prolonged clinical effect, even though its half-life is short.
- An intravenous form of aspirin is available (Aspri-Ject Injection, Vedco, St. Joseph, MO), and the recommended dose rate is 35 mg/kg, given every 6 to 8 hours.
- The most common oral form is a large tablet or bolus containing 15.6 g aspirin (Aspirin Boluses, Butler, Dublin, OH; Farmtech, Kansas City, MO; Vedco, Agri Laboratories, Phoenix, St. Joseph, MO; RX Veterinary Products, Porterville, CA).
- Aspirin has a prolonged effect on clotting time, and this should be remembered if the drug is given prior to surgery.
- We have found aspirin useful for controlling minor abdominal pain, for low-grade lameness, as an antipyretic agent, and for treatment of uveitis. It is relatively inexpensive and is available as a bolus that can be administered with a balling gun or ground up to permit a paste to be made.
- Because of its antithrombotic effects, aspirin also has been used for attempted prevention of laminitis.
- Other NSAIDs that have been used in horses include meclofenamic acid, indomethacin, and naproxen, but none of these drugs is commonly used in equine practice. There is less clinical experience with these NSAIDs, which appear to produce a less reliable result than phenylbutazone, flunixin, or aspirin. Furthermore, most of the NSAIDs are considerably more expensive than phenylbutazone.

Nonsteroidal Anti-Inflammatory Drug Toxicity

KEY POINT ► Phenylbutazone has been used widely in equine practice for the last 30 years, and there have been few reports of ill effects.

However, during the last 10 years, reports of toxicity, particularly affecting the gastrointestinal tract and to a lesser extent the kidneys, have appeared in the scientific literature.

Ponies have been thought to be particularly susceptible to the toxic effects of phenylbutazone, but this is probably related to relative overdosage because of overestimation of body weight. Our experience indicates that because the granule or tablet formulations are in 1-g lots, many small ponies are given 2 g per day, which can translate into dose rates around 12 to 15 mg/kg, well above the upper limit of acceptable therapeutic range, which is around 8 to 9 mg/kg.

The more difficult clinical situation is the horse with severe laminitis that may require large doses of phenylbutazone for prolonged periods to provide analgesia. While the doses of phenylbutazone required (4–6 mg/kg daily) may produce signs of gastrointestinal dysfunction, lower doses will not result in sufficient analgesia, and the horse may suffer great discomfort.

Signs of toxicity relate to gastrointestinal dysfunction, ulceration being a common finding. Clinical signs include anorexia, colic, lethargy, weight loss, diarrhea, melena, and terminally, death from shock. There is invariably a protein-losing enteropathy in cases of phenylbutazone toxicity because of the gastrointestinal ulceration. Toxicity has been reported rarely with the other NSAIDs, but the possibility of similar problems with phenylbutazone could be anticipated if dosages above those recommended are given. Care must be taken with concurrent administration of NSAIDs and aminoglycoside antibiotics because they may increase the nephrotoxic effects of aminoglycosides. Phenylbutazone is also very irritant if injected perivascularly.

KEY POINT ▶ If large doses of phenylbutazone are required, the possibility of toxicity can be monitored by measurement of total plasma or serum protein (TPP).

Before any clinical abnormalities are found, blood biochemistry will show a decrease in TPP. Therefore, intermittent blood sampling can be used to determine whether phenylbutazone is producing adverse effects on gastrointestinal function if prolonged or high dosage is required.

Toxicity appears to be less of a problem with the other anti-inflammatory drugs, although adverse signs have been reported with high doses of meclofenamic acid. Flunixin has been administered at dose rates of 3.3 mg/kg daily for 10 days without signs of toxicity or adverse effects on blood or urinary values. However, foals may be more susceptible, and therefore, flunixin should be used with care.

Dose Rates

Recommended dose rates for nonsteroidal anti-inflammatory drugs are provided in Table 17-4. These dose rates are only a guide, but care should be taken if higher dose rates than those recommended are used.

DIMETHYLSULFOXIDE (DMSO)

- While the physiologic effects of DMSO are incompletely understood, the clinical usefulness of DMSO is well established in the treatment of acute musculoskeletal injuries, acute traumatic and inflammatory disorders of the central nervous system, and septic arthritis.

- DMSO appears to be of most use in acute inflammatory conditions and has little or no effect in chronic conditions.
- The anti-inflammatory effect of DMSO is associated with its role as a scavenger of free radicals, together with inhibition of the influx of inflammatory cells into the sites of inflammation.
- While toxicity of DMSO is low, rapid IV administration can induce seizures, and hemolysis may be observed with high concentrations because of the high osmolality of DMSO. Topical DMSO may produce local skin irritation and "blistering" because of histamine release.
- DMSO is also used as a carrier in combination with other drugs (particularly corticosteroids) because it increases absorption through the skin. Because of this, care should be taken when using DMSO with any other drugs and also in avoiding contact of DMSO with the skin of the person applying the product. Preferably, local application should be performed using gloves.
- DMSO enhances the skin and blood–brain barrier penetration of nonionized molecules of low molecular weight, such as corticosteroids and some antibiotics.
- In horses, a 20% solution of DMSO in normal saline can be given safely as an intravenous infusion at a dose rate of 0.5 to 0.9 g/kg for the treatment of cranial or spinal cord trauma and some septic conditions.

KEY POINT ▶ More recently, a 20% solution of DMSO also has been found useful in the local treatment of septic arthritis.

- After placement of indwelling drains under general anesthesia, 4 to 5 L of DMSO solution is infused into the joint, followed by 5 to 6 L of a povidone-iodine solution (see Disinfectants).

CORTICOSTEROIDS (TREATMENT Nos. 12, 13, 29, 30, 74, 92, 106)

Mode of Action

- Two classes of corticosteroid esters are available for parenteral administration. Prednisolone is the most widely used corticosteroid for oral administration.
- The short-acting succinate and phosphate preparations are used to attain high plasma and tissue concentrations, but the effect is short lasting. Conditions in which short-acting corticosteroids can be considered include shock, anaphylaxis, and allergic reactions.
- The insoluble esters such as acetate are absorbed and excreted more slowly, thus producing prolonged clinical effects. These "depot" type corticosteroids are used widely in equine practice, particularly for intraarticular medication.

TABLE 17–4. Dose Rates and Routes of Administration of Nonsteroidal Anti-Inflammatory Drugs in the Horse

Drug	Form	Route	Recommended Dose and Use
Phenylbutazone	Tablets, paste, granules, powder	PO	Loading dose on 1st day of 4.4 mg/kg followed by 2.2 mg/kg q12h for 4 days and maintenance dose of 2.2 mg/kg daily thereafter. Used for musculoskeletal problems and perioperatively to minimize the extent of swelling.
Phenylbutazone	Solution	IV	Used to establish initial therapeutic blood levels. Dose rate varies from 2.2 to 4.4 mg/kg.
Flunixin meglumine	Solution, granules, paste	IV, IM or PO	Highest recommended dose rate is 1.1 mg/kg. This is the dose used in colic cases. For endotoxemia, dose is 0.2 mg/kg given q6–8h.
Meclofenamic acid	Granules	PO	2.2 mg/kg daily for 5–7 days, and if further treatment needed, 2.2 mg/kg every second day. Most useful for horses with chronic laminitis. More expensive than phenylbutazone.
Naproxen	Powder	PO	10 mg/kg daily. Few clinical indications and seldom used.
Dipyrone monohydrate	Solution	IM or IV	10–20 mg/kg given once or twice only. Useful as a spasmolytic agent in some colic cases and as an antipyretic.
Phenylbutazone and isopyrin	Solution	IV only	4 mg/kg of phenylbutazone component of preparation, given once daily. Combination with isopyrin more than doubles the plasma half-life. Must be given very slowly (30–60 s) IV, since rapid injection causes excitement and ataxia. Useful to achieve prolonged response.
Aspirin	Solution and tablets	IV or PO	30–100 mg/kg q8h or q6h. Useful for some musculoskeletal problems, uveitis, laminitis, and mild abdominal pain.
Ketoprofen	Solution	IV	1–2 mg/kg q24h. Useful for musculoskeletal problems and endotoxemia.

■ The corticosteroids act by stabilizing cellular, lysosomal, and mitochondrial membranes. They also inhibit phospholipase A_2, which is involved in the formation of arachidonic acid.

KEY POINT ▶ The corticosteroids have a profound negative effect on wound healing, unlike the NSAIDs, and therefore should not be used perioperatively.

■ Clinical experience with horses that required arthrotomies within 1 to 2 months of administration of a long-acting corticosteroid intraarticularly is that wound breakdown was common. With the advent of arthroscopic surgery, this has become less of a problem.

Indications for Corticosteroid Use

■ Corticosteroids act nonspecifically, and there are many undesirable side effects, particularly delayed healing, increased susceptibility to infection, and in joints some cartilage degradation. These possible adverse effects have to be weighed against the therapeutic benefits.

KEY POINT ▶ Particular care must be taken in decisions about topical corticosteroid use in ocular disease (possibility of corneal rupture if an ulcer is present), pulmonary disease (may worsen a low-grade infection), and joint disease (may aggravate preexisting cartilage damage).

■ Corticosteroids are useful for the treatment of various autoimmune disorders, the most common of which is probably pemphigus foliaceus.

■ One of the contentious areas of corticosteroid use is in the treatment of shock. Most cases of shock do not require corticosteroids. However, in severe endotoxic shock, there may be a role for short-acting corticosteroid administration. High dose rates (0.5–1 mg/kg of dexamethasone) have been advocated.

■ Corticosteroids are probably of most use in the treatment of some skin disorders (see Chap. 12). Oral prednisolone is inexpensive and effective. The usual dose rate is 1 mg/kg twice daily for the first 2 to 4 days, followed by 1 mg/kg once daily in the morning for 5 to 7 days, after which an every-other-day dosage (in the morning) is given to effect. This regimen has been shown to produce little adverse effect on adrenal function.

■ Intraarticular use of corticosteroids is valuable where there is an acute synovitis (see Chap. 3). The main drugs used are methylprednisolone acetate (Treatment No. 74) and the combination of betamethasone acetate and betamethasone phosphate (Treatment Nos. 12 and 13). The possible negative effects of corticosteroids on joint function have probably been overemphasized, and clinical experience with the corticosteroids indicates that few adverse effects are encountered.

KEY POINT ▶ In states with controlled medication in performance horses, it should be remembered that when used intraarticularly, the long-acting corticosteroids can remain detectable for up to 6 weeks.

Other conditions where corticosteroids can be considered are rhabdomyolysis, some ocular conditions, some central nervous system diseases, and some chronic pulmonary diseases. Chapters on individual body systems should be consulted for further details.

Adverse Effects of Corticosteroids

■ Inhibition of fibroblasts and increase in collagen breakdown resulting in detrimental effects on wound healing.

■ Inhibition of bone growth, matrix formation, and calcification can occur.

■ Suppression of the hypothalamic–pituitary–adrenal system. Soluble forms of the corticosteroids result in adrenal suppression for 1 to 2 days. In contrast, the long-acting corticosteroids may produce adrenal suppression for up to 1 month.

■ Great care must be used with sterile technique when injecting corticosteroids intraarticularly. Introduction of infection when corticosteroids are injected will result in septic arthritis with severe long-term consequences for joint function, even if the infection is treated successfully.

References

Alsup, E. M., and Debowes, R. M.: Dimethylsulfoxide. *J. Am. Vet. Med. Assoc.* 185:1011, 1984.

Bertone, J. J.: The use of nonsteroidal anti-inflammatory drugs and steroids in the equine emergency patient. *Proc. 36th Annu. Conv. Am. Assoc. Equine Pract.*, 1990, p. 239.

Blythe, L. L., Craig, A. M., Appell, L. H., and Lassen, E. D.: Intravenous use of dimethylsulfoxide (DMSO) in horses: Clinical and physiologic effects. *Proc. 33rd Annu. Conv. Am. Assoc. Equine Pract.*, 1987, p. 441.

Brayton, C. F.: Dimethylsulfoxide (DMSO): A review. *Cornell Vet.* 76:61, 1986.

Cohn, L. A.: The influence of corticosteroids on host defense mechanisms. *J. Vet. Intern. Med.* 5:95, 1991.

Conner, G. H., Riley, W. F., Beck, C. C., and Coppock, R. W.: Arquel (CI-1583): A new nonsteroidal anti-inflammatory drug for horses. *Proc. 19th Annu. Conv. Am. Assoc. Equine Pract.*, 1973, p. 81.

Hillidge, C. J.: The case for dimethylsulfoxide (DMSO) in equine practice. *Equine Vet. J.* 17:259, 1985.

Lees, P., Creed, R. F. S., Gerring, E. E. L., et al.: Biochemical and hematological effects of phenylbutazone in horses. *Equine Vet. J.* 15:158, 1983.

Lees, P., and Higgins, A. J.: Clinical pharmacology and therapeutic uses of nonsteroidal anti-inflammatory drugs in the horse. *Equine Vet. J.* 15:158, 1983.

Moore, J. N.: Nonsteroidal anti-inflammatory drug therapy for endotoxemia: We're doing the right thing, aren't we? *Compend. Contin. Educ. Pract. Vet.* 6:741, 1989.

Rose, R. J., Kohnke, J. R., and Baggot, J. D.: Bioavailability of phenylbutazone preparations in the horse. *Equine Vet. J.* 4:234, 1983.

Sandford, J.: DMSO: An alternative perspective. *Equine Vet. J.* 17:262, 1985.

Snow, D. H., Douglas, T. A., Thompson, H., et al.: Phenylbutazone toxicosis in Equidae: A biochemical and pathophysiologic study. *Am. J. Vet. Res.* 42:1754, 1981.

Tobin, T., Chay, S., Kamerling, S., et al.: Phenylbutazone in the horse: A review. *J. Vet. Pharmacol. Ther.* 9:1, 1986.

Bandaging and Casting

Bandaging of the distal limbs is necessary for restriction of movement, support, and to prevent swelling after surgery or after suturing wounds. If additional support or immobilization is required, the use of a large supporting bandage such as a Robert Jones bandage or a cast is required.

BANDAGING

A variety of bandages can be used but are usually based around three principles:

- Nonadherent dressings such as paraffin gauze to prevent the dressings adhering to the wound.
- Some form of padding such as sheet cotton to restrict movement, absorb any exudate, and allow pressure to be maintained evenly along the limb.
- A conforming bandage and/or elastic adhesive bandage to maintain the padding in position as a compressive layer.

Three main types of bandages will be demonstrated in this section.

Foot Bandage

- Bandaging the foot is required after foot surgery to protect the foot and, if necessary, to maintain a poultice in position to aid in provision of drainage (e.g., subsolar abscess).
- After a poultice has been placed over the sole (Fig. 17-2), sheet cotton (cotton wool) is used to

maintain the poultice in position (Fig. 17-3) and a cotton conforming bandage is applied as firmly as possible (Fig. 17-4). To prevent the bandage from becoming contaminated or wet, a plastic wrap can be positioned underneath the foot (Fig. 17-5) and fixed in position using elastic adhesive bandage (Fig. 17-6).

Bandaging the Carpus or Fetlock

- For a light restrictive bandage that is useful to provide support to the carpus or fetlock, if there

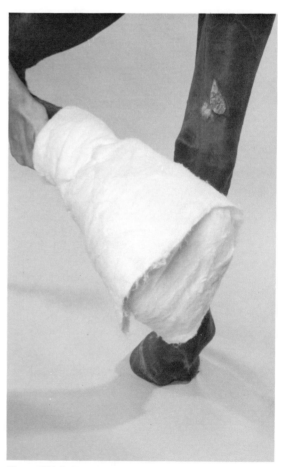

Figure 17–3. Foot bandage. After application of a poultice. sheet cotton is applied over the foot.

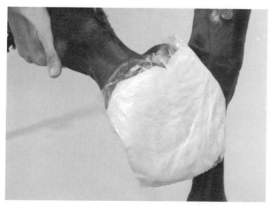

Figure 17–2. Foot bandage. Application of a poultice to encourage drainage of a subsolar abscess.

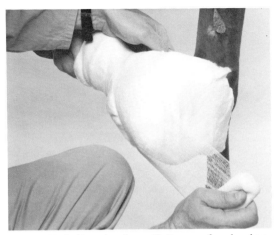

Figure 17–4. Foot bandage. Cotton conforming bandage is applied firmly to hold the sheet cotton in position.

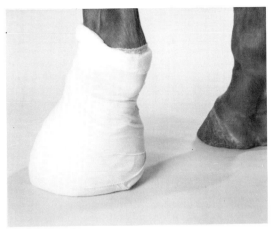

Figure 17–6. Foot bandage. Elastic adhesive bandage is used to complete the bandaging of the foot.

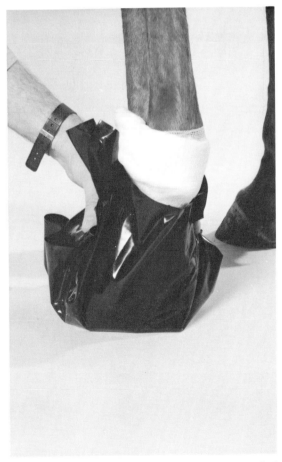

Figure 17–5. Foot bandage. Thick plastic is applied over the foot to prevent contamination of the bandage with urine and feces.

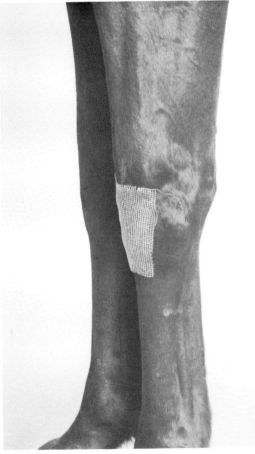

Figure 7–7. Bandaging of the carpus. Paraffin-gauze dressing applied over a wound on the dorsum of the carpus.

is a wound, a paraffin gauze dressing is applied (Fig. 17-7).

■ This is followed by polypropylene light bandage (Fig. 17-8) and a conforming bandage such as Vetwrap (3M Company, St. Paul, MN). This is best applied in a figure of 8 format (Figs. 17-9 and 17-10) so that pressure is avoided over the accessory carpal bone.

■ When the fetlock is bandaged, a similar process is used, but a figure of 8 bandage is not necessary.

■ An alternative is the use of an elastic adhesive bandage applied instead of the Vetwrap.

KEY POINT ▶ With elastic adhesive bandages, pressure over the accessory carpal bone is released by cutting through the elastic adhesive bandage with a scalpel blade (Fig. 17-11).

Robert Jones Bandage

KEY POINT ▶ For more extensive support and immobilization (e.g., in cases of severe lacerations or temporary fracture

support), a Robert Jones bandage is extremely useful.

■ This is a bandage that consists mainly of sheet cotton fixed in place with cotton conforming bandages.

■ A full-limb Robert Jones bandage commences with rolls of 10-cm (4-in) elastic adhesive bandage applied to the cranial and caudal surfaces of the limb (Fig. 17-12). These serve to prevent the bandage from slipping down the leg. Sheet cotton (four to five 500 g [1-lb] rolls) is then applied to the leg (Fig. 17-13), after which 10-cm (4-in) cotton conforming bandages are applied as tightly as possible. For a full-limb bandage, about six to eight cotton conforming bandages are required (Fig. 17-14). After the cotton conforming bandages are in place, the original elastic adhesive bandages are taken up over the front and back of the bandage (Fig. 17-15), after which the bandage is completed using elastic adhesive bandages applied over the outside (Fig. 17-16). Flicking the bandage with the fingers should result in a sound similar to a tight drum.

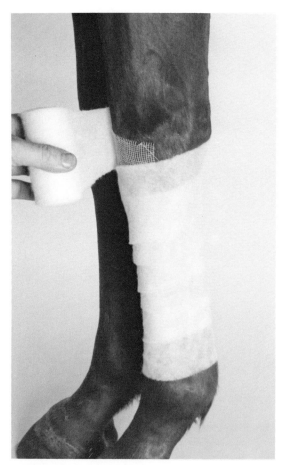

Figure 7–8. Bandaging of the carpus. Application of a light polypropylene bandage to the carpus.

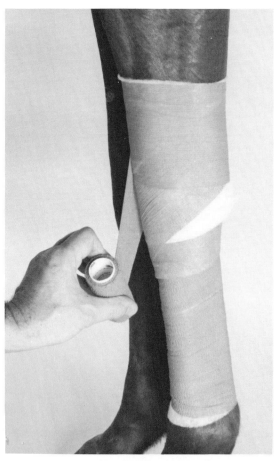

Figure 7–9. Bandaging of the carpus. A figure of 8 bandage is used to avoid pressure over the accessory carpal bone.

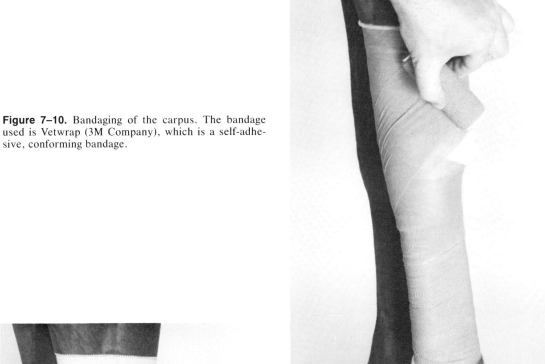

Figure 7–10. Bandaging of the carpus. The bandage used is Vetwrap (3M Company), which is a self-adhesive, conforming bandage.

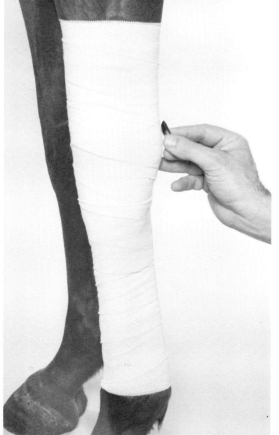

Figure 7–11. Bandaging of the carpus. An alternative to a figure of 8 bandage is an elastic adhesive bandage which is applied normally over the carpus. After bandaging, pressure over the accessory carpal bone is released by cutting the bandage over the accessory carpal bone.

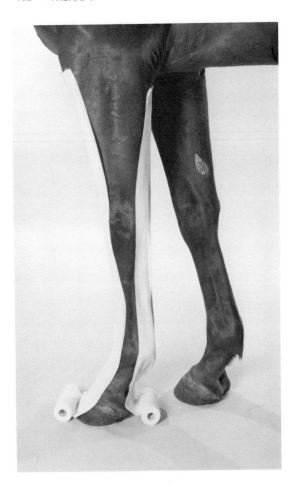

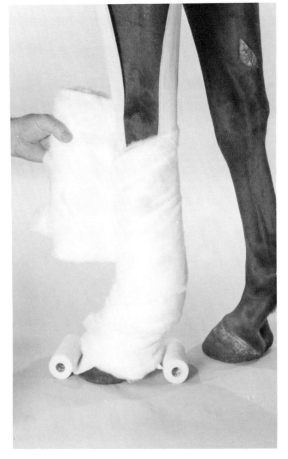

Figure 7–12. Robert Jones bandage. The bandage begins with application of elastic adhesive bandage to the front and back of the limb. While this is not essential, it is useful to prevent the bandage from slipping down.

Figure 7–13. Robert Jones bandage. Sheet cotton rolls are applied to the limb from the foot up to the proximal forearm. For a full-limb Robert Jones bandage, four to five 500-g (1-lb) rolls of sheet cotton are used.

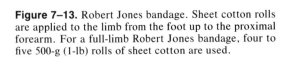

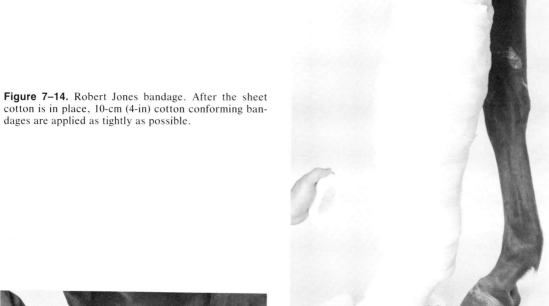

Figure 7–14. Robert Jones bandage. After the sheet cotton is in place, 10-cm (4-in) cotton conforming bandages are applied as tightly as possible.

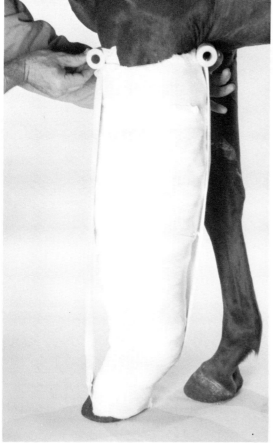

Figure 7–15. Robert Jones bandage. The elastic adhesive bandages, applied initially to the skin, are taken back over the front and back of the cotton conforming bandage layer so that the adhesive side is to the outside.

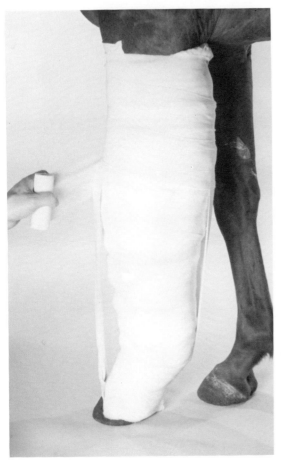

Figure 17–16. Robert Jones bandage. The bandage is completed by application of 10-cm (4-in) elastic adhesive bandages.

CASTING

Materials

- A range of casting techniques has been used with a variety of materials, including plaster of paris, thermoplastics, and fiberglass.

    KEY POINT ▶ Plaster of paris is the easiest material to work with, but it has less strength than the other materials and is extremely heavy.

- The other problem with plaster of paris is that it does not reach its full strength for approximately 24 hours after application, whereas the time that the major stress is on the cast is during recovery from anesthesia.
- Fiberglass is now the most widely used casting material, and its advantages are that it is strong, light, and impervious to water. The major disadvantage of fiberglass is that it is extremely rigid and unforgiving and can result in pressure sores if applied with uneven pressure.

Types of Casts and Indications

- Two types of casts are used: half-length and full-length casts. All casts include the foot, but half-length casts only go as far proximal as the heads of the small metatarsal or metacarpal bones, whereas full-length casts are applied up to the proximal radius or tibia.
- Half-length casts are useful for severe lacerations involving the distal limb and for phalangeal fractures.
- Full-length casts are necessary, with or without internal fixation, for metacarpal or metatarsal fractures, fractures of the radius and tibia, and tendon transection. The basic principle of fracture immobilization is to apply the cast so that the joints above and below the fracture are immobilized. However, in fractures of the radius or tibia, it is not possible to immobilize the joints above the fracture, and reliance is placed on internal fixation, with the casting giving additional support.

Cast Application

- Casts should be applied under general anesthesia with the leg to be cast uppermost.
- The cast should be applied with the leg in extension, and if reduction of fractures is necessary, this can be achieved by drilling holes and placing wires through the lateral and medial sides of the hoof wall to enable connection to a pulley system.
- It is always a compromise between good immobilization (the least amount of padding possible) and prevention of pressure sores (extra padding). We prefer the least amount of padding possible and use a single roll of polypropylene padding (Fig. 17-17) with a 10-cm-diameter stockinette (Figs. 17-18 and 17-19) applied over it. Foam rubber (Reston foam, 3M Company) can be used to prevent pressure sores at the top of the cast and over areas such as the accessory carpal bone, sesamoids, and calcaneus (Fig. 17-20).

KEY POINT ▶ To aid in easy cast removal, we include embryotomy wire underneath the cast.

- To prevent rusting and wire breakage, the wire is placed inside suitable material such as drip-set tubing and fixed on the medial and lateral sides of the limb with elastic adhesive bandage (Fig. 17-21).
- We begin the cast with one to two layers (two to three rolls) of 10-cm (4-in) plaster of paris bandage (Fig. 17-22), which helps to avoid pressure sores that can result when fiberglass is applied directly. For application of plaster of paris, we use hot water to hasten the setting time. After this, a roll of 10-cm plaster of paris is used underneath the heel of the foot to ensure that there is a level surface underneath the cast on which the horse

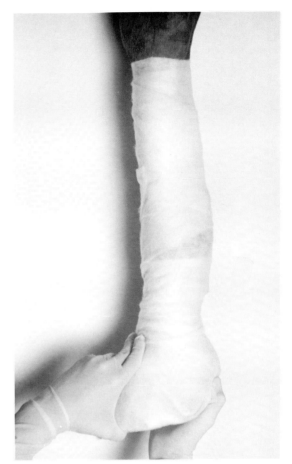

Figure 17–17. Application of a half-length cast. Casting begins with application of light padding using a polypropylene bandage.

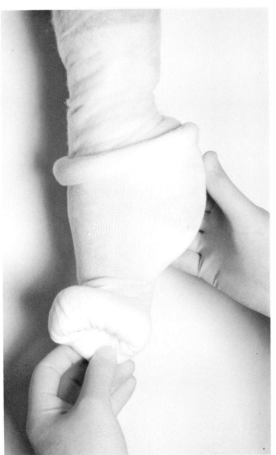

Figure 17–18. Application of a half-length cast. Stockinette (10 cm diameter) is applied over the padding.

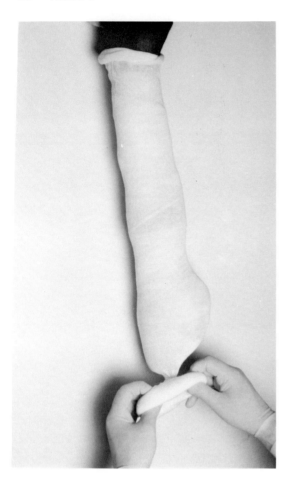

Figure 17–19. Application of a half-length cast. Stock-inette in position.

Figure 17–20. Application of a cast. Preparation of the hindleg for a full-limb cast. Note the foam rubber used to protect areas where pressure sores are likely to occur.

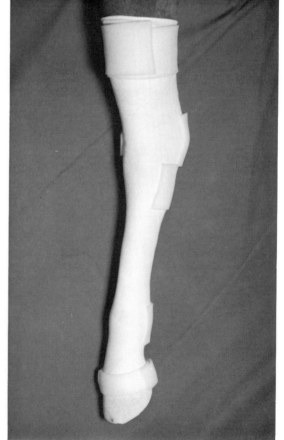

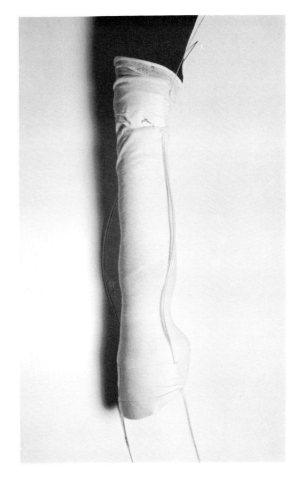

Figure 17–21. Application of a half-length cast. Prior to the casting material being applied, embryotomy wire may be applied inside drip-set tubing to provide a simple mechanism for later removal.

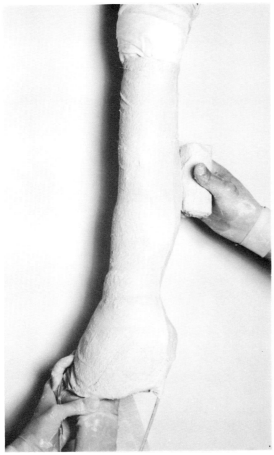

Figure 17–22. Application of a half-length cast. The cast is begun using 10-cm (4-in) rolls of plaster of paris bandage.

can walk (Fig. 17-23). An alternative is the use of a metal walking bar. Fiberglass rolls (10-cm-diameter; Vetcast, 3M Company) are then applied after immersion in lukewarm water. These rolls should not have the excess water squeezed out, unlike plaster, but rather the water should be allowed to drip from the bandage prior to its application. The rolls are applied beginning at the foot, overlapping each layer by about two-thirds of the diameter of the bandage (Fig. 17-24). Extra layers should be applied over regions where the cast is more likely to break, such as the pastern, fetlock, carpus, and tarsus. For a half-length cast, about 6 rolls of 10-cm-diameter fiberglass are needed, and for a full length cast, 10 to 12 rolls of fiberglass are needed. To prevent a sharp edge at the top of the cast, the stockinette can be pulled distally immediately after fiberglass application to ensure a smooth edge to the cast. The embryotomy wires within the drip-set tubing are taped to the cast to complete it (Fig. 17-25).

- To remove the cast, it is simple to attach handles to the embryotomy wire and saw through the medial and lateral sides of the cast (Fig. 17-26).

KEY POINT ▶ It is critical that a cast be changed at the first sign of any sudden lameness or obvious irritation, with the horse biting at the cast.

- Daily inspection should be made for signs of discharge and cracks, and the cast should be changed if a crack appears. If prolonged casting is required, the cast should be changed at least every 3 weeks.

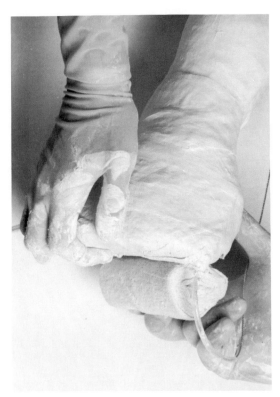

Figure 17–23. Application of a half-length cast. To ensure a level surface underneath the cast, a 10-cm (4-in) roll of plaster of paris can be placed at the heel of the cast.

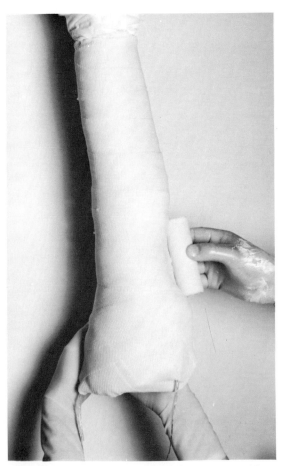

Figure 17–24. Application of a half-length cast. After the plaster of paris bandages are applied, 10-cm (4-in) fiberglass bandages are used to provide the reinforcement necessary for the cast.

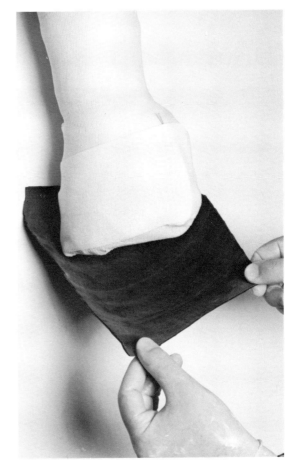

Figure 17–25. Application of a half-length cast. The cast is completed by taping the embryotomy wire to the cast and using a piece of rubber inner tube applied to the bottom of the cast. This is to prevent the cast from slipping when the horse places weight on it.

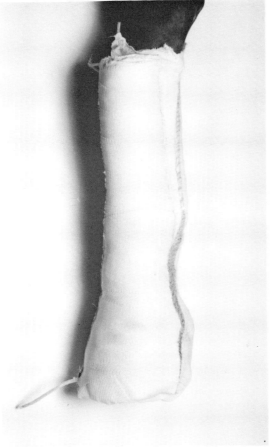

Figure 17–26. Cast removal. The cast is easily removed by attaching handles to the embryotomy wire and sawing through the medial and lateral sides of the cast.

Disinfectants

Disinfection is the elimination of some or all pathogenic microorganisms from an object so that infection is prevented. Disinfectants are used widely in equine practice for some instruments and where sterilization is not possible or impractical. Disinfectants are also used in the treatment of some wounds and irrigation of abscesses.

KEY POINT ▶ However, many disinfectants are inactivated by organic materials such as pus and blood.

More important, the disinfectants will cause considerable tissue irritation and should be used with great care around wounds or mucous membranes. Too often disinfectants are splashed into a bucket until a color is achieved that the practitioner thinks is appropriate. Accurate dilution is required to achieve the correct concentration for efficacy without tissue irritation. Some of the major disinfectants available are presented in Table 17-5. A wide variety of other disinfectants are available, and readers are referred to the *Compendium of Veterinary Products* (North American Compendiums, Port Huron, MI) for further details.

Medication Administration

Medication is administered to horses via three main routes: orally or via a nasogastric tube, intramuscularly, and intravenously. A variety of preparations such as antibiotics, anti-inflammatories, vitamins, minerals, and anthelmintics are available in paste form, and these products are easily administered by depositing on the back of the tongue via a syringe placed in the interdental space. Nasogastric tubing is also used for fluid and electrolyte administration, as well as for a range of other medications, such as mineral oil and anthelmintics. Details of the technique for nasogastric tubing are given in Chapter 6.

Intramuscular Injection

■ Intramuscular (IM) injections can be given in four main sites: the neck, pectorals, rump, and hindleg.

KEY POINT ▶ We use 18- or 19-gauge, 3.75 cm (1.5-in) needles for all IM injections, and the needle should always be inserted right up to the needle hub.

■ If the needle is inserted only part of the way, it is possible that as the injection is being given the needle may be pushed into a vessel, and therefore, some of the drug may be administered intravascularly.
■ Skin cleansing and disinfection are done using a suitable solution such as 70% alcohol. For IM injections in the neck, after a few taps with the back of the hand, the needle is inserted about 7.5 cm cranial to the line of the shoulder, in the middle of the neck (Fig. 17-27). Note that further ventral there is a risk of striking the transverse processes of the cervical vertebrae, and dorsally,

TABLE 17–5. Disinfectants: Effective Concentrations and Use

Disinfectant	Group	Trade Name	Use	Concentration	Effective Concentration
Hexachlorophane	Phenols	pHisoHex (Winthrop)	Skin	3%	Concentrate (3%) is used on skin
Chlorhexidine	Phenols	Hibiclens (Stuart)	General	4%	0.5% solution for general use (10 ml in 100 ml water) and 0.05% (1 ml in 100 ml) solution for wound cleansing
Iodine	Halogens	Tincture of iodine (mitis)	Skin		2.5% iodine and 2.5% KI in 90% ethanol
Povidone-iodine	Halogens	Betadine (Purdue-Frederick)	Skin and mucous membranes	10% povidone-iodine	10% iodine needed (equivalent to 1% available iodine)
Ethyl alcohol	Volatile solvent	—	Skin		70% alcohol is the most active form. To make up appropriate concentration using surgical spirits, take 815 ml and make up to 1 L with water
Benzalkonium chloride	Quarternary ammonium	Zephiran (Winthrop)	General	17%	0.05%–0.2% solution (5–20 ml in 1 L water)
Dialdehyde	Aldehydes	Cidex (Surgikos)	Instruments	2%	Place instruments in activated solution for 10 minutes

the injection will be made into the ligamentum nuchae, where it will be poorly absorbed.

KEY POINT ▶ The pectoral site is a good one because horses tolerate injections in this site (Fig. 17-28).

- The only disadvantage is that localized edema is often seen in the days following the injection, and this may be considered a problem by the clients.
- The middle gluteal muscle in the rump is a useful injection site because it is one of the largest muscles in the body. It is located by placing the thumb along the tuber coxa and spreading the hand so that where the small finger lies, the site is close to the center of the middle gluteal muscle. The needle is inserted at this site (Fig. 17-29).
- Injections into the semitendinosis and/or semi-membranosis muscles are useful sites in foals and also may be used in adults (Fig. 17-30).
- Prior to administration of the medication, aspiration should be performed with the syringe to ensure that the needle is not lying within a vessel. If intramuscular injections are required several times a day for several days or weeks, it is wise to alternate the injection sites as well as using the left and right sides of the horse so that the degree of inflammatory reaction is minimized at each of the locations.

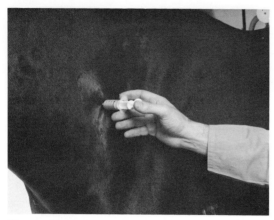

Figure 17–27. Intramuscular injection. Position of needle for injections in the neck.

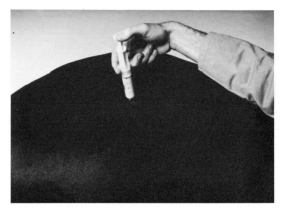

Figure 17–29. Intramuscular injection. Position of needle for injections in the middle gluteal muscle.

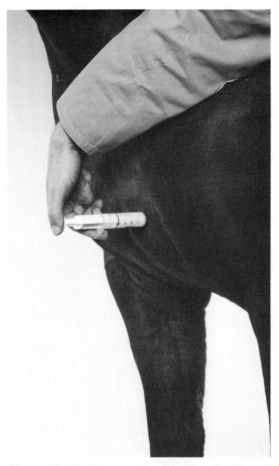

Figure 17–28. Intramuscular injection. Position of needle for injections in the pectoral muscles.

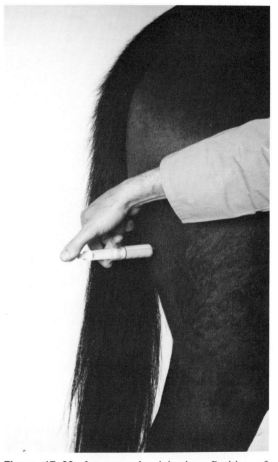

Figure 17–30. Intramuscular injection. Position of needle for injections in the semitendinosis muscle.

Intravenous Injection and Catheterization

■ Intravenous injections are necessary for administering a wide range of medications.

■ Many of the drugs given are irritating if injected perivascularly, and therefore, care must be taken to ensure that the needle is wholly within the vein.

■ While a range of veins are used for intravenous catheterization, most injections are given via the jugular vein. After the skin over the vein is cleaned and disinfected, the vein is distended by maintaining digital pressure on the vein in the lower third of the neck, and the needle is inserted (Fig. 17-31). We prefer 19-gauge, 3.75-mm (1.5-in) needles for all intravenous injections.

KEY POINT ► Catheterization must be done with care given to sterile technique.

■ Complications such as phlebitis and septicemia can arise from inadequate skin disinfection and trauma during catheterization.

■ The jugular vein is commonly used for intravenous catheterization, and the following technique is used: Hair over the vein should be clipped and shaved, after which the skin is given three 1-minute scrubs with povidone-iodine scrub (Treatment No. 91), interspersed with application of 70% alcohol. To complete disinfection, povidone-iodine solution (1% available iodine) is sprayed on the skin. Local anesthetic (0.5–1.0 ml of 2% lidocaine, mepivicaine, or prilocaine) is injected intradermally over the center of the jugular vein (Fig. 17-32), after which the skin is disinfected with povidone-iodine.

■ Sterile gloves are worn when inserting either a 12- or 14-gauge catheter, 8 to 30 cm (3–12 in) long. The longer catheter is used if long-term fluid therapy is planned, and a 12-gauge catheter

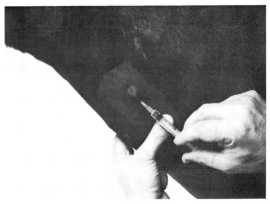

Figure 17–32. Intravenous catheterization. After skin disinfection, a bleb of local anesthetic is injected over the middle of the jugular vein.

is selected if rapid fluid infusion is required. The catheter can be inserted either up or down the vein, and for longer-term fluid administration, it may be better to insert the catheter down the vein. A 12-gauge catheter is too large to insert without a stab incision in the skin. The catheter should be inserted at a 45 degree angle to the horizontal plane of the skin (Fig. 17-33), until blood is visible in the catheter stylet, indicating that the tip of the stylet is within the vein. The catheter and stylet are straightened toward a zero angle with the skin and advanced 2 to 3 cm (1 in). The stylet is then withdrawn about 1.25 cm (0.5 in), and the catheter is advanced up to the hub of the catheter (Fig. 17-34). Extension tubing, which has previously been filled with heparinized saline (10 IU heparin per liter), is connected to the catheter, and the hub of the catheter and extension tube are fixed in place with a few drops of a rapid-setting glue such as Superglue or Crazyglue (Fig. 17-35).

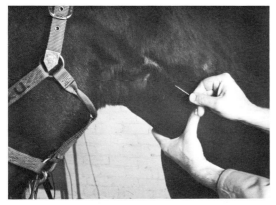

Figure 17–31. Intravenous injection. The needle is inserted at a slight angle to the jugular vein, and after blood flows from the needle, it is straightened and inserted up the lumen of the vein until the hub is reached.

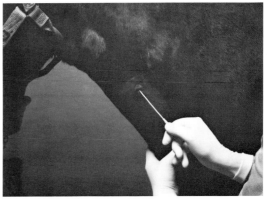

Figure 17–33. Intravenous catheterization. With the jugular vein distended, the catheter is inserted at an angle to the vein until blood appears at the end of the stylet.

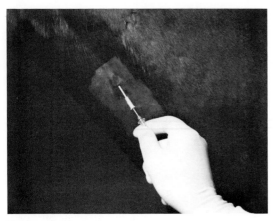

Figure 17–34. Intravenous catheterization. After the catheter and stylet are within the lumen of the vein, they are advanced for 2 to 3 cm (1 in), and the stylet is withdrawn 1 cm (0.5 in). The catheter and stylet are then inserted up the vein.

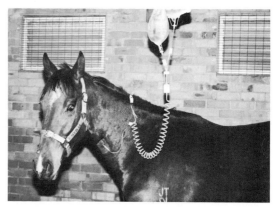

Figure 17–36. Intravenous catheterization. Connection of the extension tubing to extendable rubber or plastic tubing allows the horse to receive fluids while moving around its box stall.

- Extendable plastic or rubber tubing is connected to the extension tubing. This extendable tubing allows the horse to move around freely within its box stall (Fig. 17-36).

KEY POINT ▶ We find that the use of the Gyro Fluid Hanger and Stat Large Animal IV Set (Internation Win, Ltd., PO Box 5569, Cary, NC), shown in Figure 17-36, is helpful in the administration of large volumes of fluid with minimal supervision.

- Other veins that can be used for fluid administration include the cephalic (Fig. 17-37), saphenous (Fig. 17-38), and superficial (lateral) thoracic (Fig. 17-39) veins.

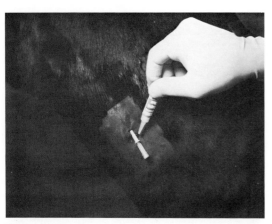

Figure 17–35. Intravenous catheterization. The catheter and extension tubing can be fixed in position with a rapidly acting glue such as Superglue or Crazyglue.

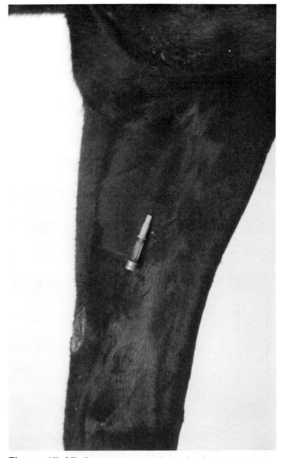

Figure 17–37. Intravenous catheterization. An alternative site to the jugular vein for intravenous catheterization is the cephalic vein. This site is particularly useful for intravenous fluid administration to foals.

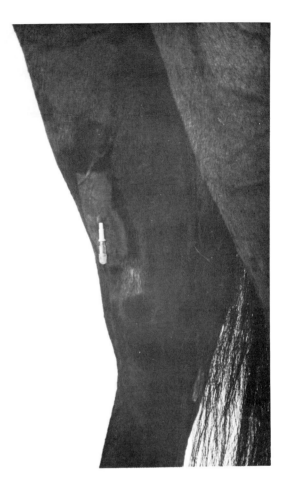

Figure 17–38. Intravenous catheterization. An alternative site to the jugular vein for intravenous catheterization is the saphenous vein. This site is more difficult and dangerous to catheterize than other available sites.

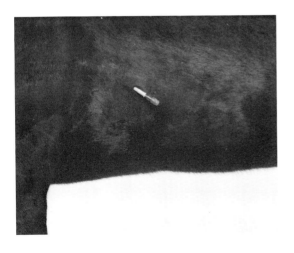

Figure 17–39. Intravenous catheterization. An alternative site to the jugular vein for intravenous catheterization is the lateral thoracic vein. Because this is a large-diameter vein, a 10- or 12-gauge catheter can be inserted if needed. The vein is located deeper than the other veins used for catheterization.

Fluid and Electrolyte Therapy

Many clinicians regard the old saying "the horse's kidney is smarter than the smartest equine clinician" as indicating that they can give whatever fluid-electrolyte solution they like and the horse will sort it all out. While there is a little truth in this, selection of the correct fluid and route and rate of administration and deciding whether or not bicarbonate is required are critical decisions that need to be made affecting the outcome of treatment. To make these decisions, laboratory data are required, together with an accurate clinical assessment of the case. A few principles are helpful when instituting fluid therapy:

KEY POINT ▶ Think in big volumes in adult horses—that is, 20 to 50 L is the usual range.

- Use a balanced electrolyte solution, usually with similar composition to plasma.
- If the peripheral pulse is weak or absent and there is a prolonged capillary refill time, rapid infusion of large volumes (>20 L in 1–2 hours) of polyionic isotonic solutions is necessary.
- Do not use bicarbonate solutions unless measurements are made and plasma values are less than 15 mmol/L (mEq/L).

KEY POINT ▶ Consider fluid administration by nasogastric tube if gastrointestinal function is normal.

Assessment of Fluid and Electrolyte Balance

Clinical assessment of hydration state can be gained from clinical examination; pulse rate and quality, capillary refill time, heart rate, and skin turgor provide a guide to the extent of fluid loss.

KEY POINT ▶ Skin turgor is best assessed by pulling up a fold of skin over the point of the shoulder to determine how quickly the skin moves back into a normal position. This site provides more reliable results than when the skin is assessed over the neck.

Five percent dehydration is the minimum degree of dehydration that can be detected, and there are few changes in clinical signs. Moderate dehydration

(7%–8%) results in a thready pulse, prolonged capillary refill time to 3 to 4 seconds, and a decrease in skin turgor. Severe dehydration (10%–12%) is evidenced by dry mucous membranes, prolonged capillary refill time (4–5 seconds), a weak or no detectable pulse, and a marked decrease in skin turgor.

Laboratory aids that are available in practice and are useful in assessing fluid and electrolyte deficits and deciding on therapy are as follows:

Hematocrit (PCV) and Total Plasma Protein (TPP)—These are simply measured using the microhematocrit technique (PCV) and refractometry (TPP) and provide a guide to extracellular fluid (ECF) balance. While extra red cells are released if the horse is excited or in pain, a high PCV (>0.45 L/L or 45%) generally indicates reduction in ECF volume and sodium loss. The TPP is unaffected by excitement and so is often a better guide to ECF volume depletion, with values greater than 75 g/L (7.5 g/dl) indicating sodium and water loss. It should be remembered, however, that in conditions where there is protein loss (e.g., diarrhea, renal disease), a horse may be dehydrated yet have a normal to low TPP. Similarly, if there is a chronic infection with increases in fibrinogen and gammaglobulins, the TPP may be elevated without dehydration being present. In general, TPP values less than 75 g/L (7.5 g/dl) indicate less than 5% dehydration. TPP values in the range 75 to 85 g/L (7.5–8.5 g/dl) indicate 5% to 8% dehydration, and values between 85 and 95 g/L (8.5 to 9.5 g/dl) signify 8% to 10% dehydration.

Serum or Plasma Electrolytes—These are essential measurements if accurate estimations of electrolyte losses are to be made. We prefer plasma samples to be collected because an estimate of bicarbonate concentration can be performed if samples are collected into Vacutainer tubes containing lithium heparin as an anticoagulant. Electrolytes that should be measured are sodium, potassium, chloride, and bicarbonate.

Significance of Fluid and Electrolyte Alterations

The total-body water (60%–70% of body weight) is divided between two main compartments, the intracellular fluid (ICF) and the extracellular fluid (ECF), which vary considerably in electrolyte composition. The ECF has high sodium and low potassium concentrations, whereas the ICF has low sodium and high potassium concentrations. It should be remembered that water moves freely between the ECF and ICF.

Sodium

The average 450- to 500-kg horse has a total exchangeable sodium of approximately 14,000 mmol (mEq) (average [Na] 140 mmol/L and ECF volume 100 L), nearly all of which is located in the ECF.

KEY POINT ▶ Plasma or serum sodium values do not indicate sodium deficits or excesses but are affected by water movement as well as changes in sodium or potassium concentrations.

This relationship has been represented by the following equation (Edelman et al., 1958):

$$\text{Serum Na (mmol/L } H_2O \text{ or mEq/L } H_2O) = \frac{\text{exchangeable Na + exchangeable K}}{\text{total body water}}$$

This equation can provide a guide to the sodium and potassium deficits and the distributions of fluid losses between compartments if the serum or plasma sodium is known and an estimate of the total body water can be made. Accurate measurement of body weight is of great value in assessing the response to therapy because fluid retention (liters) approximately equals increase in body weight (kg).

Potassium

The ECF contains only 400 mmol (mEq) or less than 2% of the total-body potassium (approximately 28,000 mmol), and therefore, plasma and serum potassium values do not indicate total-body potassium status. While hyperkalemia (serum or plasma K values > 4.5 mmol/L) in the horse is rare, hypokalemia (serum or plasma K values < 3.0 mmol/L) is more common, particularly in horses with diarrhea.

KEY POINT ▶ Serum or plasma potassium values greater than 4.5 mmol/L may be due to problems with sample handling or processing rather than to a pathologic process.

Delays in processing or storage of samples in the heat can result in potassium movement out of the erythrocytes or hemolysis with resulting increases in plasma potassium. Therefore, high plasma or serum potassium values should be regarded intially as suspicious of a laboratory error rather than of a disease state. A further blood sample should be collected to confirm hyperkalemia.

KEY POINT ▶ Hypokalemia usually indicates total-body potassium depletion, but the extent of depletion cannot be quantified from the extent of hypokalemia found.

For example, horses with diarrhea often have plasma or serum potassium values less than 2.0 mmol/L (mEq/L), but the extent of potassium loss may be less than half that of a horse that has had food and water deprivation for several days and has a plasma potassium value of 3.0 mmol/L (mEq/L). Plasma potassium values are also affected by acid–base status, with acidosis increasing and alkalosis decreasing plasma potassium. However, the extent of change is quite small in most clinical settings, usually less than 1.0 mmol/L.

Chloride and Bicarbonate

Chloride and bicarbonate are the principal anions of the ECF. Chloride is located in the ECF, and changes in plasma or serum concentrations reflect changes in whole-body status. Changes tend to occur in conditions where there is chloride loss, such as diarrhea, and in substantial sweat losses, such as occur during prolonged exercise. Plasma chloride and bicarbonate concentrations are inversely related.

KEY POINT ▶ In metabolic acidosis, plasma bicarbonate concentration is decreased and chloride increased, while the reverse is true in metabolic alkalosis.

Bicarbonate values are most commonly measured as total CO_2 in plasma using autoanalyzers. Alternatively, true bicarbonate can be measured from the pH and PCO_2 using a blood gas machine. The total CO_2 represents the bicarbonate plus dissolved CO_2, and in most situations the bicarbonate is approximately 5% lower than the total CO_2. If blood samples are collected into lithium heparin Vacutainer tubes and kept refrigerated, bicarbonate concentrations will remain stable for up to 3 days after blood collection.

Because primary respiratory acid–base alterations are rare in the conscious horse, increased total CO_2 indicates metabolic alkalosis, while decreased CO_2 is evidence of metabolic acidosis.

KEY POINT ▶ Metabolic acidosis occurs when there is bicarbonate loss (e.g., diarrhea) or increased lactate production (e.g., shock, high-intensity exercise). In contrast, metabolic alkalosis is rarely found but may occur where there is excessive loss of gastric secretions such as in anterior enteritis, where there are extensive losses of chloride in the sweat, or where horses have been administered high doses of bicarbonate prior to racing.

Calculating Fluid and Electrolyte Losses

KEY POINT ▶ A guide to the electrolyte and fluid deficits can be obtained using the equation of Edelman et al. (1958), with measurement of serum or plasma sodium and assessment of total-body water.

An example of calculations that can be made of fluid and electrolyte deficits is set out below. The symbol I refers to initial values, and D refers to dehydrated values.

A 500-kg horse is assessed from clinical findings as being 8% dehydrated due to severe diarrhea. The assessment is made on the basis of increased skin turgor, dry mucous membranes, and increased capillary refill time. Plasma sodium is 130 mmol/L (mEq/L), and plasma potassium is 3.0 mEq/L. Assumptions that are made are that the plasma sodium value prior to dehydration was the mean of the normal range (134–142 mmol/L), that is, 138 mmol/L, and that the total-body water is 60% of the body weight, that is, 300 L prior to dehydration.

If the horse was 500 kg before diarrhea, 8% dehydration would result in a loss of approximately 40 kg. We assume that 90% of the body weight loss is due to water loss, and therefore, the water loss is 36L:

$$
\begin{aligned}
\text{Water deficit} &= \text{weight loss} \times 0.9 \\
&= 40 \text{ kg} \times 0.9 \\
&= 36 \text{ L}
\end{aligned}
$$

$$
\begin{aligned}
\text{Total-body water (TBW)} \\ \text{before dehydration} &= 300 \text{ L (60\% body weight)}
\end{aligned}
$$

$$
\begin{aligned}
\text{Total-body water} \\ \text{after dehydration} &= 264 \text{ L}
\end{aligned}
$$

Serum or plasma sodium times TBW equals exchangeable Na (Na_e) plus exchangeable K (K_e) (Edelman et al., 1958), that is,

$$140 \times 300 = Na_e + K_e \ (I)$$

$$Na_e + K_e \ (I) = 42,000 \text{ mmol (mEq)}$$

$$Na_e + K_e \ (D) = 264 \times 130$$

$$= 34,320 \text{ mmol/L (mEq)}$$

$$\text{Total deficit of Na} + \text{K} = 42,000 - 32,320$$

$$= 7680 \text{ mmol (mEq)}$$

How can this deficit be apportioned between Na and K? In diarrhea, approximately 70% of Na + K loss is Na. In food and/or water deprivation, approximately 10% to 15% of Na + K loss is Na. Thus, the 7680 Na + K deficit can be apportioned as follows:

Na deficit = 5376 mmol (mEq)

K deficit = 2304 mmol (mEq)

Because virtually all the exchangeable Na is in the ECF and all the exchangeable K in the ICF, some calculations can be made concerning compartmental fluid distributions:

$$
\begin{aligned}
\text{Na content}_D &= 14,000 \text{ mmol (mEq)} \\
&\quad (140 \times 100 \text{ L of ECF}) \\
&\quad - 5376 \text{ mmol (mEq)} \\
&= 8624 \text{ mmol (mEq)}
\end{aligned}
$$

$$
\begin{aligned}
ECF_D \text{ (L)} &= \frac{\text{Na content}_D}{\text{Na mmol/L (mEq/L)}_D} \\
&= \frac{8624}{130} \\
&= 66 \text{ L}
\end{aligned}
$$

$$
\begin{aligned}
ICF_D &= TBW_D - ECF_D \\
&= 264 \text{ L} - 66 \text{ L} \\
&= 198 \text{ L}
\end{aligned}
$$

Overall Deficits

TBW deficit = 40 kg × 0.9 = 36 L
ECF deficit = 100 − 66 L = 34 L
ICF deficit = 200 − 198 L = 2 L
Na deficit = 5376 mmol (mEq)
K deficit = 2304 mmol (mEq)

KEY POINT ▶ Thus, quite substantial electrolyte deficits can exist in the face of relatively normal plasma/serum values.

■ Administration of 36 L of a balanced polyionic solution (e.g., Multisol, Normosol R, Sanofi, Overland Park, KS) would provide 5040 mmol (mEq) and almost completely replace the sodium debt, whereas only 180 mmol (mEq), or less than 10%, of the potassium debt would be corrected. This is not a major problem in the short term, but if fluid therapy is required over several days and there is little potassium replacement, substantial deficits can develop that can affect cardiac, neuromuscular, and gastrointestinal function.

KEY POINT ▶ Of major importance is the sodium deficit, because sodium controls the ECF volume.

■ With substantial sodium deficits, such as in the case illustrated above, there will be decreased peripheral perfusion and signs of shock. The sodium and volume deficit correction are the chief concerns when initiating fluid and electrolyte therapy.

KEY POINT ▶ It also should be remembered that the equine kidney has adapted to a diet rich in potassium by excreting large amounts of potassium in the urine.

■ Therefore, potassium deficits may occur when a horse is not eating or does not have access to green feed. In these circumstances, the oral or nasogastric administration of potassium chloride for several days can be effective in restoring potassium balance, since this is impossible using IV fluids. Usual doses of oral potassium chloride are 50 to 100 g (2–3.5 oz), equivalent to 675 to 1350 mmol (mEq) of potassium. These doses are usually administered in several liters of water by nasogastric tube.

Route of Fluid Administration

If rapid blood volume expansion is not needed, and if the gastrointestinal tract is functioning normally, oral fluids or fluids given by nasogastric tube should be considered. In horses with diarrhea, electrolyte solutions administered by nasogastric tube are well absorbed and are useful for maintaining hydration status in addition to potassium balance.

KEY POINT ▶ Fluids administered by nasogastric tube should not be used if the horse has ileus or positive nasogastric reflux.

We have found the use of glucose–glycine–electrolyte mixtures such as Re-Sorb (SmithKline Beecham, Exton, PA), Hy-Sorb (Sanofi, Overland Park, KS), Hydra-Lyte and Isotone A (Vet-A-Mix, Shenandoah, IA), and Revive (Fermenta, Kansas City, MO) to be effective for oral or nasogastric fluid administration. The glucose and glycine enhance the uptake of fluid and electrolytes from the small intestine. Some of these mixtures were formulated for calf diarrhea but are useful for fluid and electrolyte therapy in horses when mixed with an appropriate volume of water to make an isotonic solution. Most horses will not drink these mixtures, but in adult horses, 8 to 10 L can be administered by nasogastric tube every 30 to 60 minutes until the estimated fluid loss is replaced. Fluids administered by nasogastric tube are useful for maintenance fluid therapy.

KEY POINT ▶ Hypertonic solutions administered by nasogastric tube should be avoided in horses with hypovolemia because water will move out of other spaces into the gastrointestinal tract and worsen the hypovolemia.

Type and Volume of Fluid

Three main fluid types should be considered:

Replacement Fluids—Have a sodium composition similar to plasma. The major fluids used are polyionic, and the typical composition (mmol/L or mEq/L) would be: Na 140 mmol/L, K 5 mmol/L, Mg 3 mmol/L, Cl 98 mmol/L, and bicarbonate precursors (usually acetate and gluconate) 50 mmol/L. In the past, normal saline (0.9% sodium chloride) has been used, but the main disadvantages are a high chloride content (154 mmol/L), lack of bicarbonate precursors, and higher than desired sodium (154 mmol/L).

KEY POINT ▶ Replacement fluids should be used in situations where there has been sodium loss (hypovolemia) or where the horse is in shock.

Sterile replacement fluids are available in 3-L bags (Normosol R or Lactated Ringer's Solution Rx, Sanofi, Overland Park, KS). Alternatively, concentrated electrolyte solutions are available that can be added to sterile water to constitute 3 L of a replacement electrolyte solution. Products that are available include Lactated Ringer's Solution, Multisol-R 3X, and Equi-Lyte Concentrate (Sanofi, Overland Park, KS).

Maintenance Fluids—Have a much lower sodium but higher potassium concentration than those in replacement fluids. The typical composition (mmol/L or mEq/L) would be Na 40 mmol/L, K 13 mmol/L, Cl 40 mmol/L, acetate 16 mmol/L, and Mg 3 mmol/L, in 5% dextrose. If maintenance with intravenous fluids is required over several days, a high sodium concentration in the fluid is contraindicated. Use of a replacement fluid in these situations may not correct dehydration, owing to the excessive sodium load being excreted, together with water.

Hypertonic Fluids—In horses with severe hypovolemic shock (e.g., blood loss, bowel torsion), the intravenous administration of small volumes of fluids with a high concentration of sodium (e.g., 5% NaCl) can rapidly correct the hypovolemia. This is only a short-term measure to improve cardiac output and arterial blood pressure and should not be relied on to correct the fluid deficits. A 7% saline solution is available commercially (Hyper Saline-7, Butler, Dublin, OH).

The volume and type of fluid to be administered varies with the condition requiring treatment, and some guidelines are presented in Table 17-6. In general, the flow rate of intravenous fluids should not exceed 2 L/h unless the horse is in shock. Higher flow rates will result in increased urinary excretion of fluids with poor retention.

Bicarbonate Use

Sodium bicarbonate is used to aid in treatment of conditions that result in severe metabolic acidosis.

KEY POINT ▶ Metabolic acidosis itself causes little adverse effects; rather, it is the problem that caused the acidosis that should be treated.

Thus, in shock or ischemic colic, metabolic acidosis is the result of reduced tissue perfusion, with a resulting increase in lactate production. In such cases, therapy should focus on expansion of ECF volume rather than bicarbonate administration.

KEY POINT ▶ Bicarbonate therapy is useful in cases where there has been substantial bicarbonate loss (e.g., diarrhea) or where metabolic acidosis is severe ($HCO_3 < 15$ mmol/L).

TABLE 17–6. Likely Fluid and Electrolyte Deficits and Alterations in Laboratory Data with Conditions that Cause Fluid and Electrolyte Disturbances in a Typical Adult (500-kg) Horse

Clinical Problem	Estimated Deficits			Likely Changes in Laboratory Data†						Suggested Type and Amount of Fluid
	H₂O (L)	Na (mmol*)	K (mmol*)	PCV	TPP	Na	K	Cl	HCO₃	
Diarrhea—mild, horse drinking	15–25	800–1200	300–450	N	N	↓ ↓	↓	↓	N or ↓	15–20 L by stomach tube of a glucose–glycine-electrolyte mix (Treatment No. 57) with added KCl (50 g/10 L H₂O)
Diarrhea—severe, horse not drinking	40–60	2000–4000	800–1600	↑↑	↑↑	N or ↑	↓	↓	↓	30–40 L IV replacement fluid. 3 L of 5% NaHCO₃. Possibly IV plasma
Food and water deprivation 24–48 h	10–25	200–500	2000–3000	↑	↑	↑	N	↑	N	10–15 L of IV maintenance fluid supplemented by 10 L glucose–glycine-electrolyte mix by stomach tube with 75 g KCl
Colic—LI impaction for 2–3 days	15–30	500–1500	2000–3000	↑	↑	↑	N	N	N	No fluids by stomach tube until some gut motility. Large volumes (50–80 L) of IV fluids, preferably maintenance, to soften mass
Colic—torsion, intussusception	20–50	2000–5000	1000–2000	↑↑	↑↑	N	N	N	↓	IV replacement fluid to effect. Bicarbonate not needed in most cases. 20–40 L IV; monitor TPP; slow fluids if TPP < 50 g/L (5 g/dl)
Postexercise dehydration (fast exercise), 3–10 km	5–10	500–1000	400–800	↑	↑	↑	N	N	↓	5–10 L of glucose-glycine-electrolyte mixture by stomach tube
Postexercise dehydration, 80–160 km (endurance)	20–50	2000–5000	1000–2500	↑	↑	N or ↓	↓	↓	N or ↑	15–20 L replacement fluids IV if signs of decreased perfusion. If normal gut activity, fluids can be then given by stomach tube

PCV—packed cell volume; TPP—total plasma protein

*mmol is the same as mEq.

†N = within the normal range; ↓ = slightly decreased; ↓ ↓ = substantially decreased; ↑ = slightly increased; ↑ ↑ = substantially increased.

If bicarbonate is administered, it should be used sparingly because an equal number of milliequivalents of sodium will also be given, which may lead to additional excretion of water.

To calculate the amount of bicarbonate to be used, the following formula is generally used:

Bicarbonate required (mEq or mmol) = 0.3 × body weight (kg) × base deficit (mEq/L or mmol/L)

The amount of bicarbonate calculated is based on a deficit in the extracellular fluid (approximately 30% of body weight), which is why 0.3 is included in the formula. The base deficit is calculated by subtracting the plasma bicarbonate or total carbon dioxide from 25 mmol/L (mEq/L), which is the lower end of the normal range (25–33 mmol/L). In severe acidosis, the plasma bicarbonate concentration may fall to 10 mEq/L. Thus the calculated bicarbonate requirement in a 500-kg horse would be 0.3 × 500 × (25 − 10) = 2500 mmol (mEq). Half the calculated deficit is usually replaced so that overcorrection of the acidosis does not occur, and a further blood sample is taken for measurement of bicarbonate concentrations. Thus, in the case above, 1250 mmol (mEq) of sodium bicarbonate could be administered, which is approximately 2 L of a 5% solution.

References

Becht, J.: Fluid therapy in the acutely injured or exhausted horse. *Proc. 34th Annu. Conv. Am. Assoc. Equine Pract.*, 1988, p. 505.

Bertone, J. J.: Hypertonic saline in the management of shock in horses. *Compend. Contin. Educ. Pract. Vet.* 13:665, 1991.

Brown, C. M., Green, N., and Lamar, A. M.: Intravenous use of large volumes of commercially prepared sterile electrolyte solutions. *Equine Pract.* 8:26, 1986.

Carlson, G. P.: Fluid therapy in horses with acute diarrhea. *Vet. Clin. North Am. (Large Anim. Pract.)* 1:313, 1979.

Carlson, G. P.: Fluid and electrolyte therapy: The role of sodium bicarbonate. *Proc. 36th Annu. Conv. Am. Assoc. Equine Pract.*, 1990, p. 141.

Divers, T. J., Freeman, D. E., Ziemer, E. L., and Becht, J. L.: Interpretation of electrolyte abnormalities in clinical disease in the horse. *Proc. 32nd Annu. Conv. Am. Assoc. Equine Pract.*, 1986, p. 69.

Edelman, I. S., Leibman, J., O'Meara, M. P., and Birkenfeld, L. W.: Interrelations between serum sodium concentrations, serum osmolality and total exchangeable sodium, total exchangeable potassium and total body water. *J. Clin. Invest.* 37:1236, 1958.

Hansen, T. O., White, N. A., and Kemp, D. T.: Total parenteral nutrition in four healthy adult horses. *Am. J. Vet. Res.* 49:122, 1988.

Kemp, D. T.: A comprehensive guide to intravenous fluid therapy in horses. *Vet. Med.* 83:193, 1988.

Rose, R. J.: A physiological approach to fluid and electrolyte therapy in the horse. *Equine Vet. J.* 13:7, 1981.

Schmall, L. M.: New approaches to fluid therapy and management in the equine emergency patient. *Proc. 36th Annu. Conv. Am. Assoc. Equine Pract.*, 1990, p. 267.

Spurlock, G. H., and Spurlock, S. L.: A technique of catheterization of the lateral thoracic vein in the horse. *Equine Prac.* 9:33, 1987.

Dose Rates, Use, and Route of Administration of Some Drugs Commonly Used in Equine Practice

Name of Drug	Dose	Main Use	Route
Acepromazine	0.03–0.06 mg/kg	Tranquilization	IV
Altrenogest (allyl trenbolone)	0.044 mg/kg (1 ml/50 kg body weight)	Transitional estrus Estrus synchronization Control of aggression	PO
Amikacin sulfate	7 mg/kg q8–12h	Antibiotic—gram-negative bacteria	IV or IM
Aminophylline	4–7 mg/kg q8h	Bronchodilatation	PO
Ampicillin sodium	10–50 mg/kg q8h	Antibiotic—mostly for gram-positive bacteria	IV or IM
Aspirin	15–100 mg/kg q24h	Anti-inflammatory and antithrombotic	PO or IV
Bismuth subsalicylate suspension (1.75%)	0.6 ml/kg q6–12h	Foal diarrhea	PO
Boldenone undecyclenate	1 mg/kg repeated at 2–4 week intervals	Debility, anemia	IM
Bromhexine	3 mg/kg q12h	Respiratory disease	PO
Butorphanol	0.03–0.08 mg/kg	Analgesia, colic pain	IV
Captan	2%–3% solution	Ringworm	Topical
Ceftiofur	2–4 mg/kg q12h	Some bacterial respiratory infections	IM or IV
Cephalothin sodium	10–20 mg/kg q8h	Only if sensitivity tests indicate no alternative	IM or IV
Cimetidine HCl	6–7 mg/kg q6h	Gastroduodenal ulcer disease	PO or IV
Clenbuterol	0.8 µg/kg q12h	Respiratory disease	IV, by nebulizer, or PO
Cloxacillin sodium	30 mg/kg q6–8h	Antibiotic for beta-lactamase staphylococci	IM or IV
Detomidine HCl	0.01–0.08 mg/kg	Sedative	IV
Dexamethasone	0.04–0.4 mg/kg q24h	Corticosteroid—shock, CNS injury, autoimmune disorders	IV, IM, or PO

Name of Drug	Dose	Main Use	Route
Diazepam	0.05–0.4 mg/kg	Tranquilizer, seizures	IV or IM
Digoxin	14 μg/kg IV for digitilization 3.5 μg/kg q12h IV maintenance. Oral dose 70 μg/kg once then 35–40 μg/kg q12h	Heart failure	IV or PO
Dimethylsulfoxide (DMSO)	Available as 90% solution (9 g/ml). IV dose 0.5–1 g/kg as a 10%–20% solution in saline q12h for up to 3 days. May also be used as an intraarticular infusion for septic arthritis or synovitis	CNS trauma, gastrointestinal disorders, topical application for local inflammation, septic arthritis	Topical or IV
Dioctyl sodium sulfosuccinate	10–20 mg/kg q24h	Large bowel impactions	PO
Dipyrone	22 mg/kg q24h	Analgesic and antipyretic	IV or IM
Dobutamine	2–10 μg/kg/min	Use during anesthesia to treat hypotension	IV
Epinephrine 1:1000 (Adrenaline)	3–5 ml/450 kg	For treatment of anaphylaxis	IM or SC
Erythromycin lactobionate	10 mg/kg q8h	Antibiotic broad spectrum but bacteriostatic	IV or IM
Erythromycin estolate	25 mg/kg q8–12h	For treatment of *R. equi* in combination with rifampin	PO
Fenbendazole	5 mg/kg or 10 mg/kg q24h for 5 days for *S. vulgaris* in foals	Anthelmintic	PO
Flunixin meglumine	0.25 mg/kg q6h or 1 mg/kg q12–24h	Abdominal pain, musculoskeletal, endotoxemia	IV or PO
Fluprostenol	250–500 μg/500 kg	Luteolytic agent, induction of parturition	IM
Furosemide	0.4–1.5 mg/kg	Edema, renal failure, EIPH	IV or IM
Gentamicin	2–3 mg/kg q8–12h	Gram-negative infections	IV or IM
Glycosaminoglycan (polysulfated)	250 mg per joint, once weekly for 3 weeks or 500 mg intramuscular	Degenerative joint disease	Intraarticular or IM
Griseofulvin	10–20 mg/kg q24h	Ringworm	PO
Heparin	10–40 IU/kg q6–24h	Abdominal surgery, laminitis, DIC	IV
hCG	2000 IU/450 kg IV	Induction of ovulation	IV
Hyaluronate sodium	20–60 mg intraarticularly	Traumatic and degenerative joint disease	Intraarticular
Hydrocortisone sodium succinate	1–4 mg/kg q6–12h	Shock	Slow IV infusion
Iodochlorhydroxyquin	20 mg/kg q24h for 3 days; reduce dosing frequency thereafter	Chronic diarrhea	PO
Isoxsuprine hydrochloride	0.6–1.8 mg/kg q12h	Navicular disease	PO
Ivermectin	0.2 mg/kg once for internal parasites or 0.2 mg/kg q96h for lice and mange	Internal parasites, ectoparasites	PO
Kanamycin	5 mg/kg q8h	Gram-negative infections	IV
Ketamine	2.2 mg/kg	Anesthesia induction after IV xylazine 1 mg/kg IV	IV
Levothyroxine	20 μg/kg q24h	Hypothyroidism	PO
Lidocaine, 2% solution	As required for local anesthesia; for arrhythmias, 0.5 mg/kg repeated at 5-min intervals for total dose of 4 mg/kg	Local anesthesia or treatment of arrhythmias	SC or IV; for epidural, use 5–8 ml of 2% solution
Malathion	0.5% wash	Ectoparasites	Topical
Mannitol	0.25–2 g/kg using 20% solution	CNS trauma, renal failure	Slowly IV
Mebendazole	9 mg/kg	Internal parasites and lungworm	PO

Table continues on next page.

Name of Drug	Dose	Main Use	Route
Meclofenamic acid	2.2 mg/kg q12h	Laminitis and musculoskeletal pain	PO
Meperidine	0.5–0.8 mg/kg q8–12h	Analgesia	IV or IM
Methadone	0.05–0.15 mg/kg	Only use in combination with sedatives such as xylazine and detomidine	IV after prior sedation
Methicillin	25 mg/kg q6h	Antibiotic for beta-lactamase staphylococci	IV or IM
Methylprednisolone acetate	40–160 mg per joint	Synovitis, degenerative joint disease	Intraarticular
Methylprednisolone sodium succinate	2–4 mg/kg	Shock, anti-inflammatory, urticaria	IV
Metaclopramide	0.25 mg/kg q6–8h	Ileus	IV
Mineral oil	5–10 ml/kg q12–24h	Gastrointestinal lubrication or treatment of laminitis	PO
Morphine	0.2–0.5 mg/kg	Analgesic; only use in combination with sedatives such as xylazine and detomidine	IV
Naproxen	10 mg/kg q12–24h	Musculoskeletal pain	PO or IV
Neomycin	5–10 mg/kg q12h	Gram-negative infections	IV or IM
Neostigmine	0.02 mg/kg q30min	Ileus	SC
Omeprazole	1–2 mg/kg q12–24h	Gastroduodenal ulcer disease	PO
Oxacillin	25–40 mg/kg q12h	Antibiotic for beta-lactamase staphylococci	IV or IM
Oxfendazole	10 mg/kg	Anthelmintic	PO
Oxibendazole	10–15 mg/kg	Anthelmintic	PO
Oxytetracycline	5 mg/kg q12h	Bacteriostatic antibiotic; use only where sensitivity tests indicate only effective drug	IV
Oxytocin	5–10 IU given IV for induction of parturition; 40 IU given IM or alternatively 150 IU in 1 L of polyionic solution	Induction of parturition; retained placenta	IV or IM
Penicillin, procaine	15,000 IU/kg or 15 mg/kg q12h	Gram-positive infections	IM only
Penicillin, Na or K	20,000 IU/kg or 12 mg/kg q6h	Gram-positive infections	IM or IV
Pentazocine	0.3–0.8 mg/kg	Analgesic; only use in combination with sedatives such as xylazine and detomidine	IV
Pentosan sulfate	250 mg q7–14d	Degenerative joint disease	Intraarticular
Phenoxybenzamine hydrochloride	0.5–1.0 mg/kg in 1 L saline given IV	Diarrhea, laminitis; should not be used if already hypotensive	IV
Phenylbutazone	2.2–4.4 mg/kg q12h or q24h. Dose of 4.4 mg/kg q12h should not be used for more than 1 day	Anti-inflammatory, musculoskeletal problems, prevention of postoperative swelling	PO or IV
Phenytoin	10–12 mg/kg q12h for 3–4 days, then 10–12 mg/kg q24h for 3–4 days, then 5–6 mg/kg q24h	Chronic low-grade rhabdomyolysis, stringhalt	PO
Piperazine	67 mg/kg	Anthelmintic, for *Parascaris equorum*	PO
Potassium chloride	30–60 g (400–800 mmol or mEq K) in 4 Ls water	Potassium replacement therapy	By nasogastric tube
Prednisolone sodium succinate	0.2–3 mg/kg q6–12h	Anti-inflammatory therapy, shock, purpura	IV
Prednisolone	Commencing dose rate 1 mg/kg q12h for 3–4 days, then 1 mg/kg q24h for 3–4 days; maintenance 0.5–1 mg/kg q24h every other day	Low-grade respiratory disease, dermatitis, pemphigus, autoimmune disorders	PO
Promazine	0.25–1.0 mg/kg or 1–2 mg/kg oral form	Tranquilization	IV PO

Name of Drug	Dose	Main Use	Route
Propantheline	0.1–0.2 mg/kg	To reduce rectal straining when undertaking rectal examination	IV
Proparacaine	0.5% solution, drops	Topical analgesia for eye problems	Ophthalmic
Psyllium mucilloid	1 g/kg q24h	Sand impaction of the large bowel	PO
Pyrantel pamoate	6.6 mg/kg	Anthelmintic	PO
Quinidine sulfate	20 mg/kg q2–3h until cardioversion (not to exceed 160 mg/kg in 12 hours)	Atrial fibrillation	By nasogastric tube
Quinidine gluconate	1.5 mg/kg q10min until cardioversion (not to exceed 40 mg/kg)	Atrial fibrillation	IV
Ranitidine	6.6 mg/kg q12h	Gastroduodenal ulcer disease	PO or IV
Rifampin	5–10 mg/kg q12h	Use in combination with erythromycin to treat *R. equi*	PO
Stanozolol	0.5–1 mg/kg q7–14d	Anabolic agent for debility and anemia	IM
Streptomycin	5–10 mg/kg q12h	Antibiotic; few equine pathogens are sensitive	IM
Sucralfate	30 mg/kg q6–8h	Used as a gastric protectant in gastroduodenal ulcer disease	PO
Theophylline	1 mg/kg q6h	Bronchodilator	PO
Trichlorfon	40 mg/kg	Anthelmintic for treatment of *Gastrophilus* spp.	PO
Trimethoprim–sulfadiazine	15 mg/kg or 15–20 mg/kg q12h	Antibiotic; useful for respiratory infections	IV PO
Tripelennamine hydrochloride	1 mg/kg q8–12h	Antihistamine	Slowly IV or IM
Xylazine	0.2–1.0 mg/kg (repeated as necessary)	Sedative	IV
Yohimbine	0.12 mg/kg for reversal of xylazine or detomidine sedation	Antagonist for xylazine	Slowly IV

Reference Values for Serum or Plasma Biochemical Measurements

Plasma Biochemistry Value*	Normal Range
Sodium (mmol/L or mEq/L)	132–142
Potassium (mmol/L or mEq/L)	3.2–4.2
Chloride (mmol/L or mEq/L)	94–104
Bicarbonate or total CO_2 (mmol/L or mEq/L)	24–32
Osmolality (mosmol/kg)	276–290
Urea (mmol/L)	4–8 (24–48 mg/dl) (11.2–22.4 mg/dl for BUN)
Creatinine (μmol/L)	100–160 (1.1–1.8 mg/dl)
Glucose (mmol/L)	5–8 (90–144 mg/dl)
Bilirubin (μmol/L)	10–50 (0.6–2.9 mg/dl)
Iron (μmol/L)	14–42 (78–235 mg/dl)
Total protein (g/L)	55–75 (5.5–7.5 g/dl)
AP, alkaline phosphatase (U/L)	138–251
AST, aspartate amino transaminase (U/L)	150–400
CK, creatine kinase (U/L)	100–300
GGT, gamma glutamyl transferase (U/L)	10–40
Calcium (mmol/L)	2.7–3.3 (10.8–13.2 mg/dl)
Phosphate (mmol/L)	0.75–1.25 (2.3–3.9 mg/dl)
Cholesterol (mmol/L)	2.1–3.6 (81–139 mg/dl)
Uric acid (μmol/L)	0–60 (0–1 mg/dl)
Serum Biochemistry Value†	
Albumin (g/L)	28–36 (2.8–3.6 g/dl)
Alphaglobulin (g/L)	8–13 (0.8–1.3 g/dl)
Betaglobulin (g/L)	8–15 (0.8–1.5 g/dl)
Gammaglobulin (g/L)	7–14 (0.7–1.4 g/dl)

*Using automated techniques—SMAC Autoanalyzer, Technicon.

†Protein electrophoresis.

Treatment Numbers

TRADE NAMES AND FORMULATIONS OF COMMONLY USED DRUGS

Dose rates are provided in Appendix 1 for the drugs given in this table. Attempts have been made to include all manufacturers of products in this table, but some may be missing. Please write to us if you are aware of a product that is not included so that it can be included in the next edition. The treatment numbers in this table refer to numbers given in the text of each of the chapters, where mention of a drug is given.

No.	Drug	Trade Name	Company	Form	Concentration	Presentation	Route
1	Acepromazine maleate	Promace Injectable	Aveco Fort Dodge	Solution	10 mg/ml	50-ml vial	IV, IM, or SC
2	Acetylcysteine	Mucomist	Bristol	Solution	100 mg/ml or 200 mg/ml	4-, 10-, and 30-ml bottles	Eye, topical
3	Allyl trenbolone (altrenogest)	Regu-Mate	Hoechst-Roussel	Solution	2.2 mg/ml	1-L bottles	PO
4	Amikacin sulfate	Amiglyde-V	Aveco Fort Dodge	Solution	50 or 250 mg/ml	48-ml vials (250 mg/ml) and 50-ml bottles (50 mg/ml)	IV, intrauterine
5	Aminophylline	Aminophylline Injection	Abbott	Solution	25 mg/ml	10- and 20-ml vials	IV
6	Ampicillin sodium	AMP-Equine	SmithKline Beecham	Powder, reconstitute with saline	300 mg/ml	1- and 3-g vials	IV or IM
7	Amphotericin B	Fungizone	Squibb	Lotion, cream, or ointment	30 mg/ml or 30 mg/g	30-ml bottle, 20-g tubes	Topical
		Fungizone Intravenous	Squibb	Freeze-dried powder	50 mg/vial	Vial	IV
8	Antibiotic–corticosteroid ointments	Amphoderm Ointment	Aveco Fort Dodge	Ointment and solution	5 mg/g amphomycin, 5 mg/g kanamycin, 10 mg/g hydrocortisone	7.5- and 15-g tubes; squeeze bottles of 227 g	Topical
		Animax Derma-4 Dermalone	Pharmaderm SmithKline Beecham Vedco	Ointment	Nystatin 100,000 U/ml, neomycin 2.5 mg/ml thiostrepton 2500 U/ml triamcinolone 1 mg/ml	7.5-, 15-, and 30-ml tubes and 240-ml bottles	Topical
		Forte-Topical	Upjohn	Suspension	Hydrocortisone acetate 2 mg/ml, hydrocortisone succinate 1.25 mg/ml, neomycin 25 mg/ml, penicillin 10,000 IU/ml, polymyxin B 5000 U/ml	10-ml tubes	Topical
		Kymar Ointment	Schering-Plough	Ointment	Neomycin 3.5 mg/g, hydrocortisone	57-g tubes	Topical

No.	Generic name	Trade name	Manufacturer	Form	Concentration	Size	Route
		Liquichlor	Evsco	Ointment	2.5 mg/g, trypsin–chymotrypsin 10,000 U/g Chloramphenicol 4.2 mg/ml, prednisolone 1.7 mg/ml, tetracaine 4.2 mg/g	10-ml tubes and 12-fl oz (355-ml) bottles	Topical
		Neo-Predef Sterile Ointment	Upjohn	Ointment	Isoflupredone acetate 1 mg/g, neomycin sulfate 5 mg/g	3.5- and 5-g tubes	Topical
		Tritop	Upjohn	Ointment	Isoflupredone acetate 1 mg/g, neomycin sulfate 5 mg/g, tetracaine hydrochloride 5 mg/g	10-g tubes	Topical
9	Aspirin	Aspirin Boluses	Vedco AgriLabs Butler Farmtech Phoenix RX	Bolus/tablet	240 grains (15.6 g) per tablet	Jars of 50 boluses	PO
		Aspri-Ject Injection	Vedco	Solution	100 mg sodium salicylate/ml	30-ml vial	IV
10	Atropine eye ointment	Atrophate	Schering-Plough	Ophthalmic ointment	10 mg atropine/g	3.5-g tubes	Eye
11	Atropine	Atropine Injectable L.A.	Fort Dodge	Solution	2 mg/ml	100-ml vial	IV, SC
		Atropine L.A. Atropine Sulfate	Butler J.A. Webster	Solution Solution	15 mg/ml 0.5 mg/ml	100-ml vial 30- and 100-ml vials	IV, SC IV, SC
		Atropine Sulfate Injection L.A.	Vedco	Solution	15 mg/ml	100-ml vial	IV, SC
12	Betamethasone acetate, betamethasone sodium phosphate	Betavet Soluspan	Schering-Plough	Suspension	12 mg/ml betamethasone acetate, 2 mg/ml betamethasone sodium phosphate, total 13.8 mg betamethasone	5-ml vial	IM, IA

Table continues on next page.

Note: IA = intraarticular; IM = intramuscular; IV = intravenous; PO = oral or by nasogastric tube; SC = subcutaneous.

No.	Drug	Trade Name	Company	Form	Concentration	Presentation	Route
13	Betamethasone diproprionate, betamethasone sodium phosphate	Betasone	Schering-Plough	Suspension	5 mg/ml betamethasone as betamethasone diproprionate, 2 mg/ml betamethasone as betamethasone sodium phosphate	5-ml vial	IM, IA
14	Buprenorphine	Buprenex	Norwich Eaton	Solution	0.3 mg/ml	1-ml ampules	IV
15	Butorphanol tartrate	Torbugesic	Aveco Fort Dodge	Solution	10 mg/ml	10- and 50-ml vials	IV
16	Cefotaxime	Claforan	Hoechst	Powder		1-, 2-, and 10-g vials	IV
17	Captan	Available from agricultural and garden supply stores	Various manufacturers	Powder	45 g/100 g powder	Make up a 3% solution for topical use in dermatophytosis	Topical
18	Ceftiofur sodium	Naxcel	Upjohn	Powder	Reconstitute solution to 50 mg/ml	1- and 4-g vials	IV
19	Cefazolin	Ancef	SmithKline Beecham	Powder	Reconstitute with dextrose 5% in water	0.25-, 0.5-, 1-, 5-, and 10-g vials	IV
		Kefzol	Lilly			0.25-, 0.5-, 1-, and 10-g vials	
20	Cephalothin sodium	Keflin	Lilly	Powder	Reconstitute with dextrose 5% in water	1-g vials	IV
21	Cephapirin sodium	Cefadyl	Bristol	Powder	Reconstitute with dextrose 5% in water	500-mg, 1-, 2-, 4-, and 20-g vials	IV
22	Chloral hydrate	Chloral Hydrate	Various manufacturers	Crystals	Make up appropriate solution	1- and 5-lb containers	PO and IV
23	Chlorhexidine citrate	Chlorhex Surgical Scrub	Vedco	Solution	20 mg/ml	128-fl oz (1- gal) containers	Topical
24	Chlorhexidine diacetate	Chlorhexiderm Shampoo	DVM	Solution	5 mg/ml	8-fl oz and 1-gal containers	Topical
25	Chorionic gonadotrophin (hCG)	A.P.L.	Wyeth-Ayerst	Freeze-dried powder	5000, 10,000 or 20,000 U per vial	10-ml vial	IV
		Chorigon	Dunhall	Freeze-dried powder	10,000 U per vial	10-ml vial	IV

#	Drug	Product	Company	Form	Concentration	Package	Route
		Chorex	Hyrex	Freeze-dried powder	5000 or 10,000 U per vial	10-ml vial	IV
		Chorion-Plus	Pharmex	Freeze-dried powder	10,000 U per vial	10-ml vial	IV
		Choron 10	Forest	Freeze-dried powder	10,000 U per vial	10-ml vial	IV
		Follutein	Squibb Marsan	Freeze-dried powder	10,000 U per vial	10-ml vial	IV
		Rochoric	Rocky Mountain	Freeze-dried powder	10,000 U per vial	10-ml vial	IV
26	Cimetidine	Tagamet	SmithKline	Tablets and solution	200-, 300-, 400-, and 800-mg tablets; solution 150 mg/ml	For injection, 300 mg/2ml	PO or IV
27	Clenbuterol	Ventipulmin Granules	Boehringer Ingelheim	Granules	0.016 mg/g	500-g container	PO
		Ventipulmin Injection	Boehringer Ingelheim	Solution	0.03 mg/ml	50-ml vial	IV, IM or by nebulizer
28	Detomidine hydrochloride	Dormosedan	SmithKline Beecham	Solution	100 µg/ml	5- and 20-ml vials	IV or IM
29	Dexamethasone	Azium Powder	Schering-Plough	Powder	10 mg/packet	100 × 10-mg packets	PO
		Azium Solution	Schering-Plough	Solution	2 mg/ml	100-ml vial	IV or IM
		Dexamethasone 2.0-mg Injection	Vedco	Solution	2 mg/ml	100-ml vial	IV
		Dexamethasone Injection	Butler	Solution	2 mg/ml	30-, 50-, and 100-ml vials	IV
		Dexamethasone Injection	Durvet	Solution	2 mg/ml	30-, 50-, and 100-ml vials	IV
		Dexamethasone Injection	Webster	Solution	2 mg/ml	30-, 50-, and 100-ml vials	IV
		Dexamethasone Injection	Lextron	Solution	2 mg/ml	100-ml vial	IV
		Dexamethasone Injection	ProLabs	Solution	2 mg/ml	100-ml vial	IV
		Dexameth-A-Vet	Anthony	Solution	2 mg/ml	30-, 50-, and 100-ml vials	IV
30	Dexamethasone sodium phosphate	Dexasone	Phoenix	Solution	2 mg/ml	100-ml vial	IV
		Dexamethasone Sodium Phosphate Injection	Butler	Solution	4 mg/ml	100-ml vial	IV
		Dexamethasone Sodium Phosphate Injection	Webster	Solution	4 mg/ml	100-ml vial	IV

Table continues on next page.

No.	Drug	Trade Name	Company	Form	Concentration	Presentation	Route
		Dexamethasone Sodium Phosphate Injection	Phoenix	Solution	4 mg/ml	100-ml vial	IV
		Dexamethasone Sodium Phosphate Injection	Steris	Solution	4 mg/ml	50- and 100-ml vials	IV
		Dexamethasone Sodium Phosphate Injection	Vedco	Solution	4 mg/ml	100-ml vial	IV
		Dex-A-Vet	Anthony	Solution	4 mg/ml	100-ml vial	IV
31	Dialdehyde glutaraldehyde	Cidex	Surgikos	Solution		Quart, gallon, and 2.5-gal bottles	Instrument disinfection
		Cidex-7	Surgikos	Solution	2% solution plus vial of activator	Quart, gallon, and 5-gal bottles	Instrument disinfection
32	Diazepam	Valium Injectable	Roche	Solution	5 mg/ml	2-ml ampules and 10-ml vials	IV or IM
33	Digoxin	Lanoxin Tablets, Veterinary	Coopers	Tablet	Yellow tablet, 0.125 mg/tablet, and white tablet, 0.25 mg/tablet	Bottles of 100 and 1000 tablets	PO
		Lanoxin	Burroughs Wellcome	Solution	0.25 mg/ml	2-ml ampule	IV
34	Dimethylsulfoxide (DMSO)	Domoso Gel	Syntex	Gel	900 mg/ml	60- and 120-g collapsible tubes, and 425-g containers	Topical
		Domoso Solution	Syntex	Solution	900 mg/ml	4 fl oz with or without sprayer and 1-pt (16-fl oz) and 1-gal (128-fl oz) containers	Topical, IV (as 10%–20% solution) or PO
35	Dioctyl sodium sulfosuccinate (DSS)	Dioctynate	Butler	Solution	50 mg/ml	1-gal container	Nasogastric tube
36	Dipyrone monohydrate	Dipyrone	Lextron	Solution	500 mg/ml	250-ml vial	IM or IV
		Dipyrone 50% Injection	Phoenix	Solution	500 mg/ml	100- and 250-ml vials	IM or IV
		Dipyrone 50% Injection	RX	Solution	500 mg/ml	250-ml vials	IM or IV

No.	Drug	Product	Manufacturer	Form	Concentration	Packaging	Route
		Dipyrone 50% Injection	Vedco	Solution	500 mg/ml	100- and 250-ml vials	IM or IV
		Dipyrone Injectable	Butler	Solution	500 mg/ml	100- and 250-ml bottles	IM or IV
		Dipyrone Injection 50%	Lextron	Solution	500 mg/ml	250-ml vial	IM or IV
37	Emilconazole	Clinifarm EC	Sterwin	Solution	13.8 mg/ml	750-ml container; to use, dilute 1:100	Topical (*Note:* Product not registered for use in horses)
38	Erythromycin estolate	Ilosone	Dista	Suspension	25 or 50 mg/ml	10- and 100-ml bottles	PO
39	Erythromycin ethylsuccinate	E.E.S. Liquid–200 & 400	Abbott	Suspension	40 or 80 mg/ml	100- and 480-ml bottles	PO
		E.E.S. Granules	Abbott	Granules	40 mg/ml	60-, 100- and 200-ml bottles	PO
40	Erythromycin glucceptate	Ilotycin Gluceptate	Dista	Solution	1 g/30 ml	30-ml vials	IV
41	Eye preparations—antibiotic: bacitracin–neomycin–polymyxin	Bacitracin-Neomycin-Polymyxin Ointment	Pharmaderm	Ointment	3.5 mg/g neomycin, 400 U/g bacitracin, 10,000 U polymyxin B sulfate/g	3.5-g tube	Eye, topical
42	Eye preparations—antibiotic: chloramphenicol	Chloromycetin	Parke Davis	Eye drops and eye ointment	1% (ointment) and 5 mg/ml (drops)	3.5-g tube and 5-ml bottle	Eye, topical
		Chloroptic	Allergan	Eye drops	5 mg/ml	2.5- and 7.5-ml bottles	Eye, topical
43	Eye preparations—antibiotic: gentamicin	Garramycin Ophthalmic, Gentacin Ophthalmic	Schering-Plough	Eye drops and eye ointment	3 mg/ml or 3 mg/g	3.75-g tubes and 5-ml bottles	Eye, topical
		Genoptic Liquifilm, Genoptic SOP	Allergan	Eye drops and eye ointment	3 mg/ml or 3 mg/g	1- and 5-ml bottles and 3.5-g tube	Eye, topical
44	Eye preparations—antibiotic: tobramycin	Tobrex	Alcon	Eye drops and eye ointment	3 mg/ml, 3 mg/g	5-ml bottle and 3-g tube	Eye, topical
45	Eye preparations—antifungal: natamycin	Natacyn	Alcon	Eye drops	50 mg/ml	15-ml bottle	Eye, topical
46	Eye preparations—antifungal: miconazole	Monistat IV	Janssen	Solution	10 mg/ml	20-ml ampule	Eye, topical

Table continues on next page.

No.	Drug	Trade Name	Company	Form	Concentration	Presentation	Route
47	Eye preparations—corticosteroids: dexamethasone	Maxidex	Alcon	Eye drops	1 mg/ml of dexamethasone	5- and 15-ml bottles	Eye, topical
48	Eye preparations—nonsteroidal: flurbiprofen	Ocufen	Allergan	Eye drops	3 mg/ml	2.5-, 5-, and 10-ml bottles	Eye, topical
49	Eye preparations—corticosteroids: betamethasone + gentamicin	Gentocin Durafilm	Schering Plough	Eye drops	Gentamicin 3 mg/ml and 1 mg/ml betamethasone acetate	5-ml bottle	Eye, topical
50	Eye preparations—corticosteroids + chloramphenicol	Chlorasone	Evsco	Eye ointment	10 mg/g chloramphenicol and 2.5 mg/g prednisolone acetate	3.5-g tube	Eye, topical
51	Fenbendazole	Panacur Granules 22.2%	Hoechst-Roussel	Granules	222 mg/g	20 × 5.2 g packets per box	PO
		Panacur Paste 10%	Hoechst-Roussel	Paste	100 mg/g	25-g syringe	PO
		Panacur Suspension 10%	Hoechst-Roussel	Suspension	100 mg/ml	1-L bottle	PO
		Safe-Guard Paste 10% (Horse)	Hoechst-Roussel	Paste	100 mg/g	25-g syringe	PO
52	Flunixin meglumine	Banamine Granules	Schering-Plough	Granules	250 mg/10g	250 mg in 10-g packets and 500 mg in 20-g packets	PO
		Banamine Paste	Schering-Plough	Paste	500 mg/30g	30-g syringe	PO
		Banamine Solution	Schering-Plough	Solution	50 mg/ml	50- and 100-ml vials	IV or IM
53	Fluprostenol sodium	Equimate	Haver/Diamond	Solution	50 µg/ml	5-ml vial	IM
54	Furosemide as a monoethanolamine salt	Disal Injection	Fermenta	Solution	50 mg/ml	50- and 100-ml vials	IV or IM
55	Furosemide as a diethanolamine salt	Furos-A-Vet	Anthony	Solution	50 mg/ml	50- and 100-ml vials	IV or IM
		Furosemide Injection	Webster	Solution	50 mg/ml	30-, 50-, and 100-ml vials	IV or IM
		Furosemide Injection	Phoenix	Solution	50 mg/ml	100-ml vial	IV or IM
		Furosemide Injection 5%	Butler	Solution	50 mg/ml	50- and 100-ml vials	IV or IM
		Furosemide Injection 5%	ProLabs	Solution	50 mg/ml	100-ml vial	IV or IM
		Furosemide Injection 5%	Vedco	Solution	50 mg/ml	50- and 100-ml vials	IV or IM
		Lasix Injection 5%	Hoechst-Roussel	Solution	50 mg/ml	50-ml vial	IV or IM

No.	Drug	Brand	Manufacturer	Form	Composition	Package	Route
56	Gentamicin sulfate	Gentocin Solution (50 mg/ml)	Schering-Plough	Solution	50 mg/ml	50- and 100-ml multiple-dose vials (box of 1 or 6)	IV, IM, or intrauterine
57	Glucose–glycine and electrolytes	Hydra-Lyte	Vet-A-Mix	Soluble powder	16 mM glycine, 368 mM glucose 30 mEq/L K, 85 mEq/L Na, 60 mEq/L acetate, 45 mEq/L citrate	5.76-oz (163.4-g) two-compartment foil packets	PO
		Life-Guard	SmithKline Beecham	Soluble powder	Dextrose 56.76% and glycine 3.12%; when reconstituted, 105 mEq/L Na, 80 mEq/L bicarbonate, 51 mEq/L chloride, 26 mEq/L K, 10 mEq/L Ca, 6 mEq/L phosphate, 6 mEq/L Mg, 4 mEq/L sulfate	200-g twin pack	PO
		Re-Sorb	SmithKline Beecham	Soluble powder	Glucose 44.0 g and glycine 6.36 g and electrolytes	Boxes containing 12 packets	PO
		Revive	Fermenta	Soluble powder	Dextrose and glycine and electrolytes	5.73-oz (162.5-g) packets (cartons of 12 or 50 per pail)	PO
		Survive	Lextron	Soluble powder	Dextrose and glycine and electrolytes	5.73-oz (162.5-g) packets (48 and 50 packets)	PO
		Survive	RX	Soluble powder	Dextrose and glycine and electrolytes	5.73-oz (162.5-g) packets (48 packets)	PO
58	Gonadotropin-releasing hormone infusion—gonadorelin diacetate tetrahydrate	Cystorelin	Sanofi	Solution	50 μg/ml	Single- and multidose 10-ml vials	IM or IV (only registered for use in cattle); probably not effective in horses

Table continues on next page.

No.	Drug	Trade Name	Company	Form	Concentration	Presentation	Route
59	Heparin sodium	Heparin Sodium	Upjohn	Solution	1000 and 5000 U/ml	1- and 10-ml vials	IV
		Heparin Sodium	Winthrop	Solution	5000 U/ml	1- and 4-ml vials	IV
		Liquaemin Sodium	Organon	Solution	1000, 5000, 10,000, 20,000 and 40,000 U/ml	1- and 30-ml vials	IV
60	Hyaluronate sodium	Equron	Solvay	Solution	5 mg/ml	2-ml glass syringe	IA
		Hyalovet	Fort Dodge	Solution	10 mg/ml	2-ml syringe or 2-ml vial	IA
		Hylartin V	American Equine Products	Solution	10 mg/ml	2-ml glass syringe	IA
		Synacid	Schering-Plough	Solution	10 mg/ml	5-ml single-dose vial	IA
61	Isoxsuprine hydrochloride	Rolisox	Robinson	Tablets	10- and 20-mg tablets	Bottles of 100 tablets	PO
		Vasodilan	Mead Johnson	Tablets	10- and 20-mg tablets	Bottles of 100, 500, and 1000 tablets	PO
		Circulon	Vetsearch	Paste	40 mg/ml	230-ml jars of paste	PO
62	Ivermectin	Eqvalan Liquid	MSD-Agvet	Solution	10 mg/ml	50- and 100-ml bottles	PO
		Eqvalan Paste 1.87%	MSD-Agvet	Paste	1.87%	0.21-oz (6.08-g) syringe	PO
63	Kanamycin sulfate	Kantrim	Aveco Fort Dodge	Solution	50 and 200 mg/ml	50-ml bottle	IV and IM
64	Ketamine hydrochloride	Ketaset	Aveco Fort Dodge	Solution	100 mg/ml	10-ml vial	IV
65	Ketoconazole	Nizoral	Janssen	Tablets	200-mg tablets	Bottles of 100	PO
66	Ketoprofen	Ketofen	Aveco Fort Dodge	Solution	100 mg/ml	50- and 100-ml bottles	IV
67	Lidocaine hydrochloride	Lidocaine 2% Injectable	Butler	Solution	20 mg/ml	100-ml vial	Epidural, nerve block, infiltration
		Lidocaine Hydrochloride	ProLabs	Solution	20 mg/ml	100-ml vial	Epidural, nerve block, infiltration
		Lidocaine Hydrochloride Injectable	Phoenix	Solution	20 mg/ml	100-ml vial	Epidural, nerve block, infiltration

No.	Generic name	Trade name	Manufacturer	Form	Concentration	Container	Route
		Lidocaine Injectable 2%	Vedco	Solution	20 mg/ml	100-ml container	Epidural, nerve block, infiltration
68	Mannitol	Osmitrol	Travenol	Solution	5%, 10%, 20% solution	250- and 500-ml bottles	IV
69	Meclofenamic acid	Arquel Granules	Aveco Fort Dodge	Granules	50 mg/g	10-g packet	PO
70	Medroxyprogesterone acetate	Depo-Provera	Upjohn	Suspension	100 or 400 mg/ml	2.5- and 10-ml vials	IA
71	Meperidine hydrochloride	Demerol	Winthrop	Solution	25, 50, 75, and 100 mg/ml	0.5-, 1-, 1.5-, and 2-ml ampules	IV
72	Mepivacaine hydrochloride	Carbocaine-V	Upjohn	Solution	20 mg/ml	50-ml vial	Nerve block, epidural, IA, infiltration, topical
73	Methadone hydrochloride	Dolophine	Lilly	Solution	10 mg/ml	1-ml ampule	IV
74	Methylprednisolone acetate	Depo-Medrol	Upjohn	Suspension	20 or 40 mg/ml	20 mg/ml in 10- and 20-ml vials or 40 mg/ml in 5-ml vial	IM and IA
		Methylprednisolone Acetate Injection	Fermenta	Solution	20 or 40 mg/ml	20 mg/ml in 10- and 30-ml vials or 40 mg/ml in 5- and 30-ml vials	IM or IA
75	Metronidazole	Flagyl	Searle	Tablets	250- or 500-mg tablets	Bottles of 50, 100, 500, and 1000 tablets	PO
		Metrozole	Metro Med	Tablets	250- or 500-mg tablets	Bottles of 100 and 250 tablets	PO
		Metryl	Lemmon	Tablets	250- or 500-mg tablets	Bottles of 100 and 500 tablets	PO
76 77	Miconazole Mineral oil	Monistat Mineral Oil	Janssen AgriLabs Lextron RX Vedco	Solution	10 mg/ml	20-ml ampule 1 qt and 1-gal container	IV Nasogastric tube
78 79	Oxymorphone Orgotein	Numorphan Palosein	Dupont Coopers	Solution Powder	1 and 1.5 mg/ml 5 mg/vial or 5 mg/2 ml has saline for reconstitution of freeze-dried powder	1- and 10-ml vials Single-dose vials with 2-ml ampule of saline	IV IM or IA

Table continues on next page.

No.	Drug	Trade Name	Company	Form	Concentration	Presentation	Route
80	Oxytetracycline	Agricyl	Anthony	Solution	50 and 100 mg/ml	500-ml bottle	IV
		Agrimycin	AgriLabs	Solution	50 and 100 mg/ml	500-ml bottle	IV
		Anaject	Farmtech	Solution	50 and 100 mg/ml	500-ml bottle	IV
		Bio-Mycin	Bio-Ceutic	Solution	50 and 100 mg/ml	500-ml bottle	IV
		Duramycin	Durvet	Solution	50 and 100 mg/ml	500-ml bottle	IV
		Liquamycin	Pfizer	Solution	100 and 200 mg/ml	100-, 250-, and 500-ml bottles	IV
		Medamycin	Fermenta	Solution	50 and 100 mg/ml	500-ml bottle	IV
		Oxyject	AgriLabs Durvet Lextron RX	Solution	50 and 100 mg/ml	500-ml bottle	IV
		Oxy-Tet	Anchor	Solution	50 and 100 mg/ml	100- and 500-ml bottles	IV
		Oxytetracycline HCl	Fermenta	Solution	50 and 100 mg/ml	500-ml bottle	IV
		Promycin	Phoenix	Solution	50 and 100 mg/ml	500-ml bottle	IV
		Terramycin 100	Pfizer	Solution	100 mg/ml	100- and 500-ml bottles	IV
81	Oxytocin	Terra-Vet	Lextron	Solution	50 and 100 mg/ml	500-ml bottle	IV
		Oxytocin	Webster	Solution	20 USP U/ml	30- and 100-ml vials	IV, IM, or SC
		Oxytocin	Lextron	Solution	20 USP U/ml	100-ml vial	IV, IM, or SC
		Oxytocin Injection	Anthony	Solution	20 USP U/ml	100-ml vial	IV, IM, or SC
		Oxytocin Injection	Durvet	Solution	20 USP U/ml	100-ml vial	IV, IM, or SC
		Oxytocin Injection	Lextron	Solution	20 USP U/ml	100-ml vial	IV, IM, or SC
		Oxytocin Injection	Phoenix	Solution	20 USP U/ml	100-ml vial	IV, IM, or SC
		Oxytocin Injection	ProLabs	Solution	20 USP U/ml	100-ml vial	IV, IM, or SC
		Oxytocin Injection	RX	Solution	20 USP U/ml	100-ml vial	IV, IM, or SC
		Oxytocin Injection	Vedco, Butler	Solution	20 USP U/ml	100-ml vial	IV, IM, or SC
		Ambi-Pen	Butler	Suspension	150,000 U/ml penicillin G benzathine and 150,000 U/ml penicillin G procaine	100-ml vial	IM
82	Penicillin G benzathine, penicillin G procaine	Benza-Pen	SmithKline Beecham	Suspension	150,000 U/ml penicillin G benzathine and 150,000 U/ml penicillin G procaine	100- and 250-ml vials	IM
		Crystiben	Solvay	Suspension	150,000 U/ml penicillin G	100-ml vial	IM

#	Drug	Product	Manufacturer	Form	Concentration	Package	Route
		Dual-Pen	Fermenta	Suspension	benzathine and 150,000 U/ml penicillin G procaine	100- and 250-ml vials	IM
		Durapen	Vedco	Suspension	150,000 U/ml penicillin G benzathine and 150,000 U/ml penicillin G procaine	100- and 250-ml vials	IM
		Flo-Cillin	Fort Dodge	Suspension	150,000 U/ml penicillin G benzathine and 150,000 U/ml penicillin G procaine	100- and 250-ml vials	IM
83	Penicillin G procaine	Agri-Cillin	Agri Laboratories	Suspension	300,000 U/ml	100-, 250-, and 500-ml vials	IM
		Aquacillin	Vedco	Suspension	300,000 U/ml	100-, 250-, and 500-ml vials	IM
		Crysticillin 300 A.S.	Solvay	Suspension	300,000 U/ml	100- and 250-ml bottles	IM
		Fermicillin Aqueous	Fermenta	Suspension	300,000 U/ml	100- and 250-ml vials	IM
		Pen-Aqueous	Durvet	Suspension	300,000 U/ml	100- and 250-ml vials	IM
		Pen-Aqueous	Fermenta	Suspension	300,000 U/ml	100- and 250-ml vials	IM
		Pen-Aqueous	Professional Veterinary Pharmaceuticals	Suspension	300,000 U/ml	250-ml vial	IM
		Penicillin G Procaine	Hanford	Suspension	300,000 U/ml	100- and 250-ml vials	IM
		Penicillin G Procaine Suspension	Butler	Suspension	300,000 U/ml	100- and 250-ml vials	IM
		Penicillin G Procaine Suspension	SmithKline Beecham	Suspension	300,000 U/ml	100- and 250-ml vials	IM
		PFI-Pen G	Pfizer	Suspension	300,000 U/ml	100- and 250-ml vials	IM

Table continues on next page.

No.	Drug	Trade Name	Company	Form	Concentration	Presentation	Route
		Sterile Penicillin G Procaine	Farmtech	Suspension	300,000 U/ml	100- and 250-ml bottles	IM
		Vetpro-G	Coopers Animal Health	Suspension	300,000 U/ml	100- and 250-ml vials	IM
84	Penicillin G, potassium	Pfizerpen for Injection	Roerig	Buffered powder	1,000,000, 5,000,000 or 20,000,000 U	Vials	IV or IM
85	Penicillin G, sodium	Various manufacturers	—	—	1,000,000 or 5,000,000 U	Vials	IV or IM
86	Pentazocine lactate	Talwin-V	Upjohn	Solution	30 mg/ml	10-ml multiple-dose vial	IV
87	Phenobarbital	Luminal Injection	Winthrop	Solution	130 mg/ml	1-ml ampule	IV
		Solubarb	Forest	Tablets	16-mg tablets (0.25 grains)	Bottles of 24 tablets	PO
88	Phenylbutazone	Bizolin Gel	Bio-Ceutic Division Boehringer Ingelheim	Gel	4 g/30 g gel	30 g gel in calibrated oral syringe	PO
		Butatron Oral Gel	Sanofi	Gel	4 g/30 g gel	30-g dose in syringe	PO
		Butazolidin	Coopers	Tablet or solution	1 g/tablet or 200 mg/ml solution	1-g tablets in bottles of 100, solution in 100-ml vials	PO or IV
		Butazolidin Paste	Coopers	Paste	6 g/syringe or 12 g/syringe	Syringe	PO
		Phen-Buta-Vet	Anthony	Tablet or solution	1 g/tablet or 200 mg/ml solution	Bottles of 100 tablets or 100-ml vials	PO or IV
		Phenylbutazone	Butler	Tablet or solution	1 g/tablet or 200 mg/ml	Bottles of 100 tablets or 100-ml vials	PO or IV
		Phenylbutazone	Webster	Tablet or solution	1 g/tablet or 200 mg/ml	Bottles of 100 tablets or 30-, 50-, or 100-ml vials	PO or IV
		Phenylbutazone	Phoenix	Tablet or solution	1 g/tablet or 200 mg/ml	1.0-g tablets in bottles of 100 or 100-ml vials	PO or IV
		Phenylbutazone Injection 20%	Butler	Solution	200 mg/ml	100-ml vial	IV
		Phenylbutazone Injection 20%	Vedco	Solution	200 mg/ml	100-ml bottle	IV
		Phenylbutazone Tablets (Horses)	Vedco	Tablet	1 g/tablet	100-tablet bottles	PO

No.	Generic Name	Trade Name	Manufacturer	Form	Concentration	Packaging	Route
		Phenylzone Paste	Phoenix	Paste	1 g/mark on plunger	30- and 60-g syringes	PO
		Pro-Bute Injection	ProLabs	Solution	200 mg/ml	100-ml vial	IV
		Pro-Bute Tablets	ProLabs	Tablets	1 g/tablet	Bottles of 100 tablets	PO
89	Phenytoin sodium	Extended Phenytoin	Aveco	Capsule	100 mg/capsule	Bottles of 1000 capsules	PO
		Extended Phenytoin	Fort Dodge	Capsule	100 mg/capsule	Bottles of 1000 capsules	PO
90	Polysulfated glycosaminoglycans	Adequan I.A.	Luitpold	Solution	250 mg/ml	1-ml glass vial	IA
		Adequan I.M.	Luitpold	Solution	100 mg/ml	5-ml glass vial	IM
91	Povidone-iodine	Betadine Aerosol Spray	Purdue Frederick	Solution	50 mg/ml	3-fl oz (89-ml) aerosol bottles	Topical
		Betadine Solution	Purdue Frederick	Solution	50 mg/ml	16- and 32-oz bottles and 1-gal bottles	Topical
		Betadine Surgical Scrub	Purdue Frederick	Solution	75 mg/ml	16- and 32-oz bottles and 1-gal bottles	Topical
		Groom Rite Iodine Shampoo	Pro Vet	Solution	20 mg/ml	8-oz and 1-gal bottles	Topical
		Iodine Shampoo	Evsco	Solution	20 mg/ml	12-fl oz (355-ml) bottle	Topical
		Lanodine	Butler	Solution	100 mg/ml	8- and 16-oz bottles	Topical
		Pro Vet Povidone-Iodine Ointment	Pro Vet	Ointment	100 mg/ml	8- and 16-oz jars	Topical
		Pro Vet Povidone-Iodine Solution	Pro Vet	Solution	100 mg/ml	1-gal plastic jug	Topical
		Pro Vet Povidone-Iodine Surgical Scrub	Pro Vet	Solution	75 mg/ml	1-gal plastic jug	Topical
		Prodine Scrub	Phoenix	Solution	75 mg/ml	1-gal bottle	Topical
		Prodine Solution	Phoenix	Solution	100 mg/ml	1-gal bottle	Topical
		Vetadine Scrub	Vedco	Solution	75 mg/ml	1-gal bottle	Topical
		Vetadine Solution	Vedco	Solution	100 mg/ml	1-gal containers	Topical
92	Prednisolone	Cordrol	Vita Elixir	Tablets	5-, 10-, or 20-mg tablets	Bottles of 100 tablets	PO
		Delta-Cortef	Upjohn	Tablets	5-mg tablets	Bottles of 100 and 500 tablets	PO
		Orasone	Solvay	Tablets	1-, 5-, 10-, 20-, and 50-mg tablets	Bottles of 100 tablets	PO
		Ulacort	Fellows	Tablets	5-mg tablets	Bottles of 1000 tablets	PO

Table continues on next page.

No.	Drug	Trade Name	Company	Form	Concentration	Presentation	Route
93	Prilocaine hydrochloride	Citanest	Astra	Solution	4% solution	1.8-ml cartridge	Nerve blocks, infiltration, IA
94	Promazine hydrochloride	Promazine Granules	Fort Dodge	Granules	8 g/10.25 oz	10.25-oz containers	PO
		Tranquazine	Anthony Products	Solution	50 mg/ml	30- and 100-ml bottles	IV
95	Propantheline bromide	Pro-Banthine	Searle	Tablets	15 mg/tablet	100 and 500 tablets per bottle	Only oral form available in U.S.; sterile powder available in some countries allowing IV use
96	Proparacaine	Ophthaine hydrochloride	Squibb	Solution	5 mg/ml	15-ml bottle with dropper	Eye, topical
97	Psyllium mucilloid	Metamucil	Procter and Gamble	Powder	7-, 14-, and 21-oz jars	Jars	PO
98	Quinidine sulfate	Cin-Quin	Reid Rowell	Tablets	100-, 200-, and 300-mg tablets	Bottles of 100 and 1000 tablets	PO
		Quinidex Extentabs	Robins	Tablets	300-mg tablets	Bottles of 100 and 250 tablets	PO
		Quinora	Key	Tablets	300-mg tablets	Bottles of 100 and 1000 tablets	PO
99	Ranitidine hydrochloride	Zantac Syrup	Glaxo	Syrup	15 mg/ml	1-pt bottle	PO
		Zantac Tablets	Glaxo	Tablets	150- or 300-mg tablets	Bottles of 30 or 60 tablets	PO
		Zantac Injection	Glaxo	Solution	25 mg/ml	2-, 10-, and 40-ml vials	IV
100	Rifampin	Rifadin	Marion Merrell Dow	Capsules	150- and 300-mg capsules	Bottles of 30, 60, and 100 capsules	PO
		Rimactane	Ciba	Capsules	300-mg capsules	Bottles of 30, 60, and 100 capsules	PO
101	Sucralfate	Carafate	Marion Merrell Dow	Tablets	1-g tablets	Bottles of 100	PO
102	Terbutaline sulfate	Brethine	Geigy	Solution	1 mg/ml	1-ml ampule	IV
		Brethine	Geigy	Tablets	2.5-mg tablets	Bottles of 100 and 1000 tablets	PO

	Drug	Product	Manufacturer	Form	Concentration/Preparation	Container	Route
103	Topical insecticides—coumaphos	Co-Ral 1% Shaker Can	Cutter	Powder	10 mg/g powder; shake on as a dusting powder	2-lb can	Topical
		Co-Ral 25% Wettable Powder	Cutter	Powder	10 mg/g powder; make up solution of 125 g (¼ lb) in 45 L (12 gals) water	4-lb bag	Topical
104	Topical insecticides—permethrin	Atroban 11% EC Insecticide	Coopers	Solution	110 mg/ml; make up solution of 1 pt/25 gals (1 ml/200 ml)	1-pt container	Topical
		Ectiban EC	Durvet or RX	Solution	57 mg/ml; make up as 1 qt/25 gals (10 ml/L)	8-oz, 1-qt, and 1-gal containers	Topical
		Permectrin 25% WP	Anchor	Powder	250 mg/g powder; make up as 1 oz/3 gals water (2.5 g/L)	6-oz containers	Topical
		Permectrin Horse and Stable Spray	Anchor	Solution	100 mg/ml; make up as 0.5 oz/3 gals (1.3 ml/L)	8-oz and 1-qt containers	Topical
105	Topical insecticides—pyrethrins	Derma-Sect Shampoo	Anchor	Solution, shampoo	0.6 mg/ml	8-oz and 1-gal containers	Topical
106	Triamcinolone acetate (acetonide)	Triamcinolone Acetonide Injection	Fermenta	Solution	2 and 6 mg/ml	2 mg/ml in 30- and 100-ml vials or 6 mg/ml in 5- and 30-ml vials	IM, SC, or IA
		Vetalog Parenteral	Solvay	Suspension	2 and 6 mg/ml	6 mg/ml in 3-, 5-, and 25-ml vials or 2 mg/ml in 25- and 100-ml vials	IM, SC, or IA
107	Trimethoprim—sulfadiazine	Di-Trim 48% Injection	Syntex	Solution	Trimethoprim 80 mg/ml and sulfadiazine 400 mg/ml	100-ml bottle	IV
		Di-Trim 400	Syntex	Paste	Trimethoprim 67 mg/g paste and sulfadiazine 333 mg/g paste	37.5-g Dial-A-Dose syringe	PO
		Tribrissen 48% Injection	Coopers	Solution	Trimethoprim 80 mg/ml and sulfadiazine 400 mg/ml	100-ml bottle	IV

Table continues on next page.

No.	Drug	Trade Name	Company	Form	Concentration	Presentation	Route
		Tribrissen 400 Oral Paste	Coopers	Paste	Trimethoprim 67 mg/g and sulfadiazine 333 mg/g	37.5-g Dial-A-Dose syringe	PO
108	Xylazine hydrochloride	Anased Injection (Horses)	Lloyd	Solution	100 mg/ml	50-ml bottle	IV or IM
		Rompun 100 mg/ml Injectable	Haver/Diamond	Solution	100 mg/ml	50-ml bottle	IV or IM
		Rugby Gemini Equine Injectable	Burns	Solution	100 mg/ml	50-ml bottle	IV or IM
		Xylazine HCl Injection	Butler	Solution	100 mg/ml	50-ml bottle	IV or IM
		Xylazine HCl Injection	Fermenta	Solution	100 mg/ml	50-ml bottle	IV or IM

VACCINES AND ANTITOXINS
Encephalomyelitis Vaccines: Treatment No. 109

Cephalovac VEW (Coopers)—Trivalent killed virus vaccine from cell lines infected with eastern and western encephalomyelitis viruses and attenuated strain of Venezuelan equine encephalomyelitis virus; *vaccination:* 2-ml dose repeated 21 to 28 days after initial dose using a different injection site; *revaccination:* single annual 2-ml booster; 10-dose vials, IM.

Encephloid IM (Fort Dodge)—Killed vaccine from chicken tissue culture infected with eastern and western encephalomyelitis viruses; *vaccination:* inject 1 ml IM followed by second dose 21 days later using a different injection site; *revaccination:* annual 1-ml booster dose; 25 × 1-ml disposable syringes with needles or 10-ml vials, IM.

Encephalomyelitis Vaccine (Colorado Serum)—Killed vaccine from cell culture infected with eastern and western encephalomyelitis viruses; *vaccination:* inject 1 ml IM followed in 21 to 28 days by second dose IM in different site; *revaccination:* annual 1-ml booster or when outbreak; 10 × 1-ml vials or 10-ml vials, IM.

Encephol TC with Spur (Cutter)—Killed vaccine from tissue culture infected with eastern and western encephalomyelitis viruses; *vaccination:* inject 1 ml IM followed in 21 to 28 days by second dose IM in different site; *revaccination:* annual 1-ml booster or when outbreak; 10 × 1-ml syringes with needles or 10-ml vials, IM.

Encevac with Havlogen (Haver/Diamond)—Killed vaccine from tissue culture infected with eastern and western encephalomyelitis viruses; *vaccination:* inject 1 ml IM followed in 21 to 28 days by second dose IM in different site; *revaccination:* annual 1-ml booster or when outbreak; 10-ml vials, IM.

Triple E (Solvay)—Trivalent killed-virus vaccine grown in cell cultures infected with eastern, western, and Venezuelan equine encephalomyelitis viruses; *vaccination:* 1-ml dose repeated 21 to 28 days after initial dose using a different injection site; *revaccination:* single annual 1-ml booster or in the event of an outbreak; 10 × 1-ml syringes or 10-dose vial, IM.

Herpesvirus Vaccines: Treatment No. 110

Equine Herpesvirus Type 1 Antigens

Rhinomune (SmithKline Beecham)—Freeze-dried; *vaccinate* 3 months of age or older; administer 2 doses 4 to 8 weeks apart, and *revaccinate* every 3 months; 1- and 5-ml vials, IM.

Pneumabort K (Fort Dodge)—Killed vaccine; suspension; *vaccinate* pregnant mares and maiden or barren mares sharing the paddock: 2 ml during fifth, seventh, and ninth months of pregnancy; *vaccinate* young horses: 2-ml dose after weaning and 3 to 4 weeks later; *revaccinate* with 2-ml dose 6 months after secondary primary dose and annually thereafter; *vaccinate* mares more than 5 months pregnant on arrival on the stud farm and at 2-month intervals until foaling; *vaccinate* pregnant mares in contact with mares that have aborted EHV-1 infected foals; 2-ml syringes and 20-ml bottle, IM.

Equine Herpesvirus Types 1 and 4

Prestige II (Haver/Diamond)—Killed vaccine for both EHV-1 and EHV-4; *vaccination* of young and mature horses; because of the use of antigen purification system, few cases show reaction to vaccination; 1-ml dose, IM.

Influenzavirus Vaccines: Treatment No. 111
Equine Influenza A/Equine 1 and A/Equine 2

Equicine II with Havlogen (Haver/Diamond)—Inactivated, purified, adjuvanted, tissue culture origin of EIV A_1 and A_2 (Kentucky 81, Fountainbleau 79, Kentucky 87, and other pertinent U.S. and European strains); suspension; primary immunization: inject 1 ml and repeat dose 3 to 4 weeks later; *revaccination:* 1-ml booster dose annually or on imminent exposure; 10-ml (10 dose) vials, IM.

Equi-Flu (Coopers)—Killed equine influenza virus A/Eq_1 and A/Eq_2; *primary immunization:* inject 2 ml and repeat dose 3 to 4 weeks later; *revaccination:* 2-ml annual booster and prior to anticipated exposure; 10 × 1-dose (2-ml) syringes, 10-dose (20-ml) vials, IM.

Flucine TC with Spur (Cutter)—Inactivated, adjuvanted equine influenza virus A_1 and A_2; suspension; primary immunization: inject 1 ml and repeat dose 3 to 4 weeks later; *revaccination:* annual booster or in epidemic conditions or when exposure is imminent; 1-ml (1-dose) syringes with separate sterile needles and 10-ml (10-dose) vials, IM.

Flumune (SmithKline Beecham)—Inactivated, liquid, adjuvanted equine influenza virus A_1 and A_2; *primary immunization:* 1 ml initially and 1 ml 3 weeks later; *revaccination:* 1-ml annual booster or in epidemic conditions; 1-dose and 10-dose vials, IM.

Fluvac (Fort Dodge)—Liquid, adjuvanted equine influenza virus A_1 and A_2 (including Kentucky 81); *primary vaccination:* 1 ml initially and 1 ml 2 to 4 weeks later; *revaccination:* 1-ml annual booster or in epidemic conditions; 25 × 1-ml (25-dose) prefilled disposable plastic syringes with needles, IM.

Inflogen (Solvay)—Purified, liquid, inactivated equine influenza virus A/Eq$_1$ and A/Eq$_2$; *primary vaccination:* 1 ml initially and 1 ml 2 to 4 weeks later; *revaccination:* 1-ml annual booster or in epidemic conditions; 10 × 1-ml doses and 10-ml vials, IM.

Potomac Horse Fever Vaccines: Treatment No. 112

PHF-Vax (Schering-Plough)—*Ehrlichia risticii* bacterin; *primary vaccination:* 1 ml initially, repeated after 3 to 4 weeks in horses older than 3 months of age; *revaccination:* administer booster every 6 to 12 months; 1-ml vials, IM.

Potomovac (Rhone Merieux)—*Ehrlichia risticii* bacterin; *primary vaccination:* 1 ml initially, repeated after 3 to 4 weeks in horses older than 3 months of age; *revaccination:* administer booster every 6 to 12 months; 1- and 10-ml vials, IM.

Rabies Vaccines: Treatment No. 113

Imrab (Rhone Merieux)—Killed virus from hamster embryo cell line; *vaccination:* IM or SC administration of 2-ml dose in horses older than 3 months; *revaccination:* 2-ml dose annual booster; local reaction at site of injection following subcutaneous injection; 10-ml vials, IM.

Rabvac 3 (Solvay)—Killed virus from cell line culture; *vaccination:* 2-ml dose in horses over 3 months of age; *revaccination:* 2-ml dose annual booster; 10-ml vials, IM.

Rabguard-TC (SmithKline Beecham)—Killed virus from porcine cell line; *vaccination:* 2-ml dose in horses over 3 months of age; *revaccination:* 1-ml dose annual booster; 1-dose, 10-dose, and 25-dose vials, IM.

Strangles Vaccines: Treatment No. 114

Streptococcus equi

Equibac II (Fort Dodge)—Killed suspension; administer three 2-ml doses at 2–4-week intervals; 20-ml vials, IM.

Strep. equi M-Protein

Strepvax II (Coopers)—Suspension of purified antigens; *primary vaccination:* administer three 1-ml doses at 3-week intervals; *revaccination:* 1-ml annual booster or prior to anticipated exposure; 1- and 10-ml vials, IM.

Strep. equi Purified Enzyme Extract

Stranglevac (Cutter)—Suspension; *primary immunization:* 1 ml initially and 1 ml 3 to 4 weeks later; *revaccination:* 1-ml annual booster or foals at 6 months (or at weaning); 1-ml syringes, IM.

Strepguard with Havlogen (Haver/Diamond)—Suspension; *primary immunization:* 1 ml initially and 1 ml 3 to 4 weeks later; *revaccination:* 1-ml annual booster or foals at 6 months (or at weaning); 10-ml vials, IM.

Tetanus Antitoxin: Treatment No. 115

Tetanus Antitoxin (Colorado Serum)—Solution; 10 × 1500-U vials, SC or IM.

Tetanus Antitoxin (Coopers)—Solution; 10 × 1500-U vials and 10,000-U vials, SC or IM.

Tetanus Antitoxin (Fort Dodge)—Solution; 5 × 10,000-U, 10,000-U, and 1,500-U vials, SC or IM.

Tetanus Antitoxin (Franklin)—Solution; 1500-U, 10 × 1500-U, 10,000-U, and 5 × 10,000-U vials, SC, IV, or intraperitoneally.

Tetanus Antitoxin (Haver/Diamond)—Solution; 1500-U vials (10 per box), SC.

Tetanus Antitoxin (Sanofi)—Solution; 1500-U vial, IM and SC.

Tetanus Vaccination: Treatment No. 116

Super-Tet with Havlogen (Haver/Diamond)—Suspension; *primary immunization:* 1 ml initially and 1 ml 3 to 4 weeks later; *revaccination:* 1-ml annual booster, 10-ml vials, IM.

Tetanus Toxoid (Colorado Serum)—Suspension; *primary immunization:* two doses of 10 ml each at 30-day intervals; *revaccination:* at least annual booster; 1- and 5-dose (50-ml) vials, IM.

Tetanus Toxoid (Fort Dodge)—Suspension; *primary immunization:* 1 ml initially and revaccination after 30 days; *revaccination:* 1-ml annual booster; prefilled syringes with needles (25 doses) and 10-ml (10-dose) vials, IM.

Tetanus Toxoid–Concentrated (Colorado Serum)—Suspension; *primary immunization:* 1 ml initially and 1 ml 30 days later; *revaccination:* 1-ml annual booster; 10 × 1-dose (10 × 1-ml) and 10-dose (10-ml) vials, IM.

Tetnogen (Solvay Animal Health)—Suspension; *primary vaccination:* 1 ml initially and 1 ml 30 days later; *revaccination:* 1-ml annual booster; 10 × 1-ml and 1 × 10-ml vials, IM.

T-Toxol with Spur (Cutter)—Suspension; *primary immunization:* 1 ml initially and 1 ml 3 to 4 weeks later; *revaccination:* 1-ml annual booster; 1-ml syringes with separate sterile needles and 10-ml vials, IM.

Unitox (Coopers)—Suspension; *primary immunization:* 1 ml initially and 1 ml 30 days later; *revaccination:* 1-ml annual booster; 10-ml vials and 10 × 1-ml syringes, SC or IM.

Viral Arteritis Vaccine: Treatment No. 117

Arvac (Fort Dodge)—Desiccated, viable, tissue culture origin, modified equine arteritis virus; *vaccinate* 3 months prior to breeding, administer 1 ml; 10-ml vials, IM.

Combined Vaccines: Treatment No. 118

For most encephalomyelitis vaccines, combined vaccines with tetanus toxoid and influenza are also available.

Combined Encephalomyelitis and Tetanus

Cephalovac EWT (Coopers)—Killed vaccine for eastern and western encephalomyelitis and tetanus; *vaccination:* 2-ml dose followed by second dose 4 to 6 weeks later using a different site; *revaccination:* single 2-ml annual booster; 1-ml syringes or 10-dose vial, IM.

Cephalovac VEWT (Coopers)—Killed multivalent vaccine for eastern, western, and Venezuelan encephalomyelitis and tetanus; *vaccination:* 2-ml dose followed by second dose 4 to 6 weeks later using a different site; *revaccination:* single 2-ml annual booster; 1-ml syringes or 10-dose vials, IM.

Double-E-T (Solvay)—Killed vaccine for eastern and western encephalomyelitis and tetanus; *vaccination:* 1-ml dose followed by second dose 2 to 4 weeks later using a different site; *revaccination:* single 1-ml annual booster or in outbreak; 1-ml syringes or 10-ml vials, IM.

Encephalomyelitis Vaccine–Tetanus Toxoid (Colorado Serum)—Killed vaccine for eastern and western encephalomyelitis and tetanus; *vaccination:* 2-ml dose followed by second dose 3 to 4 weeks later using a different site; *revaccination:* single 2-ml annual booster or in outbreak; 2-ml syringes or 20-ml vials, IM.

Encephol-Tet with Spur (Cutter)—Killed vaccine for eastern and western encephalomyelitis and tetanus; *vaccination:* 1-ml dose followed by second dose 3 to 4 weeks later using a different site; *revaccination:* single 1-ml annual booster or in outbreak; 10 × 1-ml dose syringes or 10-ml vials, IM.

Encevac-T with Havlogen (Haver/Diamond)—Killed vaccine for eastern and western encephalomyelitis and tetanus; *vaccination:* 1-ml dose followed by second dose 3 to 4 weeks later using a different site; *revaccination:* single 1-ml annual booster or in outbreak; 1- or 10-ml vials, IM.

Equiloid (Fort Dodge)—Killed vaccine for eastern and western encephalomyelitis and tetanus; *vaccination:* 1-ml dose followed by second dose 4 to 8 weeks later using a different site; *revaccination:* single 1-ml annual booster or in outbreak; 1- or 10-ml vials, IM.

Triple-E-T (Solvay)—Killed multivalent vaccine for eastern, western, and Venezuelan encephalomyelitis and tetanus; *vaccination:* 1-ml dose followed by second dose 2 to 4 weeks later using a different site; *revaccination:* single 1-ml annual booster; 1-ml syringes or 10-ml vials, IM.

Vax-Pac EW-T (Franklin)—Killed vaccine for eastern and western encephalomyelitis and tetanus; *vaccination:* 1-ml dose followed by second dose 4 to 8 weeks later using a different site; *revaccination:* single 1-ml annual booster or in outbreak; 1-ml dose syringe, IM.

Combined Influenza, Encephalomyelitis, and Tetanus

Double-E FT (Solvay)—Killed vaccine for eastern and western encephalomyelitis, equine influenza, and tetanus; *vaccination:* 1-ml dose followed by second dose 2 to 4 weeks later using a different site; *revaccination:* single 1-ml annual booster or in outbreak; 1-ml syringes or 10-ml vials, IM.

Encephol-Plus TC with Spur (Cutter)—Killed vaccine for eastern and western encephalomyelitis, equine influenza, and tetanus; *vaccination:* 1-ml dose followed by second dose 3 to 4 weeks later using a different site; *revaccination:* single 1-ml annual booster or in outbreak; 10 × 1-ml dose syringes or 10-ml vials, IM.

Encevac TC-4 with Havlogen (Haver/Diamond)—Killed vaccine for eastern and western encephalomyelitis, equine influenza, and tetanus; *vaccination:* 1-ml dose followed by second dose 3 to 4 weeks later using a different site; *revaccination:* single 1-ml annual booster or in outbreak; 1-ml syringes, IM.

Equi-Flu EWT (Coopers)—Killed vaccine for eastern and western encephalomyelitis, equine influenza, and tetanus; *vaccination:* 2-ml dose followed by second dose 4 to 6 weeks later using a different site; *revaccination:* single 2-ml annual booster or in outbreak; 2-ml syringes or 20-ml vials, IM.

Fluvac EWT (Fort Dodge)—Killed vaccine for eastern and western encephalomyelitis, equine influenza, and tetanus; *vaccination:* 1-ml dose followed by second dose 4 to 8 weeks later using a different site; *revaccination:* single 1-ml annual booster or in outbreak; 1-ml syringes or 10-ml vials, IM.

Triple-E FT (Solvay)—Killed multivalent vaccine for eastern, western, and Venezuelan encephalomyelitis, equine influenza, and tetanus; *vaccination:* 1-ml dose followed by second dose 2 to 4 weeks later using a different site; *revaccination:* single 1-ml annual booster; 1-ml dose syringes or 10-dose vials, IM.

Vax-Pac EW-T-Flu (Franklin)—Killed vaccine for eastern and western encephalomyelitis, equine influenza, and tetanus; *vaccination:* 1-ml dose followed by second dose 4 to 8 weeks later using a different site; *revaccination:* single 1-ml annual booster or in outbreak; 1-ml dose syringe, IM.

Combined Influenza and Herpesvirus Vaccines

Fluvac EHV-1 (Fort Dodge)—Liquid, adjuvanted equine influenza virus A_1 and A_2 (including Kentucky 81) and equine herpesvirus 1 cell line culture; *primary vaccination:* 1 ml initially and 1 ml 4 to 6 weeks later and for young horses a third dose 4 to 6 weeks after second dose; *revaccination:* 1-ml annual booster or in epidemic conditions; 1-ml disposable syringes or 10-ml vials, IM.

Rhino-Flu (SmithKline Beecham)—Freeze-dried preparation of attenuated EHV-1 plus inactivated, liquid, adjuvanted equine influenza virus A_1 and A_2; *primary vaccination:* 1 ml initially and 1 ml 3 weeks later; *revaccination:* 1 ml annually or in epidemic conditions; 1-dose and 5-dose vials, IM.

Influenza and Tetanus

Fluvac-T (Fort Dodge)—Liquid, adjuvanted equine influenza virus A_1 and A_2 (including Kentucky 81) and tetanus toxoid; *primary vaccination:* 1 ml initially and 1 ml 4 to 8 weeks later; *revaccination:* 1-ml annual booster or in epidemic conditions; 1-ml disposable syringes or 10-ml vials, IM.

Inflogen-T (Solvay)—Inactivated equine influenza virus A/Eq_1 and A/Eq_2 and tetanus toxoid; *primary vaccination:* 1 ml initially and 1 ml 2 to 4 weeks later; *revaccination:* 1-ml annual booster or in epidemic conditions; 1-ml syringes and 10-ml vials, IM.

COMPANY ADDRESSES

Abbott Laboratories, One Abbott Road, Abbott Part, IL 60064

Agri Laboratories Ltd., 6221 North K Highway, P.O. Box 3101, St. Joseph, MO 64505

Allergan Pharmaceuticals, 2525 DuPont Drive, Irvine, CA 92714-1599

American Equine Products, 372 Ely Avenue, South Norwalk, CT 06854

Anchor Division, Boehringer Ingelheim Animal Health, Inc., 2621 North Belt Highway, St. Joseph, MO 64506

Anthony Products Co., 5600 Peck Road, Arcadia, CA 91006

Astra Pharmaceutical Products, 50 Otis, Westborough, MA 01581

Aveco Co. Inc., Division American Home Products, 800 5th Street N.W., Fort Dodge, IA 50501

Bioceutic Division of Boehringer Ingelheim Animal Health, Inc., 2621 North Belt Highway, St. Joseph, MO 64506

Boehringer Ingelheim, Inc., 90 East Ridge, Ridgefield, CT 06877

Burns Veterinary Supply, 2019 McKenzie Drive, Suite 109, Carrollton, TX 75006

Burroughs Wellcome Co., 3030 Cornwallis Road, Research Triangle Pk, NC 27709

The Butler Company, 5000 Bradenton Avenue, Dublin, OH 43017-0753

Ciba Pharmaceutical, 556 Morris Avenue, Summit, NJ 07901

Colorado Serum Company, 4950 York Street, P.O. Box 16428, Denver, CO 80216

Coopers Animal Health Inc., A Pitman-Moore Company, 421 East Hawley Street, Mundelein, IL 60060

Cutter Animal Health, Mobay Corporation, Animal Health Division, 12707 West 63rd Street, P.O. Box 390, Shawnee, KS 66201.

Dermatologics for Veterinary Medicine, Inc., 8785 N.W. 13th Terrace, Miami, FL 33172-3013

Dista Products Co., Bldg. 11/3 Lilly Corp. Centre, Indianapolis, IN 46285

Dunhall Pharmaceuticals, P.O. Box 100, Gravette, AR 72736

Durvet, Inc., P.O. Box 279, Highway 40 Eastbound, Blue Springs, MO 64015

Evsco Pharmaceuticals, Affiliate of IGI, Inc., P.O. Box 209 (Harding Hwy.), Buena, NJ 08310

Farmtech, Premier Farmtech, 10380 North Executive Hills, P.O. Box 7305, Dept. 120, Kansas City, MO 64116

Fermenta Animal Health Company, 10150 N. Executive Hills Blvd., Kansas City, MO 64153

Forest Pharmaceutical, Inc., 2510 Metro Blvd., Maryland Heights, MO 63043-9979

Fort Dodge Laboratories, Division American Home Products, P.O. Box 518, Fort Dodge, IA 50501

Franklin Laboratories, Inc., Division of American Home Products, P.O. Box 669, Amarillo, TX 79105

Geigy Pharmaceuticals, 556 Morris Avenue, Summit, NJ 07901

Glaxo, Inc., Five Moore Dr., Research Triangle Pk, NC 27709

G. C. Hanford Manufacturing Company, 304 Oneida St., P.O. Box 1017, Syracuse, NY 13201

Haver/Diamond Scientific, Mobay Corporation, Animal Health Division, 12707 West 63rd Street, P.O. Box 390, Shawnee, KS 66201

Hoechst-Roussel Agri-Vet Company, Animal Health Products, Route 202-206, Somerville, NJ

Hyrex Pharmaceuticals, P. O. Box 18385, Memphis, TN 38181-0385

J.A. Webster, Inc., 86 Leominster Road, Sterling, MA 01564

Janssen Pharmaceutic, Inc., 40 Kingsbridge, Road, Piscataway, NJ 08854

Key Pharmaceuticals, Galloping Hill Road, Kenilworth, NJ 07033

Lemmon Company, P. O. Box 30, Sellersville, PA 18960

Lextron, Inc., 630 "O" Street, P. O. Box BB, Greeley, CO 80632

Lloyd Laboratories, A Division of Vet-A-Mix, 604 West Thomas Avenue, Shenandoah, IA 51601

Marion Merrell Dow Inc., P. O. Box 8480, Kansas City, MO 64114

Mead Johnson Laboratories, 2404 Pennsylvania Street, Evansville, IN 47721

MSD-Agvet, Division of Merck and Co., Inc., P.O. Box 2000, WBF 475, Rahway, NJ 07065-0912

Organon, Inc., 375 Mt. Pleasant Avenue, West Orange, NJ 07052

Parke-Davis, 201 Tabor Road, Morris Plains, NJ 07950

Pfizer Inc., Animal Health Division, 235 East 42nd Street, New York, NY 10017-5755

Pharmaderm, A Division of Altana Inc., 60 Baylis Road, Melville, NY 11747

Phoenix Pharmaceutical, Inc., 3336 Pear Street, P. O. Box 7, Fairleigh Station, St. Joseph, MO 64506-0007

The Procter and Gamble Company, P. O. Box 599, Cincinnati, OH 45201-0599

Professional Veterinary Pharmaceuticals, 301 N. Hockett, Suite B, Porterville, CA 93257

ProLabs Ltd., c/o Agri Laboratories, Ltd., 6221 North K Highway, P. O. Box 3101, St. Joseph, MO 64505

Pro Vet Companies, P. O. Box 2286, Loves Park, IL 611311

The Purdue Frederick Company, 100 Connecticut Avenue, Norwalk, CT 06850-3590

Reid-Rowell, 901 Sawyer Road, Marietta, GA 30062-2224

A.H. Robins Company, Inc., P. O. Box 8299, Philadelphia, PA 19101-1245

Roche Laboratories, 340 Kingsland St., Nutley, NJ 07110-1199

J. B. Roerig Division, 235 E. 42nd St., New York, NY 10017

RX Veterinary Products, 15 West Putnam, Porterville, CA 93257

Sanofi Animal Health, Inc., 7101 College Blvd., Overland Park, KS 66210

Schering-Plough Animal Health, P.O. Box 529, Kenilworth, NJ 07033

Searle & Company, Box 5110, Chicago, IL 60680

SmithKline Beecham Animal Health, Whiteland Business Park, 812 Springdale Drive, Exton, PA 19341

SmithKline Beecham Pharmaceutical, P.O. Box 7929, Philadelphia, PA 19103

Solvay Animal Health, Inc., 1201 Northland Drive, Mendota Heights, MN 55120-1139

Squibb-Marsam, P.O. Box 1022, Cherry Hill, NJ 08034

Squibb Pharmaceutical Corp., P. O. Box 52330, Durham, NC 27717

Steris Laboratories, Inc., 620 North 51st Avenue, P.O. Box 23160, Phoenix, AZ 85063-3160

Syntex Animal Health, Inc., Subsidiary of Syntex Agribusiness, Inc., 4800 Westown Parkway, Suite 200, West Des Moines, IA 50265

The Upjohn Company, Animal Health Division, 7000 Portage Road, Kalamazoo, MI 49001

Vedco, Inc., Route 6, Box 35A, St. Joseph, MO 64504

Vet-A-Mix Animal Health, 604 West Thomas Avenue, Shenandoah, IA 51601

Vetsearch International, 6 Lenton Place, North Rocks, NSW 2151, Australia

Winthrop Pharmaceuticals, 90 Park Avenue, New York, NY 10016

Wyeth-Ayerst Laboratories, P.O. Box 8299, Philadelphia, PA 19101

References

Bennett, K.: *Compendium of Veterinary Products*. Port Huron, Mich.: North American Compendiums, 1991.

Billups, N. F., and Billups, S. M. *American Drug Index*. St. Louis: Facts and Comparisons, 1992.

Plumb, D. C.: *Veterinary Drug Handbook*. White Bear Lake, Minn.: PharmaVet Publishing, 1991.

Index

Note: Page numbers in *italics* refer to illustrations; page numbers followed by the letter "t" refer to tables.

ISBN 0-7216-3739-6